Contemporary Issues
in Fetal and Neonatal
Medicine

4

Bronchopulmonary
Dysplasia

GENERAL SERIES EDITORS

NEIL N. FINER, M.D., F.R.C.P.(C.)
Professor of Pediatrics
Director of Newborn Medicine
Royal Alexander Children's Pavilion
Edmonton, Alberta, Canada

MALCOLM L. CHISWICK, M.D.
St. Mary's Hospital
Manchester, England

NOTE FROM THE PUBLISHER
Due to the number of illustrations used in Chapter 12, "The Radiology of Bronchopulmonary Dysplasia and Its Complications" by David K. Edwards III, we have published this book in a trim size larger than that used for the other books in this series.

VOLUMES IN THE SERIES
1. Scanlon, J.W. Perinatal Anesthesia (1985)
2. Silverman, W.A., and Flynn, J.T. Retinopathy of Prematurity (1985)
3. Weil, W.B., Jr., and Benjamin, M. Ethical Issues at the Outset of Life (1987)

FORTHCOMING VOLUMES
5. Pape, K., and Wigglesworth, J. Perinatal Brain Damage (1988)

Contemporary Issues in Fetal and Neonatal Medicine

4

Bronchopulmonary Dysplasia

EDITED BY
T. ALLEN MERRITT, M.D.
WILLIAM H. NORTHWAY, JR., M.D.
BRUCE R. BOYNTON, M.D.

Blackwell Scientific Publications

BOSTON OXFORD LONDON

EDINBURGH MELBOURNE PALO ALTO

Blackwell Scientific Publications
Editorial Offices
Three Cambridge Center, Suite 208, Cambridge, Massachusetts 02142, USA
Osney Mead, Oxford, OX20EL, England
8 John Street, London, WC1N 2 ES, England
23 Ainslie Place, Edinburgh, EH3 6AJ, Scotland
107 Barry Street, Carlton, Victoria, 3053, Australia
667 Lytton Avenue, Palo Alto, California 94301, USA

Distributors
USA and Canada
   Year Book Medical Publishers, Inc.
   200 North LaSalle Street
   Chicago, Illinois 60601
Australia
   Blackwell Scientific Publications, Pty., Ltd.
   107 Barry Street
   Carlton, Victoria, 3053
Outside North America and Australia
   Blackwell Scientific Publications, Ltd.
   Osney Mead
   Oxford OX2 0EL
   England

Typeset by The William Byrd Press.
Printed and bound by Hamilton Printing Company.

Blackwell Scientific Publications, Inc. © 1988 by Blackwell Scientific Publications, Inc.
Printed in the United States of America
88 89 90 91 5 4 3 2 1

All rights reserved. No part of this book may be reproduced in any form or by any electronic or mechanical means, including information storage and retrieval systems, without permission in writing from the publisher, except by a reviewer who may quote brief passages in a review.

Library of Congress Cataloging in Publication Data

Bronchopulmonary dysplasia/edited by T. Allen Merritt, William H. Northway, Jr., Bruce R. Boynton.
  p. cm. — (Contemporary issues in fetal and neonatal medicine; 4)
  Includes index.
  ISBN 0-86542-047-5
  1. Bronchopulmonary dysplasia. I. Merritt, T. Allen, 1946- . II. Northway William H., 1932- III. Boynton, Bruce R., : 1948- . IV. Series.
    [DNLM: 1 . Bronchopulmonary Dysplasia. W1 CO769MQP v. 4 / WS 280 B8691]
RJ320.B75B76 1988b
618.92'2—dc19
DNLM/DLC
for Library of Congress   88-14563
                                CIP

Contents

Contributors, ix

Foreword, xiii
DOROTHY BERLIN GAIL AND SUZANNE S. HURD

Preface, xv

PART I. INTRODUCTION AND OVERVIEW

1. Historical Perspectives in Bronchopulmonary Dysplasia, 3
   WILLIAM H. NORTHWAY, JR.

PART II. PATHOGENESIS AND PATHOPHYSIOLOGY

2. Epidemiology of Bronchopulmonary Dysplasia, 19
   BRUCE R. BOYNTON

3. Pathogenesis of Bronchopulmonary Dysplasia, 33
   DIONYSIS S. BONIKOS AND KLAUS G. BENSCH

4. Tracheal Aspirate Cytology in Neonatal Respiratory Distress Syndrome and Bronchopulmonary Dysplasia, 59
   CHARLES NEAVE

   COMMENT BY T. ALLEN MERRITT

5. Mechanisms and Pathobiologic Effects of Barotrauma, 79
   DONALD W. THIBEAULT AND MICHAEL J. LANG

   COMMENT BY BRUCE R. BOYNTON

6   Development of Antioxidant Systems, 103
    JONATHAN R. WISPE AND ROBERT J. ROBERTS

    COMMENT BY WILLIAM H. NORTHWAY, JR.

7   Interactions in the Immature Lung: Protease-Antiprotease Mechanism of
    Lung Injury, 117
    T. ALLEN MERRITT AND MIKKO HALLMAN

8   Alterations in Surfactant Composition, 131
    MICHAEL OBLADEN

    COMMENT BY T. ALLEN MERRITT

9   Pulmonary Edema in Respiratory Distress Syndrome and Bronchopulmonary
    Dysplasia, 143
    HUGH M. O'BRODOVICH AND GEOFFREY COATES

    COMMENT BY BRUCE R. BOYNTON

10 Bronchopulmonary Dysplasia: Can the Laboratory Duplicate Factors That Influence Its
    Pathogenesis and Evolution? 161
    JACQUELINE J. COALSON

    COMMENT BY WILLIAM H. NORTHWAY, JR.

PART III.   CLINICAL MANIFESTATIONS AND MANAGEMENT OF
            BRONCHOPULMONARY DYSPLASIA

11 Clinical Presentation of Bronchopulmonary Dysplasia, 179
    T. ALLEN MERRITT AND BRUCE R. BOYNTON

12 The Radiology of Bronchopulmonary Dysplasia and Its Complications, 185
    DAVID K. EDWARDS III

    COMMENT BY WILLIAM H. NORTHWAY, JR.

13 Contribution of the Patent Ductus Arteriosus to Lung Injury, 235
    ROBERT B. COTTON

    COMMENT BY T. ALLEN MERRITT

CONTENTS

14 Cor Pulmonale, 251
    FREDERICK S. SHERMAN

    COMMENT BY T. ALLEN MERRITT

15 Assessment of Pulmonary Function in the PostNeonatal Period, 263
    ROBERT S. TEPPER

    COMMENT BY BRUCE R. BOYNTON

16 Diuretic Therapy in Bronchopulmonary Dysplasia, 277
    T. F. YEH

    COMMENT BY T. ALLEN MERRITT

17 Bronchodilators and Anti-Inflammatory Agents, 293
    ROBERT KATZ AND SHIRLEY MURPHY

    COMMENT BY T. ALLEN MERRITT

18 Nursing Care of the Infant with Bronchopulmonary Dysplasia, 313
    CAROLE A. BOYNTON AND BARBARA JONES

19 Home Respiratory Care, 331
    HENRY L. DORKIN

    COMMENT BY BRUCE R. BOYNTON

PART IV. NEW APPROACHES TO TREATMENT AND PREVENTION OF BRONCHOPULMONARY DYSPLASIA

20 Impact of Surfactant Therapy for Respiratory Distress in Preventing or Reducing Bronchopulmonary Dysplasia, 343
    T. ALLEN MERRITT AND MIKKO HALLMAN

21 High-Frequency Ventilation, 351
    BRUCE R. BOYNTON AND IVAN D. FRANTZ III

22 Pharmacologic Intervention: Use of the Antioxidant Superoxide Dismutase, 365
    WARREN ROSENFELD AND LUZMINDA CONCEPCION

    COMMENT BY WILLIAM H. NORTHWAY, JR.

23 Use of Steroids, 375
RONALD L. ARIAGNO

COMMENT BY WILLIAM H. NORTHWAY, JR.

PART V.   OUTCOME OF BRONCHOPULMONARY DYSPLASIA

24 Growth and Neurodevelopmental Outcome of Infants Who Had Bronchopulmonary Dysplasia, 403
ELSA J. SELL AND YVONNE E. VAUCHER

COMMENT BY BRUCE R. BOYNTON

25 Pulmonary Status of Infants and Children with Bronchopulmonary Dysplasia, 421
GREGORY P. HELDT

COMMENT BY BRUCE R. BOYNTON

26 Prevention of Bronchopulmonary Dysplasia: The Challenge, 439
WILLIAM H. NORTHWAY, JR.

INDEX, 445

Contributors

RONALD L. ARIAGNO, M.D.
Associate Professor of Pediatrics
Associate Director of Nurseries
Associate Director, Premature Research Center
Stanford University School of Medicine
Stanford, California

KLAUS G. BENSCH, M.D.
Professor of Pathology and Chairman
Department of Pathology
Stanford University Medical Center
Stanford, California

DIONYSIS S. BONIKOS, M.D.
Professor and Chairman
Department of Pathology
University of Patra School of Medicine
Rion, Patra, Greece

BRUCE R. BOYNTON, M.D., M.P.H.
Assistant Professor of Pediatrics
Tufts University School of Medicine;
Assistant Pediatrician
New England Medical Center
Boston, Massachusetts

CAROLE A. BOYNTON, B.S.N., R.N.
The Children's Hospital
Boston, Massachusetts

JACQUELINE J. COALSON, Ph.D
Professor of Pathology
University of Texas Health Science Center
 at San Antonio
San Antonio, Texas

GEOFFREY COATES, M.B., B.S., F.R.C.P.(C.)
Professor of Radiology
McMaster University
Hamilton, Ontario, Canada

LUZMINDA CONCEPCION, M.D.
Assistant Professor of Pediatrics
Winthrop–University Hospital
SUNY-Health Science Center at Brooklyn
Brooklyn, New York

ROBERT B. COTTON, M.D.
Professor of Pediatrics
Department of Pediatrics
Vanderbilt University School of Medicine
Nashville, Tennessee

HENRY L. DORKIN, M.D.
Chief of Service
Pediatric Pulmonology and Allergy Division
New England Medical Center;
Assistant Professor, Pediatrics
Tufts University School of Medicine
Boston, Massachusetts

DAVID K. EDWARDS III, M.D.
Associate Professor and Chief
Pediatric Radiology
University of California at San Diego
San Diego, California

IVAN D. FRANTZ III, M.D.
Professor of Pediatrics
Tufts University School of Medicine;
Chief, Division of Newborn Medicine
New England Medical Center;
Director, Boston Perinatal Center
Boston, Massachusetts

MIKKO HALLMAN, M.D.
Professor of Pediatrics
University of Helsinki Children's Hospital
Helsinki, Finland

GREGORY P. HELDT, M.D.
Associate Professor of Pediatrics
University of California
San Diego Medical Center
San Diego, California

BARBARA LEE JONES, R.N., M.N., C.P.N.P.
Instructor in Pediatrics
Nurse Coordinator
Neonatal Follow-Up Program
University of California at San Diego
San Diego, California

ROBERT KATZ, M.D.
Assistant Professor, Pediatrics
University of New Mexico School of Medicine
Albuquerque, New Mexico

MICHAEL J. LANG, M.D.
Neonatal Fellow
University of Missouri at Kansas City
Children's Mercy Hospital
Kansas City, Missouri

T. ALLEN MERRITT, M.D.
Professor of Pediatrics
Division of Neonatal-Perinatal Medicine
University of California at San Diego;
Neonatologist, Children's Hospital and Health Center
San Diego, California

SHIRLEY MURPHY, M.D.
Associate Professor
Director, Pediatric Pulmonary/Critical Care Division;
Department of Pediatrics
University of New Mexico School of Medicine
Albuquerque, New Mexico

CHARLES NEAVE, M.D., Dr.P.H.
Assistant Professor of Pathology
Sir Isaac Walton Killiam Hospital
Dalhousie University
Halifax, Nova Scotia, Canada

WILLIAM H. NORTHWAY, JR., M.D., F.A.C.R.
Professor of Radiology and Pediatrics
Department of Radiology and Nuclear Medicine
Stanford University Medical Center
Stanford, California

MICHAEL OBLADEN, M.D.
Professor of Pediatrics
Director, Division of Neonatology
Free University of Berlin
Children's Hospital
West Berlin, Federal Republic of Germany

HUGH M. O'BRODOVICH, M.D., F.R.C.P.(C.)
Associate Professor of Pediatrics
Chest Division
The Hospital for Sick Children
University of Toronto
Toronto, Ontario, Canada

ROBERT J. ROBERTS, M.D., Ph.D.
Professor and Chairman
Department of Pediatrics
Children's Medical Center
Charlottesville, Virginia

WARREN ROSENFELD, M.D.
Chairman of Pediatrics
Winthrop—University Hospital
Associate Professor of Clinical Pediatrics
SUNY/Health Science Center at Brooklyn

ELSA JOYCE SELL, M.D.
Associate Professor Pediatrics
Arizona Health Sciences Center
University of Arizona
Tucson, Arizona

CONTRIBUTORS

FREDERICK S. SHERMAN, M.D.
Assistant Professor of Pediatrics
Division of Pediatric Cardiology
University of California
San Diego Medical Center
San Diego, California

ROBERT S. TEPPER, M.D., Ph.D.
Associate Professor of Pediatrics
Indiana University Medical Center
James Whitcomb Riley Hospital for Children
Indianapolis, Indiana

DONALD W. THIBEAULT, M.D.
Professor of Pediatrics
University of Missouri at Kansas City
Children's Mercy Hospital
Kansas City, Missouri

YVONNE E. VAUCHER, M.D.
Associate Professor of Pediatrics
University of California, San Diego;
Neonatalogist
Children's Hospital and Health Center
San Diego, California

JONATHAN R. WISPE, M.D.
Assistant Professor of Pediatrics
Division of Neonatology
University of Cincinnati College of Medicine
Children's Hospital Medical Center
Cincinnati, Ohio

T. F. YEH, M.D., F.A.A.P., F.C.C.P.
Professor of Pediatrics
College of Medicine
University of Illinois;
Deputy Director. Division of Neonatology
Cook County Children's Hospital
Chicago, Illinois

Foreword

This book on bronchopulmonary dysplasia deals with a topic of considerable importance. Dr. Boynton points out in his chapter on epidemiology that the costs of medical care for infants with bronchopulmonary dysplasia are substantial, with approximately $25 million a year required to cover only the costs of initial hospitalization. Yet the etiology and pathogenesis of bronchopulmonary dysplasia are not understood. Indeed there is still no agreement on what criteria should be included in its definition, and the long-term consequences for survivors of bronchopulmonary dysplasia as children, adolescents, and adults are not yet known. The scope of this book by Dr. Merritt and his colleagues reflects the multidisciplinary approach that will likely be required to unravel the fundamental causes of bronchopulmonary dysplasia, and to devise effective strategies for its prevention and management. Of course the prevention of premature births remains a most critical need.

The 20 years since bronchopulmonary dysplasia was first described have been a time of remarkable progress in pulmonary research, especially in lung cell-biology. These gains were rapidly translated into improved care and survival of premature infants, and were accompanied by major technological advances in neonatal intensive care.

Since the Workshop on Bronchopulmonary Dysplasia, sponsored by the National Heart, Lung, and Blood Institute in 1978, there have been considerable improvements in the clinical management of infants with bronchopulmonary dysplasia. Research efforts have suggested new and exciting approaches that have the potential to lead to further gains. Many of the chapters in this book address these important new directions, and point out that several promising approaches to ameliorating or preventing bronchopulmonary dysplasia are, as yet, unproven. It is clear that much more needs to be done.

Our knowledge of basic immune and defense functions of the developing lung is very incomplete; the effects of injury on these fundamental processes and on alveolar development in the postnatal lung are virtually unknown. The optimal nutritional requirements for premature infants are not completely understood. How the pulmonary response to prematurity and bronchopulmonary dysplasia affects the cardiovascular system is unclear, and the sequelae of the cardiovascular complications associated with bronchopulmonary dysplasia are not yet understood. It is crucial to continue to monitor the survivors of bronchopulmonary dysplasia to develop data on long-term sequelae and outcomes. The importance of controlling and preventing premature labor remains paramount.

This book organizes and assesses results

from disparate studies concerned with bronchopulmonary dysplasia. It will undoubtedly stimulate new ideas and encourage new collaborations. It is certain to challenge both basic and clinical research scientists to continue their important pursuit of understanding the complexities of bronchopulmonary dysplasia from many different perspectives.

Dorothy Berlin Gail, Ph.D.
Suzanne S. Hurd, Ph.D.
Division of Lung Diseases
National Heart, Lung, and Blood Institute
Bethesda, Maryland.

Preface

Anniversaries provide an admirable opportunity to take stock of past experience and to resolve to do better in the future. It has now been 20 years since the first description of bronchopulmonary dysplasia by Dr. William H. Northway, Jr., and associates. It is therefore an appropriate time to review the state of the art in bronchopulmonary dysplasia research. Toward that end Drs. T. Allen Merritt and Bruce R. Boynton have joined with Dr. Northway to summarize what is known about the epidemiology, pathophysiology, biochemistry, treatment, and prevention of bronchopulmonary dysplasia. Because the consequences of neonatologists' actions may affect their patients for a lifetime, we have stressed the important issues of residual pulmonary and neurodevelopmental handicap. It is usual for physicians to be somewhat severe in assessing the ignorance and errors of their medical predecessors. We trust that in 20 more years, a greater understanding of bronchopulmonary dysplasia will enable the next generation of physicians to be similarly critical of current therapy and that, by then, bronchopulmonary dysplasia will have joined the ranks of the extinct diseases.

The preparation of any monograph requires the labor of many contributors. The editors have been blessed with dedicated coworkers and understanding colleagues. We especially would like to thank Ron Coen, David K. Edwards, Ivan D. Frantz III, Klaus G. Bensch, M.D., Rita Petriceks, Robert C. Rosan, M.D., and David Y. Porter, M.D. Emily Jones organized the chapters and typed or retyped many of them. She encouraged contributors to be prompt and has served as an important liaison between editors and publisher. Finally, the patience and understanding of our wives, Maryanne, Carole, and Linda, deserve our acknowledgment and loving thanks.

I

Introduction and Overview

1

Historical Perspectives in Bronchopulmonary Dysplasia

WILLIAM H. NORTHWAY, JR.

Introduction

The disease process later named bronchopulmonary dysplasia was first observed in October 1964. In August 1964 I had finished a pediatric radiology fellowship with Professor Jacques Lefebvre at Hôpital des Enfants Malades in Paris, which had included a project at the Center for Premature Infants at Hôpital Baudeloque. Upon arriving at Stanford University Medical Center as an instructor in pediatric radiology, I was asked to review a series of chest radiographs of an infant with severe hyaline membrane disease who had been treated with the then new therapy of intermittent positive pressure ventilation and high-concentration supplemental oxygen. These chest radiographs showed the gradual development of an unusual cystic appearance of the lungs which I had not seen before. Dr. Philip Sunshine, associate director of the newborn nurseries, indicated that there were several other severely ill infants whose lungs had developed the same radiographic appearance. Shortly thereafter two colleagues from the Department of Pathology, Drs. Robert Rosan and David Porter, and I began to review the clinical, radiologic, and pathologic findings in these infants.

In 1967 we reported a series of 32 newborn infants with a previously undescribed chronic pulmonary disease that developed during treatment for severe hyaline membrane disease (HMD) (1). This new disease process was called bronchopulmonary dysplasia (BPD). The infants had not responded to the initial conservative treatment of control of body temperature, intravenous administration of glucose and sodium bicarbonate to combat acidosis, and antibiotics. They were cyanotic in 100% oxygen, appeared moribund, and had undergone one or more prolonged apneic spells. These infants were subsequently treated with prolonged intermittent positive pressure ventilation and warm humidified supplemented oxygen, and in spite of their severe respiratory distress, 41% survived. The remarkable finding in this series of severely ill infants was not only that many of them survived, but also that some of them developed chronic lung disease. Prior to this report survival with a clear chest radiograph at 1 week of age or death at 5 days had been the expected course of infants with HMD (2). An idealized picture of the clinical, radiologic, and pathologic development of BPD was proposed, and four characteristic radiographic and pathologic stages were described. The readily recognizable late stage of the disease, Stage IV, was associated with receiving 80% to 100% concentrations of supplemental oxygen and intermittent positive pressure ventilation for more than 150 hours. It was postulated that BPD could result from the following: pulmonary healing in infants with severe HMD, who ordinarily do not survive; the toxic effect of oxygen on the lung, superimposed upon pulmonary healing in infants with severe HMD; or a combination of the effects of pulmonary oxygen toxicity, healing severe HMD, intermittent positive pressure ventilation, and poor bronchial drainage secondary to endotracheal intubation. The problem of associated persistent patent ductus and development of cor pulmonale was recognized. The continued development of potentially functional parenchymal tissue during the disease and the reversibility of the chest radiographic findings, even with diffuse severe pulmonary involvement, were stressed.

Several historical paths joined to produce the setting for the development and recognition of BPD. These were advances in the care of the premature infant including the development of modern incubators, sophisticated resuscitation and artificial ventilation techniques, the use of supplemental oxygen therapy, identification of HMD as a distinct clinical and pathologic entity, and development of x-ray equipment that allowed the diagnosis of HMD to be affirmed in the living infant and the changes of BPD to be appreciated.

Care of Premature Infants

Prior to the Middle Ages congenitally debilitated infants and premature infants were often allowed to die because they were assumed to be of no value to the state (3). A general sentiment of pity for these infants gradually spread in Europe during the Middle Ages. But for centuries homes for abandoned infants were the only places where infants received care outside the family, and the death rates in these homes approached 100% (4). As late as 1780 half the infants born in France were said to have died before they were 2 years old (3). High infant mortality was considered inevitable, and the premature infant was only a small part of the problem. The world's first hospital devoted to the treatment of sick infants and children, Hôpital des Enfants Malades, was established in Paris in 1802. Children from 2 to 15 years of age were admitted there for care (4). Care of infants was provided primarily at home by their mothers, midwives, and wet nurses. Most physicians avoided caring for newborn infants, as they were unable to prevent their high morbidity and mortality (5). Before 1872, when Guéniot first described the diagnosis of prematurity on the basis of birth weight (6), newborn infants were rarely weighed (7), and special care of the premature infant had hardly been considered.

The foundation for modern care of the premature infant began in the nineteenth century, and was initiated in Paris by the obstetrician Stephane Tarnier and his pupil Pierre Constant Budin (8). A declining birth rate, high infant mortality, and humanitarian concerns led to an investigation of the causes and prevention of infant mortality in France. Proper warming of premature infants was addressed for the first time in the medical literature in 1829, when Villermé and Milne-Edwards noted the influence of environmental temperature on neonatal mortality (9). In 1857 Denucé first described a double-walled tub for use as an incubator (10), but Tarnier was the first physician to develop a closed incubator, which he introduced at the Maternité at Port Royal in Paris in 1881 (Fig. 1.1) (11). With use of the closed incubator, the mortality of infants weighing less than 2000 grams at birth fell from 66% to 38% during the years 1879 to 1881 (11). Budin set forth the principles of special care for premature infants: "With weaklings we shall then have to consider three points: 1) their temperature and their chilling; 2) their feeding; 3) the diseases to which they are prone" (12). The Maternité and the Clinique Tarnier were the

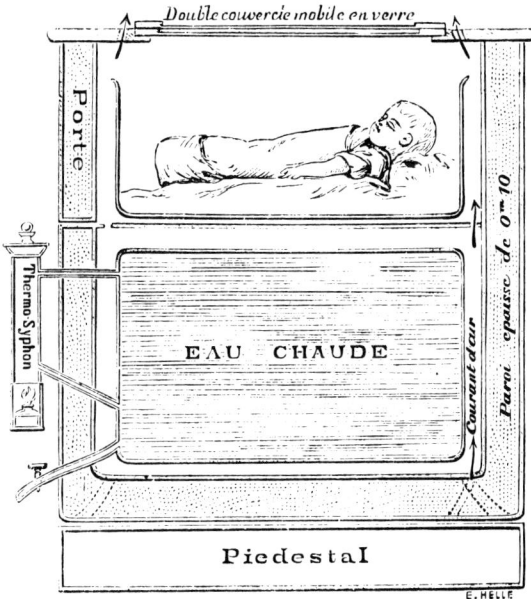

Figure 1.1. The first closed incubator developed by Tarnier, introduced at the Maternité at Port Royal in Paris in 1881. (Reprinted from Auvard A. De la couveuse pour enfants. Arch de Tocologie 1883;10: 579).

first centers in the world for clinical research and teaching of premature infant care (12).

Tarnier and Budin were interested in improving the feeding of, and preventing infection in, the premature infant. In 1884 Tarnier introduced gavage feeding of premature infants, described in 1850 by Marchant (13), at the Maternité (11). Budin daily weighed the infants in his care, to determine both their intake and the amount of milk required for weight gain. In 1896 he designed a special unit to prevent the spread of infection in premature infants. The fundamental features of this unit, the first of its kind in the world, were that it grouped together healthy premature infants, separated ill infants, and provided a place where wet nurses could wash their hands and faces and put on gowns before handling their patients (14).

Budin sent his student, Martin Cooney, to the 1896 Berlin Exposition to demonstrate the effectiveness of the incubator. Cooney borrowed six premature infants from the Berlin Charite Hospital and placed them in six incubators in his booth. Since their chance of survival was considered remote, the borrowing of the infants to demonstrate the incubators caused little concern (15). The demonstration was a great scientific as well as financial success, and not a single infant died during the Exposition. Cooney developed similar demonstrations for other expositions even though the medical community attacked the showmanship aspects of the proceedings. He came to America in 1898 and participated in many incubator exhibitions at various annual fairs and expositions and even opened a permanent incubator exhibition at Coney Island Amusement Park (16). By the time of Cooney's death in 1950, the use of incubators in caring for premature infants had become accepted medical practice.

Beginning in the early 1900s increasing numbers of women in the United States and Europe were delivering babies in hospitals rather than at home. The increase in hospitalization for childbirth coincided with the elimination of puerperal fever and the development of obstetrics (5). Less than 5% of American women delivered in hospitals in 1900, but by 1921 more than half the deliveries in large cities occurred in hospitals (17). As a result more newborn nurseries were being developed in hospitals, and a few pediatricians were beginning to study the disorders of the neonatal period in order to improve the medical care of the newborn infant.

The studies by Max Rubner and Otto Heubner on the metabolism and average daily caloric requirements of the infant published in 1898 began the modern investigation of infant metabolism (18). Between 1912 and 1920 Arvo H. Ylppo, working at the Kaiserin-Auguste-Victoria-Haus in Berlin, published several classic monographs on the physiology and pathology of prematurity (19–21). In 1922 Julius H. Hess, founder of the first continuously operated premature infant center in the United States, published the first book dealing solely with premature and "congenitally diseased" infants (22). The most common of these diseases were rickets, syphilis, anemia, and sepsis. Prematurity was the most important cause of death in infants under 1 year of age in the 1930s and 1940s in the United States (8). Over half of the deaths due to prematurity occurred in the first 24 hours of life (23, 24). In 1947 Chappel introduced a closed, transparent incubator of the Isolette^R type. This meant that the pediatrician could view the unclothed (previously swaddled) infant continuously during this critical period (8). Further developments in the feeding of premature infants and the introduction of sulfonamides (1935), penicillin (1944), and other antibiotics contributed to decreasing rates of mortality among premature infants. But from the 1920s to the 1960s, most textbooks on care of the premature infant recommended minimal handling, strict isolation, and the exclusion of all visitors from the nursery (5).

Artificial Ventilation

The history of resuscitation can be traced to the Old Testament of the Holy Bible (25) and is probably older than this written record. Cannulation of the trachea to support ventilation was first mentioned by Hippocrates in approximately 400 B.C. (26). Some form of intermittently applied positive pressure is the oldest type of artificial ventilation. In 1472, in the first printed book on diseases of children, Bagellardus described the use of mouth-to-mouth resuscitation in the newborn infant (27). By 1543 Andreas Vesalius had described in detail the use of tracheostomy, intubation, and ventilation to maintain the life of a pregnant sow (28). In 1667 Robert Hook repeated the experimental procedures of Vesalius, added the use of a mechanical bellows to provide continuous inspiration and expiration and described the gross physiologic effects (29). During the eighteenth century there was great interest in techniques for resuscitation of asphyxiated humans. The publications of the Royal Humane Society between 1774 and 1776 recommended mouth-to-mouth resuscitation of stillborn infants (26). By the end of the eighteenth century artificial ventilation utilizing mechanical devices and tubes passed into the mouth, nose, or trachea for the purpose of supporting rhythmic breathing was established.

The intralaryngeal tube for resuscitation of infants was developed by Chaussier, a professor of obstetrics, in 1806. The advocacy of this technique by his successor at the Maternité, De Paul, in 1845 (30), began a new era in resuscitation and ventilation of asphyxiated infants. The broad end of Chaussier's curved intralaryngeal tube was used for insufflation by the physician (Fig. 1.2). Gairal (1879) added a rubber bulb to the end of the tube to replace the physician's lungs (31). Truehead described in 1869 an intubation cannula and bellows respirator machine for newborn infants that automatically pumped and aspirated air in and out of the trachea in rhythmic fashion (31). Truehead's work was not widely recognized but preceded the simpler and more widely acclaimed Fell-O'Dwyer ventilating apparatus (31). Champneys in 1882 characterized the pressures required to produce interstitial emphysema and pneumothorax in stillborn human infants (32). In 1887 O'Dwyer reported the first successful use of extended intermittent positive pressure ventilation in a large series of children with croup (33). In 1889 Alexander Graham Bell of Canada (34) and Egon Braun of Vienna (35) developed intermittent negative pressure ventilation for use in infants and children.

The development of a reliable intermittent positive pressure ventilator capable of long-term clinical application probably stems from modifications of a design developed by Giertz of Sweden in 1916 (36). Drinker and Shaw in 1929 developed the first negative pressure ventilator capable of prolonged artificial ventilation of humans (37). The polio epidemics of the early 1950s spurred development of mechanical ventilating devices in Europe. At the same time advances in design of intermittent positive pressure ventilators in the United States led to the development of the Bird^R and Bennett^R respirators. Donald and Lord in 1953 reported the first series of newborn infants treated for respiratory failure by mechanical ventilation using a negative pressure ventilator designed in their hospital (Fig. 1.3) (38, 39) and began the modern era of prolonged artificial ventilation of the newborn infant.

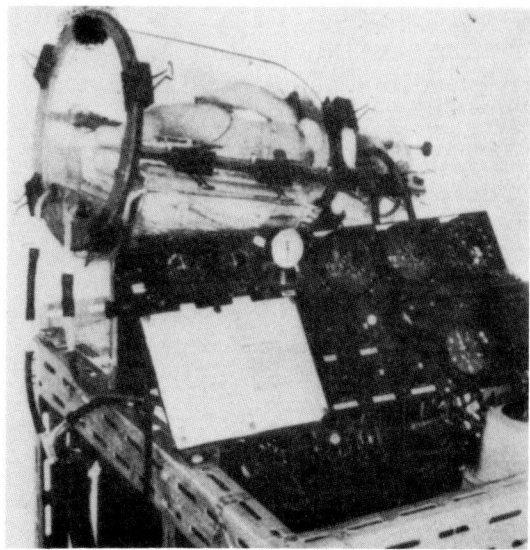

Figure 1.3. The negative pressure ventilator used by Donald and Lord in 1953, which began the modern era of prolonged artificial ventilation of the newborn infant. (Reprinted, with permission, from Donald I, Lord J. Augmented respiration: studies in atelectasis neonatorum. Lancet 1953;1:13.)

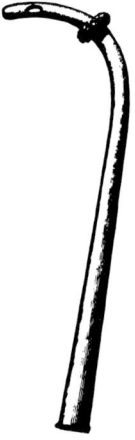

Figure 1.2. The first intralaryngeal tube for resuscitation of infants, developed by Chaussier in 1806. (Reprinted from DePaul JAH. Nouveau-né. In: DeChambre A, ed. Dictionnaire encyclopédique des sciences médicale 1879; Deuxieme series, Tome Treizieme. Paris: Masson G, Asselin P, p 601.

Supplemental Oxygen Treatment

One of the first things Joseph Priestley did after isolating oxygen (1771) was to test its effect on living things. In experiments conducted on mice and on himself, he demonstrated that oxygen was essential to life, suggested its possible use as a therapeutic agent, and commented on the possible danger of such use (40). The first adverse effects of oxygen to be observed were those described by Lavoisier, who in 1785 noted an "inflammatory" action on the lungs of guinea pigs (41). Paul Bert was the first to document scientifically the toxicity of oxygen. His studies culminated in the classic book, *La Pression Barometrique*, published in 1878 (42). His observations on birds, mammals, reptiles, fish, fungi, bacteria, and plants proved the universality of oxygen toxicity. Interestingly he did not discover pulmonary oxygen toxicity, because almost all of his work in animals was carried out at hyperbaric pressures at which central nervous system abnormalities occur before those in the lung. J. Lorrain Smith in 1899 definitively described pulmonary oxygen toxicity in mice in the absence of seizures (43). These pulmonary changes were studied in greater detail by many subsequent investigators, who demonstrated that supplemental concentrations of oxygen could cause edema, hepatization, pleural effusions, extravasation of red blood cells, atelectasis, hyaline membranes, and consolidation to a degree where pulmonary function failed and the experimental animals died (44).

Oxygen was first used experimentally in newborn infants with respiratory difficulty in 1780 by Chaussier (45). Bonnaire published the first detailed clinical report of oxygen therapy in premature infants with cyanosis in France in 1891 (46). Bakwin, in 1923, postulated "anoxemia" as a cause of irregularity in rate and depth of breathing by premature infants and was able to relieve cyanosis and increase the oxygen saturation of two premature infants by giving them supplemental oxygen (47). Oxygen therapy did not become common practice in the care of premature infants until the 1930s and 1940s. In 1942 Smith and Kaplan demonstrated that oxygen inhalation increased hemoglobin saturation in a series of infants and noted that several who had the biochemical measurements of cyanosis were not cyanotic in appearance (48). Wilson *et al.* in 1942 (49) and Graham *et al.* in 1950 (50) reported on the favorable effect of oxygen on periodic breathing. Although asphyxia had been related to brain damage as early as 1861 by Little (51), it was not until the 1940s that perinatal asphyxia was appreciated as a major cause of neurologic damage and death in the newborn (52). The high mortality rate among premature infants and the association of these deaths with problems of respiration also contributed to the rationale for routine use of supplemental oxygen in the care of all premature infants. By the late 1940s liberal use of supplemental oxygen therapy was thought to be a major advance in the care of premature infants (8).

Although considerable research documented the potential toxic effects of supplemental oxygen on the lung, the first clinical evidence of the dangerous effects of oxygen administered at atmospheric pressure to newborn infants was seen in the development of retrolental fibroplasia (RLF). The preliminary results of a national cooperative study published in 1954 (53) confirmed the finding of the prior study published by Patz and coworkers in 1952 (54) that a high-concentration of supplemental oxygen is a factor in the pathogenesis of RLF. Thereafter the use of supplemental oxygen was severely curtailed, and the incidence of RLF fell dramatically. By 1962 a standard pediatric textbook recommended that no more than 40% oxygen be given to premature infants (55).

Hyaline Membrane Disease

The initial description of hyaline membranes in the lungs of newborns dying of respiratory disease was by Hochheim in 1903 (56). He described two cases and attributed the membranes to the aspiration of amniotic sac contents. Between 1903 and 1940 only a few reports describing or analyzing pulmonary hyaline-like membranes in infants appeared in the literature (57). Very little attention was given to pulmonary hyaline membranes as a primary cause of death. Potter's books on pathology of the fetus and newborn did not include "hyaline membrane with resorption atelectasis" until 1952 (58).

The etiologic attitude that prevailed for many years was set by Hochheim and reaffirmed by Farber and Sweet (59), and by Farber and Wilson (60) (1931–1932), who also attributed pulmonary hyaline membranes to the peripheralization of aspirated amniotic sac contents. The critical review of this theory by Miller and Hamilton in 1949 set the stage for intensified investigation of the problem (61). At about the same time a generally recognized clinical pattern emerged and was crystallized by the observations of Potter (62) and Miller and Jennison (63) (1950). It became apparent that HMD principally affected liveborn premature infants and that there was an association with fetal anoxia, maternal diabetes, and caesarean section with premature delivery. The diagnosis, however, was made at postmortem examination; antemortem diagnosis was not possible. An extensive review of hyaline-like membranes associated with diseases of the newborn published in 1953 by De and Anderson still noted that many authorities described the onset of respiration as spontaneous with continuation of normal behavior for 1 or 2 hours (57). The maximum survival for infants with hyaline membranes, summarized from several published autopsy studies in this review, was 5 days. As late as 1957 HMD was not included in the *Standard Nomenclature of Disease* (64).

Diagnostic Radiology

Conrad Roentgen announced the discovery of x-rays in December 1895 (65). In February 1896 Kriedle published in the Vienna letter a roentgen print of the arm of an infant, the first pediatric diagnostic x-ray (66). The first radiology department in the United States devoted exclusively to diagnosis of infants and children was established at the Boston Children's Hospital in 1899 (67). By 1910 there was sufficient interest in the use of x-ray for diagnosis in children that Dr. Thomas Rotch, a pediatrician, published the first book, in any language, devoted exclusively to pediatric x-ray diagnosis, *The Diagnosis of Disease in Early Life by the Roentgen Method* (68). Dr. Arial Wellington George furnished the illustrations for the book and could be regarded as the first pediatric radiologist in the United States (67). In this book Dr. Rotch indicated his concern about improved x-ray technique by noting the difference in diagnostic quality of a 1 second breath-held exposure and a 6 second uncontrolled-breathing exposure of the chest. The youngest patient whose radiograph is printed in this book is a 27-month-old infant, whose pulmonary vessels are not readily identified. In 1913 Coolidge developed the hot cathode high-vacuum x-ray tube with a tungsten target that revolutionized diagnostic radiology (69). It markedly improved accuracy of adjustment and allowed stability, exact duplication and flexibility of technique, and high output. The rotating anode x-ray tube, introduced by Phillips of Holland in 1929, increased the x-ray output per projected unit of focal area (70). This allowed continued reduction in focal spot size and subsequent improvement in radiographic detail. By 1929 most of the x-ray machines were completely shockproof, with transformer and valve tubes immersed in oil and high-tension wires and x-ray tubes in shockproof cables and housings. Power supplies were no longer the limiting factor in the generation of x-rays. The conversion from glass plates to film with emulsion on both sides accelerated during World War I. Intensifying screens appropriate for these films with emulsion on both sides were introduced in 1916 by Carl V. S. Patterson (71). In 1924 a film with a safety base of celluose acetate was introduced to replace the highly inflammable celluose nitrate base (71). Further improvements in x-ray film with increased sensitivity to light from finer grain intensifying screens and increased sensitivity to x-rays were made in the late 1920s and early 1930s. With these technical advances radiology entered a period of rapid development of an incredibly broad range of new diagnostic procedures. These included air encephalography and ventriculography (1918–1919), use of contrast media for visualization of veins and arteries (1919), contrast visualization of the gall bladder (1924), iodinated oil myelography (1923), contrast bronchography (1925), and the use of contrast medium and catheterization to visualize the heart (1922) (72). With further technical improvements in x-ray tubes, film, intensifying screens, and equipment, it became possible to visualize fine anatomic detail in the lungs of newborn infants with respiratory distress.

In 1953 Donald and Lord described for the first time radiologic changes in the lungs of infants with HMD in an article on augmented respiration for therapy of neonatal atelectasis (38). They hoped to identify the disease antemortem so that therapy by artificial ventilation could be tried. Later that same year Donald and Steiner demonstrated the now classic reticular granular pattern of density in the lungs with air bronchogram, which they found associated with proven HMD in 11 infants in a series of chest radiographs of 28 newborn infants at the Hammersmith Hospital (73). In 1955 Peterson and Pendleton differentiated the radiologic pattern of HMD from aspiration pneumonia with radiologic and pathologic correlation (2). This clarification of the radiologic diagnosis allowed pediatricians working in the nursery to establish firm diagnoses in nonfatal cases. In addition Peterson and Pendleton described the usual radiologic course of HMD as either progressive opacification of the lungs with death within 3 to 5 days or complete radiographic clearing and clinical improvement by 7 to 10 days. Gregg and Bernstein reported in 1961 that when recovery occurred it was apparently complete (74).

Prologue to the Discovery of Bronchopulmonary Dysplasia

Between 1955 and 1962 there was continued improvement in the equipment and techniques of artificial ventilation and a re-evaluation of the approach to therapy for HMD. This was stimulated in 1959, following the earlier work of Pattle (75) and Clements (76), by the demonstration by Avery and Mead that the atelectatic lungs of infants dying of HMD behaved as though they lacked surface active material (77). The possibility that additional supplemental oxygen above a 40% concentration might be a useful therapeutic aid for these premature infants with atelectatic lungs was supported by the observations of Avery and Oppenheimer in 1960 (78). They found that deaths from the disease were greater during a 5 year period in which no or very little supplemental oxygen was given to premature infants than during an earlier 5 year period in which oxygen was used in higher concentration. In an effort to treat premature infants with HMD with assisted ventilation, pediatricians began to use concentrations of oxygen higher than 40% and to control the artificial ventilation and ambient oxygen levels by monitoring the arterial PO_2 with blood from umbilical artery catheters, even though the "safe" level of arterial PO_2 was not known.

In 1962 Boss and Craig described proliferative reparative phenomena in lungs of neonates with hyaline membranes and noted that only 2 of 24 infants who died after 60 hours of age did not have proliferative activity in the involved alveoli (79). The highest degree of regeneration (grade IV) occurred most commonly in the lungs of those infants with the longest survival times, who were presumably exposed to high-oxygen tensions for longer periods. They postulated that this diffuse response might be related to oxygen toxicity. The longest survivor lived 7 days. Radiographs of a small number of these infants presented no special features. This was the first report in the literature on HMD to refer directly to regenerative and reparative activity of alveolar septal cells.

In 1964 Shepard, Gray, and Stahlman reported, in an abstract, a series of 52 infants with HMD, 23 of whom, when examined at ages 6 months to 6½ years, had radiographic findings said to be compatible with pulmonary fibrosis (80). During the discussion period a series of chest x-rays was shown of an infant with severe HMD who, the authors said, had developed emphysematous changes in both lung fields by 3 weeks of age. The validity of their findings was questioned by Dr. Silverman and others in the discussion that followed, and a more complete presentation was not published.

Robertson, Tunell, and Rudhe in 1964 reported on the late stages of pulmonary hyaline membranes of the newborn in four infants with the disease (81). They found thickened alveolar walls showing an increase of fibroblasts and excess of reticulin or collagen fibers in three infants who died at 13, 21, and 23 days of life and in one studied by lung biopsy in the eighth week of life. They considered such changes compatible with the process of repair described in the first postnatal week by Boss and Craig but noted that two of their own patients had received prolonged intermittent positive pressure ventilation, with high concentrations of oxygen. In their oldest living patient, treated initially with 100% oxygen and high positive pressure by an Engstrom respirator, "emphysematous blebs and patchy infiltrate" developed on early films of the chest and changed to "small areas of atelectasis" by 2 months of life. Artificial ventilation was discontinued at 1 month of age, but signs of pulmonary disease persisted at 2 months of age. The radiographic findings in this case may well have been those of BPD.

In 1962 the first premature infant research center sponsored by the National Institutes of Health was established at Stanford University Medical Center, and the first baby was admitted to the unit in 1963. That same year, using the Bird^R Mark VII respirator and an orotracheal tube, Drs. Vernon Thomas and Joe Daily began intermittent positive pressure ventilation with supplemental oxygen therapy in a moribund infant with severe HMD. The child survived, and this success led to further use and development of artificial ventilation therapy. Initially, the Bird^R Mark VII respiratory provided only two concentration settings for supplemental oxygen, 100% and 40%. The laboratory tests of respiratory effectiveness then available were the pH and $PaCO_2$ of arterialized capillary blood. The clinical condition of the patient, as judged by skin color, was also used to guide treatment. By 1964 arterial oxygen tension could be measured by a micromethod and more accurate monitoring and control of oxygen administration obtained. A description of the artificial ventilation technique developed at Stanford and the results of its use on 26 severely ill infants, with 18 survivors, was published in 1965 (82). This report emphasized the use of the endotracheal tube and suggested that with its use earlier and more prolonged artificial ventilation could be possible.

Bronchopulmonary dysplasia was initially recognized in the nursery at Stanford University Medical Center, probably because the meticulous attention paid to the details of artificial ventilation and airway maintenance allowed severely ill, small premature infants to survive long enough to develop chronic lung disease. The use of intermittent positive pressure ventilation was also critical since, as later became evident, it was a more effective technique than negative pressure ventilation for supporting the respiration of small premature infants. As these moribund premature infants with severe HMD began to survive longer than 1 or 2 weeks with the support of artificial ventilation, it became clear that the expected course of the disease had been significantly altered. The results of the review of these infants undertaken by Drs. Robert Rosan, David Porter, and myself, documenting and evaluating these changes, were commented on critically and with great concern both at Stanford and nationally prior to their publication in 1967 in the *New England Journal of Medicine* (1).

Epilogue

Since the initial description of BPD, it has been recognized worldwide in the setting of artificial ventilation and supplemental oxygen treatment of premature infants (83). Concerted efforts have been made to learn more about its pathogenesis and to develop effective methods for its prevention and treatment. These are well documented in this book. The short history of BPD has coincided with a remarkable increase in the "intensity" of care provided not only to immature infants with respiratory failure, but also to children and adults with respiratory failure. The improvements in artificial ventilation technique which followed the recognition of BPD contributed to a general lowering of the oxygen concentration used therapeutically and would have more significantly reduced the incidence of BPD had these changes not been accompanied by treatment of increasingly immature infants. The improvements in the treatment of respiratory failure and their extension to more immature infants resulted in some modifications of the clinical course and radiographic appearance of BPD as originally described. The lung pathology of BPD has, however, remained the same. This pathology has now also been seen with prolonged artificial ventilation and supplemental oxygen therapy of adults with respiratory failure who developed adult respiratory distress syndrome (ARDS) (84). Children with ARDS should be expected to develop BPD pathology as well. This history has focused on the occurrence of BPD in the premature infant. In the future that focus may well have to be broadened.

References

1. Northway WH Jr, Rosan RC, Porter DY. Pulmonary disease following respirator-therapy of hyaline membrane disease: bronchopulmonary dysplasia. N Engl J Med 1967;276:357–368.
2. Peterson HG Jr, Pendleton ME. Contrasting roentgenographic pulmonary patterns of the hyaline membrane and fetal aspiration syndromes. Am J Roentgen 1955;74:800–817.
3. Holt LE. Infant mortality, ancient and modern: an historical sketch. Trans Am Assoc Study Prevention Infant Mortality 1913;4:24–54.
4. Radbill SX. A history of children's hospitals. Am J Dis Child. 1955;90:411–416.
5. Cone TE Jr. Perspectives in neonatology. In: Smith GF, Vidyasagar D, eds. Historical review and recent advances in neonatal and perinatal medicine. Vol 1, Neonatal medicine. Mead Johnson Nutritional Division, 1983, pp 9–34.
6. Guéniot M. Sur la faiblesse congenitale et son traitement. Gaz Hôp (Paris) 1872; 45:1161–1162,1171–1172.
7. Haven HC. The systematic weighing of infants. Boston Med Surg J 1881;105:222–224.
8. Cone TE Jr. History of the care and feeding of the premature infant. Boston: Little, Brown, 1985.
9. Villermé MM, Milne-Edwards H. De l'influence de la temperature sur la mortalité des infants nouveau-nés. Ann Hyg Publique 1829; 2:291–307.
10. Denucé P. Berceau incubateur pour les enfants nés avant terme. J Med Bordeaux 1857;2:723–724.
11. Auvard A. De la couveuse pour enfants. Arch de Tocologie 1883;10:577–609.
12. Dunham EC. Evolution of premature infant care. Ann Paediatr Fenn 1957;3:170–184.
13. Marchant M. Soins a donner aux nouveau-nés. Gaz Med (Paris) 1851;6(3rd series):824.
14. Budin P. The nursling: the feeding and hygiene of premature and full-term infants. Maloney WJ, tr. London: Caxton Publishing, 1907.
15. Liebling AJ. Patron of the premies. New Yorker Magazine, June 3, 1939, pp 20–24.
16. Stern L. The newborn infant and his thermal environment. Curr Probl Pediatr 1970;1:1–29.
17. Wertz RW, Wertz DC. Lying in: a history of childbirth in America. New York: The Free Press, 1977.
18. Rubner M, Heubner O. Die natürliche ernährung eines säuglings. Z Biol 1898;36:1–55.
19. Ylppo A. Pathologisch-anatomische stuben bei frühgeborenen. Z Kinderheilkd 1919;20:212–432.
20. Ylppo A. Das wachstrum der frühgeborenen von der geburt biszum schulaltzer. Z Kinderheilkd 1919;24:111–178.
21. Ylppo A. Zur physiologie, klinik und zum schicksal der frühgeborenen. Z Kinderheilkd 1919;24:1–110.
22. Hess JH. Premature and congenitally diseased infants. Philadelphia: Lea and Febiger, 1922.
23. Hoch LA, Weymuller CA, James E. Reduction of mortality from premature birth: some practical measures. J Am Med Assoc 1948;136:217–221.
24. Hess JH. Experiences gained in a 30 year study of prematurely born infants. Pediatrics 1953; 11:425–434.
25. Holy Bible: 1 Kings 17:17 and 2 Kings 4:34.
26. Daily WJR, Smith PC. Mechanical ventilation of the newborn infant, I. Curr Probl Pediatr 1970;1:1–29.
27. Bagellardus a Flumine, P. Libellus de egritudinibus infantium. Part 1, On the care of infants during the first month. Padua: Valdezocchio and Septem Arboribus, 1472. English translation in: Ruhrah, J. *Pediatrics of the Past*. New York: Paul B. Hoeber Inc, 1925, p. 34.
28. Vesalius A. De humani corporis fabrica. Libri septem. Basel: Oporinus, 1543, p 658.
29. Hook R. An account of an experiment made by M Hook, of preserving animals alive by blowing through their lungs with bellows. Philosoph Trans Roy Soc Lond 1667;2:539–540.
30. De Paul JAH. Bulletin de l'academie de med-

icine, September 4, 1977. Quoted in Matas R. Intralaryngeal insufflation. J Am Med Assoc, 1900;34:1371–1375, 1468–1473.
31. Cited in Matas R. Intralaryngeal insufflation. J Am Med Assoc 1900;34:1271–1375, 1468–1473.
32. Champneys FH. Artificial respiration in still-born children. Mediastinal emphysema and pneumothorax in connection with tracheostomy. An experimental inquiry. Med Chir Tr (Lond) 1882;65:75–86.
33. O'Dwyer J. Fifty cases of croup in private practice treated with intubation of the larynx with a description of the method and the danger incident thereto. Med Rec 1887;32:557–561.
34. Stern L, Angeles RD, Outerbridge EW, Beaudry PH. Negative pressure artificial respiration: use in treatment of respiratory failure of the newborn. Can Med Assoc J 1970;102:595–601.
35. Doe OW. Apparatus for resuscitating asphyxiated children. Boston Med Surg J 1889;120:9.
36. Giertz KH. Studier över tryckdifferinsandning enligt sauerbruck och över konstjord andning (rhythmisk luftin blastning) vid intrathoracala operationer. Uppsala läkareför. Forhandl. 1916;Suppl 22.
37. Drinker P, Shaw LA. An apparatus for the prolonged administration of artificial respiration. I. A design for adults and children. J Clin Invest 1929;7:229–247.
38. Donald I, Lord J. Augmented respiration. Studies in atelectasis neonatorum. Lancet 1953;1:9–17.
39. Donald I, Young IM. An automatic respiratory amplifier. J Physiol 1952;116:41P–43P.
40. Lavoisier AL. Recherches de M Priestley sur les differentes especes d'air, 1773. Reprinted in: Oeuvres de Lavoisier. Tome premier. Chapter 15. Paris: Imprimerie Imperiale, 1864, pp 512–535.
41. Lavoisier AL. Alterations qu'éprouve l'air respiré, 1785. Reprinted in: Oeuvres de Lavoisier. Tome 2. Paris: Le Ministre d'l'instruction publique et des cultes, Imprimerie Imperiale, 1862, pp 676–687.
42. Bert P (1878). La pression barometrique. Recherches de physiologie expérimentale. Hitchcock MA, Hitchock FA, trs. Columbus, Ohio: College Book Company, 1943.
43. Smith JL. The pathological effects due to increase of oxygen tension in the air breathed. J Physiol (Lond) 1899;24:19–35.
44. Clark JM, Lambertsen CJ. Pulmonary oxygen toxicity—a review. Pharmacol Rev 1971;23:37–133.
45. Campbell A, Poulton EP. Oxygen and carbon dioxide therapy. London: Oxford University Press, 1934, p 4.
46. Bonnaire E. Des inhalations d'oxygène chez les nouveau-nés. J Med (Paris) 1891;3(2nd series):312–314.
47. Bakwin H. Oxygen therapy in premature babies with anoxemia. Am J Dis Child 1923;25:157–162.
48. Smith CA, Kaplan E. Adjustment of blood oxygen levels in neonatal life. Am J Dis Child 1942;64:843–859.
49. Wilson JL, Long SB, Howard PJ. Respiration of premature infants: response to variations of oxygen and to increased carbon dioxide in inspired air. Am J Dis Child 1942;63:1080–1085.
50. Graham BD, Reardon HS, Wilson JL, et al. Physiologic and chemical response of premature infants to oxygen-enriched atmosphere. Pediatrics 1950;6:55–71.
51. Little WJ. On the influence of abnormal parturition, difficult labours, premature birth and asphyxia neonatorum on the mental and physical condition of the child, especially in relation to deformities. Trans Obstet Soc Lond 1861;3:293–344.
52. Clifford SH, Cole WCC, Smith CA. Round table discussion of neonatal asphyxia. J Pediatr 1941;19:258–273.
53. Kinsey VE. Retrolental fibroplasia: cooperative study of retrolental fibroplasia and the use of oxygen. Arch Ophthalmol 1956;56:481–529.
54. Patz A, Hoeck LE, De la Cruz E. Studies on the effect of high oxygen administration in retrolental fibroplasia. I. Nursery observations. Am J Ophthalmol 1952;35:1248–1252.
55. Holt LE Jr, McIntosh R, eds. Pediatrics, 13th ed. New York: Appleton-Century-Crofts, 1962, p 159.
56. Hochheim K. Ueber einige befunde in den

lungen von neugeborenen und die beziehung derselben zur aspiration von fruchtwasser. Centralbl Pathol 1903;14:537–538.
57. De TD, Anderson GW. Hyaline-like membranes associated with diseases of the newborn lungs; a review of the literature. Obstet Gynecol Surv 1953;8:1–44.
58. Potter EL. Pathology of the fetus and newborn. Chicago: Year Book Medical Publishers, 1952.
59. Farber S, Sweet LK. Amniotic sac contents in the lungs of infants. Am J Dis Child 1931;42:1372–1383.
60. Farber S, Wilson JL. The hyaline membrane in the lungs. I. A descriptive study. Arch Pathol 1932;14:437–449.
61. Miller HC, Hamilton TR. The pathogenesis of "vernix membrane." Relationship to aspiration pneumonia in stillborn and newborn infants. Pediatrics 1949;3:735–748.
62. Potter EL. Pathology of prematurity. J Am Med Wom Assoc 1950;5:391–396.
63. Miller HC, Jennison MH. Study of pulmonary hyaline-like material in 4117 consecutive births: incidence, pathogensis, diagnosis. Pediatrics 1950;5:7–20.
64. Curtis P. Hyaline membrane disease. J Pediatr 1957;51:726–741.
65. Röntgen WC. Ueber eine neue Art von Strahlen (Vorläufige Mittheilung), Sitzber Physik—Med Ges, Wurzburg, December 1895, 9:132–141.
66. Caffey J. Pediatric x-ray diagnosis. Chicago: Year Book Medical Publishers, 1945, preface.
67. Caffey J. The first 60 years of pediatric roentgenology in the United States, 1896 to 1956. Am J Roentgen 1956;76:437–454.
68. Rotch TM. Living anatomy and pathology, the diagnosis of disease in early life by the roentgen method. Philadelphia: JB Lippincott, 1910.
69. Coolidge WD. US patent application filed May 9, 1913, patent number 1,203,495. Cited in: Brecher R, Brecher E. The rays: a history of radiology in the United States and Canada. Baltimore: Williams and Wilkins, 1969, pp 191–199.
70. Grigg ERN. The trial of the invisible light. Springfield, Illinois: Charles C. Thomas, 1905, p 158.
71. Fuchs A. Evolution of roentgen film. Am J Roentgen 1956;75:30–48.
72. Brecher R, Brecher E. The rays: a history of radiology in the United States and Canada. Baltimore: Williams and Wilkins, 1969; pp 219–257.
73. Donald T, Steiner RE. Radiography in the diagnosis of hyaline membrane. Lancet 1953;2:846–849.
74. Gregg RH, Bernstein J. Pulmonary hyaline membranes and the respiratory distress syndrome. Am J Dis Child 1961;102:871–890.
75. Pattle RE. Properties, function, and origin of the alveolar lining layer. Nature 1955;175:1125–1126.
76. Clements JA. Surface tension of lung extracts. Proc Soc Exp Biol Med 1957;95:170–172.
77. Avery ME, Mead J. Surface properties in relation to atelectasis and hyaline membrane disease. Am J Dis Child 1959;97:517–523.
78. Avery ME, Oppenheimer EH. Recent increase in mortality from hyaline membrane disease. J Pediatr 1960;57:553–559.
79. Boss JH, Craig JM. Reparative phenomena in lungs of neonates with hyaline membranes. Pediatrics 1962;29:890–898.
80. Shepard F, Gray J, Stahlman M. The occurrence of pulmonary fibrosis in children who had ideopathic respiratory distress syndrome. J Pediatr 1964;65:1078–1079.
81. Robertson B, Tunell R, and Rudhe U. Late stages of pulmonary hyaline membranes of newborn. Acta Paediatr 1964;53:433–446.
82. Thomas VD, Fletcher G, Sunshine P, Schafer IA, Klaus MH. Prolonged respirator use in pulmonary insufficiency of newborn. J Am Med Assoc 1965;193:183–190.
83. Northway WH Jr. Bronchopulmonary dysplasia. In: Raivio KO, Hallman N, Kouvalainen K. Valimaki I, eds. Respiratory distress syndrome. London: Academic Press, 1984.
84. Churg A, Golden J. Fliegiel S, Hogg JC. Bronchopulmonary dysplasia in the adult. Am Rev Respir Dis 1983;127:117–120.

II
Pathogenesis and Pathophysiology

2

The Epidemiology of Bronchopulmonary Dysplasia

BRUCE R. BOYNTON

Introduction

Clinical epidemiology deals with the distribution and determinants of disease frequency in human populations (1). Although the unit of interest is a well-defined population rather than an individual, the information gathered in epidemiologic studies is of great importance to clinicians (2).

There are many controversies about bronchopulmonary dysplasia (BPD) that are well suited for epidemiologic investigation. Unfortunately many of the studies have been so limited in scope or flawed in design that their results cannot be generalized in any useful way. Because of this our epidemiologic understanding has scarcely advanced since Northway's original description of the disease. This review covers what is known about the epidemiology of BPD along with the special problems encountered in conducting and interpreting research in this area.

Diagnostic Criteria

The lack of standardized diagnostic criteria for BPD has been a major impediment to research (3, 4). Without a uniform definition of what constitutes a case and consistent application of that definition, the results of different studies cannot be compared. The original definition of BPD was based on a sequence of changes observed in radiographs of neonates with respiratory distress syndrome (RDS) (5). This sequence was divided into four stages. Stage I occurred between 2 and 3 days of life and was indistinguishable from severe RDS. Stage II followed between 4 and 10 days of life and consisted of complete opacification of the lung fields. During Stage III (10 to 20 days) small round cystic areas of radiolucency developed, alternating with areas of irregular density. In Stage IV (beyond 1 month of life) the small bubbles of radiolucency enlarged to form hyperaerated cysts. We now know that BPD can follow other diseases besides RDS, so Stage I and II radiographs may not occur in all cases of BPD. Moreover all infants with Stage I or II radiographs do not progress to Stages III and IV. For these reasons many investigators restrict their study populations to patients with Stage III or IV radiographs. However, this classic sequence of radiographic changes is rarely seen today (6, 7). Parenchymal opacification (corresponding to Northway's Stage II) is more likely to be caused by fluid overload, pulmonary hemorrhage, or a left-to-right shunt through a patent ductus arteriosus. Bubbly lungs (Northway's Stage III) more likely indicates pulmonary interstitial emphysema than BPD. At many medical centers patients with Stage IV radiographs are rarely seen. Unlike the classic form of the disease, the new BPD has an insidious onset with the gradual appearance of persisting abnormalities that become radiographically unequivocal after 20 to 30 days of life. The salient characteristics include generalized hyperinflation and a persistent haze followed by multiple lacy infiltrates that obscure the pulmonary vessels. If the diagnostic criteria are restricted to those originally described by Northway and his coworkers, many cases of what is now considered to be BPD will be missed. These temporal changes in the radiographic appearance of BPD raise the question of whether the new BPD is a different disease from that described by Northway. An alternative explanation is that the differences are caused by changes in the neonatal population or in intensive care practices.

There are other drawbacks to diagnostic criteria based solely on radiographs. Infants with other chronic lung diseases, such as Wilson-Mikity syndrome and viral pneumonia, may be erroneously included in the BPD group (8). These infants often require treatment with supplemental oxygen and mechanical ventilation for weeks to months. Consequently lung changes caused by these therapies (*e.g.*, interstitial emphysema) may be superimposed upon those of the underlying disease, making radiographic interpretation difficult.

For the reasons outlined above many investigators have adopted operational definitions that include nonradiographic characteristics of BPD. One of the most common is that of Bancalari (9), who proposed the following criteria: 1) a requirement for intermittent positive pressure ventilation during the first week of life and for a minimum of 3 days; 2) tachypnea, auscultatory rales, and retractions persisting for longer than 28 days; 3) a requirement for supplemental oxygen for more than 28 days to maintain a PaO_2 over 50 torr; and 4) a chest radiograph showing persistent strands of density in both lungs, alternating with areas of normal or increased lucency.

Although this is one of the better operational definitions, it has some important shortcomings. Some infants with apnea of prematurity or "immature lungs" require prolonged mechanical ventilation and develop BPD (10). Many of these infants are not mechanically ventilated within the first week of life and therefore will be excluded under this definition. All infants treated solely with negative pressure ventilators will be excluded, although some are known to have developed BPD. More elaborate criteria have been proposed, but they are unwieldy and have not been widely accepted.

There is a tendency for investigators to design diagnostic criteria that are either overly exclusive or overly inclusive. If exclusive criteria are adopted, the investigator can ensure that all patients who meet the criteria actually have the disease. Restriction of the study group to infants with Stage IV chest radiographs is an example of an exclusive criterion. The disease will appear to be less common (since mild cases are excluded) but more severe. If the criteria are overly inclusive (*e.g.*, all infants who receive supplemental oxygen at 1 month of life), the investigator may detect all patients with the disease, but the study group will be diluted by patients with other disorders. The disease will appear to be more common but less severe.

Recently Farrell made an informal survey of criteria used in 17 medical centers to diagnose BPD (11). Although different criteria were used at each center, all but one listed abnormalities in the chest radiograph. Fourteen centers listed a requirement for supplemental oxygen beyond 3 or 4 weeks in addition to radiographic changes as a basis for diagnosis. Seven centers included dependence on mechanical ventilation beyond 2, 3, or 4 weeks. Farrell noted that many centers base diagnostic criteria on a perceived need for treatment (*e.g.*, mechanical ventilation or supplemental oxygen) and not on the signs and symptoms of disease (*e.g.*, respiratory rate, abnormal blood gas values). The use of therapeutic decisions as diagnostic criteria will inevitably lead to variations in diagnosis from center to center.

Thus far there is no agreement on what criteria should be included in a definition of BPD. Since the symptoms of respiratory distress are not specific, radiographic changes and blood gas data should also be considered. Toce and coworkers have proposed a set of diagnostic criteria that include signs of respiratory distress, prior treatment with either supplemental oxygen or positive pressure ventilation, abnormal blood gas values, and radiographic changes (12). They recommend that neonates at risk for BPD be examined between 14 and 28 days of life, preferably on day 21 for uniformity. The examination concentrates on signs of respiratory distress, including an abnormal respiratory rate (>40/min), intercostal retractions, a requirement for supplemental oxygen, or elevation of PCO_2. Infants without signs of respiratory distress are considered not to have BPD. If respiratory distress is present further evaluation is indicated, including a review of the medical history and thorough physical examination. A history of support with positive pressure ventilation or supplemental oxygen for at least 24 hours is needed to make a diagnosis of BPD. An anteroposterior chest radiograph and a blood gas determination complete the assessment. Radiographic changes consistent with BPD are required to confirm the diagnosis.

To improve the diagnostic criteria further information is needed about the joint distribution of BPD signs and symptoms. It would be helpful to follow a large cohort of infants from birth and record their clinical symptoms, dependence upon supplemental oxygen and mechanical ventilation, and radiographic changes. This information is essential to eliminate nondiscriminating, redundant, and overlapping diagnostic criteria and would assist in constructing a simple and accurate operational definition of BPD.

Prevalence and Incidence

Prevalence and incidence are the two basic measures of disease frequency (1). The number of cases of disease present at a given time is the disease prevalence. Incidence is a measurement of the rate at which new cases of disease occur in a given population; thus incidence is an expression of the risk of acquiring the disease. An incidence figure has a numerator (the number of new cases) and a denominator (the population in which they occurred). In strict usage incidence figures refer to risk over a given period of time, for example, new cases per 100,000 persons at risk per year. However, since the risk of acquiring BPD is negligible after the newborn period, the time is usually omitted in discussions of BPD incidence.

In order for incidence to reflect the risk of acquiring disease, every case in the numerator must have come from the population in the denominator. Likewise everyone in the denominator must be at risk for the disease. The reported incidence of a disease will be affected by changes in either numerator or denominator. Bancalari illustrated this point with the following example (9). During a 10 month period 10 neonates developed BPD. In the same period 235 infants were treated with mechanical ventilation. If the latter group is considered the population at risk, the incidence is 10/235 or 4.2%. If the population is restricted to the 182 infants with RDS who received mechanical ventilation, the incidence rises to 5.5%. Finally, if the population is restricted to the 69 infants who were ventilated for more than 3 days and who survived more than 30 days, the incidence becomes 14.5%.

The population of infants at risk for BPD has not been defined formally, and investigators have differed widely in their selection of study populations. Because estimates of BPD incidence depend both upon cases and the population in which those cases occur, every effort must be made in the future to study homogeneous and well defined populations of infants. Infants not treated with either mechanical ventilation or supplemental oxygen have a negligible risk of developing BPD so the study population should be limited to infants receiving these therapies. Incidence figures that use a denominator based on total nursery admissions are less useful because of regional differences in neonatal populations. Some diagnostic criteria require assessment of the infant at 1 month of age. If these criteria are adopted, only infants who survive till that time should be considered at risk. Infants who die in the first few days of life do not have BPD. Some diseases, such as RDS, carry a higher risk of BPD than others. It would be helpful to have incidence figures for infants with each underlying disease, using as a denominator only infants ventilated for the same disease.

There has been no prospective cohort study of newborn infants to determine the incidence of BPD. The incidence reported in retrospective studies ranges from 0% to 70% (7–24). This variability may be caused by differences in diagnostic criteria and in composition of the patient populations, by temporal changes in the survival rate of low birth weight infants, or by differences in the clinical management of infants with respiratory disease.

The risk of BPD is greatest in very low birth weight infants. The combined data from two studies (22, 23) of infants mechanically ventilated for RDS reveal an incidence of 14% (birth weight 501–1000 g), 6% (birth weight 1001–1500 g), 4% (birth weight 1501–2000 g), and 2% (birth weight >2000 g). In a study of infants who were mechanically ventilated over 24 hours for any reason, the incidence of BPD was 72% in infants weighing less than 1000 g but was only 22% in infants weighing between 1250 and 1500 g (25). In an analysis of BPD frequency between 1969 and 1978, the incidence of BPD in survivors of RDS was 25% to 40% in infants with birth weights between 750 and 1500 g but was less than 10% in infants weighing over 1500 g (8).

Although BPD is usually associated with RDS, it has also been reported in infants with pneumonia, meconium aspiration, cyanotic congenital heart disease, and apnea (26, 27). The disease specific incidence of BPD has been calculated for only a few of these underlying disorders. Data from seven retrospective studies of infants ventilated for RDS are summarized in Table 2.1. Approximately 18% of the infants developed BPD. Lindroth and coworkers found a 20% incidence of BPD in infants who were ventilated for apnea and survived to 28 days of life (10). About 6% of infants mechanically ventilated for persistent pulmonary hypertension develop BPD (28). This low rate may reflect the greater birth weight of infants with persistent pulmonary hypertension.

Improvement in the survival rate of very low birth weight infants might be expected to increase the incidence of BPD (18). On the

Table 2.1. Incidence of Bronchopulmonary Dysplasia in Infants with Respiratory Distress Syndrome

Study	Dates	Diagnostic Criteria	No. of Infants	Cases of BPD (%)
Harrod et al. (17)	1974	Radiographic–Northway Stage III and IV	22	15 (68%)
Truog et al. (18)	1970–75	Radiographic–Northway Stage IV	100	6 (6%)
Wung et al. (7)	1970–77	Radiographic plus clinical history	109	20 (18%)*
Bancalari et al. (9)	1978	Radiographic plus chronic oxygen requirement	69	10 (14%)
Lindroth et al. (10)	1980	Radiographic–Northway Stage III and IV	44	11 (25%)
Boynton et al. (23)	1977–82	Radiographic plus chronic oxygen requirement	221	13 (6%)
Toce et al. (12)	?	Radiographic plus clinical signs and symptoms	55	34 (62%)
			620	109 (18%)

Infants were mechanically ventilated and survived 3 or more weeks.
*Incidence recomputed for surviving infants.

other hand refinements in neonatal care might be expected to lower the incidence. Wung et al. reported that the incidence of BPD fell between 1970 and 1977 in neonates with RDS (7). However, reanalysis of the data in this study suggests that there was no real change. A transient increase in incidence from 5% to 21% occurred in 1972–1973, followed by a return to the 6% baseline incidence only 3 years later. Two other studies have shown no change in incidence between 1967 and 1977 (8, 18). It is not known whether the incidence of BPD has changed since then.

The reported incidence of BPD differs substantially among medical centers. Some of the differences can be attributed to variability in the diagnostic criteria for BPD and in the composition of the patient population. For example nurseries with a large proportion of outborn patients might be expected to have high incidence of BPD. However, outborn infants do not appear to have a higher incidence of BPD if the data are expressed as a fraction of the cases of RDS (11). The effect of differences in the ventilatory management of respiratory failure is difficult to interpret. Several investigators have reported a decrease in the incidence of BPD after they changed some aspect of their ventilatory management (22, 29, 30). However, these reports have not been verified in a prospective randomized trial.

Certain population groups may have an increased biologic susceptibility to BPD. The incidence of HLA-A2 antigen is increased among infants who develop BPD (31). An increased risk of BPD has been reported in infants with a family history of reactive airway disease (32, 33). The effects of other variables, such as sex, ethnic group, and socioeconomic status, have not been investigated.

Bancalari has estimated that there are about 1300 new cases of BPD in the United States each year (34). This figure is conservative since it was calculated using an incidence of only 15%. Assuming that 80% of these infants survive and that full recovery does not occur until 3 years of age, the prevalence of BPD is at least 3100 cases. Thus BPD is a problem of major medical importance. I know of no data on the cost of medical care for infants with BPD, but it must be enormous. Assuming that the initial hospitalization is prolonged by 4 weeks and that hospital costs average $700 per day, BPD costs over $25 million a year for the initial care of new cases.

Natural History

The natural history of BPD is incompletely understood. We do know that affected infants have an excessive postneonatal mortality rate and suffer from continued pulmonary dysfunction, recurrent lower respiratory tract infections, and delays in growth and development (35). In survivors pulmonary dysfunction decreases with time, and the patient may appear to be clinically well by age 3 or 4 (35). Abnormal pulmonary function tests and decreased exercise tolerance have been reported in school-age children (36). Almost nothing is known about pulmonary function in adolescents who survive BPD, although there are individual patients as old as 12 years with demonstrable abnormalities in gas exchange. BPD was first described in 1967, so the earliest cases have just reached adulthood. These patients may have an increased risk of developing chronic obstructive or reactive airway disease (37, 38).

The reported mortality of infants with BPD varies from 11% to 73%. Of course these figures depend upon the criteria for diagnosis and the length of follow-up, neither of which are standardized. The combined data from 11 studies of infants with BPD who survived the neonatal period reveal the deaths of 107 of 462 patients (23%) within the first few years of life (7, 10, 14, 18, 19, 26, 39–43). Most nonsurviving patients die in the first year of life (26, 42). The incidence of sudden infant death syndrome is reported to be seven times higher in infants with BPD than in normal infants (44).

Children who survive BPD often have continuing pulmonary disability. Approximately one-half of these infants require readmission to the hospital during the first 2 years of life (14, 17, 19, 26, 42). Most admissions are for respiratory illnesses such as pneumonia and bronchiolitis (19, 26, 42, 43). Some infants require multiple hospitalizations. In one study infants with BPD were readmitted an average of five times during the first 2 years of life (range, 1–13 admissions) (42).

The radiographic abnormalities of BPD persist for variable lengths of time. Mayes reported that 5 of 11 infants with BPD had abnormal chest radiographs at 6 months of age (14). Harrod *et al.* (17) found radiographic abnormalities in 15 of 15 patients at 1 to 5 years, and Smyth *et al.* (36) found persistent atelectasis and hyperinflation in 8 of 9 children between 7 and 9 years of age. It is probable that the patients studied by Harrod and Smyth were more severely affected than those reported by Mayes. If this is true, it might explain the difference in radiographic outcome.

Children with BPD may have continued abnormalities of pulmonary mechanics and gas exchange even in the absence of clinical symptoms. Expiratory flow limitation, decreased dynamic compliance, and abnormal airway reactivity have all been reported (10, 36, 45). Harrod et al. demonstrated abnormal oxygenation in 12 infants with BPD who were between 1 and 2 years of age (17). The mean PaO_2 was 70 torr in room air and 372 in 100% O_2. The mean alveolar-arterial oxygen gradient in 100% O_2 was 279 torr (normal < 100 torr). Elevations in $PaCO_2$ are also common. Both lung mechanics and gas exchange appear to improve with age, probably as a result of increases in airway size and chest wall strength (46). Increased airways resistance has been reported in infants treated with positive pressure ventilation who have no clinical or radiographic evidence of BPD (47). These changes may persist for months to years and have not been observed in infants who receive supplemental oxygen but do not receive positive pressure ventilation. These infants make up a population with chronic subclinical lung disease. Although these infants will be excluded by all current definitions of BPD, it is likely that they suffer mechanistically similar, though less severe, airway damage. Consequently the BPD prevalence may grossly underestimate the number of infants with mild pulmonary damage.

In addition to chronic pulmonary dysfunction, many infants with BPD develop cardiovascular disease. Harrod et al. found right ventricular hypertrophy in 10 of 12 infants with BPD (17). In three children the EKG returned to normal after the first year of life while seven were persistently abnormal. In some infants pulmonary hypertension and elevated pulmonary vascular resistance were documented at cardiac catheterization. Severe systemic hypertension (systolic pressure > 113 mm Hg) has also been reported and is associated with a high mortality rate (48). There is little known about the incidence of these cardiovascular sequelae.

Delays in growth are common among infants with BPD. Over half the infants studied by Vohr et al. were at the third percentile or below for height and weight at 4 months of age (49). These abnormalities may persist for 2 or more years (41, 42, 49). Four of 11 children followed by Mayes et al. fell below the fifth percentile for height, weight, and head circumference at 3 to 5 years of age (14). These infants have many reasons for poor growth. The work of breathing is increased in BPD, and more than 120 kcal per kilogram of body weight per 24 hours may be needed for normal weight gain. However, the volume of feedings may have to be restricted to prevent exacerbation of pulmonary symptoms. Chronic hypoxia also may impair growth. When the infant's respiratory status improves, there is frequently an acceleration in linear growth (41). The eventual height attained by infants with BPD is not known but is probably within the normal range.

Both developmental delays and neurologic abnormalities have been described in infants with BPD. Mayes et al. found that 8 of 10 children with severe BPD had a developmental quotient (DQ) or IQ below 80 at 2 to 5 years of age (14). A similar frequency of developmental delay was reported by Ruiz et al. and Vohr et al. (24, 49). In contrast four other studies reported abnormal DQs in 20% to 30% of their BPD patients (26, 41, 42, 50). Harrod et al. found no definite developmental delays in 15 infants with BPD, although five had minor abnormalities and were classified as suspect (17). Some of these differences may have been caused by the use of different assessment scales. Harrod *et al.* used the Denver Developmental Screening Test (51), whereas the other investigators chose the Bayley Scales of Infant Development (52), a more sensitive psychometric tool. Two groups have reported a 19% incidence of severe motor weakness (mono- or hemiplegia) in infants that developed BPD (42, 49). However, no cases of cerebral palsy were found in two other studies (14, 41). Sensory loss is often found in infants with BPD. Combined data from four studies reveal 10 occurrences of blindness from retrolental fibroplasia in 189 patients (14, 26, 42, 49). Yu *et al.* found severe hearing loss in 2 of 16 infants (42). Infants with BPD clearly are at high risk for neurodevelopmental impairment. However, it is probable that outcome is related to perinatal events other than the presence or absence of BPD (26, 41). Studies in unselected populations of ventilated neonates have found neurologic sequelae in 4% to 30% of survivors (53). Detailed information on outcome is discussed in Chapter 24 by Sell and Vaucher.

Pathogenesis

Although the pathogenesis of BPD is incompletely understood, there is general agreement that exposure to high concentrations of inspired oxygen and barotrauma from positive pressure ventilation are major etiologic factors. Many other factors that have been suggested as contributing causes are listed in Table 2.2. Figure 2.1 shows the interaction of several factors believed to be important in the pathogenesis of BPD.

In his initial report Northway proposed that oxygen toxicity plays a major role in the

Table 2.2. Risk Factors for Bronchopulmonary Dysplasia

Immaturity of the pulmonary parenchyma
Surfactant deficiency
Exposure to elevated concentrations of inspired oxygen
Barotrauma from positive pressure ventilation
Systemic-to-pulmonary shunt through a patent ductus arteriosus
Pulmonary edema
Pulmonary air leak
Protease–antiprotease imbalance
Family history of reactive airway disease
Tissue type HLA-A2
Vitamin A deficiency

pathogenesis of BPD (5). There is now abundant evidence to support this hypothesis. BPD does not develop in infants who are not treated with supplemental oxygen. Numerous studies have shown that infants who develop BPD are treated for longer periods with higher concentrations of oxygen than infants who have normal outcomes (17, 40, 49). Oxygen is also known to be toxic for many animal species. Lambs ventilated with 100% oxygen die in 2 to 4 days with severe lung damage whereas those ventilated with air suffer no significant pulmonary damage (54). However, most infants exposed to elevated concentrations of inspired oxygen do not acquire BPD. Term infants with small pneumothoraces frequently are treated with 100% oxygen for 8 to 12 hours. These infants almost never develop BPD. BPD is rarely found in infants who are treated with supplemental oxygen but not with positive pressure ventilation. Moreover BPD is found in some infants with either brief exposure to oxygen or else exposure to relatively low concentrations. Hodson reported BPD in nine infants who never received oxygen in concentrations

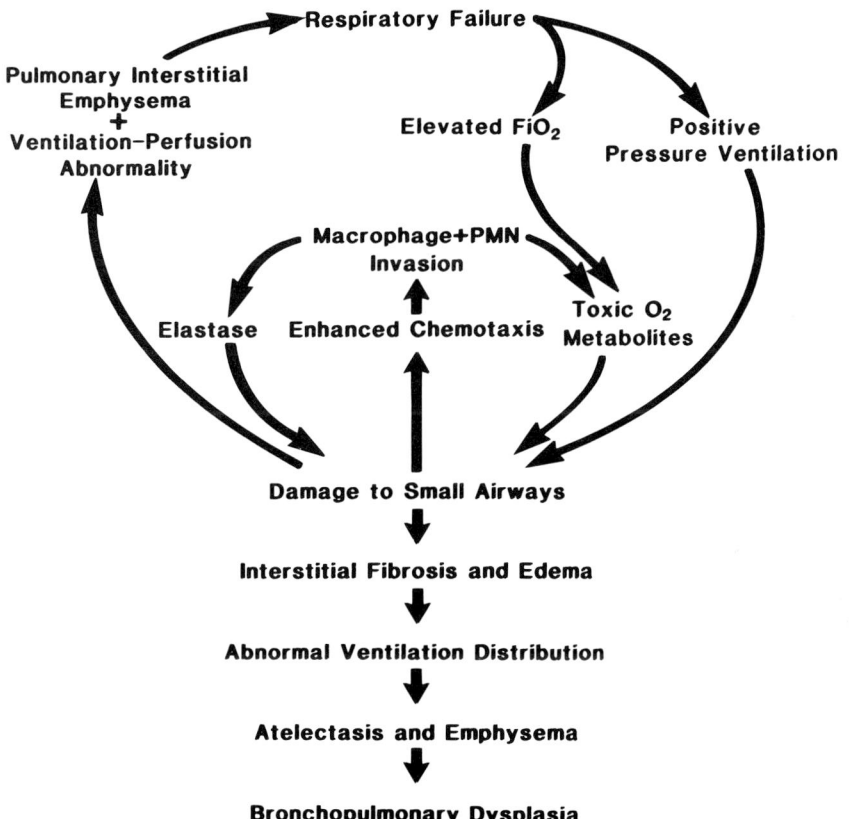

Figure 2.1. Interaction of factors involved in the pathogenesis of bronchopulmonary dysplasia. Adapted from Bancalari, 1985 (34).

over 60% (55). In summary, oxygen appears to be a necessary, but not a sufficient, stimulus for the development of BPD.

Some investigators have argued that barotrauma from intermittent positive pressure ventilation, rather than oxygen toxicity, is the major cause of BPD (56). BPD is rare in infants treated solely with negative pressure ventilators or continuous positive airway pressure (CPAP) (57). There is a strong association between the occurrence of pulmonary air leak syndrome (a group of disorders known to be caused by high inflation pressures) and the development of BPD. Moylan et al. studied 99 infants treated for RDS with intermittent positive pressure ventilation (58). Forty infants suffered air leaks (pulmonary interstitial emphysema, pneumothorax, and pneumomediastinum). BPD developed in 27 of 40 infants with air leaks but in only 3 of 59 without air leaks. Taghizadeh and Reynolds reported a strong correlation between the use of high peak-inspiratory pressures (>35 cm H_2O) and the most serious lesions of BPD, damage to airways followed by repair and fibrosis (56). Several workers have reported an association between the use of lower peak-inspiratory pressures and a decreased incidence of BPD (16, 29). Not all studies have found an association between high peak airway pressures and BPD. Bancalari *et al.* found no difference in the incidence of BPD between infants ventilated with high peak pressures and short inspiratory times and those ventilated with lower peak pressures and long inspiratory times (59). Similar findings were reported by Heicher *et al.* (60). Brown and her colleagues described six infants with BPD who were never ventilated with pressures above 30 cm H_2O (15). Most infants treated with intermittent positive pressure ventilation do not develop BPD. Like oxygen exposure, positive pressure ventilation appears to be necessary, but not sufficient, for the development of BPD.

Many of the remaining risk factors in Table 2.2 are difficult to dissociate from oxygen exposure and barotrauma. Infants with pulmonary edema or a patent ductus arteriosus often have decreased lung compliance and may require treatment with increased ventilatory pressures and oxygen concentrations. However, the role played by surfactant deficiency deserves special consideration. RDS is the most common underlying disease of infants who develop BPD. This is partly because RDS is a very common cause of respiratory failure. However, the immature, surfactant deficient lung may be predisposed to barotrauma. In one study premature newborn rabbits were mechanically ventilated with ambient air for 10 minutes with a peak pressure of 35 cm H_2O with or without prior instillation of natural surfactant into the airways (61). Bronchial epithelial lesions were found in 9 of 10 control animals but in only 4 of 11 surfactant treated animals. Lesions in the surfactant treated animals were less severe than those in controls. The investigators proposed that the observed bronchial epithelial lesions were caused by an abnormal lung expansion pattern with overdistention of terminal bronchioles, caused in turn by surfactant deficiency. Taghizadeh and Reynolds studied the inflation of lungs excised from infants dying of RDS in the first 5 days of life. When distending pressures as high as 60 cm H_2O were applied, there was remarkable overexpansion of the terminal airways even though the saccules remained collapsed (56). Using premature baboons with RDS, Ackerman *et al.* demonstrated that pulmonary air leaks originate from the terminal bronchioles rather than the saccules (62).

It is probable that BPD has multiple causes. Philip proposed that the injurious effects of oxygen and pressure are additive (63). In other words the causative factors are oxygen plus pressure plus time. Perhaps the stretching and shearing forces of conventional mechanical ventilation potentiate the toxic effects of oxygen by tearing bronchial epithelium and exposing subepithelial connective tissue.

Recently, Goetzman brought the various risk factors together in a nice model of BPD pathogenesis (see ch 18, fig 18.4) (64). In this model a susceptible host (immature respiratory system, genetic predisposition, asphyxia) suffers acute pulmonary injury from barotrauma and surfactant deficiency. The initial lung injury causes the release of toxic oxidants and proteolytic enzymes leading to secondary lung injury. The lung then heals in an abnormal manner, perhaps complicated by continued hyperoxia, inadequate nutrition, and vitamin A deficiency. Little is known about the interaction of pulmonary immaturity with the effects of oxygen toxicity and barotrauma. The immature lung is surfactant deficient, underdeveloped in its antioxidant defenses, and is probably more prone to pressure injury. Thus the effects of pulmonary immaturity may be additive with those of oxygen and pressure. Perhaps Philip's equation should be amended to: immaturity + oxygen + pressure + time = BPD.

Our understanding of the pathogenesis of BPD is still elementary. As Sir Ronald Ross once commented, "To say that a disease depends upon certain factors is not saying much, until we can also form an estimate as to how largely each factor influences the whole result" (65). Thus far we are unable to do this.

Prevention

The best therapy for any disease is prevention. Prevention is usually thought of as the interruption of pathogenetic mechanisms in order to prevent the appearance of clinical disease. However, there are several levels of prevention (Table 2.3). In primary prevention both clinical disease and subclinical pathologic changes are blocked. For example BPD could be prevented by eradicating those forms of respiratory distress that require treatment with supplemental oxygen and mechanical ventilation. The introduction of less toxic treatments for respiratory distress constitutes secondary prevention. Several innovative approaches have been proposed including high-frequency ventilation (66); exogenous surfactants (67, 68), and various antioxidants (69, 70). The development of techniques for early diagnosis is another example of secondary prevention. With early case finding therapy might be altered to prevent the appearance of clinical disease. In tertiary prevention the emphasis is on optimal treatment for infants with established BPD. What is being prevented at this level is long-term disability.

Table 2.3. Bronchopulmonary Displasia: Levels of Prevention

Primary prevention
  Prevention of preterm birth
  Prevention of respiratory distress
Secondary prevention
  Use of less toxic therapies
    Exogenous surfactants
    High-frequency ventilation
    More insightful use of conventional ventilation
  Antidotes for toxic therapies
    Antioxidants
      Vitamins A and E
      Superoxide dismutase
    Corticosteroids
Tertiary prevention
  Optimal treatment of BPD
  Screening for complications
  Early detection of neurodevelopmental delay

Summary

Our understanding of the clinical epidemiology of BPD is still inadequate. Reliable information about the incidence and distribution of disease is difficult to obtain because there has been no agreement on diagnostic criteria or on an appropriate denominator for comparative studies (55). These parameters must be standardized in order to assess the efficacy of new therapies. Since the original description there have been changes in the clinical and radiographic manifestations of BPD. It is not known whether these are the result of changes in neonatal care or whether BPD is now occurring in a different population of infants. Considerable information has been gathered about the short-term (2–3 year) outcome of infants with BPD, but almost nothing is known about the long-term (10–20 year) prognosis. Prematurity, RDS, oxygen toxicity, and intermittent positive pressure ventilation are all associated with the occurrence of BPD. Many other factors, such as vitamin A deficiency (71), may increase individual susceptibility to pulmonary damage. The ultimate goal for both epidemiologist and clinician must be the prevention of disease. The reduced incidence of BPD observed in recent therapeutic trials suggests that this goal may be within our grasp.

References

1. Lillienfeld AM. Foundations of epidemiology. New York: Oxford University Press, 1976.
2. Morris JN. Uses of epidemiology. 3rd ed. Edinburg: Churchill Livingstone, 1975.
3. Workshop on Bronchopulmonary Dysplasia. J Pediatr 1979;85:920.
4. O'Brodovich HM, Mellins RB. Bronchopulmonary dysplasia—unresolved neonatal lung injury. Am Rev Respir Dis 1985;132:694–709.
5. Northway WH Jr, Rosan RC, Porter DY. Pulmonary disease following respirator therapy of hyaline membrane disease: bronchopulmonary dysplasia. N Engl J Med 1967;276:357–368.
6. Edwards DK. Radiographic aspects of bronchopulmonary dysplasia. J Pediatr 1979;95:823–829.
7. Wung J-T, Koons AH, Driscoll JM, James LS. Changing incidence of bronchopulmonary dysplasia. J Pediatr 1979;95:845–847.
8. Tooley WH. Epidemiology of bronchopulmonary dysplasia. J Pediatr 1979;95:851–858.
9. Bancalari E, Abdenour GE, Feller R, Gannon J. Bronchopulmonary dysplasia: clinical presentation. J Pediatr 1979;95:819–823.
10. Lindroth M, Svenningsen NW, Ahlström H, Jonson B. Evaluation of mechanical ventilation in newborn infants. II. Pulmonary and neurodevelopmental sequelae in relation to original diagnosis. Acta Paediatr Scand 1980;69:151–158.
11. Farrell PM, Palta M. Bronchopulmonary dysplasia. In: Bronchopulmonary dysplasia. Report of the 90th Ross Conference on Pediatric Research. Columbus, Ohio: Ross Laboratories, 1986.
12. Toce SS, Farrell PM, Leavitt LA, Edwards DK. Clinical and roentgenographic scoring systems for assessing bronchopulmonary dysplasia. Am J Dis Child 1984;138:581–585.
13. Reynolds EOR. Management of hyaline membrane disease. Br Med Bull 1975;31:18.
14. Mayes L, Perkett E, Stahlman MT. Severe bronchopulmonary dysplasia: a retrospective review. Acta Paediatr Scand 1983;72:225–229.
15. Brown ER, Stark A, Sosenko I, Lawson EE, Avery ME. Bronchopulmonary dysplasia: possible relationship to pulmonary edema. J Pediatr 1978;92:982–984.
16. Berg TJ, Pagtakhan RD, Reed MH, Langston C, Chernick V. Bronchopulmonary dysplasia and lung rupture in hyaline membrane disease: influence of continuous distending pressure. Pediatrics 1975;55:51–54.
17. Harrod JR, L'Heureux P, Wangensteen OD, Hunt CE. Long-term follow-up of severe respiratory distress syndrome treated with IPPB. J Pediatr 1974;84:277–286.
18. Truog WE, Prueitt JL, Woodrum DE. Unchanged incidence of bronchopulmonary dysplasia in survivors of hyaline membrane disease. J Pediatr 1978;92:261–264.
19. Truog WE, Jackson JC, Badura RJ, Sorensen GK, Murphy JH, Woodrum DE. Bronchopulmonary dysplasia and pulmonary insufficiency of prematurity—lack of correlation of outcome with gas exchange abnormalities at 1 month of age. Am J Dis Child 1985;139:351–354.
20. de Kleine MJ, Peters GJ, Deen L, Koppe JG. Behandelingsresultaten bij 951 pasgeborenen in de periode 1967 tot en met 1981. Tijdschr Kindergeneeskd 1984;52(3):71–81.
21. Pezzani FM, Montali S, Lazzerini M, Bini F. Bronchopulmonary dysplasia in very low birth weight infants. Pediatr Med Chir 1982;4(5):497–500.
22. Rhodes PG, Graves GR, Patel DM, Campbell SB, Blumenthal BI. Minimizing pneumothorax and bronchopulmonary dysplasia in venti-

lated infants with hyaline membrane disease. J Pediatr 1983;103:634–637.
23. Boynton BR, Mannino FL, Randel RC, et al. Minimizing bronchopulmonary dysplasia in VLBW infants (letter). J Pediatr 1984;104:962.
24. Ruiz MD, LeFever JA, Hakanson DO, Clark DA, Williams ML. Early development of infants of birth weight less than 1,000 grams with reference to mechanical ventilation in newborn period. Pediatrics 1981;68:330–335.
25. Finer N, Peters K, Barrington K, Hayek Z. Risk factors for bronchopulmonary dysplasia (abstr). Pediatr Res 1985;19:341A.
26. Sauve RS, Singhal N. Long-term morbidity of infants with bronchopulmonary dysplasia. Pediatrics 1985;76:725–733.
27. Rhodes PG, Hall RT, Leonidas JC. Chronic pulmonary disease in neonates with assisted ventilation. Pediatrics 1975;55:788–796.
28. Hageman JR, Adams MA, Gardner TH. Pulmonary complications of hyperventilation therapy for persistent pulmonary hypertension. Crit Care Med 1985;13:1013–1014.
29. Sosulski R, Heneghan MA. Comparison of risk factors associated with bronchopulmonary dysplasia (abstr). Pediatr Res 1985;19:417A.
30. Avery ME, Tooley WH, Keller JB, et al. Is chronic lung disease in low birth weight infants preventable? A survey of eight centers. Pediatrics 1987;79:26–30.
31. Clark DA, Pincus LG, Oliphant M, Hubbell C, Oates RP, Davey FR. HLA-A2 and chronic lung disease in neonates. J Am Med Assoc 1982;248:1868–1869.
32. Nickerson BG, Taussig LM. Family history of asthma in infants with bronchopulmonary dysplasia. Pediatrics 1980;65:1140–1144.
33. Fineberg M, Stabile MW, Lew CD, Platzker ACG, Keens TG. Bronchial hyperreactivity in parents of infants with bronchopulmonary dysplasia. Am Rev Respir Dis 1985;131:A265.
34. Bancalari E. Bronchopulmonary dysplasia. In: Milner AD, Martin RJ, eds. Neonatal and pediatric respiratory medicine. London: Butterworths, 1985.
35. Northway WH. Observations on bronchopulmonary dysplasia. J Pediatr 1979;95:815–817.
36. Smyth JA, Tabachnik E, Duncan WJ, Reilly BJ, Levison H. Pulmonary function and bronchial hyperreactivity in long-term survivors of bronchopulmonary dysplasia. Pediatrics 1981;68:336–340.
37. Burrows B, Knudson R, Lebowitz M. The relationship of childhood respiratory illness to adult obstructive airways disease. Am Rev Respir Dis 1977;115:751–760.
38. Tepper RS. Chronic respiratory disturbances in bronchopulmonary dysplasia. In: Bronchopulmonary dysplasia. Report of the 90th Ross Conference on Pediatric Research. Columbus, Ohio: Ross Laboratories, 1986.
39. Perlman JM, Moore V, Siegel MJ, Dawson J. Is chloride depletion an important contributing cause of death in infants with bronchopulmonary dysplasia? Pediatrics 1986;77:212–216.
40. Edwards DK, Dyer WM, Northway WH. Twelve years' experience with bronchopulmonary dysplasia. Pediatrics 1977;59:839–846.
41. Markestad T, Fitzhardinge PM. Growth and development in children recovering from bronchopulmonary dysplasia. J Pediatr 1981;98:597–602.
42. Yu VYH, Orgill AA, Lim SB, Bajuk B, Astbury J. Growth and development of very low birthweight infants recovering from bronchopulmonary dysplasia. Arch Dis Child 1983;58:791–794.
43. Bryan MH, Hardie MJ, Reilly BJ, Swyer PR. Pulmonary function studies during the first year of life in infants recovering from the respiratory distress syndrome. Pediatrics 1973;52:169–178.
44. Werthammer J, Brown ER, Neff RK, Taeusch HW. Sudden infant death syndrome in infants with bronchopulmonary dysplasia. Pediatrics 1982;69:301–304.
45. Tepper RS, Morgan W, Cota K, Taussig L. Forced expiratory flow in infants: a simple non-invasive test of airways obstruction in infants with bronchopulmonary dysplasia (abstr). Am Rev Respir Dis 1983;127(4):213.
46. Morray JP, Fox WW, Kettrick RG, Downes JJ. Improvement in lung mechanics as a function of age in the infant with severe bronchopulmonary dysplasia. Pediatr Res 1982;16:290–294.
47. Stocks J, Godfrey S, Reynolds EO. Airway

resistance in infants after various treatments for hyaline membrane disease: special emphasis on prolonged high levels of inspired oxygen. Pediatrics 1978;61:178–183.
48. Perlman J, Moore V, Siegel M, Dawson J. Factors associated with fatal outcome in premature infants with prolonged bronchopulmonary dysplasia (abstr). Pediatr Res 1985; 19:413A.
49. Vohr BR, Bell EF, Oh W. Infants with bronchopulmonary dysplasia—growth pattern and neurologic and developmental outcome. Am J Dis Child 1982;136:443–447.
50. Koops BL, Abman SH, Accurso FJ. Outpatient management and follow-up of bronchopulmonary dysplasia. Clin Perinatol 1984;11:101–122.
51. Frankenburg WK, Dodds JB. The Denver Developmental Screening Test Manual, rev. Denver: University of Colorado Press, 1970.
52. Bayley N. Bayley Scales of Infant Development. New York: The Psychological Corporation, 1969.
53. Marriage KJ, Davis PA. Neurological sequelae in children surviving mechanical ventilation in the neonatal period. Arch Dis Child 1977;52: 176–182.
54. deLemos R, Wolfsdor J, Nachman R, et al. Lung injury from oxygen in lambs: the role of artificial ventilation. Anesthesiology 1969;30: 609.
55. Hodson WA, Truog WE, Mayock DE, Lyrene R, Woodrum DE. Bronchopulmonary dysplasia: the need for epidemiologic studies. J Pediatr 1979;95:848–851.
56. Taghizadeh A, Reynolds EOR. Pathogenesis of bronchopulmonary dysplasia following hyaline membrane disease. Am J Pathol 1976;82:241–264.
57. Stern L. The role of respirators in the etiology and pathogenesis of bronchopulmonary dysplasia. J Pediatr 1979;95:867–868.
58. Moylan FMB, Walker AM, Krammer SS, Todres ID, Shannon DC. Alveolar rupture as an independent predictor of bronchopulmonary dysplasia. Crit Care Med 1978;6:10–13.
59. Bancalari E, Feller R, Gerhardt T, Abdenour G, Gannon J, Melnick G. Prospective evaluation of different IPPV settings in infants with RDS (abstr). Clin Res 1980;28:870A.
60. Heicher DA, Kasting DS, Harrod JR. Prospective clinical comparison of two methods for mechanical ventilation of neonates: rapid rate and short inspiratory time versus slow rate and long inspiratory time. J Pediatr 1981;98: 957–961.
61. Nilsson R, Grossmann G, Robertson B. Pathogenesis of neonatal lung lesions induced by artificial ventilation: evidence against the role of barotrauma. Respiration 1980;40:218–225.
62. Ackerman NB, Kuehl TJ, Coalson JJ, et al. Distal airway rupture during high frequency ventilation (HFV) in the premature baboon with hyaline membrane disease (HMD) (abstr). Crit Care Med 1983;11:223.
63. Philip AGS. Oxygen plus pressure plus time: the etiology of bronchopulmonary dysplasia. Pediatrics 1975;55:44–50.
64. Goetzman BW. Understanding bronchopulmonary dysplasia. Am J Dis Child 1986;140: 332–334.
65. Ross, Sir R. The prevention of malaria. 2nd ed. New York: EP Dutton, 1910.
66. Special conference report—high frequency ventilation for immature infants. Pediatrics 1983;71:280–287.
67. Hallman M, Merritt TA, Jarvenpaa A, et al. Exogenous human surfactant for treatment of severe respiratory distress syndrome: a randomized prospective clinical trial. J Pediatr 1985;106:963–969.
68. Merritt TA, Hallman M, Bloom BT, et al. Prophylactic treatment of very premature infants with human surfactant. N Engl J Med 1986;315:785–790.
69. Rosenfeld W, Evans H, Concepcion L, Jhaveri R, Shaeffer H, Friedman A. Prevention of bronchopulmonary dysplasia by administration of bovine superoxide dismutase in preterm infants with respiratory distress syndrome. J Pediatr 1984;105:781–785.
70. Ehrenkranz RA, Ablow RC, Warshaw JB. Prevention of bronchopulmonary dysplasia with vitamin E administration during the acute stages of respiratory distress syndrome. J Pediatr 1979;95:873–878.
71. Shenai JP, Chytil F, Stahlman MT. Vitamin A status of neonates with bronchopulmonary dysplasia. Pediatr Res 1985;19:185–189.

3

Pathogenesis of Bronchopulmonary Dysplasia

DIONYSIS S. BONIKOS AND KLAUS G. BENSCH

Introduction

The pathologic abnormalities of bronchopulmonary dysplasia (BPD) have been presented in detail in several reports (1–11). These reports have demonstrated a steady chronologic progression of changes from the initial typical alterations of the exudative stage of diffuse alveolar damage of the respiratory distress syndrome (RDS) to a regenerative and fibroproliferative reparative stage. In the original description of BPD, Northway *et al.* (1) distinguished four radiologic and pathologic stages. Each one of these is characterized by histopathologic changes which consist of a broad spectrum of alterations ranging from barely recognizable abnormalities at Stage I to profound lesions at Stage IV. However, it should be emphasized that one of the main observations made in most of the studies of the pathology of BPD is that, in the individual patient, there is a great deal of overlapping of the pathologic stages and several pathologic states characteristically exist at the same time.

On inspection the lungs in Stage IV BPD are heavy and their external surface usually shows indented fissures representing underlying tissue condensation and scarring. A frequently observed cobblestone appearance is brought about by a network of finer scarring and by thickening of interlobular connective tissue septa. The cut surface of such lungs has a variegated appearance and shows irregularities in density and aeration (6, 11). Examination by light microscopy, as well as ultrastructural (6, 10) study of the lungs in BPD, reveals a variable admixture of alterations in bronchi, bronchioli, alveoli, and vessels. However, the pulmonary alterations in BPD vary with the stage. In mild cases of BPD the initial typical histopathologic changes, with membranous inspissated exudates lining mainly dilated alveolar transitional ducts and respiratory bronchioles, is followed by early attempts at organization and/or resorption of these protein-rich hyaline membranes. In patients that had received supplemental oxygen at high concentration, there is a concomitant patchy loss of cilia accompanied by focal mucosal denudation of the airway lining (Fig. 3.1). A dominant feature of this exudative early reparative stage of BPD (10) is edema of the interstitial space of bronchi, vessels, and lobular and alveolar septa. This early reparative response of the pulmonary tissue is also characterized by epithelialization of hyaline membranes by type II pneumocytes (6–10). Also not uncommon at this stage is the incorporation of fibrin into the alveolar septa. Cases of BPD of moderate severity, such as Stage III, are characterized by an extensive loss of cilia and bronchial and bronchiolar lining cells, the presence of intramucosal (Fig. 3.2) as well as intraluminal inflammatory cells, necrosis of alveolar lining cells, and marked edema of the peribronchial and perivascular spaces, as

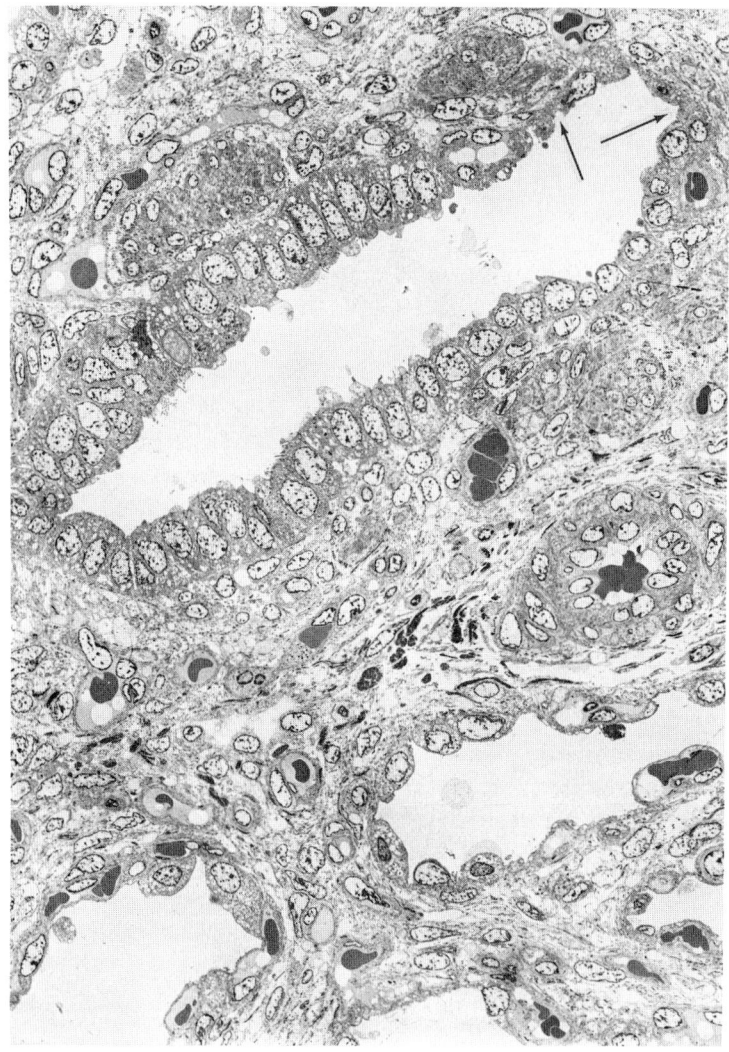

Figure 3.1. This micrograph from an infant that survived 23 days and had had 547 hours of supplemental oxygen shows focal sloughing of the bronchiolar mucosa (arrows) and loss of cilia. ×900. (Reprinted, with permission from W. B. Saunders Co., From Bonikos DS, Bensch KG, Northway WH Jr, Edwards DK. Bronchopulmonary dysplasia. Human Pathol 1976;7:643–666.)

well as the alveolar septa. Small foci of atelectasis can also be present. In addition a striking finding is the appearance of squamous metaplasia of the cells lining the conductive airways (Figs. 3.3 and 3.4). In cases of severe BPD, Stage IV, the marked necrosis of the airway lining results in intraluminal accumulation of excessive amounts of dense eosinophilic debris containing necrotic epithelial cells, mucus, and inflammatory cells (Fig. 3.3). The alveolar lumina contain increased numbers of alveolar macrophages, while the overall al-

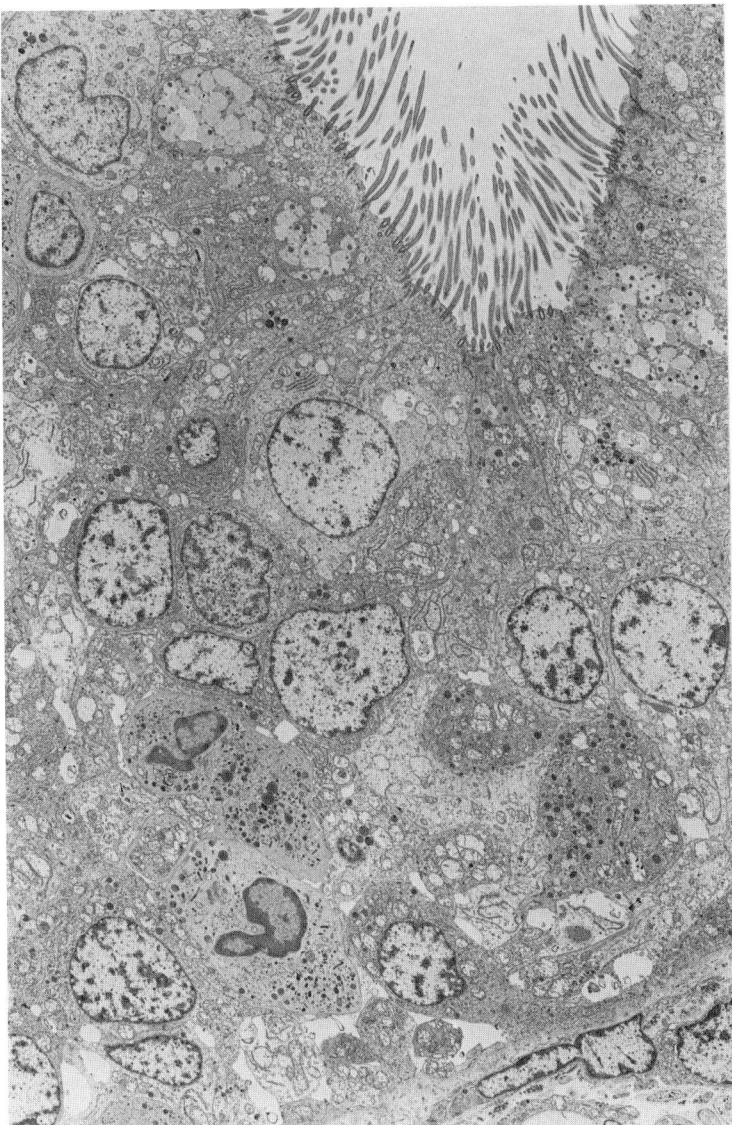

Figure 3.2. This micrograph shows polymorphonuclear leukocytes among the mucosal cells of a major segmental bronchus. ×5800. (Reprinted, with permission from W. B. Saunders Co., From Bonikos DS, Bensch KG, Northway WH Jr, Edwards DK. Bronchopulmonary dysplasia. Human Pathol 1976;7:643–666.)

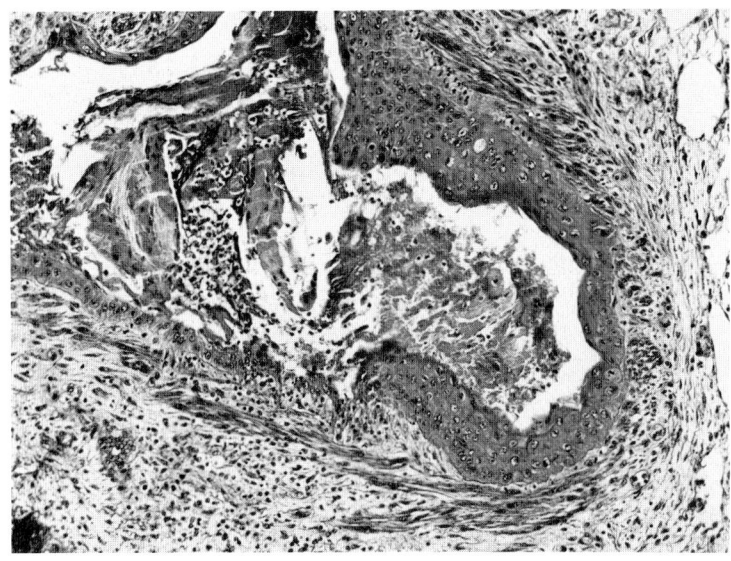

Figure 3.3. In this bronchiole from the lung of an infant that survived 33 days and had had 796.5 hours of supplemental oxygen, necrosis of the epithelial lining is accompanied by marked squamous metaplasia of the mucosa. Within the bronchiolar lumen an inflammatory exudate, intermingled with epithelial cell debris and mucus, can be identified. Hematoxylin-eosin; ×120. (Reprinted, with permission from W. B. Saunders Co., From Bonikos DS, Bensch KG, Northway WH Jr, Edwards DK. Bronchopulmonary dysplasia. Human Pathol 1976;7:643–666.)

veolar architecture is markedly disturbed with foci of atelectasis alternating with areas of hyperinflated air sacs. In addition there is marked squamous metaplasia of bronchial and bronchiolar epithelium and vascular medial hypertrophy of the hypertensive type. A very conspicuous feature in such cases is the presence of patchy interstitial alveolar fibrosis (Fig. 3.5) as well as foci of organizing intra-alveolar exudates containing fibroblasts and newly formed connective tissue elements. Eventually in severe, advanced cases of BPD, the changes described above are more widespread and very pronounced. The overall picture in such cases is dominated by peribronchial and peribronchiolar fibrosis, obliterative fibroproliferative bronchiolitis, and severe derangement of the alveolar architecture characterized by widely dispersed foci of severe hyperinflation and bullous emphysema (Fig. 3.6) alternating with irregularly distributed dense scars and areas of atelectasis. Severe vascular changes with prominent medial hypertrophy, endothelial cell hyperplasia, and adventitial fibrosis are usually present (Fig. 3.7), as well as a reduction in the volume of the capillary and precapillary vascular beds. In summary, the pathology of BPD comprises a broad spectrum of simultaneous acute and chronic lung changes that begin with an exudative and early reparative stage and ultimately progress to a chronic fibroproliferative process, the main features of which are obliterative airway disease and a widespread parenchymal fibrosis with alternating areas of

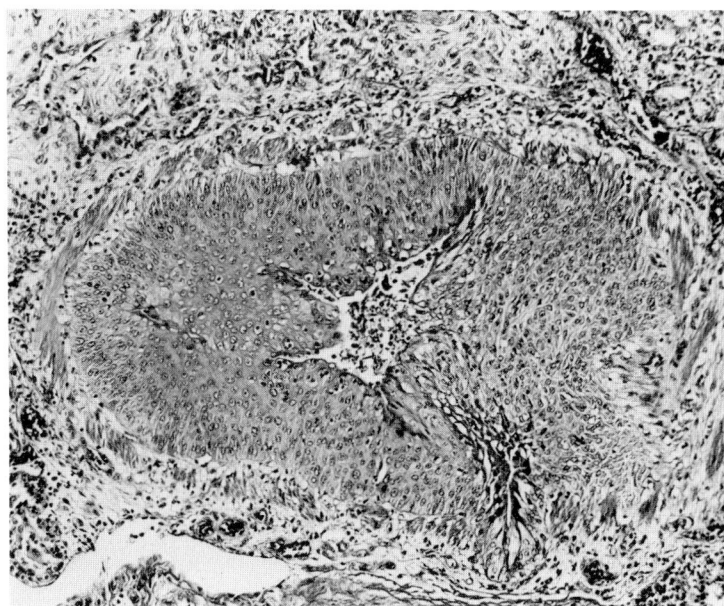

Figure 3.4. Squamous metaplasia in this bronchiole is so pronounced that it has led to an almost complete occlusion of the bronchiole lumen. This infant survived 137 days and had had 2083 hours of supplemental oxygen. Hematoxylin-eosin; ×120. (Reprinted, with permission from W. B. Saunders Co., From Bonikos DS, Bensch KG, Northway WH Jr, Edwards DK. Bronchopulmonary dysplasia. Human Pathol 1976;7:643–666.)

atelectasis and emphysema and capillary vascular damage leading to diminished alveolization in the developing lung of the newborn.

The relative contribution of several factors to the pathogenesis of BPD is still a matter of intense dispute. However, several predisposing conditions greatly determine the development, severity, and course of the syndrome: the immaturity of the newborn, its birth weight, and the initial severity of the RDS ("hyaline membrane disease") (12). These parameters in turn dictate the concentration of supplemental oxygen that will have to be delivered by artificial ventilation as well as the mode by which oxygen is given. The duration of ventilation with supplemental oxygen is another major factor influencing the development and the severity of BPD. In addition there are not infrequently coincidental aggravating circumstances present, such as a patent ductus arteriosus with congestive heart failure (13), excessive intravenous fluid administration (14), the development of pulmonary interstitial emphysema, pneumomediastinum and/or pneumothorax (15), and pulmonary infections, any one of which could contribute to the development of the disease by prolonging the need for supplemental oxygen therapy. Since BPD can occur in infants with respiratory distress from causes other than RDS (16–20)—as seen in adults (21, 22)—the etiology of BPD is believed to be mainly iatrogenic. Thus it is not surprising that the major controversy has been over the relative contributions of oxygen toxicity (12, 23), artificial ventilation, and

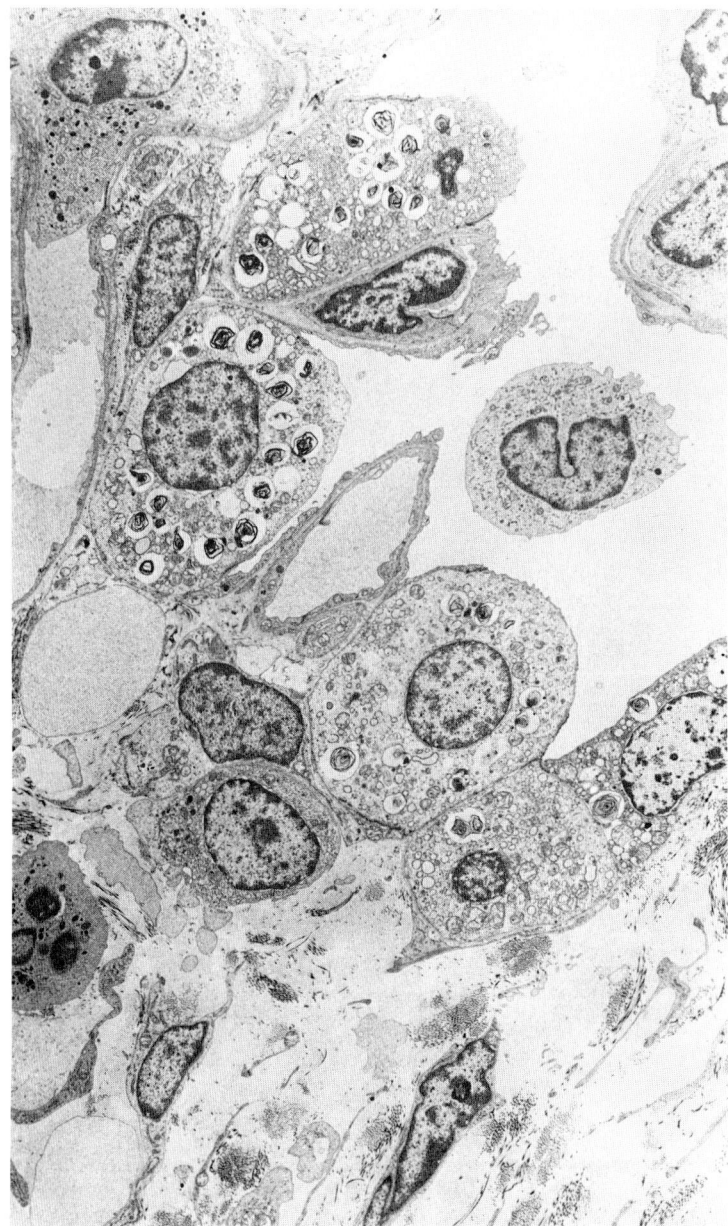

Figure 3.5. In infants in whom the overall pulmonary damage is severe and especially in those with the longest survival on high oxygen concentrations, large areas of previously denuded basement membranes are eventually covered by sheets of granular pneumocytes. Increased amounts of collagen are not infrequently seen. This infant survived 156 days and had had 2666.5 hours of supplemental oxygen. ×4830. (Reprinted, with permission from W. B. Saunders Co., From Bonikos DS, Bensch KG, Northway WH Jr, Edwards DK. Bronchopulmonary dysplasia. Human Pathol 1976;7:643–666.)

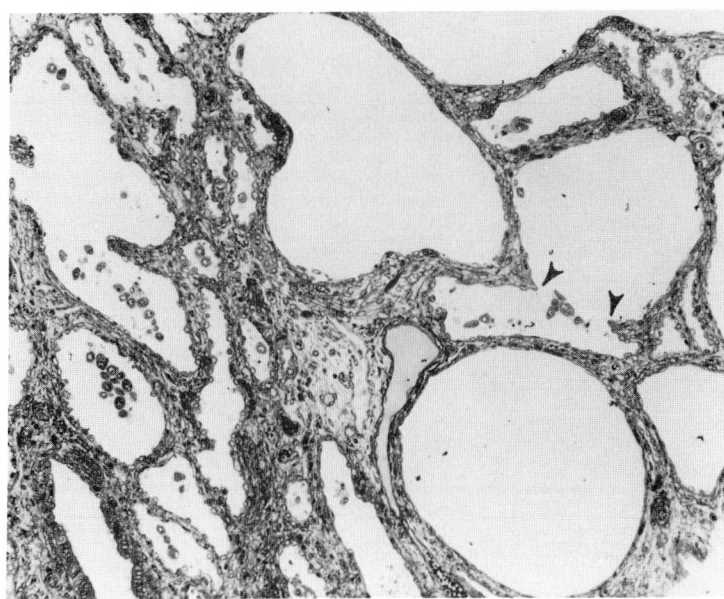

Figure 3.6. This picture from an infant that survived 217 days and had had 5221 hours of supplemental oxygen shows huge irregular air spaces adjacent to alveoli, some of which are smaller than normal. Arrowheads indicate possible remnants of rupture of alveolar walls. Alveolar macrophages are noted within some of the alveolar lumina. Hematoxylin-eosin; ×120. (Reprinted, with permission from W. B. Saunders Co., From Bonikos DS, Bensch KG, Northway WH Jr, Edwards DK. Bronchopulmonary dysplasia. Human Pathol 1976;7:643–666.)

barotrauma (7, 24–26) to the development of BPD.

Pulmonary Oxygen Toxicity

Data from clinical studies (1, 4, 6, 12) as well as experimental studies (27–31) are providing support for the argument advanced by some investigators that the most important etiologic factor in the development of BPD is the deleterious effect of high concentrations of supplemental oxygen on the lungs. This contention is supported by the observation that BPD has occurred in infants who received supplemental oxygen therapy without being on an intermittent positive pressure apparatus (32–34), and by animal model studies that showed striking histopathologic similarities between the human BPD lung and lungs of newborn animals used in the oxygen toxicity experiments (29, 31). The detrimental effect of oxygen on the lung has been thoroughly documented in the clinical and experimental literature (35–38). It has been shown that there is a limited variation in the resistance of different species to high concentrations of oxygen and an age related effect, with newborn and very young animals being more resistant to oxygen induced lung damage (39, 40). This age related resistance to oxygen can

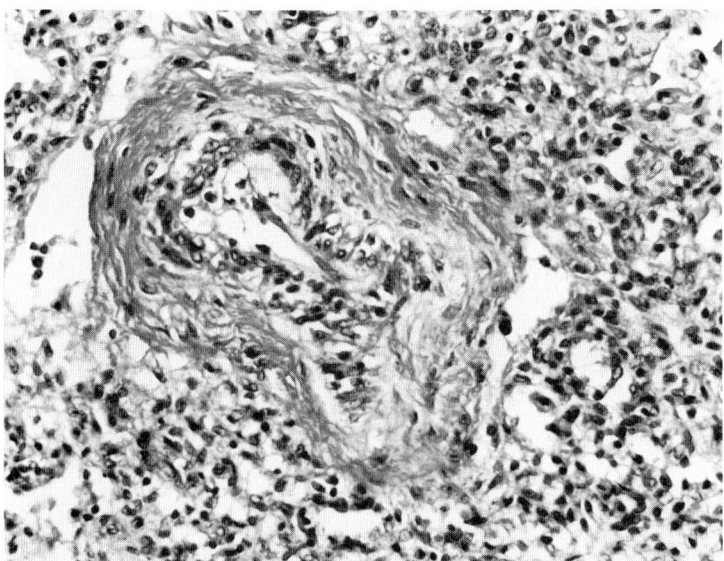

Figure 3.7. A marked accentuation of the periarteriolar fibroconnective tissue resulting in an "onionskin" concentric thickening, particularly of the adventitia, is seen. There is also a moderate increase in the intimal cells, some of which are distinctly edematous. This infant survived 156 days and had had 2666.5 hours of supplemental oxygen. Note the pronounced cellular infiltrate in the tissue surrounding the vessel. Hematoxylin-eosin; ×480. (Reprinted, with permission from W. B. Saunders Co., From Bonikos DS, Bensch KG, Northway WH Jr, Edwards DK. Bronchopulmonary dysplasia. Human Pathol 1976;7:643–666.)

be traced to a more rapid response in the synthesis rate of several enzymes, the most important of which appear to be superoxide dismutase, catalase, and glutathione peroxidase. Under normal circumstances these enzymes inactivate toxic oxygen metabolites. Most important among these are free radicals, which are produced during the univalent reduction of molecular oxygen; they damage the lung by initiating lipid peroxidation chain reactions, inactivating sulfhydryl enzymes, altering nucleic acids, and depleting cells of their reducing capacities (41–44). A hypothesis based on the free radical theory of oxygen toxicity has been advanced that explains the unusual vulnerability of preterm infants with RDS to increased concentrations of oxygen. According to this hypothesis the premature infant with RDS who requires vigorous hyperoxic respiratory support has a lung that is biochemically ill adapted for protecting itself against increased concentrations of oxygen metabolites because of the immaturity of its pulmonary antioxidant system (45). This hypothesis is supported by the findings of Rosenfeld *et al.* (46), who reported on the effectiveness of superoxide dismutase (SOD) in the amelioration of BPD in preterm infants with RDS.

Lung Growth and Maturation

In the original description of the syndrome, Northway and his coworkers stated that the term BPD was selected in order to emphasize the involvement of all the tissues of the lung in the pathologic process (1). What has to be emphasized in this respect is the fact that the pathologic picture of BPD is not only the result of injury and repair of the various components of the newborn lung, but also the result of the marked inhibitory effect of hyperoxia on lung growth and development. In this regard the term dysplasia also denotes the interrupted and abnormal development of the bronchopulmonary system. The lung of the newborn is in a stage of rapid growth and maturation because the formation of adult-like terminal air ducts and alveoli is primarily a postnatal event. Conducting airways are formed by the 16th week of gestational age, whereas multiplication of alveoli continues throughout gestation, infancy, and early childhood (47–50). Experimental studies with newborn animals exposed to hyperoxia have shown marked impairment of lung growth and maturation, resulting in a smaller lung, with fewer alveoli, and a diminished alveolar and vascular surface area for diffusion (29, 51–55). A recent morphometric study of human infants with BPD who died later in life illustrates most convincingly the adverse effect of hyperoxia on alveolar growth and development. This study showed that, compared with age matched control infants, infants with oxygen induced lung injury had a markedly reduced number of alveoli and an alveolar surface area that was only one-third to one-half that of normal (54).

It should be stressed that the vascular development in these lungs is also severely affected by the toxic actions of oxygen. Studies of the effect of hyperoxia on pulmonary vascular development of newborn and young rats have revealed decreased growth rates (55, 56). This effect is additive to the extensive direct structural damage of the pulmonary capillary bed by elevated oxygen concentrations (57, 58). In addition experimental evidence has been presented that hyperoxia causes a rapid structural remodeling of larger vessels, particularly the pulmonary arteries, and pulmonary hypertension.

It should be recalled at this point that medial hypertrophy of small pulmonary arteries is not an infrequent finding in BPD (6). Jones and her coworkers, in their morphometric studies on the pulmonary microvasculature, have demonstrated that hyperoxia induced intimal thickening of intra-acinar arteries, muscular hypertrophy of the normally muscular arteries, and neomuscularization of nonmuscular arterial segment (59, 60). These investigators propose that the newly formed muscle in pulmonary arterial walls probably represents a phenotypic conversion of precursor cells, such as the intermediate cell and pericyte to smooth muscle cells. They further suggest that this transition could be in response to an acute or continuing injury of the vessel wall by oxygen metabolites, or could possibly be caused by specific growth factors released from the platelets or granulocytes that are sequestered in increased numbers in the oxygen damaged pulmonary tissues (28, 29) (Figs. 3.8 and 3.9). Thus the observations of these investigators are not only entirely in keeping with, but also provide an additional interpretation of, the spectrum of vascular changes identified in BPD. This hyperoxia induced vascular remodeling and its hemodynamic consequences lead to an increased pulmonary vascular resistance.

The contribution of vasoconstrictor agents to the increased pulmonary vascular resistance should also be taken into consideration in this context. Johnson *et al.* (61) found a

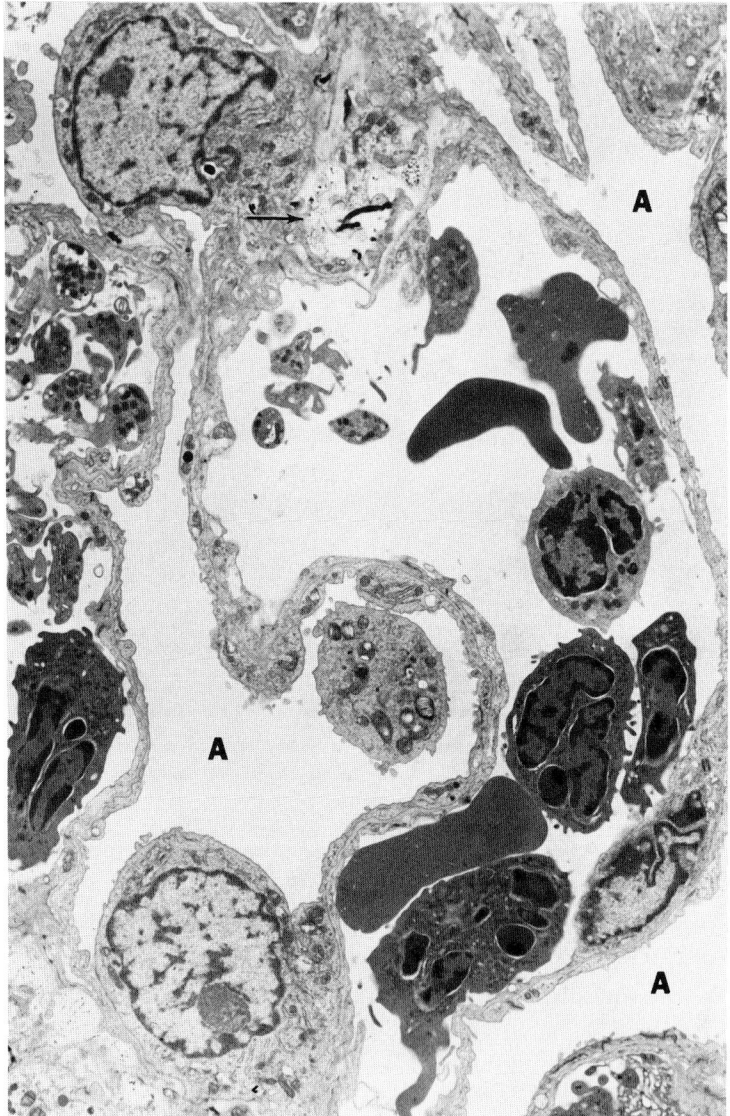

Figure 3.8. Lung from newborn mouse after 5 days of continuous exposure to 100% oxygen at normal atmospheric pressure for 7 days. There is marked dilatation of alveolar capillaries. Present within these vessels are increased numbers of platelets and polymorphonuclear leukocytes. Interstitial edema is also apparent (arrow). A = alveolar lumina. ×7000. (Reprinted, with permission, from Bonikos DS, Bensch KG, Ludwin SK, Northway WH Jr. Oxygen toxicity in the newborn. Lab Invest 1975;32:619–635. Copyright by the US–Canadian Division of the IAP.)

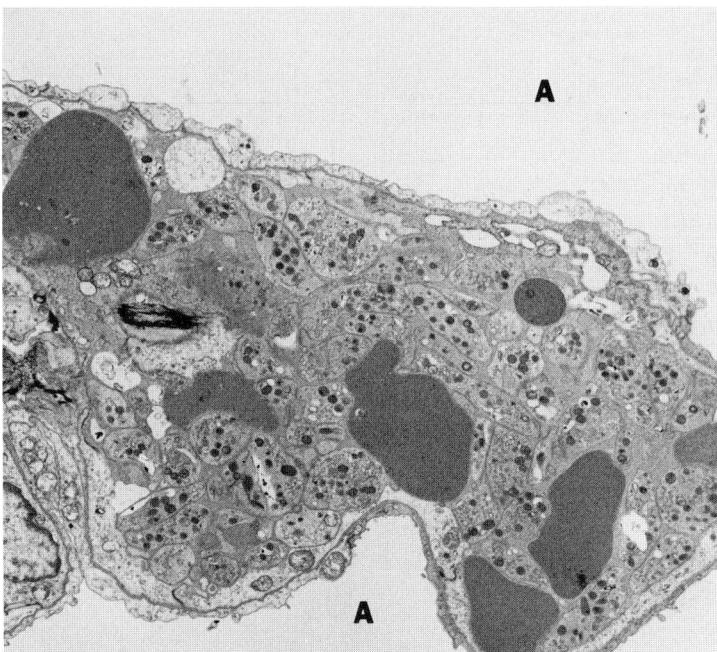

Figure 3.9. Lung from newborn mouse after 5 days of continuous exposure to 100% oxygen at normal atmospheric pressure for 7 days. The alveolar capillary lumina (A) are packed with platelets. ×6000. (Reprinted, with permission, from Bonikos DS, Bensch KG, Ludwin SK, Northway WH Jr. Oxygen toxicity in the newborn. Lab Invest 1975;32:619–635. Copyright by the US–Canadian Division of the IAP.)

marked increase in the number of bombesin-immunoreactive pulmonary neuroendocrine cells in infants with BPD. Since bombesin (actually its mammalian analogue, gastrin-releasing protein) and other substances regulate the smooth muscle tone, it is likely that this increase in the number of these neuroendocrine cells in the lung participates in pulmonary vascular and airway resistance associated with BPD.

It has already been stated that there are numerous factors which appear to contribute to the bronchopulmonary alterations seen in BPD. The precise interplay between the immaturity of the lung, pulmonary surfactant deficiency, the duration and intensity of oxygen exposure, type and depth of mechanical ventilation, patency of the ductus arteriosus, and other factors in the pathogenesis of these alterations is unknown; however, it should be re-emphasized that the toxicity of oxygen alone can be responsible for virtually the entire spectrum of these changes, as borne out by numerous studies on pulmonary oxygen toxicity both in humans (62–66) and in experimental animal models (27–31, 67–72).

Blood Vessels

A cell type particularly sensitive to elevated oxygen concentrations is the endothelial cell. One of the hallmarks of BPD and an early finding in the disease is an extensive interstitial edema which is a result of widespread damage to the capillary endothelium. The extraordinary vulnerability of endothelial cells to hyperoxia has been well documented (28, 67, 68, 73–76). The findings of two *in vitro* studies are of particular interest in this respect because they clearly document the interference of metabolic aberrations with specialized cell functions. Endothelial cells derived from aortas or pulmonary arteries show evidence of an impaired uptake of serotonin or alpha-aminoisobutyric acid after 24–72 hours of exposure to 80%–95% O_2 (77). Similarly hyperoxia has been shown to impair the ability of the perfused lung to remove various compounds including 5-hydroxytryptamine and prostaglandins from the pulmonary circulation (78, 79).

Attempts have also been made to identify the cytoplasmic organelles that are damaged by high oxygen concentrations. A recent study by Lee *et al.* concludes that the initial early structural injury of endothelial cells occurs in lysosomes and that mitochondria are relatively resistant to oxygen injury (80). The extensive endothelial damage in conjunction with the delayed endothelial regeneration caused by the antimitotic effect of oxygen has severe consequences for the host. Most detrimental to pulmonary function is the development of fibrosis, which appears to be related to a disruption of the normal relationships and channels of communication between epithelial and endothelial lining cells and the supporting extracellular mesenchymal components including the cells of the pulmonary interstitium (81). Studies on radiation induced endothelial injury have shown that acute endothelial injury can be rapidly repaired with little fibroblastic stimulation, whereas severe or prolonged injury and delayed regeneration disturb the normal endothelial-mesenchymal relationships and lead to fibrosis (82). Similarly changes in the interaction between epithelial and interstitial elements appear to be key factors in promoting fibroblast proliferation and the deposition of abnormal amounts of collagen.

Other mechanisms, aside from the endothelial injury induced by toxic levels of oxygen, in the genesis of pulmonary edema in BPD are thought to be excessive and inappropriate fluid administration (14) and ductus arteriosus patency with left-to-right shunting (13). Merritt *et al.* found that a patent ductus arteriosus with left-to-right shunting usually results in pulmonary edema necessitating protracted assisted ventilation and higher oxygen concentrations, and higher incidence of BPD and death (83). Failure or delay in the resorption of particularly the intra-alveolar edema fluid with its subsequent organization is a contributory mechanism in the development of fibrosis. In this respect the possible role of barotrauma in interfering with the resolution of edema through entry of air into the pulmonary lymphatic vessels ("pneumatosis pulmonalis") and obstruction of the drainage of interstitial fluid (15, 84) should be taken into consideration.

Airways and Alveoli

The bronchial and bronchiolar lesions of BPD have been attributed to a variety of mechanisms. Taghizadeh and Reynolds have suggested that these lesions are related to mechanical ventilator trauma or the endotracheal intubation (7). On the other hand Nilsson *et al.* (85) favor the concept that the bronchiolar epithelial lesions reflect an abnormal expansion pattern due to the surfactant deficiency. It is postulated that overdistention of airways and irregular aeration of the alveolar compartment produce shear forces in the airway mucosa which lead to disruption of the epithelium. Although barotrauma and surfactant deficiency cannot be disregarded as possible contributory factors in the pathogenesis of the necrotizing bronchiolitis of BPD, experimental data are strongly in favor of the bronchiolar (27, 71, 86) as well as the bronchial (27, 29, 86) lesions being directly related to hyperoxia. It is of particular importance to note that the experimental oxygen induced necrotizing bronchiolitis reported by Harrison et al. (71) was associated with an atypical regeneration of bronchiolar epithelium in the form of squamous metaplasia. The extent of this squamous metaplasia was in proportion to the duration of oxygen exposure.

Similar changes have been noticed in the lungs of infants with severe BPD (6).

The bronchiolitis and peribronchiolar fibrosis of the type associated with the oxygen induced injury of the small airways in experimental animals, which is also present in the lungs of infants with BPD, can have a devastating long-term effect on lung function. Monkeys chronically exposed to ozone develop a bronchiolitis characterized by peribronchiolar inflammation and marginal fibrosis (87); although there was a substantial resolution of the inflammation 3 months after the ozone exposure, progression in the peribronchiolar fibrosis continued (88). In another study, in which peribronchiolar inflammation and fibrosis developed in the lungs of cats chronically exposed to the exhaust of diesel engines, it was shown that the peribronchiolar fibrosis progressed in severity during the subsequent 6 months of "recovery" in clean air (89). These studies imply that once the process of peribronchiolar fibrosis is set into motion, its course may persist and progress long after the precipitating factors have been removed. These data are of additional significance since inflammation and fibrosis of the small airways are considered important initiating factors in the development of emphysema (90). Finally, the bronchiolar changes observed in BPD may severely affect the subsequent growth of the lungs in these neonates. It has been demonstrated in the cat that postnatal alveolar growth may also take place from outpouchings in the walls of the terminal bronchioles (91). Thus bronchiolar injury of the degree observed in some infants with severe BPD could seriously compromise further lung development.

Alveolar type II cell hyperplasia, interstitial and intra-alveolar fibrosis, alveolar wall rupture, and emphysema have been emphasized as basic components of the pathology of BPD (6, 10). It is known that alveolar type II cell hyperplasia is triggered by necrosis of type I alveolar cells (Fig. 3.10). The new type II cells temporarily reline the damaged alveolar wall and subsequently transform into functional gas-exchanging type I cells (92–94) (Fig. 3.11). It is assumed that type II cells proliferate when alveolar epithelial cell damage is mild or moderate, but when the damage is severe the type II cells also die and are then replaced by epithelial cells of bronchiolar origin (95). This phenomenon has been frequently observed in cases of severe BPD in which there is also considerable destruction of the relatively injury resistant type II alveolar epithelial cells.

Inflammatory Response

Of all the pathologic alterations seen in the lungs of infants with BPD, the marked de-

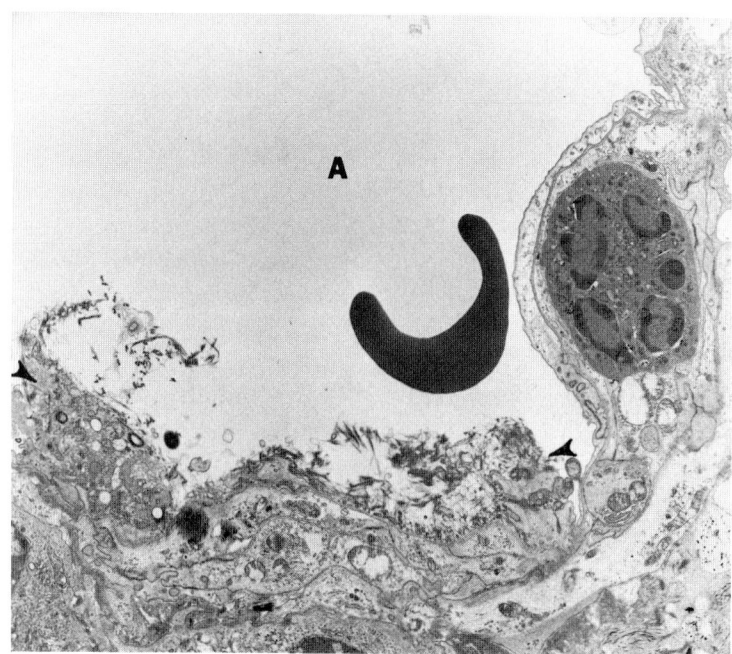

Figure 3.10. Lung from newborn mouse after 5 days of continuous exposure to 100% oxygen at normal atmospheric pressure for 7 days. There is destruction and necrosis of the cytoplasmic processes of a membranous pneumocyte (between arrowheads). Over the basement membrane at this point is amorphous heterogeneous material of increased density, consisting of fibrin strands and fragments of the disrupted or necrotic cells. A marginating leukocyte is seen within the alveolar capillary lumen. The adjacent interstitial tissue is edematous. A = alveolar lumen ×6800. (Reprinted, with permission, from Bonikos DS, Bensch KG, Ludwin SK, Northway WH Jr. Oxygen toxicity in the newborn. Lab Invest 1975;32:619–635. Copyright by the US–Canadian Division of the IAP.)

rangement of the pulmonary tissue with almost total effacement of its normal architecture associated with extensive interstitial and intralveolar fibrosis is the most impressive. This structural damage with coalescence of alveolar walls and extensive irregular fibrosis has been described in every reported pathologic study of BPD (6–8, 10). It is now recognized that the development of pulmonary fibrosis is almost always preceded by an accumulation of inflammatory cells in the alveolar walls (96) (Fig. 3.12). The oxygen induced acute alveolitis is associated with a variable degree of alveolar injury and necrosis. It appears therefore that by virtue of their ability to injure the normal alveolar components, the inflammatory cells amplify the structural damage, and thus greatly influence the recruitment and extent of proliferation of fibroblasts and the subsequent development of fibrosis (96, 97).

Either surfactant deficiency such as is present in RDS or treatment modalities for RDS (high oxygen exposure, particularly in

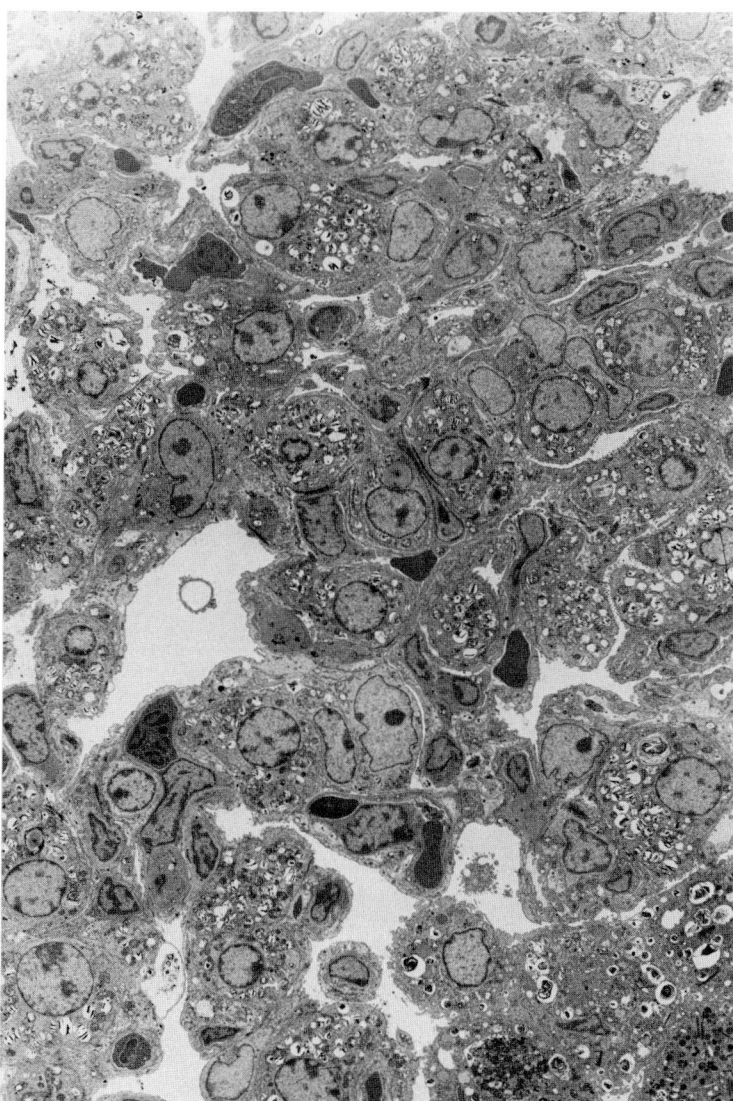

Figure 3.11. Lung from newborn mouse after 2 weeks of continuous exposure to 100% oxygen at normal atmospheric pressure. Notice the extensive proliferation of granular pneumocytes and partial alveolar collapse. ×1750. (Reprinted, with permission, from Bonikos DS, Bensch KG, Northway WH Jr. Oxygen toxicity in the newborn. Am J Pathol 1976;85:623–650.)

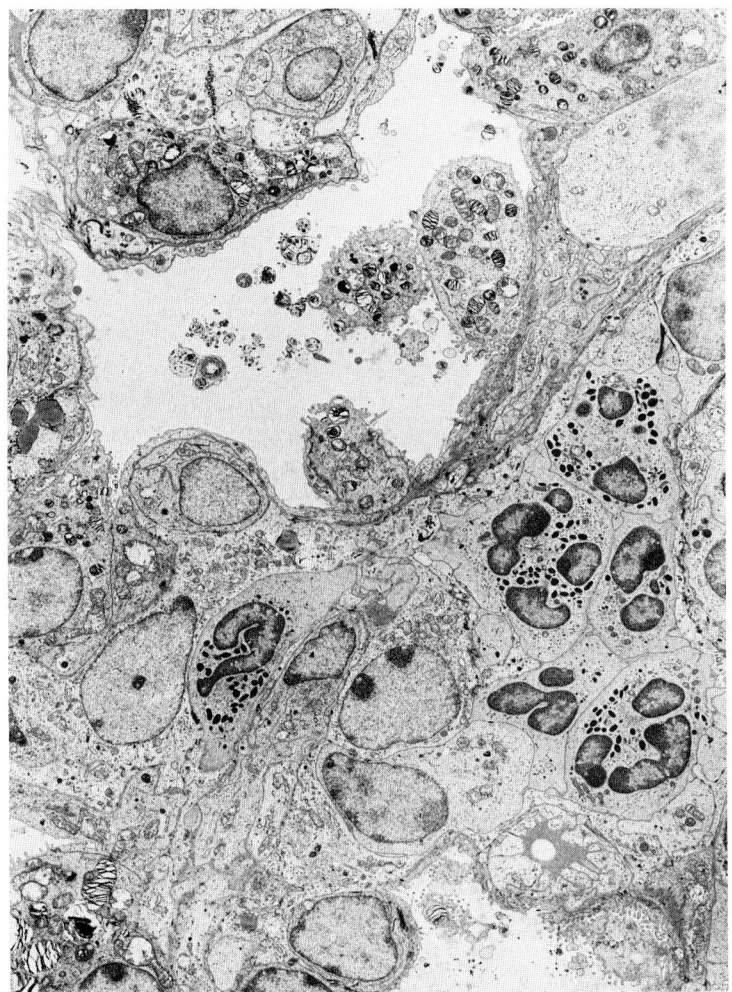

Figure 3.12. Lung from newborn mouse after 3 weeks of continuous exposure to 100% oxygen at normal atmospheric pressure. The lining of the alveolus in the upper half of the illustration consists mainly of granular pneumocytes. Note that the alveolar septum is markedly thickened due to the presence of large numbers of polymorphonuclear leukocytes and an increase of undifferentiated mononuclear septal cells, one of which is in mitosis. ×4160. (Reprinted, with permission, from Bonikos DS, Bensch KG, Northway WH Jr. Oxygen toxicity in the newborn. Am J Pathol 1976;85:623–650.)

conjunction with intermittent ventilation) may result in pulmonary inflammation; indeed increased numbers of polymorphonuclear leukocytes are invariably present in the lungs during the early exudative stage of pulmonary injury in BPD. This has been documented both morphologically (6, 8) and in serial bronchoalveolar lavage fluid of newborn infants with RDS who subsequently developed BPD (98, 99). These studies revealed that infants with RDS destined to develop BPD had persistently elevated neutrophil counts in pulmonary effluents and low α_1-protease inhibitor levels in their bronchoalveolar lavage fluid during a prolonged phase of polymorphonuclear leukocyte influx and sustained high elastase levels producing an imbalance between these substances. These investigators suggested that a significant pulmonary inflammatory reaction coupled with the inability of some infants to mount sufficient protective anti-inflammatory responses may contribute to the development of BPD.

Two major mechanisms of neutrophil recruitment to the lung have been experimentally demonstrated. The first involves the elaboration of chemotaxins by alveolar macrophages; and the second, the production of other, distinct factors by hyperoxia activated alveolar macrophages that stimulate neutrophil adhesivity to endothelial cells and neutrophil superoxide generation (100). Neutrophils, particularly when present in larger numbers, can severely damage the alveolar walls by releasing highly reactive oxygen metabolites in quantities sufficient to cause injury to parenchymal cells and by discharging their lysosomal proteases capable of degrading all components of the normal extracellular connective tissue matrix (96, 101). In polymorphonuclear leukocyte mediated cell and tissue injury of the lung, the oxidant molecules generated by the neutrophils appear to play a more important role in fibrogenesis than the proteolytic enzymes that are released by inflammatory cells. However, experimental exclusion of neutrophils from an inflammatory response in the lung appears to result in an increase in pulmonary fibrosis for unknown reason (102).

Emphysema

The severity and focal nature of an inflammatory reaction and the ensuing scar formation have relevance to the pathogenesis of the emphysematous changes in BPD. A disruption of the balance between the fibro- and elastolytic and the antiproteolytic forces in the lung is considered to play a major role in the pathogenesis of pulmonary emphysema (103). α_1-Protease inhibitor, the predominant inhibitor of neutrophil elastase (104), can also be inactivated by highly reactive oxygen metabolites produced by the same cell type. Furthermore these oxidants can directly alter the biochemical and biophysical properties of structural proteins of tissues including elastin and collagen, as well as mucopolysaccharides (101). Thus the short-lived oxygen derived free radicals and lysosomal proteases of polymorphonuclear leukocytic origin may function synergistically to initiate tissue injury leading to pulmonary emphysema. The implication of a pathogenetic role of these oxygen metabolites in the production of emphysema and impaired lung growth associated with BPD is supported by the observations of Bruce et al., who found that premature infants with RDS, ventilated with greater than 60% O_2 for more than 72 hours, excreted significantly more elastin degradation products (demosine and isodesmosine) in their urine at the end of the first week of life than did infants exposed to oxygen supplementation with 40% O_2 (105). Since elastin is thought to play a critical role in alveolar septal development, elastolytic destruction and/or impaired synthesis of elastin could contribute to the impaired alveolar growth and air space enlargement observed in the lungs of infants with BPD. Neutrophil elastase activity can also be modulated by the alveolar macrophage, because alveolar macrophage injury (including damage by O_2) accelerates the release of elastase into the extracellular space from human neutrophils (106).

Fibrosis and Repair

The above described findings indicate that injury to the pulmonary tissue in BPD is mediated either directly by the etiologic agents (oxygen or, less likely, barotrauma, or both) or indirectly through the recruitment and activation of inflammatory cells, which may result in severe and extensive damage of the pulmonary epithelial and endothelial cells as well as disruption of the extracellular matrix of the lung. Invariably, extensive injury and the associated marked derangement of the alveolar framework result in widespread interstitial and intra-alveolar fibrosis (107) with structural remodeling of the gas-exchanging part of the lung. Contributing to these changes are a number of cell types that can stimulate fibroblast proliferation and accelerate collagen synthesis. In BPD, specific chemoattractants capable of mediating fibroblast recruitment and growth factors for fibroblasts are released from alveolar macrophages, platelets, circulating monocytes, leukocytes, and lymphocytes (96). Thus several types of inflammatory cells frequently encountered in the lung of BPD patients act in concert to bring about the pronounced fibroblast recruitment and proliferation seen in this disease. This usually leads to interstitial and intra-alveolar fibrosis, long-lasting changes with great impact on architecture and function. Intra-alveolar fibrosis appears to be more important than interstitial fibrosis in structural remodeling of the lung; it has been experimentally demonstrated that migration of interstitial connective tissue cells through gaps in the epithelial basement membranes into the air spaces is responsible for this occurring (108). Finally to be mentioned is recent experimental evidence that extensive alveolar damage resulting in a disruption of the normal relationships and channels of communication between epithelial and endothelial lining cells and the supporting or mesenchymal cells of the pulmonary interstitium predisposes to the development of pulmonary fibrosis (29, 82, 108–114) (Figs. 3.13 and 3.14).

Cellular regeneration and repair of the alveoli is in many ways analogous to the events taking place during organogenesis of the lung, in which an orderly progression of events is dependent upon the transmission of messages between epithelial, endothelial, and mesenchymal cells (115–121). Delayed or abnormal regeneration of the alveolar epithelium and endothelium with an accompanying disruption of intercellular communication eventually leads to an abnormal development of the neonatal lung and a disordered repair of the injured alveolar structures.

Summary

We have discussed the relationship of pulmonary oxygen toxicity to the pathogenetic mechanisms underlying the development of BPD with an emphasis on the clinical, labo-

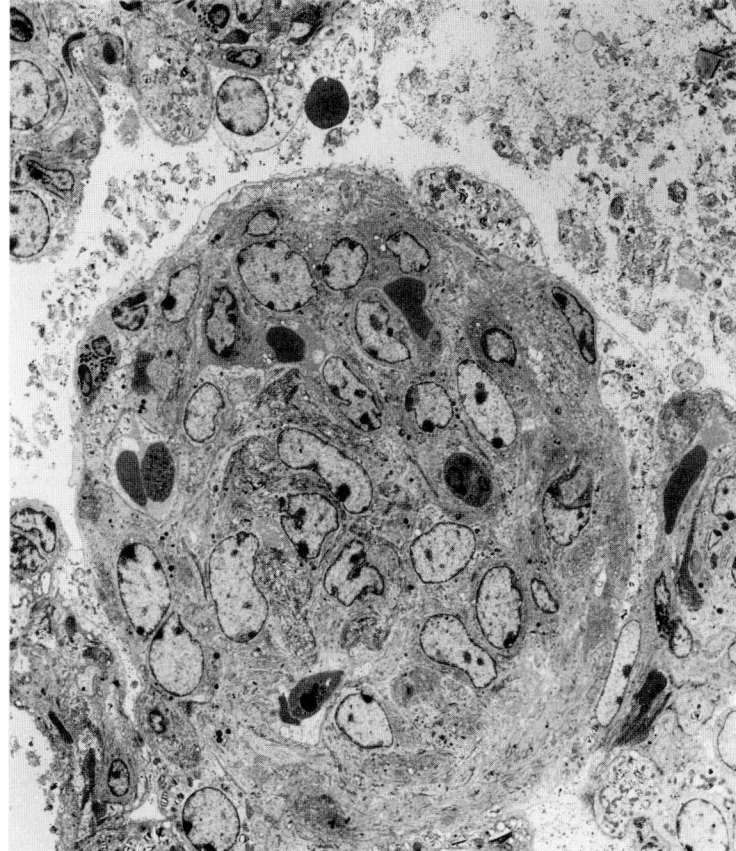

Figure 3.13. Lung from newborn mouse after 4 weeks of continuous exposure to 100% oxygen at normal atmospheric pressure. Alveolar space, protruding into which there is a heterogeneous cellular conglomerate consisting of tightly held together undifferentiated cells, polymorphonuclear leukocytes, bundles of collagen, and remnants of alveolar capillaries. ×1960. (Reprinted, with permission, from Bonikos DS, Bensch KG, Northway WH Jr. Oxygen toxicity in the newborn. Am J Pathol 1976;85:623–650.)

ratory, and experimental findings encountered in this disease. Previous data were re-evaluated in the light of recent clinical and experimental findings and particularly in regard to mechanisms of pulmonary injury. Details of these studies can be found on the referred to key publications. These provide specific data on the grading of the disease, the evolution of histopathologic abnormalities, the inflammatory mechanisms that come into play, abnormalities of lung development and growth, and the major etiologic agents. The apparent decrease in the incidence and severity of this disease is without question attributable to the reduction in the use of lower supplemental oxygen concentration and the length of oxygen therapy. Severe cases of BPD are now encountered only in

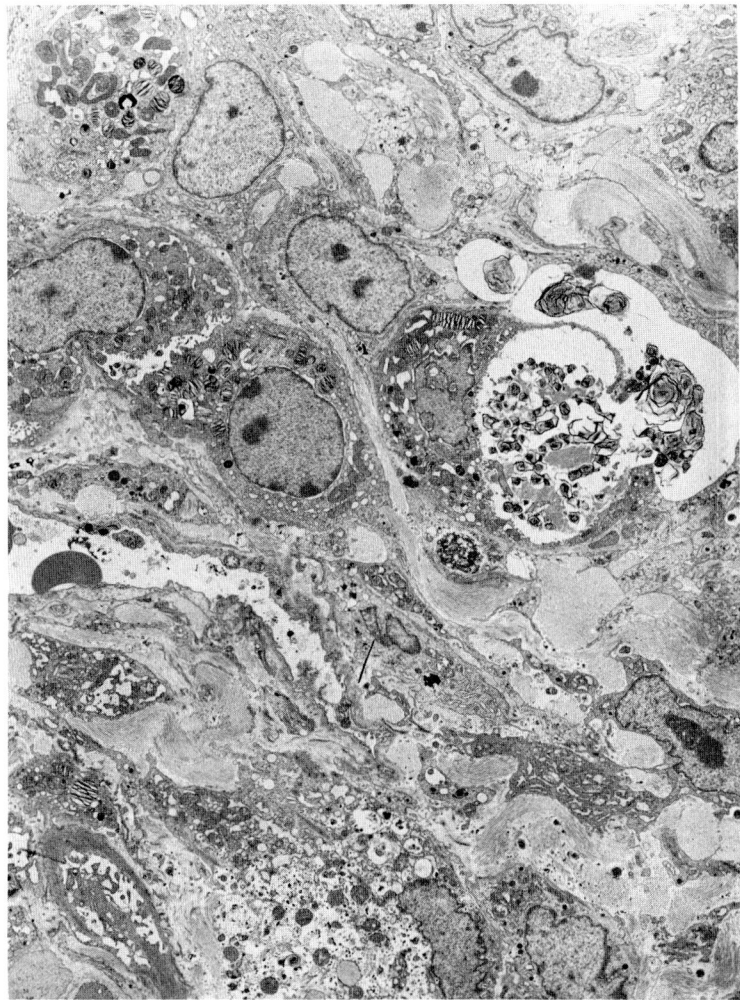

Figure 3.14. Lung from newborn mouse after 6 weeks of continuous exposure to 100% oxygen at normal atmospheric pressure. Total destruction of the alveolar architecture by a tremendous overgrowth of dense fibrous tissue. Occasional granular pneumocytes are randomly embedded within this collagenous strand. An abundance of lamellar whorls intermingled with a finely fibrillar material displaying a distinct periodicity and occasionally a latticework pattern is noted within an alveolar space. ×3840. (Reprinted, with permission, from Bonikos DS, Bensch KG, Northway WH Jr. Oxygen toxicity in the newborn. Am J Pathol 1976;85:623–650.)

premature babies that would have succumbed soon after birth a decade ago. In contrast, full-term infants with this disease are no longer seen by the pathologist. This improvement in therapy has also led to a much more subtle histopathologic expression of the disease, which may not be appreciated as being BPD by an inexperienced pathologist. Therefore, on examining the lungs of a neonate, particularly of a premature or immature baby with prolonged survival in an intensive care unit, the modalities of therapy ought to be carefully assessed. The response to a modified clinical treatment (steroids, surfactant, high-frequency ventilation which leads to focal jet injuries, etc.) may be reflected in an unusual histopathologic pattern. It also should be kept in mind that the development (maturation) of the immature lung after birth is highly susceptible to environmental factors. Thus the stage of histologic lung development and the more subtle morphologic changes in BPD have to be taken into consideration before a nonspecific diagnosis such as "lung immaturity" is made (6, 48).

References

1. Northway WH Jr, Rosan RC, Porter DY. Pulmonary disease following respirator therapy of hyaline membrane disease. N Engl J Med 1967;276:357–368.
2. Becker MJ, Koppe JG. Pulmonary structural changes in neonatal hyaline membrane disease treated with high pressure artificial respiration. Thorax 1969;24:689–694.
3. Anderson WR, Strickland MB. Pulmonary complications of oxygen therapy in the neonate. Postmortem study of bronchopulmonary dysplasia with emphasis on fibroproliferative obliterative bronchitis and bronchiolitis. Arch Pathol 1971;91:506–514.
4. Banerjee CK, Girlin DJ, Wigglesworth JS. Pulmonary fibroplasia in newborn babies treated with oxygen and artificial ventilation. Arch Dis Child 1972;47:509–518.
5. Rosan RC. Hyaline membrane disease and a related spectrum of neonatal pneumonopathies. In: Rosenberg HS, Bolande RP, eds. Perspectives in pediatric pathology. Chicago: Yearbook Medical Publishers, 1975.
6. Bonikos DS, Bensch KG, Northway WH Jr, Edwards DK. Bronchopulmonary dysplasia: the pulmonary pathologic sequel of necrotizing bronchiolitis and pulmonary fibrosis. Hum Pathol 1976;7:643–666.
7. Taghizadeh A, Reynolds EOR. Pathogenesis of bronchopulmonary dysplasia following hyaline membrane disease. Am J Pathol 1976;82:241–258.
8. Edwards DK, Colby TV, Northway WH Jr. Radiographic-pathologic correlation in bronchopulmonary dysplasia. J Pediatr 1979;95:834–836.
9. Takemura T. Histopathological study of the adverse effects of prolonged respiratory therapy on the neonate lung. Acta Pathol Jpn 1981;31:199–210.
10. Anderson WR, Engel RR. Cardiopulmonary sequelae of reparative stages of bronchopulmonary dysplasia. Arch Pathol Lab Med 1983;107:603–608.
11. Tomashefski JF, Vawter GF, Reid LM. Pathologic observations on infants who do not survive the respiratory distress syndrome. In: Nelson GH, ed. Pulmonary development. Transition from intrauterine to extrauterine life. New York: Markel Dekker, 1985.
12. Edwards DK, Dyer WH, Northway WH Jr. Twelve years' experience with bronchopulmonary dysplasia. Pediatrics 1977;59:839–846.
13. Brown ER. Increased risk of bronchopulmonary dysplasia in infants with patent ductus arteriosus. J Pediatr 1979;95:865–866.
14. Brown ER, Stark A, Sosenko I, Lawson EE, Avery ME. Bronchopulmonary dysplasia: possible relationships to pulmonary edema. J Pediatr 1978;92:982–984.
15. Stahlman MT, Cheatham W, Gray ME. The role of air dissection in bronchopulmonary dysplasia. J Pediatr 1979;95:878–882.
16. Barnes ND, Glover WJ, Hull D, Milner AD. Effects of prolonged positive pressure ventilation in infants. Lancet 1969;2:1096–1099.
17. Pusey VA, MacPherson RI, Chernick V. Pulmonary fibroplasia following prolonged artificial ventilation of newborn infants. Can Med Assoc J 1969;100:451–457.
18. Rhodes PG, Hall RT, Leonidas JC. Chronic pulmonary disease in neonates with assisted ventilation. Pediatrics 1975;55:788–796.
19. Fitzhardinge PM, Pape K, Arstikaitis M, et al. Mechanical ventilation of infants of less than 1501 grams birth weight: health, growth and

neurologic sequelae. J Pediatr 1976;88:531–541.
20. Arnold J, O'Brodovich H, Whyte R, Coates G. Pulmonary thromboemboli following neonatal asphyxia. J Pediatr 1985;106:806–809.
21. Dyck DR, Zylak CJ. Acute respiratory distress in adults. Radiology 1973;106:497–501.
22. Churg A, Golden J, Fligiel S, Hogg JC. Bronchopulmonary dysplasia in the adult. Am Rev Respir Dis 1983;127:117–120.
23. Northway WH Jr. Bronchopulmonary dysplasia. In: Raivio KO, Hallman N, Kouvalainen K, Valimaki I, eds. Respiratory distress syndrome. London: Academic Press, 1984.
24. Reynolds EOR, Taghizadeh A. Improved prognosis of infants mechanically ventilated for hyaline membrane disease. Arch Dis Child 1974;49:505–515.
25. Stern L, Ramos AD, Outerbridge EW, Beandry PH. Negative pressure artificial respiration: use in treatment of respiratory failure of the newborn. Can Med Assoc J 1970;102:595–601.
26. Stocks J, Godfrey S, Reynolds EOR. Airway resistance in infants after various treatments for hyaline membrane disease: special emphasis on prolonged high levels of inspired oxygen. Pediatrics 1978;61:178–183.
27. Ludwin SK, Northway WH Jr, Bensch KG. Oxygen toxicity in the newborn. Necrotizing bronchiolitis in mice exposed to 100 percent oxygen. Lab Invest 1974;31:425–435.
28. Bonikos DS, Bensch KG, Ludwin SK, Northway WH Jr. Oxygen toxicity in the newborn. The effect of prolonged 100 percent O_2 exposure on the lungs of newborn mice. Lab Invest 1975;32:619–635.
29. Bonikos DS, Bensch KG, Northway WH Jr. Oxygen toxicity in the newborn. The effect of chronic continuous 100 percent oxygen exposure on the lungs of newborn mice. Am J Pathol 1976;85:623–650.
30. Pappas CTE, Obara H, Bensch KG, Northway WH. Effect of prolonged exposure to 80% oxygen on the lung of the newborn mouse. Lab Invest 1983;48:735–748.
31. Coalson JJ, Kuehl TJ, Escobedo MB, et al. A baboon model of bronchopulmonary dysplasia. II. Pathologic features. Exp Mol Pathol 1982;37:335–350.
32. Lamarre A, Linsao L, Reilly BJ, Swyer PR, Levison H. Residual pulmonary abnormalities in survivors of idiopathic respiratory distress syndrome. Am Rev Respir Dis 1973;108:56–61.
33. Ahlström H. Pulmonary mechanics in infants surviving severe neonatal respiratory insufficiency. Acta Paediatr Scand 1975;64:69–80.
34. Chernick V. Epidemiology of BPS: discussion. J. Pediatr 1979;95:855–858.
35. Clark JM, Lambersten CJ. Pulmonary oxygen toxicity: a review. Pharm Rev 1971;23:37–133.
36. Deneke SM, Fanburg BL. Normobaric oxygen toxicity of the lung. N Engl J Med 1980;303:76–86.
37. Frank L, Massaro D. Oxygen toxicity. Am J Med 1980;69:117–126.
38. Small A. New perspectives on hyperoxic pulmonary toxicity: a review. Undersea Biomed Res 1984;11:1–24.
39. Frank L, Bucher JR, Roberts RJ. Oxygen toxicity in neonatal and adult animals of various species. J Appl Physiol 1978;45:699–704.
40. Yam J, Frank L, Roberts RJ. Oxygen toxicity: comparison of lung biochemical responses in neonatal and adult rats. Pediatr Res 1978;12:115–119.
41. Gilbert DL. The role of pro-oxidants and antioxidants in oxygen toxicity. Radiat Res 1963;3(suppl):44–53.
42. Freeny L, Berman ER. Oxygen toxicity: membrane damage by free radicals. Invest Ophthalmol 1976;15:789–792.
43. Fisher AB, Bassett DJP, Forman HJ. Oxygen toxicity of the lung. Biochemical aspects. In: Fishman AP, Renkin EM, eds. Pulmonary edema. Bethesda, Md: American Physiological Society, 1979.
44. Frank L, Massaro D. The lung and oxygen toxicity. Arch Intern Med 1979;139:347–350.
45. Frank L. Effects of oxygen on the newborn. Fed Proc 1985;44:2328–2334.
46. Rosenfeld W, Evans H, Concepcion L, Jhaveri R, Schaeffer H, Friedman A. Prevention of bronchopulmonary dysplasia by administration of bovine superoxide dismutase in

47. Thurlbeck WM. Postnatal growth and development of the lung. Am Rev Respir Dis 1975;111:803–844.
48. Boyden EA. Development and growth of the airways. In: Hodson AW, ed. Development of the lung. New York: Marcel Dekker, 1977.
49. Polgar G, Weng TR. The functional development of the respiratory system. From the period of gestation to adulthood. Ann Rev Respir Dis 1979;120:625–695.
50. Inselman LS, Mellins RB. Growth and development of the lung. J Pediatr 1981;98:1–15.
51. Bartlett D Jr. Postnatal growth of the mammalian lung. Influence of low and high oxygen tensions. Respir Physiol 1970;9:58–64.
52. Resnick JS, Brown DM, Vernier RL. Oxygen toxicity in fetal organ culture. II. The developing lung. Lab Invest 1974;31:665–677.
53. Bucher JR, Roberts RJ. The development of the newborn rat lung in hyperoxia. A dose-response study of lung growth, maturation and changes in antioxidant enzyme activities. Pediatr Res 1981;15:999–1008.
54. Sobonya RE, Logvinoff MM, Taussig LM, Theriault A. Morphometric analysis of the lung in prolonged bronchopulmonary dysplasia. Pediatr Res 1982;16:969–972.
55. Wilson WL, Mullen M, Olley PM, Rabinovitch M. Hyperoxia-induced pulmonary vascular and lung abnormalities in young rats and potential for recovery. Pediatr Res 1985;19:1059–1067.
56. Roberts RJ, Weesner KM, Bucher JR. Oxygen-induced alterations in lung vascular development in the newborn rat. Pediatr Res 1983;17:368–373.
57. Snow RL, Davies P, Pontoppidan H, Zapol WM, Reid L. Pulmonary vascular remodeling in adult respiratory distress syndrome. Am Rev Respir Dis 1982;126:887–892.
58. Tomashefski JF Jr, Davies P, Boggis C, Greene R, Zapol W, Reid L. The pulmonary vascular lesions of the adult respiratory distress syndrome. Am J Pathol 1983;112:112–126.
59. Jones R, Zapol WM, Reid L. Hyperoxia-induced hypertrophy of intimal precursor smooth muscle cells in pulmonary arteries. Fed Proc 1984;43:884.
60. Jones R, Zapol WM, Reid L. Pulmonary artery remodeling and pulmonary hypertension after exposure to hyperoxia for seven days. A morphometric and hemodynamic study. Am J Pathol 1984;117:273–285.
61. Johnson DE, Lock JE, Elde RP, Thompson TR. Pulmonary neuroendocrine cells in hyaline membrane disease and bronchopulmonary dysplasia. Pediatr Res 1982;16:446–454.
62. Castleman B, McNeely BV. Case records of the Massachusetts General Hospital. Case 7-1967. N Engl J Med 1967;276:401–411.
63. Nash G, Blennerhassett JB, Pontoppidan H. Pulmonary lesions associated with oxygen therapy and artificial ventilation. N Engl J Med 1967;74:276–368.
64. Kafer ER. Pulmonary oxygen toxicity. A review of the evidence for acute and chronic oxygen toxicity in man. Br J Anaesth 1971;43:687–695.
65. Gould VE, Tosco R, Wheelis RF, Gould NS, Kapansi Y. Oxygen pneumonitis in man. Ultrastructural observations on the development of alveolar lesions. Lab Invest 1972;26:499–508.
66. Davis WB, Rennard SI, Bitterman PB, Crystal RG: Pulmonary oxygen toxicity. Early reversible changes in human alveolar structures induced by hyperoxia. N Engl J Med 1983;309:878–883.
67. Kistler GS, Caldwell PRB, Weibel ER. Development of fine structural damage to alveolar and capillary lining cells in oxygen-poisoned rat lungs. J Cell Biol 1967;32:605–628.
68. Kapanci Y, Weibel ER, Kaplan HP, Robinson FR. Pathogenesis and reversibility of the pulmonary lesions of oxygen toxicity in monkeys. II. Ultrastructural and morphometric studies. Lab Invest 1969;20:101–118.
69. Bowden DH, Adamson IYR, Wyatt JP. Reaction of the lung cells to a high concentration of oxygen. Arch Pathol 1968;86:671–675.
70. Rosenbaum RM, Wittner M, Senger M. Mitochondrial and other ultrastructural changes in great alveolar cells of oxygen-adapted and poisoned rats. Lab Invest 1969;20:516–528.
71. Harrison G, Rosan RC, Sloane A. Bronchio-

litis induced by experimental acute and chronic oxygen intoxication in young adult rats. J Pathol 1970;102:115–122.
72. Crapo JD, Peters-Golden M, Marsh-Salin J, Shelburne JS. Pathologic changes in the lungs of oxygen-adapted rats. A morphometric analysis. Lab Invest 1978;39:640–653.
73. Meyrick B, Miller J, Reid L. Pulmonary edema induced by ANTU, or by high or low oxygen concentrations in rat: an electron microscopic study. Br J Exp Pathol 1972;53:347–358.
74. Bowden DH, Adamson IYR. Endothelial regeneration as a marker of the differential vascular responses in oxygen-induced pulmonary edema. Lab Invest 1974;30:350–357.
75. Lee SL, Douglas WJH, Deneke SM, Fanburg BL. Ultrastructural morphology of bovine artery endothelial cells exposed to hyperoxia in vivo. Clin Res 1982;30:434A.
76. Crapo JD, Barry BE, Foscue HA, Shelburne J. Structural and biochemical changes in rat lungs occurring during exposure to lethal and adaptive doses of oxygen. Am Rev Respir Dis 1980;122:123–143.
77. Block ER, Stalcup SA. Depression of serotonin uptake by cultured endothelial cells exposed to high O_2 tension. J Appl Physiol 1981;50:1212–1219.
78. Block ER, Fisher AB. Depression of serotinin clearance by rat lungs during oxygen exposure. J Appl Physiol 1977;42:33–38.
79. Klein LS, Fisher AB, Soltoff S, Coburn RF. Effect of O_2 exposure on pulmonary metabolism of prostoglandin E_2. Ann Rev Respir Dis 1978;118:622–625.
80. Lee SL, Douglas WHJ, Deneke SM, Fanburg BL. Ultrastructural changes in bovine pulmonary artery endothelial cells exposed to 80% O_2 in vitro. In Vitro 1983;19:714–722.
81. Bowden DH. Alveolar response to injury. Thorax 1981;36:801–804.
82. Adamson IYR, Bowden DH. Endothelial injury and repair in radiation-induced pulmonary fibrosis. Am J Pathol 1983;112:224–230.
83. Merritt TA, Harris JP, Roghmann K, et al. Early closure of the patent ductus arteriosus in very-low-birth-weight infants: a control trial. J Pediatr 1981;99:281–286.
84. Brewer LL, Moskowitz PS, Carrington CB, Bensch KG. Pneumatosis pneumonalis. A complication of the idiopathic respiratory distress syndrome. Am J Pathol 1979;95:171–190.
85. Nilsson R, Grossmann G, Robertson B. Pathogenesis of neonatal lung lesions induced by artificial ventilation: evidence against the role of barotrauma. Respiration 1980;40:218–225.
86. Northway WH Jr, Rosan RC, Shahinian L, Castelino RA, Gyepes MT, Durbridge T. Radiologic and histologic investigation of pulmonary oxygen toxicity in newborn guinea pigs. Invest Radiol 1969;4:148–155.
87. Fujinaka LE, Hyde DM, Plopper CG, Tyler WS, Dungworth DL, Lollini LO. Respiratory bronchiolitis following long-term ozone exposure in bonnet monkeys: a morphometric study. Exp Lung Res 1985;8:167–190.
88. Harkema J, Plopper CG, St. George J, et al. Persistent centriacinar lesions in bonnet monkeys following cessation of exposure to ambient levels of ozone. Am Rev Respir Dis 1984;129:137.
89. Hyde DM, Plopper CG, Weir AJ, et al. Peribronchiolar fibrosis in lungs of cats chronically exposed to diesel exhaust. Lab Invest 1985;52:195–206.
90. Niewoehner DE, Kleinerman J, Rice DB. Pathologic changes in the peripheral airways of young cigarette smokers. N Engl J Med 1974;291:755–758.
91. Burri PH. The postnatal growth of the rat lung. III. Morphology. Anat Rec 1974;180:77–98.
92. Evans MJ, Cabral LJ, Stephens RF, Freeman G. Renewal of alveolar epithelium in the rat following exposure to NO_2. Am J Pathol 1973;70:175–198.
93. Adamson IYR, Bowden DH. The type 2 cell as progenitor of alveolar epithelial regeneration. Lab Invest 1974;30:35–40.
94. Evans MJ, Cabral LJ, Stephens RJ, Freeman G. Transformation of alveolar type 2 cells to type 1 cells following exposure to NO_2. Exp Mol Pathol 1975;22:142–150.
95. Kawanami O, Ferrans VJ, Crystal RG. Structure of alveolar epithelial cells in patients

with fibrotic lung disorders. Lab Invest 1982;46:39–53.
96. Rennard SI, Bitterman PB, Crystal RG. Current concepts of the pathogenesis of fibrosis: lessons from pulmonary fibrosis. In: Berk PD, Castro-Malaspina H, Wasserman LR, eds. Myelofibrosis and the biology of connective tissue. Progress in clinical and Biological Research, vol 154. New York: Alan R. Liss, 1984.
97. Rennard SI, Bitterman PB, Crystal RG. Mechanisms of fibrosis. Am Rev Respir Dis 1984;130:492–496.
98. Merritt TA, Cochrane CG, Holcomb K, Bohl B, Hallman M, Strayer D. Elastase and alpha-1-proteinase inhibitor activity in tracheal aspirates during respiratory distress syndrome. Role of inflammation in the pathogenesis of bronchopulmonary dysplasia. J Clin Invest 1983;72:656–666.
99. Ogden BE, Murphy SA, Saunders GC, Pathak D, Johnson JD. Neonatal lung neutrophils and elastase/proteinase inhibitor imbalance. Am Rev Respir Dis 1984;130:817–821.
100. Tate RM, Repine JE. Neutrophils and the adult respiratory distress syndrome. Am Rev Respir Dis 1983;128:552–559.
101. Fantone JC, Ward PA. Polymorphonuclear leukocyte-mediated cell and tissue injury. Oxygen metabolites and their relations to human disease. Hum Pathol 1985;16:973–979.
102. Snider GL. Interstitial pulmonary fibrosis: which cell is the culprit? Ann Rev Respir Dis 1983;127:535–539.
103. Janoff A. Proteases and lung injury. A state of the art minireview. Chest 1983;83(suppl):54–58.
104. Gadek JE, Fells GA, Zimmerman RL, Rennard SI. Antielastases of the human alveolar structures: implications for the protease–antiprotease theory of emphysema. J Clin Invest 1981;68:889–898.
105. Bruce MC, Wedig KE, Jentoft N, Martin RJ, Cheng PW, Boat TF. Altered urinary excretion of elastin cross-links in premature infants who develop bronchopulmonary dysplasia. Am Rev Respir Dis 1985;131:568–572.
106. Cambell EJ, Wald MS. Hypoxic injury to human alveolar macrophages accelerates release of previously bound neutrophil elastase. Implications for lung connective tissue injury including pulmonary emphysema. Am Rev Respir Dis 1983;127:631–635.
107. Basset F, Ferrans VJ, Soler P, Takemura T, Fukuda Y, Crystal RG. Intraluminal fibrosis in interstitial lung disorders. Am J Pathol 1986;122:443–461.
108. Fukuda Y, Ferrans VJ, Schoenberger CI, Rennard SI, Crystal RG. Patterns of pulmonary structural remodeling after experimental paraquat toxicity. The morphogenesis of intra-alveolar fibrosis. Am J Pathol 1985;118:452–475.
109. Adamson IYR, Bowden DH. Pulmonary injury and repair: organ culture studies of murine lung after oxygen. Arch Pathol Lab Med 1976;100:640–643.
110. Terzaghi M, Netterheim P, Williams ML. Repopulation of denuded tracheal grafts with normal, preneoplastic and neoplastic epithelial cell populations. Cancer Res 1978;38:4546–4553.
111. Haschek WM, Meyer KR, Ulrich RL, Wittschi HP. Potentiation of chemically induced lungbrosis by thoracic irradiation. Int J Radiat Oncol Biol Phys 1980;6:449–455.
112. Brody AR, Soler P, Basset F, Haschek WM, Hanspeter W. Epithelial-mesenchymal associations of cells in human pulmonary fibrosis and BHT-oxygen-induced fibrosis in mice. Exp Lung Res 1981;2:207–220.
113. Witschi HR, Haschek WM, Klein-Szanto AJP, Hakkinen PJ. Potentiation of diffuse lung damage by oxygen-determining variables. Am Rev Respir Dis 1981;123:98–103.
114. Tanswell AK. Cellular interactions in pulmonary oxygen toxicity in vitro. I. Hyperoxic induction of fibroblast factors which alter growth and lipid metabolism of pulmonary epithelial cells. Exp Lung Res 1983;5:23–36.
115. Taderera JV. Control of lung differentiation in vitro. Dev Biol 1967;16:489–512.
116. Dameron F. An experimental study of the organogenesis of the lung: the nature and specificity of the epithelio-mesenchymatous interactions. J Embryol Exp Morphol 1968;20:151–167.

117. Masters JR. Epithelial-mesenchymal interaction during lung development. The effect of mesenchymal mass. Dev Biol 1976;51:91–108.
118. Smith BT. Lung maturation in the fetal rat: acceleration by injection of fibroblast-pneumocyte factor. Science 1979;204:1094–1095.
119. Smith BT, Fletcher WA. Pulmonary epithelial-mesenchymal interactions: beyond organogenesis. Hum Pathol 1979;10:248–250.
120. Tanswell AK, Smith BT. Human fetal lung type II pneumocytes in monolayer cell culture. The influence of oxidant stress, corticol environment and soluble fibroblast factors. Pediatr Res 1979;13:1097–1100.
121. Leung CK, Adamson IY, Bowden DH. Uptake of ^{3}H prednisolone by fetal lung explants: role of intercellular contacts in epithelial maturation. Exp Lung Res 1980;1:111–120.

4

Tracheal Aspirate Cytology in Neonatal Respiratory Distress Syndrome and Bronchopulmonary Dysplasia

CHARLES NEAVE

Introduction

Since 1975 reports have described the cytologic features of tracheal aspirates from newborns with respiratory distress (1–7). Sequential aspirates via endotracheal tube show a progression of cytologic changes that start with epithelial cell sloughing and acute inflammatory exudate and proceed through advancing degrees of metaplasia and repair. The regeneration of injured epithelium coexists with continued epithelial injury in a dynamic state for as long as the infant receives oxygen through a mechanical ventilator. Oxygen concentration, barotrauma, and the newborn's immaturity, infection, acidosis, heart failure, and nutrition influence both the injurious and regenerative processes and, of course, each other. Usually within a week of continuous mechanical ventilation, cytologic changes occur that appear to have prognostic value in terms of future pulmonary development and health. This chapter reviews the cytologic observations, the correlations of cytology with concurrent clinical, radiographic, and histologic findings, and some of the questions that remain to be answered about the use of cytology in this context.

Cytologic Observations

Technical Considerations and General Comments

Tracheobronchial secretions are obtained at the time of endotracheal tube toiletry by gentle suction after instilling 1–3 mL isotonic saline and brief manual ventilation. Some have collected the secretions in traps or containers with alcohol preparatory to centrifugation, resuspension, and transfer to glass slides (1, 3); others have spread the secretions directly onto glass slides that are plain (5), fully frosted (6), or albuminized (1, 3), followed by immediate immersion in alcohol (5, 6). Readers should consult the references for details. Papanicolaou's strain is generally used; special stains have included Gram's, iron, periodic acid–Schiff (PAS), Wright-Giemsa, Alcian blue, Sudan black, and neuron-specific enolase. Some 20% of the smears are technically unsatisfactory because of the paucity of diagnostic cells or cellular degeneration (1, 6). The quantity of the aspirates from the same infant varies greatly as does the amount of degenerative change, and it is highly desirable to obtain sequential, daily aspirates.

Tracheobronchial epithelium is complex and includes ciliated, mucous (goblet), neurosecretory, brush, and reserve (short, basal) cells. While ciliated cells are readily identified, the others are virtually impossible to differentiate from each other with Papanicolaou's stain, particularly when the cells are injured or degenerate. Since it has not yet been possible to quantitate these various cell forms in aspirates, the sequence of regeneration of the different cell forms is unclear. Animal studies suggest that ciliated and mucous cells regenerate together (8). Little is known of the regeneration of neurosecretory cells, although autopsy studies indicate they may be of great importance (9).

Tracheal aspirates also contain neutrophils and histiocytes (macrophages), hyaline membrane debris, mucus, Curschmann's spirals, blood, hemosiderin, meconium, and micro-organisms of various kinds (5, 10, 11). These are important parts of the aspirate and can be used to infer various aspects of the infant's condition.

Progressive Changes in Tracheal Aspirates

While each report uses slightly different terms to summarize the stages in the progression, the observations and descriptions are comparable (Table 4.1). In this chapter Merritt's classification (3) is modified in order 1) to categorize subgroups of epithelial repair cells, 2) to allow for a transitional class in which cellular atypia cannot be firmly diagnosed, and 3) to include changes in the aspirates of infants who have been on prolonged mechanical ventilation (6). The cytologic changes in tracheal aspirates are additive, probably because fresh areas of bronchial epithelium are constantly being exposed to oxygen by increasing endogenous surfactant production and lung expansion. Classification of the aspirate as a whole is based on the most advanced stage seen. While the progression is orderly, the speed of change from one stage to the next appears to vary with oxygen dose—that is, the product of oxygen concentration and hours of administration, expressed in hours % (12)—and whatever conditions prevail in the infant that promote its increase.

During the first 4 days of intubation from birth, Class I tracheal aspirates are usually copious and contain sloughed epithelial cells, much mucus, and numerous neutrophils. Ciliated and nonciliated cells appear as single cells, small groups, and irregular sheets; detached ciliary tufts are also present (Fig. 4.1). When there has been chorioamnionitis or fetal pneumonia, neutrophils are more numerous and micro-organisms can sometimes be seen. Degenerate, mature squamous cells observed during these early days probably result from aspirated amniotic fluid, as may some of the neutrophils. Fragments of hyaline membrane debris are usually seen after day 2.

Class II changes can occur as early as day 3 but usually start between days 4 and 7. Regenerative changes are added onto the sloughed epithelial cells and neutrophils of Class I. Class II is characterized by metaplastic and "repair" epithelial cells and by histiocytes (Fig. 4.2). Cells with squamous metaplasia are flattened, have oral or elongate nuclei, and sometimes have orangeophilic cytoplasm. Mature metaplastic cells are monomorphic with crisp borders and are arranged like cobblestones in sheets of various sizes. Repair cells presumably derive from the reserve cells next to the basal lamina of residual epithelium. Nuclear size and chromatin pattern serve to separate repair cells into early,

Table 4.1. Comparison of Different Classifications of Tracheal Cytology Findings

Neave & Masura (6)	Merritt et al. (3)	Doshi et al. (5)	D'Ablang et al. (1)

Class I
  Bronchial cells, single & groups
  Acute inflammation
  Hyaline membrane debris
	Class I (1–4d)
	  Well-preserved single cells
	  Bronchial epithelium in sheets
	  Acute inflammation
		Early
		  Columnar cell sheets
		  Ciliary tufts
		  Hyaline membrane debris
		  Metaplasia
			Well-preserved columnar cells

Class II
  Above plus . . .
  Metaplasia
  Repair (early, moderate)
  Histiocytes
  Curschmann's spirals
	Class II (4–10d)
	  Chromocenters, nucleoli, karyomegaly
	  Metaplasia
	  Histiocytes
	  Curschmann's spirals
		Intermediate
		  Dysplastic cells
		  More metaplasia
			(a) Pyknotic smudged nuclei; loss of cilia & terminal bars
			(b) Isolated nests with small nuclei; chromocenters & nucleoli

Class II-III
  Above plus . . .
  Atypical metaplasia ?
  Repair (all degrees)
  Bronchial cells: tight groups
  Nuclear irregularity
	Class III (>10d)
	  Above plus . . .
	  More sheets of cells
	  More prominent nucleoli
		Late
		  Progressive phase
		    Metaplasia & dysplasia
		    Curschmann's spirals
		    Dirty background
			Irregular clusters; sheets; vacuoles with compressed nuclei
			No cilia or bars
			Coarse chromatin & nucleoli
			Mitoses

Class III
  Above plus . . .
  Definite nuclear atypia
  Repair (moderate, late)
		Regressive phase
		  Above plus . . .
		  Clean background
			Above plus . . .
			Bizarre cells
			More histiocytes

Class IV Metaplasia; histiocytes; no atypia			

moderate, and late grades. Early repair cells have large, smooth, oval nuclei with fine salt-and-pepper chromatin (Fig. 4.3); moderate repair cells have somewhat smaller nuclei (still smooth) with coarser chromatin and chromocenters (Fig. 4.4); and late repair cells (often in tight nests) have still smaller nuclei with nucleoli and coarse chromatin (Fig. 4.5). Metaplastic and repair cells are often found together, and there may be several grades of repair in the same aspirate. Class II aspirates usually contain only early and moderate repair cells along with metaplastic cells.

Between days 6 and 12 (but earlier if the oxygen dose has risen rapidly) there is a qualitative change in tracheal aspirates that is of prognostic significance. Many infants move from Class II into a transitional category called Class II-III, which may be cytologically indefinite but is prognostically useful. These aspirates show a preponderance of moderate repair mixed with metaplasia and many histiocytes. The nuclei of both repair and metaplastic cells tend to be hyperchromatic; the cells are often in tight balls, sometimes resembling blunt papillae. Neutrophils

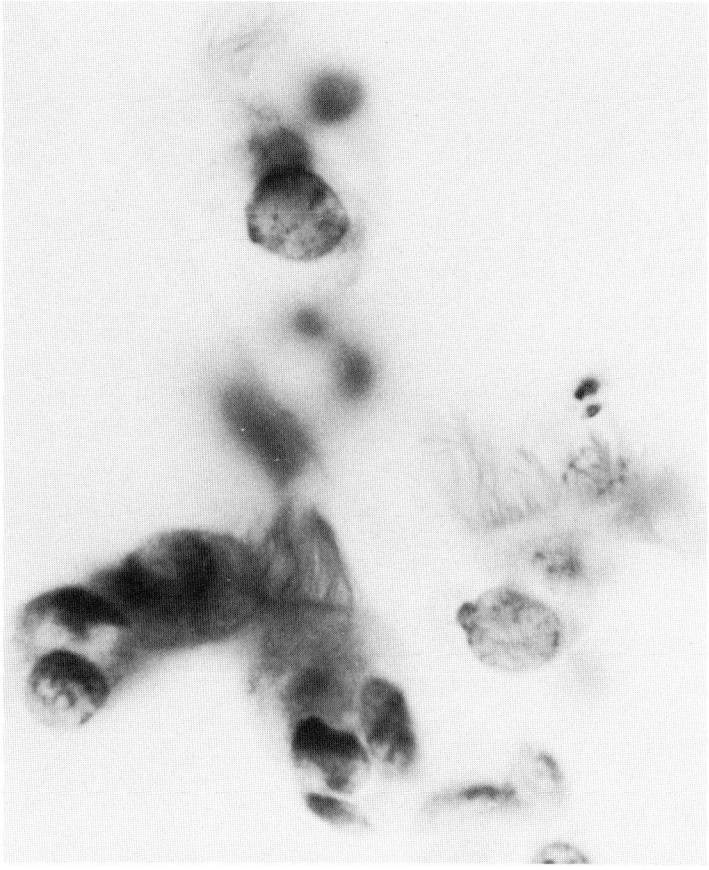

Figure 4.1. Class I tracheal aspirate with ciliated epithelial cells and detached ciliary tufts. Papanicolaou's stain; ×1000.

may be increased. Some of these infants develop further changes (Class III), with definite atypia in repair and metaplastic cells characterized by small, irregular, sometimes molded, hyperchromatic nuclei with prominent nucleoli and/or very coarse, crumbly chromatin (Figs. 4.6, 4.7, 4.8). These atypical changes have been correlated with bronchopulmonary dysplasia (BPD) by most observers (3, 5, 6). Repair cells that are not atypical tend to be of moderate or late grades. The tracheal aspirates of other infants reflect a different course, called Class IV, which is characterized by sheets of mature squamous metaplasia and histiocytes; no nuclear atypia is seen, and there is usually little acute inflammatory exudate (Fig. 4.9). Generally Class IV changes are found in infants who have been intubated for over 30 days; but rarely an infant will pass from Class II or Class II-III to Class IV (omitting Class III) if he has been extubated, as for trial on nasal continuous positive airway pressure, and then reintubated. The author has not observed an infant to pass from Class III to Class IV. It appears that the infant with Class IV cytology usually has a large accumulated oxygen dose resulting from prolonged intubation rather than high oxygen concentration, while the infant with Class III cytology

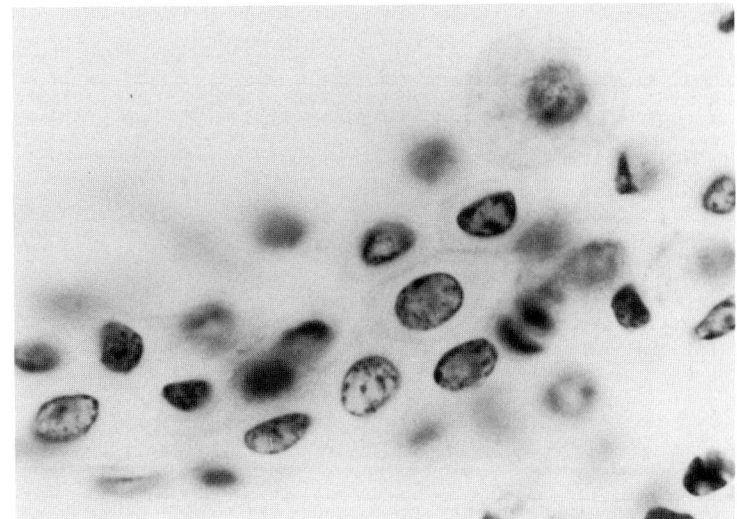

Figure 4.2. Class II tracheal aspirate. A small sheet of cells showing squamous metaplasia with crisp borders. A histiocyte is above the metaplastic cells. Papanicolaou's stain; ×1000.

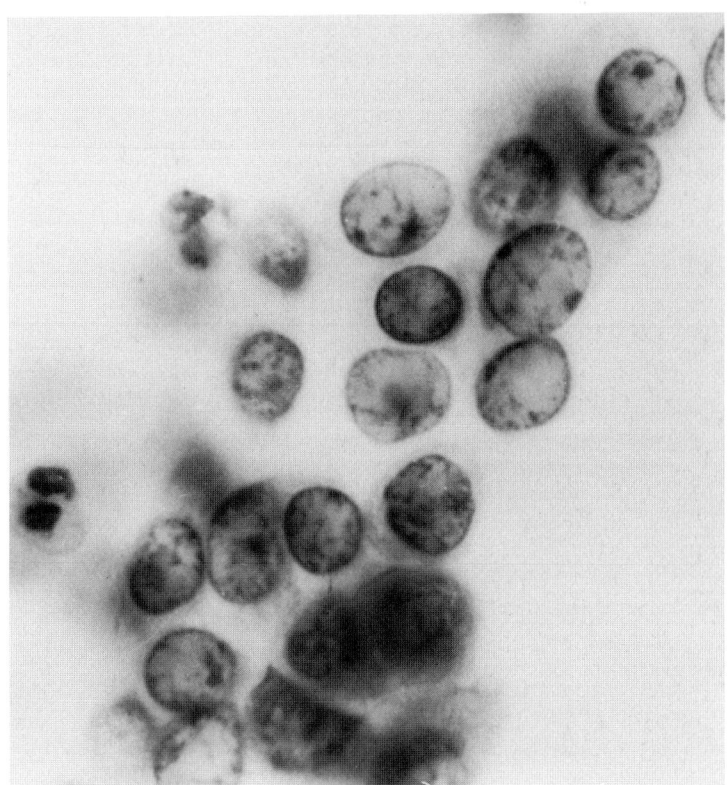

Figure 4.3. Early repair. Nuclei of these epithelial cells have smooth borders and salt-and-pepper chromatin. The cells are usually loosely grouped. Papanicolaou's stain; ×1000.

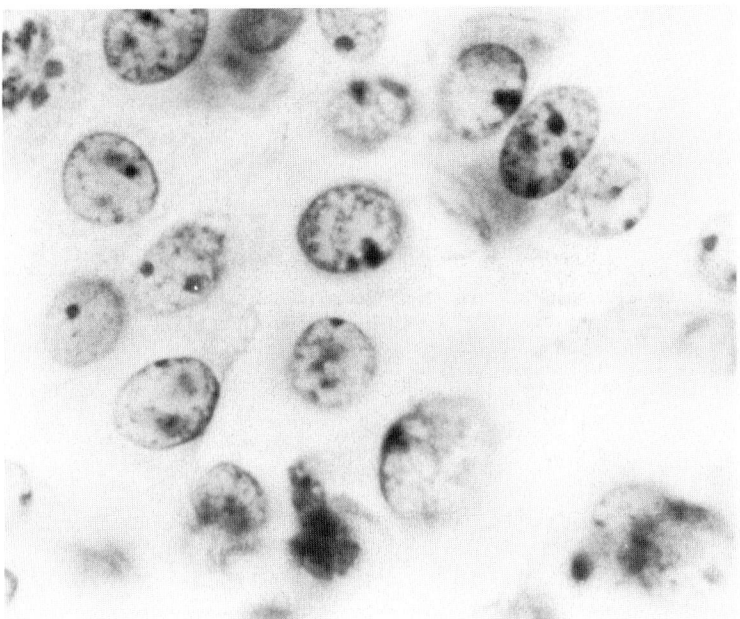

Figure 4.4. Moderate repair. Nuclei have heavier chromatin with chromocenters. A mitotic figure is at the edge of the group. Papanicolaou's stain; ×1000.

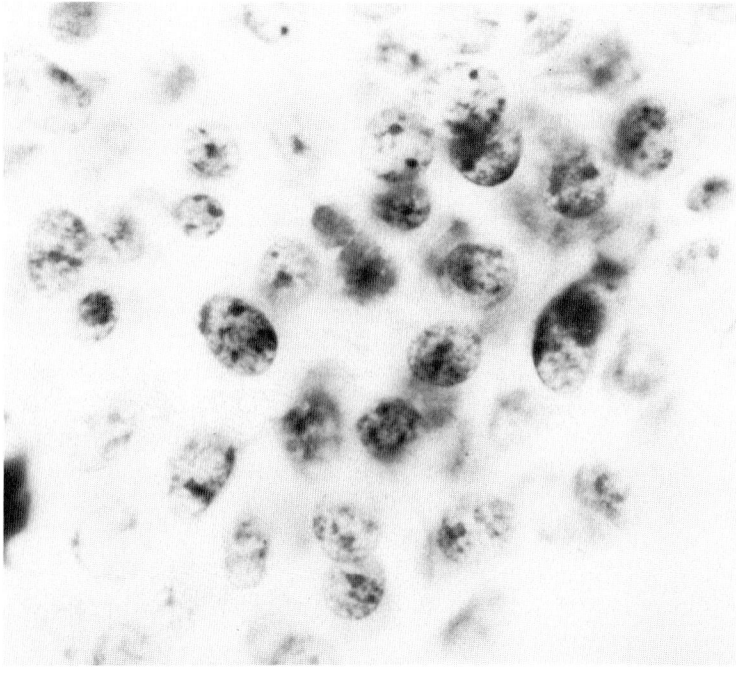

Figure 4.5. Late repair. Nuclei are smaller but still have smooth borders. Chromatin is heavy with chromocenters and occasional nucleoli. Papanicolaou's stain; ×1000.

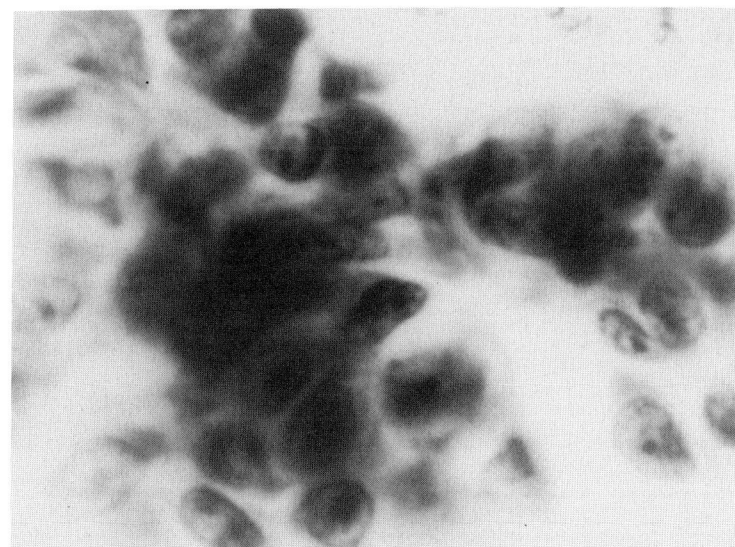

Figure 4.6. Class III. Atypical metaplastic and repair nuclei with irregular borders, variable size, prominent nucleoli, and nuclear molding. Papanicolaou's stain; ×1000.

tends to have a large oxygen dose from high FiO_2 delivered over a short period of time.

Histiocytes (Macrophages)

Histiocytes are seen in almost all aspirates obtained after day 3. Most are probably alveolar macrophages, but some may be recruited from blood monocytes as part of the inflammatory process. It should be possible to differentiate "resident" macrophages by immunohistochemical means (13), but this has not yet been done in newborn tracheal aspirates. The histiocytes are of variable size, often multinucleated, and usually less degenerate that epithelial cells in the same aspirate. Iron-

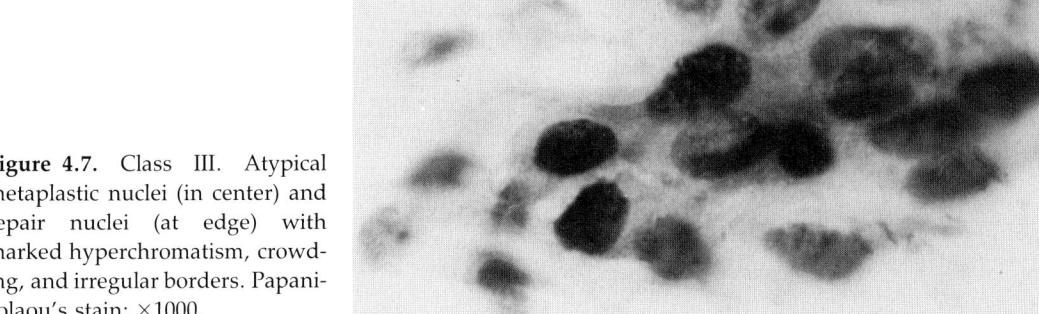

Figure 4.7. Class III. Atypical metaplastic nuclei (in center) and repair nuclei (at edge) with marked hyperchromatism, crowding, and irregular borders. Papanicolaou's stain; ×1000.

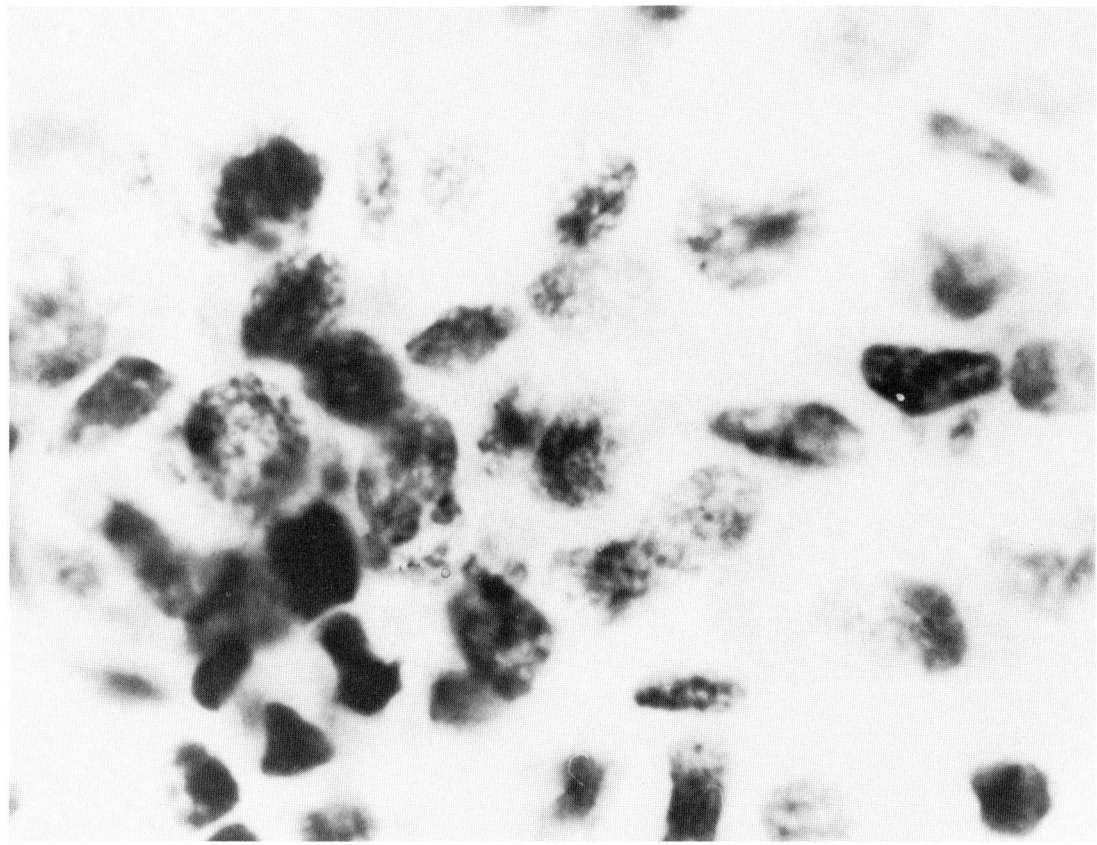

Figure 4.8. Class III. Atypical, pleomorphic nuclei with hyperchromatism, large nucleoli, and chaotic arrangement. This tracheal aspirate was from Baby BP on day 9 (see Fig. 4.12 and text) and should be compared with tissue sections from the same infant (Fig. 4.11). Papanicolaou's stain; ×1000.

stain-positive hemosiderin granules and fragments of hyaline membrane debris in the cytoplasm of these cells indicate phagocytic activity. Foamy cytoplasm has been observed in aspirates from infants receiving intravenous lipid infusions; these histiocytes are large and contain intracytoplasmic lipid on Sudan black stain (14). Foamy histiocytes were also seen in 69% of aspirates obtained from babies in congestive heart failure with patent ductus arteriosus who were not on intravenous lipid infusions or oral feeds (6).

Neutrophils

In contrast to histiocytes the frequency with which neutrophils are observed in tracheal aspirates is bimodal. Neutrophils are usually seen from the first day of intubation, and by day 4 over 90% of aspirates contain them. The frequency declines to 43% on day 7, and then increases again to 85% of aspirates obtained between days 11 and 15 from infants with Class II-III and Class III aspirates (6). Ogden *et al.* counted the numbers of neutro-

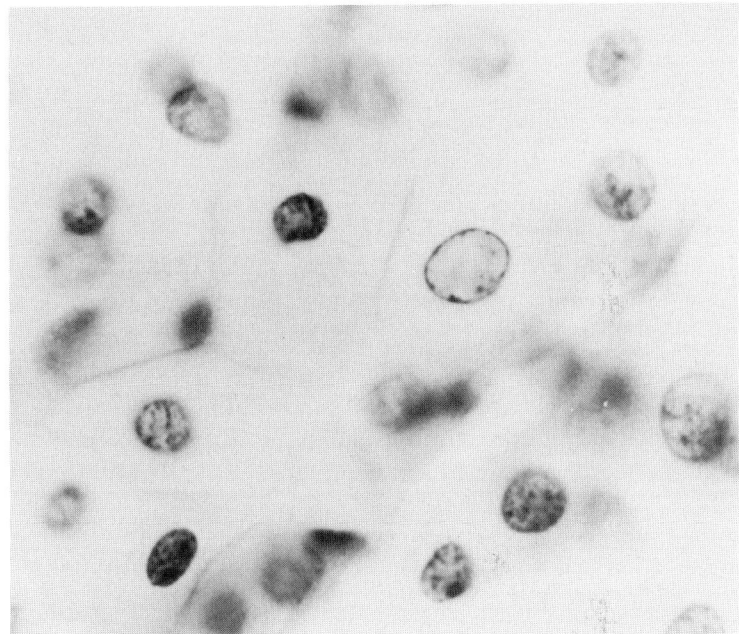

Figure 4.9. Class IV tracheal aspirate with sheets of cells showing mature squamous metaplasia. Numerous histiocytes are usual, although not in this photograph. There is no nuclear atypism. Papanicolaou's stain; ×1000.

phils in repetitive pulmonary lavages of newborns with respiratory distress syndrome (RDS) (15). Infants with RDS alone had peak ratios of neutrophil count to body weight at about 4 days, with marked decline by day 7; infants who subsequently developed BPD peaked at about day 7 and then had gradually declining ratios for the next month. The slopes of the ratios of both groups were essentially identical for only the first 2 days. These observations suggest that the initially observed neutrophils are the result of acute injury to epithelium and, in some infants, of the ridding of neutrophils aspirated *in utero*. The prolonged "influx" of neutrophils is presumed to be the result of continued injury and may, in part, be mediated through chemotactic agents released by alveolar macrophages (16). Neutrophils probably contribute to the injury by releasing proteolytic agents and free oxygen radicals (17, 18). Yet the number of neutrophils seen in Class III aspirates is often less than one would expect in the presence of so many histiocytes. In my experience many neutrophils in Class III aspirates strongly suggests intercurrent pneumonia, which invariably increases the oxygen dose. Necrotizing tracheobronchitis would also be expected to produce large numbers of neutrophils. Tracheal aspirates containing micro-organisms on Gram's stain always contain neutrophils, in contrast with less than half of Gram's-stain-negative aspirates (10).

Mucus and Curschmann's Spirals

Practically nothing is known about the composition, characteristics, or production of tracheobronchial mucus of preterm infants. Mucous cells are sloughed along with other epithelial cells, accounting for the copious and mucoid quality of aspirates obtained in the first few days of life. Thereafter aspirates are generally smaller and less mucoid. Histologic sections of lung tissue obtained at autopsy show PAS-positive, mucin-containing cells in uninjured, regenerating, or regenerated epithelium only in conjunction with cells having cilia or terminal bars. Severly injured epithelium, composed of markedly atypical cells that correlate with Class III cytology (see Fig. 4.11, C) do not contain PAS-positive material even though apparently unaffected mucous glands in subjacent submucosa do. McDowell *et al.* studied the regeneration of hamster tracheal epithelium after *one-time* induced mechanical injury (8). They noted the joint development of cytoplasmic mucin granules and early cilia about 72 hours after injury on the luminal surface of the regenerating epithelium composed, at the time, of mitotically active metaplastic cells. In the hamster model complete regeneration occurs in about 96 hours. The situation is clearly different in the human neonate exposed to *sustained* injury. However, as discussed below, neither the injury nor the regeneration of the bronchial epithelium of these neonates is spatially uniform, and the hamster model data may apply over short segments of epithelium where, for unknown reasons, healing can occur in spite of continued injury elsewhere. Even with special stains it may be extremely hard in tracheal aspirates to differentiate mucous cells from degenerative vacuolation.

Curschmann's spirals are readily identified and are found in some 10% of tracheal aspirates (6). These corkscrew-shaped objects (Fig. 4.10) are inspissated mucus extruded from submucosal mucous glands. Associated in adults with asthma, chronic bronchitis, and smoking, and occasionally found in cervical cytology, Curschmann's spirals are considered by Koss to be evidence of abnormal mucus composition (19). They tend to be seen repeatedly in the same infants, usually between days 4 and 14, and are associated with Class II and Class II-III aspirates. Some affected infants have a strong family history of allergies and asthma. There has been insufficient follow-up to determine if these infants are manifesting an early marker of airway hyperactivity, which in itself has been associated with HLA-A2 phenotype (20) and particular liability to BPD (21, 22). Creola bodies, sometimes seen in the sputa of asthmatics, have not yet been reported in neonatal tracheal aspirates.

Hyaline Membrane Debris

At autopsy, lung sections show hyaline membranes after about 3 hours of life, sometimes earlier if the infant has hypoplastic lungs. In tracheal aspirates, hyaline membrane debris starts to appear on day 2, when it has come within reach of the suctioning catheter. It continues to be found in aspirates of all classes except Class IV. The debris is usually fibrillary and rust-colored on Papanicolaou's stain and is PAS-positive presumably because of its high alpha-1-antitrypsin content (23). It is often mixed with blood. Small fragments of debris are seen as cytoplasmic inclusions in histiocytes. Doshi *et al.* report that the presence of yellow hyaline membranes in tracheal aspirates correlates with subsequent histologic changes of BPD and with kernicterus (5, 24).

Correlating Tracheal Aspirate Cytology with Histologic, Radiologic, and Clinical Findings

The original description of BPD by Northway *et al.* in 1967 correlated clinical, radiologic, and pathologic data and proposed radiologic and pathologic staging criteria (25). Even

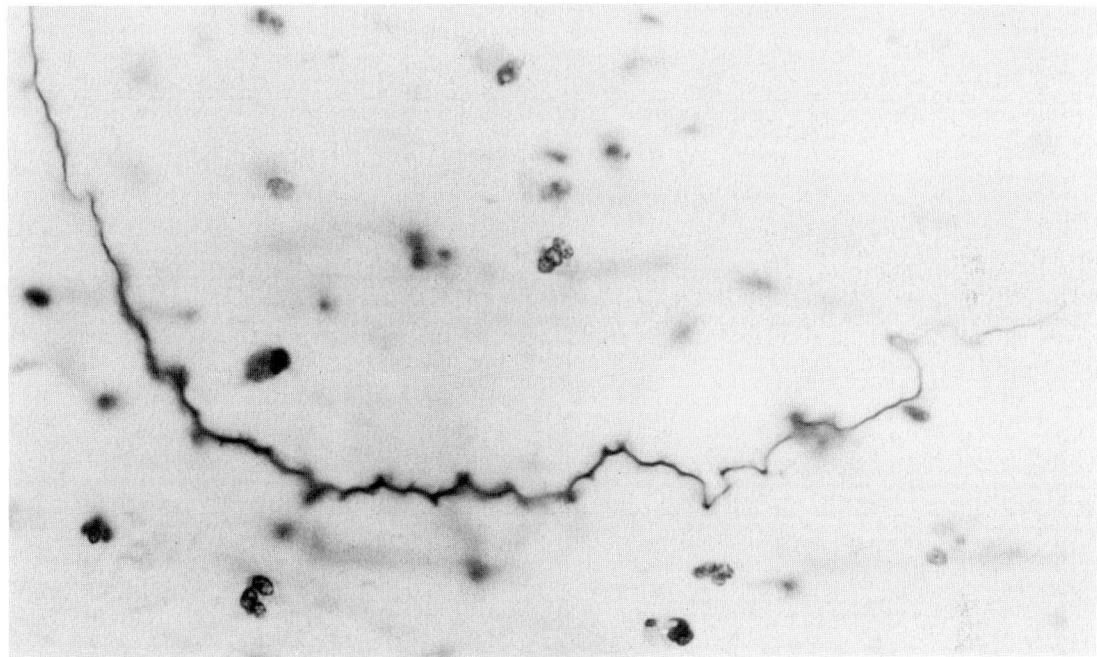

Figure 4.10. Curschmann's spiral in Class II tracheal aspirate with numerous neutrophils. Papanicolaou's stain; ×400.

earlier autopsy studies of the nature and pathogenesis of hyaline membranes, such as that of Boss and Craig (26), clearly illustrate the concurrent destructive and reparative changes in airway and alveolar epithelium so evident in the tracheal aspirates of infants with severe disease. Correlations of epithelial changes with alterations in interstitium, blood vessels, and lymphatics are detailed by Rosan (12); and blood vessel morphometry by Tomashefski et al (27). Thus there is ample evidence from autopsy material that epithelium can reflect the injury of adjacent tissues. It is equally clear, however, that the epithelium is not uniformly altered. A single bronchiole may show a segment of regenerated epithelium merging into a segment with moderate changes, which then merges into a segment with severe cellular atypia (Fig. 4.11). In my experience the most severe changes have always been distal to the least severe, and no instances of isolated atypical epithelium (skip areas) have been seen. Subepithelial tissues tend to be more uniformly damaged even beneath regenerated epithelium, as if the epithelium is the first damaged and first repaired of all pulmonary tissues. It is not clear if this is from an inherent resilience of epithelium or represents uneven, localized challenge or response. The spatial direction of regeneration from proximal to distal and the lack of skip areas favor the former explanation. The nonuniformity of epithelial change is reflected in the variety of epithelial cell-forms seen in tracheal aspirates and is the major reason for classifying an

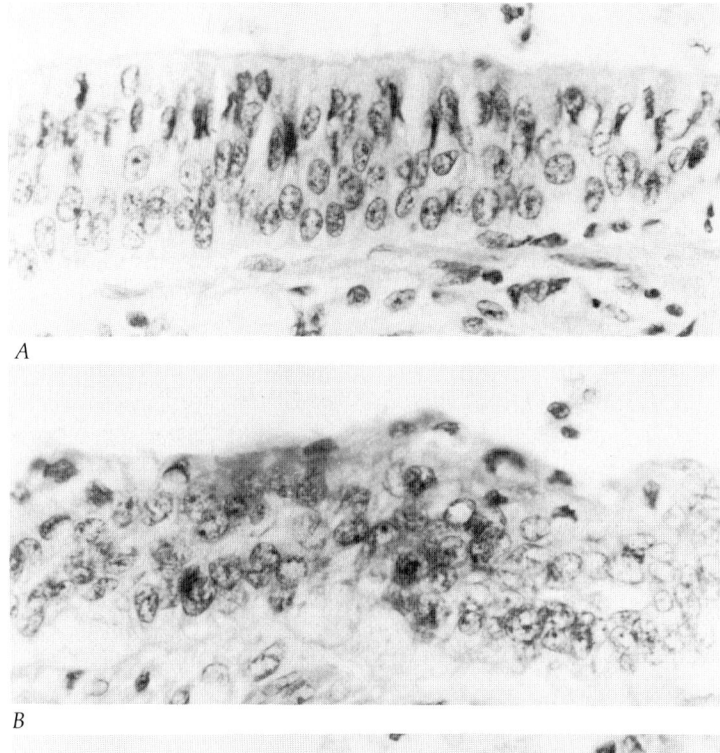

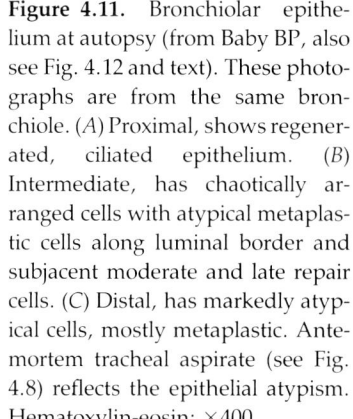

Figure 4.11. Bronchiolar epithelium at autopsy (from Baby BP, also see Fig. 4.12 and text). These photographs are from the same bronchiole. (*A*) Proximal, shows regenerated, ciliated epithelium. (*B*) Intermediate, has chaotically arranged cells with atypical metaplastic cells along luminal border and subjacent moderate and late repair cells. (*C*) Distal, has markedly atypical cells, mostly metaplastic. Antemortem tracheal aspirate (see Fig. 4.8) reflects the epithelial atypism. Hematoxylin-eosin; ×400.

aspirate on the basis of its most abnormal features. Nonrepresentative sampling, that bugaboo of exfoliative cytology, is a constant concern and emphasizes the need to obtain repetitive aspirates.

Estimating the time of onset of BPD depends on the diagnostic modality and on concepts of etiology and tissue resilience. D'Ablang *et al.* observed changes in aspirate cytology that appeared to be more advanced than in the concurrent chest x-rays (1). This asynchrony between tissue and radiologic changes has been confirmed in tracheal aspirates (4) and at autopsy (12, 28), and it is now accepted that changes correlating with BPD occur in tissue before they can be discerned by conventional x-ray. In fact recent recommendations for radiologic assessment of BPD are to evaluate the infant at about 21 days of age, when the most specific changes of BPD are least likely to be confused with other pulmonary conditions (29). Rosan, a pathologist, feels that the etiology of BPD is so intimately associated with oxygen toxicity that hyaline membrane disease is Stage I of BPD, because it represents the beginning of the process that, if continued, will result in BPD. He states: "With administration of 80–100% oxygen to the lung by endotracheal catheter for 4 days, 100% of patients will develop clinical, radiologic and cytologic signs of oxygen intoxication" (12). Some neonatologists expect BPD to be present when an infant has been ventilated for 7 days; and generally, the longer the ventilation is required, the more severe will be the subsequent pulmonary morbidity. Both the pathologist's and the clinician's views are correct within their own frames of reference; the situation is conceptually analogous to defining the beginning of a neoplasm at the time of tumor induction at the cellular level or at the time of first symptoms. Unlike a neoplasm, however, BPD is a syndrome due to biophysical injury that is self-limiting; when the injurious agents are removed, the tissue-destroying processes stop, reparative processes gain the upper hand, and healing occurs through regeneration, scarring, and remodeling. The degree of residual pulmonary disability depends on the severity of the injury (perhaps represented by oxygen dose), on the amount of lung that is injured, and on the ability of the various tissues to "normalize" themselves through regeneration and remodeling.

Epithelium is the fixed tissue sampled by tracheal aspirate cytology. Epithelium is undergoing repair and regeneration at the same time that it is being injured, although in different places. The destructive process is reflected by the severity of cellular atypia, and this in turn correlates fairly well with oxygen dose (4, 6). The correlation, however, is imperfect, with much overlapping of the class specific oxygen dose ranges (Table 4.2), even though the mean oxygen dose rises steadily with advancing cytologic class (6). The lack of precision is due to nonrepresentative sampling of the exfoliated cells and to imperfect cytologic interpretation. Other clinical attributes are so overwhelmed by the effect of oxygen dose that they cannot be analytically segregated to show their independent effects, if any. Furthermore means and ranges do not express the variations in the early clinical courses of these babies. The cytologic classes observed in the sequential tracheal aspirates of four infants illustrate the relationship of their clinical courses to cumulative oxygen dose (Fig. 4.12) (6). In the individual patient, the speed of progression to Class II-III or to Class III also indicates severity.

Baby BP (Fig. 4.12) had Class III cytology on day 6 with an accumulated oxygen dose of 11,262 hours %; unfortunately no smears were obtained on days 4 or 5, but one suspects that they would have shown a progression from Class I. Although the heaviest at birth of the four babies depicted here (1370 g), he had congenital *Haemophilus influenzae* sepsis with pneumonia and has been reported elsewhere (30). His chest x-ray on day 1 showed extensive bilateral consolidation with air bronchograms consistent with severe hyaline membrane disease. Increasing pulmonary interstitial emphysema was seen on each subsequent film without pneumothorax. Cardiac dilatation was observed on films after day 3. His clinical course was very stormy, and he died on day 9 shortly after the last aspirate was obtained. At autopsy he had Stage II-III BPD with pneumonia and residual hyaline membranes (some of which were yellow), massive intraventricular hemorrhage, kernicterus, and in-

Table 4.2. Selected Clinical Characteristics by Cytologic Class

Characteristic	Class I (9 cases)	Class II (28 cases)	Class II-III (12 cases)	Class III (10 cases)	Unclassified (10 cases)
			Means		
Birth weight (g)	1173	961	801	1027	1463
Day of life	2.7	6.4	10.1	10.2	7.7
Hours % O_2	2028	4610	7532	11316	6601
PEEP pressure	25.8	13.6	12.2	17.5	13.1
			Ranges		
Birth weight (g)	660–2080	630–2080	630–980	630–1370	630–2080
Day of life	2–4	3–15	6–14	6–16	2–11
Hours % O_2	590–5047	1651–11017	4245–12796	6211–18792	1429–17043
PEEP pressure	12–42	11–21	10–16	11–29	0–20

From Neave and Masura (6).

trahepatic cholestatic jaundice. Bronchiolar epithelium is illustrated in Fig. 4.11. Yellow hyaline membranes were plainly seen in the lung sections but could not be found on his tracheal aspirates. This patient illustrates 1) that it is extremely difficult to diagnose BPD early in a baby's course by x-ray in the presence of other severe disease processes, 2) that tissue changes characteristic of BPD occur quickly with rapidly rising oxygen dose, and 3) that the material in tracheal aspirates may not be representative.

Baby LS (Fig. 4.12) weighed 810 g when born at 30 weeks' gestation; the growth retardation may have been due to the mother's habitual use of diazepam (Valium). Her initial chest films showed bilateral granularity consistent with hyaline membrane disease and right upper lobe atelectasis; on day 4 mild interstitial emphysema was noticed. Tracheal aspirates progressed to Class II-III on day 9 and were notable for extensive squamous metaplasia without definite nuclear atypia, and foamy histiocytes before receiving indomethacin to induce ductus closure. Her course was slow but generally uncomplicated. On day 40 the tracheal aspirate showed sheets of mature metaplastic cells and histiocytes consistent with Class IV. She was extubated on day 86, weaned to room air on day 126, and discharged on day 152 weighing 3160 g. Chest films confirmed the clinical diagnosis of BPD. When examined at age 11 months (4678 g) she still had tachypnea, intercostal retractions, and scattered squeaks and wheezes in spite of metaproterenol treatment. Muscle tone and strength were slightly diminished, but there were no abnormal reflexes or ocular changes. This infant illustrates 1) that BPD can develop without nuclear atypia in the tracheal aspirate when associated with Class IV cytology, 2) that prolonged mechanical ventilation may promote such extensive squamous metaplasia as to inhibit complete epithelial regeneration, and 3) that follow-up after discharge can help to interpret changes that occurred early in life.

Baby LW (Fig. 4.12) weighed 710 g when born at 26 weeks' gestation. There was maternal history of recurrent vaginal bleeding from placenta previa, rupture of membranes 48 hours before delivery, and failure of tocolysis. The initial chest x-ray revealed very mild signs of hyaline membrane disease. On day 3 the tracheal aspirate (Class II) showed numerous foamy histiocytes coincident with a loud ductus murmur. On day 4, still Class II with an accumulated oxygen dose of 2557 hours %, the chest x-rays showed more pronounced changes of cardiac dilatation and hyaline mem-

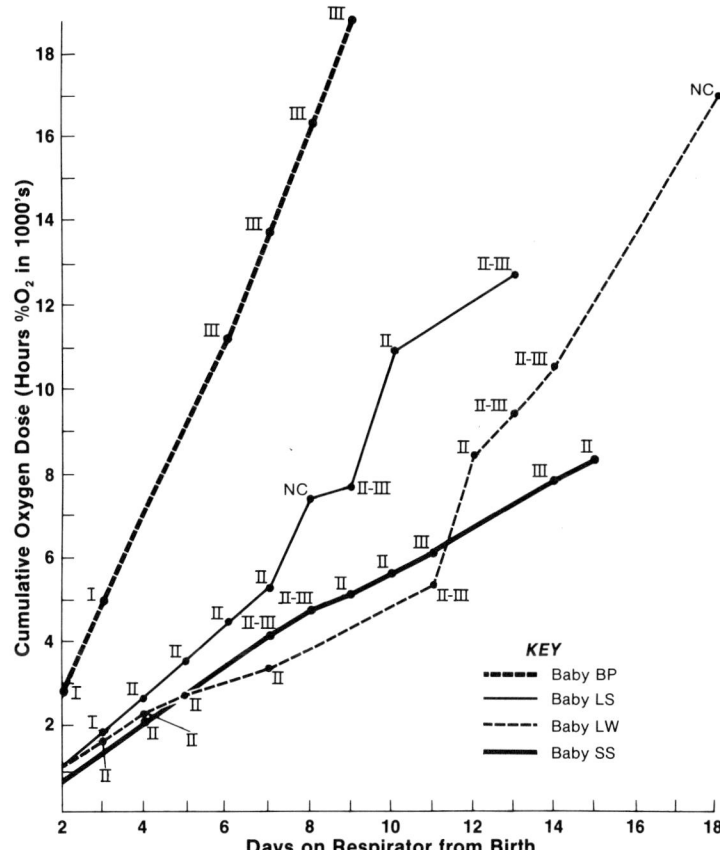

Figure 4.12. Classes of tracheal aspirates from four infants arranged by days of mechanical ventilation from birth and by cumulative oxygen dose. Cytologic classes are indicated by Roman numerals; NC means "not classified" because of cellular paucity. See text.

brane disease. The ductus was ligated on day 8 with clinical improvement until days 11–13, when she developed recurrent episodes of apnea and acidosis subsequently thought to be due to a grade 3 intraventricular cerebral bleed. Oxygen need increased abruptly. Chest x-ray on day 14 showed interstitial emphysema and, by day 17, possible fibrosis consistent with BPD. With one exception tracheal aspirates during this period showed Class II-III cytology. Her condition stabilized, and she was discharged on day 108. When re-examined at age 5½ months, she measured below the third percentile in all growth parameters. Her respiratory rate was 40 per minute; no wheezes were heard. Deep tendon reflexes were asymmetric, no stepping reflex was present, and there were equivocal Babinski signs. No visual defect was found.

At age 7 months she was briefly hospitalized for bronchiolitis. This patient illustrates 1) that a major intercurrent illness, such as intraventricular hemorrhage, can alter the oxygen dose so as to result in BPD even when the original polmonary disease was mild, 2) that subsequent pulmonary morbidity may be less if the increase in oxygen dose occurs late in the infant's course than if it occurs early, 3) that epithelial changes seen on tracheal cytology correlate best with the infant's early clinical attributes, and 4) that once having progressed to advanced stages, tracheal aspirate cytology loses specificity.

Baby SS (Fig. 4.12) had congenital *Haemophilus influenzae* sepsis and is included in a previous report (30). Unlike Baby BP, however, he did not have demonstrable congenital pneumonia. He weighed 860 g when born at 29 weeks' gestation. Placental membranes had been ruptured for a week prior to delivery, and the placenta showed severe chorioamnionitis with three-vessel umbilical vasculitis. The baby's initial chest film had minimal signs of hyaline membrane disease. His course was marked by transient episodes of apnea and bradycardia of unknown etiology that occurred after his blood cultures had become negative and disappeared after theophylline treatment. He was weaned to continuous positive airway pressure on day 14, extubated on day 16, and in room air by day 37. In spite of this relatively rapid progress, tracheal aspirates showed Class III changes on day 11 and on day 14. On physical examination just prior to discharge on day 94, he weighed 2120 g and had "clear lungs"; ophthalmologic examination showed grade I retinitis. He was not considered clinically or radiologically to have BPD. The mother subsequently refused to bring the baby to follow-up appointments. In a telephone conversation with the grandmother, when the baby was 7 months of age, it was learned that he had a "pulmonary problem" and had been hospitalized elsewhere for pneumonia. This infant illustrates 1) that residual pulmonary morbidity can occur after what appears to have been a relatively benign course, 2) that tracheal aspirate cytology early in the baby's course may be prognostically valuable even in the absence of clinical and radiologic pulmonary signs, and 3) that post-discharge follow-up is necessary to define BPD.

These vignettes suggest a close correlation between tracheal aspirate cytology and the infant's clinical status concurrently and in the near future (Fig. 4.13). Infants with Class I or Class II cytology by the time of extubation appear to have no residual pulmonary damage. Class II-III aspirates are the most difficult to interpret cytologically and the most speculative as to outcome. When the infants with Class II-III aspirates do well, one retrospectively suspects that the cytologic changes were due to degeneration; when the infants have residual pulmonary morbidity, one suspects a cytologic undercall. Unequivocal nuclear atypia (Class III) or sheets of mature metaplastic cells without atypia (Class IV) correlate with concurrent and future pulmonary deficits. The determinants of long-term restoration of pulmonary growth and function are unclear. The severity of the initial damage might be judged by tracheal aspiration cytology, but cytology cannot assess the extent of damage, because of vagaries in cell sampling. Radiologic and pulmonary function studies are more helpful and certainly less invasive than tracheal aspirate cytology in following extubated infants after discharge from hospital. Cytologic examination and microbiologic culture of material removed by bronchial suction after lavage or by transthoracic fine-needle aspiration offer alternatives to open-lung biopsy in the identification of specific organisms.

Use of Tracheal Aspiration Cytology to Monitor Clinical Trials

It has been hoped that tracheal aspirate cytology could be used to judge the effectiveness of exogenous surfactant or antioxidant medications given to preterm newborns to prevent or ameliorate BPD (3, 5, 6). The expectation is that "effective" medication will arrest or retard the progression of cytologic change and that nuclear atypia will not occur, while babies receiving "ineffective" medication or placebos will have cytologic changes that progress as usual. Of the many clinical trials that have been done, only one has reported the results of tracheal aspirate cytology in study and control infants. Merritt *et al.* (31) found that infants who received human surfactant had Class I and Class II changes

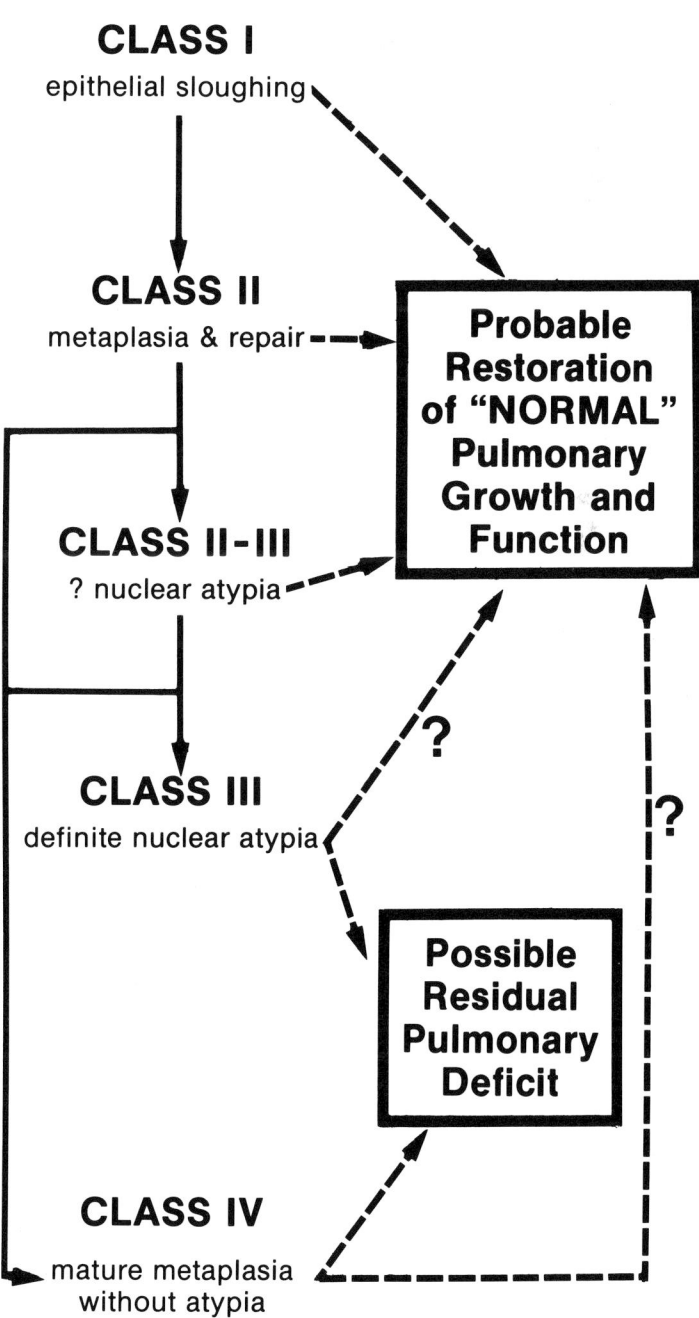

Figure 4.13. Progression of epithelial changes in tracheal aspirates of newborns on mechanical ventilation with proposed outcomes. See text.

and did not progress to Class III, while 8 of 18 control infants developed Class III cytology. Interestingly each of the babies with radiographic diagnosis of BPD by day 10 had Curschmann's spirals, suggesting that the spirals may indicate an underlying condition in the infants whose RDS might not have been helped by surfactant. These results, clearly in the expected direction, need confirmation and comparison with clinical findings at post-discharge follow-up.

Summary

The advantages of tracheal aspirate cytology in newborns are 1) that they are easy to obtain while the infant is intubated, 2) that they appear to represent fairly the condition of tracheobronchial epithelium and underlying pulmonary tissues, and 3) that they are useful in predicting the infant's near-future pulmonary morbidity. The disadvantages include (1) that, like all exfoliative cytology, these aspirates suffer from uneven sampling errors, 2) that distinguishing cellular degeneration from atypia can be very difficult, and 3) that obtaining aspirate becomes "invasive" after the infant has been extubated. At present tracheal aspirate cytology seems to be most valuable in the first 15 days of life; after that other modalities, particularly radiologic, are more helpful. Whether or not exfoliative cytology is sufficiently sensitive to assess the effects of anti-BPD medications remains to be seen.

The full potential of tracheal aspirate cytology will not be realized until the different types of nonciliated epithelial cells can be accurately identified and counted during the various stages of regeneration. While considerable knowledge has been gained when specific cell types can be identified and counted, such as foamy histiocytes (14) and neutrophils (15), virtually nothing is known of neurosecretory epithelial cells in living infants, and little is known of mucous cells. Immunohistochemical staining has been insufficiently explored in this regard. There is also much to learn of neonatal tracheobronchial mucus, the major noncellular component of these aspirates.

References

1. D'Ablang G, Bernard B, Zaharov I, Barton L, Kaplan B, Schwinn CP. Neonatal pulmonary cytology and bronchopulmonary dysplasia. Acta Cytol 1975;19(1):21–27.
2. Kanbour A, Doshi N, Fujikura T. Neonatal tracheobronchial cytology of bronchopulmonary dysplasia (abstr). Acta Cytol 1980;24(1):60.
3. Merritt TA, Puccia JM, Stuard ID. Cytologic evaluation of pulmonary effluent in neonates with respiratory distress syndrome and bronchopulmonary dysplasia. Acta Cytol 1981;25(6):631–639.
4. Merritt TA, Stuard ID, Puccia J, et al. Newborn tracheal aspirate cytology: classification during respiratory distress syndrome and bronchopulmonary dysplasia. J Pediatr 1981;98(6):949–955.
5. Doshi N, Kanbour A, Fujikura T, Klionsky B. Tracheal aspiration cytology in neonates with respiratory distress: histopathologic correlation. Acta Cytol 1982;26(1):15–21.
6. Neave C, Masura V. Cytology of tracheal aspirates in newborns with respiratory distress syndrome. Unpublished reports, Department of Pathology, Women and Infants Hospital, Providence, RI, 1985.
7. Neave C, Masura V. Cytology of tracheal aspirates from newborns with respiratory distress syndrome (abstr). Acta Cytol 1985;29(5):923.
8. McDowell EM, Becci PJ, Schurch W, Trump BF. The respiratory epithelium. VII. Epidermoid metaplasia of hamster epithelium during regeneration following mechanical injury. J Natl Cancer Inst 1979;62(4):995–1008.

9. Johnson DE, Lock JE, Elde RP, Thompson TR. Pulmonary neuroendocrine cells in hyaline membrane disease and bronchopulmonary dysplasia. Pediatr Res 1982;16(A2):446–454.
10. Sherman MP, Goetzman BW, Ahlfors CE, Wennberg RP. Tracheal aspiration and its clinical correlates in the diagnosis of congenital pneumonia. Pediatrics 1980;65(2):258–263.
11. Dute RM, Dute R. Congenital herpes simplex virus infection diagnosed by cytology of aspirated tracheobronchial material. Acta Cytol 1985;29(5):712–713.
12. Rosan RC. Hyaline membrane disease and a related spectrum of neonatal pneumopathies. Perspect Pediatr Pathol 1975;2:15–60.
13. Kobzik L, Godleski JJ, Brain JD. Ultrastructural analysis of a specific hamster alveolar macrophage antigen. Lab Invest 1985;53(5):526–533.
14. Recalde AL, Nickerson BG, Vegas M, Scott CB, Landing BH, Warburton D. Lipid-laden macrophages in tracheal aspirates of newborn infants receiving intravenous lipid infusions: a cytologic study. Pediatr Pathol 1984;2(1):25–34.
15. Ogden BE, Murphy S, Saunders GC, Johnson JD. Lung lavage of newborns with respiratory distress syndrome. Prolonged neutrophil influx is associated with bronchopulmonary dysplasia. Chest 1983;83(5 suppl):31S–33S.
16. Kazmierowski JA, Gallin JI, Reynolds HY. Mechanism for the inflammatory response in primate lungs. Demonstration and partial characterization of an alveolar macrophage-derived chemotactic factor with preferential activity for polymorphonuclear leukocytes. J Clin Invest 1977;59(2):273–281.
17. Weiss SJ, LoBuglio AF. Phagocyte-generated oxygen metabolites and cellular injury. Lab Invest 1982;47(1):5–18.
18. Merritt TA. Oxygen exposure in the newborn guinea pig lung lavage cell populations, chemotactic and elastase response: a possible relationship to neonatal bronchopulmonary dysplasia. Pediatr Res 1982;16(9):798–805.
19. Koss LG. Diagnostic cytology and its histopathologic bases. 3rd ed. Philadelphia: JB Lippincott, 1979, pp 546–547.
20. Clark DA, Pincus LG, Oliphant M, Hubbell C, Oates RP, Davey FR. HLA-A2 and chronic lung disease in neonates. J Am Med Assoc 1982;248(15):1868–1869.
21. Nickerson BG, Taussig LM. Family history of asthma in infants with bronchopulmonary dysplasia. Pediatrics 1980;65(6):1140–1144.
22. Bertrand J, Riley SP, Popkin J, Coates AL. The long-term pulmonary sequelae of prematurity: the role of familial airway hyperactivity and the respiratory distress syndrome. N Engl J Med 1985;312(12):742–745.
23. Mathis RK, Freier EF, Hung CE, Krivit W, Sharp HL. Alpha-1-antitrypsin in the respiratory-distress syndrome. N Engl J Med 1973;288(2):59–64.
24. Doshi N, Klionsky B, Fujikura T, MacDonald H. Pulmonary yellow hyaline membranes in neonates. Hum Pathol 1980;11(suppl):520–527.
25. Northway WH, Rosan RC, Porter DY. Pulmonary disease following respirator therapy of hyaline-membrane disease: bronchopulmonary dysplasia. N Engl J Med 1967;276(7):357–368.
26. Boss JH, Craig JM. Reparative phenomena in lungs of neonates with hyaline membranes. Pediatrics 1962;29(6):890–898.
27. Tomashefski JF, Oppermann HC, Vawter GF, Reid LM. Bronchopulmonary dysplasia: a morphometric study with emphasis on the pulmonary vasculature. Pediatr Pathol 1984;2(4):469–487.
28. Edwards DK, Colby TV, Northway WH. Radiographic-pathologic correlation in bronchopulmonary dysplasia. J Pediatr 1979;95(5, part 2):834–836.
29. Toce SS, Farrell PM, Leavitt LA, Samuels DP, Edwards DK. Clinical and roentgenographic scoring systems for assessing bronchopulmonary dysplasia. Am J Dis Child 1984;138(6):581–585.
30. Campognone P, Singer DS. Neonatal sepsis due to nontypable *Haemophilus influenzae*. Am J Dis Child 1986;140(2):117–121.
31. Merritt TA, Hallman M, Holcomb K, et al. Human surfactant treatment of severe respiratory distress syndrome: pulmonary effluent indicators of lung inflammation. J Pediatr 1986;108(5, part 1):741–748.

Comments

T. Allen Merritt

Dr. Neave presents a clear rationale for, and extends previous observations documenting, the predictive power of cytopathologic examination of exfoliated airway epithelia and inflammatory cell patterns.

Aside from repeated chest radiographs and complex pulmonary function testing of inspiratory and expiratory flow resistances, staging of tracheal effluent cytology predicts near future pulmonary morbidity in the vast majority of cases. Other findings, including bacterial or fungal proliferative or even talc or powder in the effluent, can prompt closer clinical examination. It is unfortunate that this technique is not utilized more in intensive care nurseries. Successful examination of tracheal aspirate cytology requires a close working relationship between the cytopathologist, the cribside nurse, and the neonatologist. Tracheal aspiration techniques should be standardized; effluent suctioned must be immediately fixed and rapidly transported to the cytology laboratory.

Therapies designed to interrupt lung injury (steroids, antioxidants, superoxide dismutase, catalase, etc.) must be based upon a high probability that BPD will develop. This probability and the efficacy to new therapies on airway epithelial cytology are best monitored by *serial* tracheal effluent examination.

With all the benefits of cytologic evaluation, interestitial fibrosis muscularization of small vessels cannot be monitored using this technique. Nonetheless routine cytologic examination of tracheal aspirates should provide additional evidence to make thoughtful early diagnoses and to monitor new therapies.

5

Mechanisms and Pathobiologic Effects of Barotrauma

DONALD W. THIBEAULT AND MICHAEL J. LANG

Introduction and Definition of Barotrauma

Pulmonary barotrauma can be defined as any response of the lung to pressure or force that results in pathologic changes in the lungs. The applied pressure may originate from the infant's own respiratory system or be exogenous. The pressure induced trauma may last less than a second or months. The applied pressure can result in functional changes both in the lung and elsewhere without obvious structural damage. An example of a functional change would be excessive positive end-expiratory pressure (PEEP) in a compliant lung, leading to a decrease in the cardiac output. Structural changes can also occur outside the lung, such as with a pneumoperitoneum. An applied pressure may be excessive and damage the lung in one situation, and in another situation the same pressure may be appropriate and safe. For example a continuous positive airway pressure (CPAP) of 10 cm H_2O would be appropriate in an infant with severe RDS whereas the same pressure in an infant partially recovered from RDS could result in lung rupture. The duration, shape, and amplitude of the applied pressure waveform are potentially important variables in the generation of barotrauma. It is clear that barotrauma needs to be assessed not only from the applied pressure but also from the tissue response.

Although pulmonary barotrauma may occur spontaneously, the overwhelming cause is related to mechanical ventilation. Pulmonary interstitial emphysema (PIE) markedly aggravates any underlying lung disease; indeed, it is associated with a high mortality rate. In addition to its acute deleterious effects, barotrauma is a recognized predisposing factor to bronchopulmonary dysplasia (BPD). Precisely what position barotrauma commands in the hierarchy of causative BPD factors is a debatable issue and to some extent is the subject of this chapter. Specifically this chapter investigates the mechanisms and sites of lung damage resulting from barotrauma, and from these considerations addresses the prevention of barotrauma.

Theoretical Analysis of Mechanical Factors That Increase the Susceptibility of the Immature Lung to Barotrauma

This section discusses the structural and mechanical qualities of the immature lung that make it so susceptible to airway damage and pulmonary interstitial emphysema. The mechanical properties of the mature lung will be described first.

Lung Structure and Mechanics in the Mature Lung

To appreciate the mechanical properties that make immature lungs vulnerable to baro-

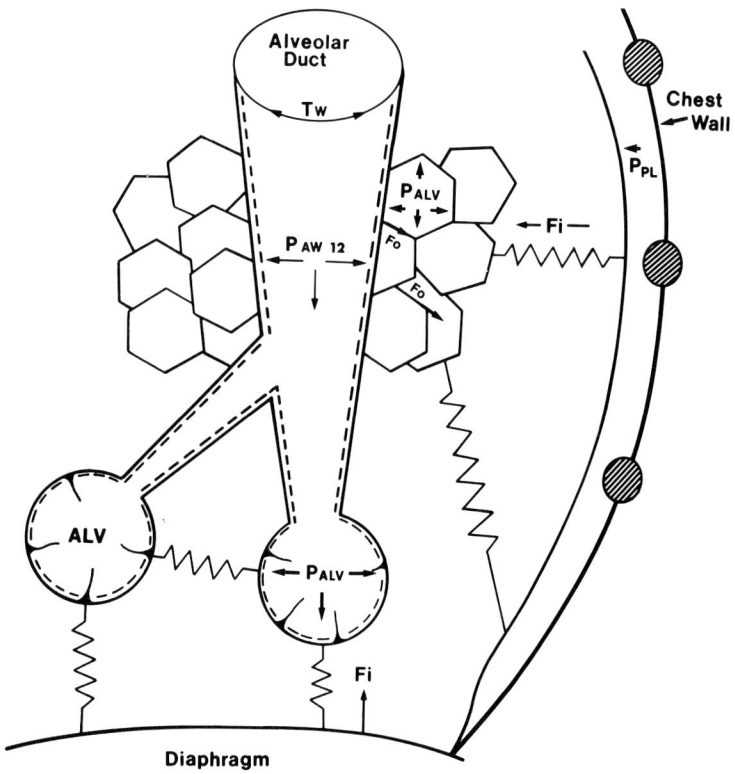

Figure 5.1. Schematic of a mature alveolar duct and alveoli. The dotted line represents surfactant. Tw is the wall tension or recoil pressure. P_{AW} is the airway pressure and P_{ALV} is the alveolar pressure. Fo is the tissue force directed outward, and Fi is the tissue force (stretched springs) acting inward. P_{PL} is the pleural pressure.

trauma and rupture, it is instructive to understand the properties of mature lungs. Figure 5.1 illustrates the lung forces in the peripheral airways and alveoli of the mature lung. The distal airway is receiving a peak positive pressure (P_{aw}) of 12 cm H_2O via the trachea. Surfactant lines the alveoli and small airways and lowers the surface tension forces so that the opening pressure of the distal airways and alveoli is very low, on the order of a few cm H_2O (1). The airway in Figure 5.1 is in continuity with the alveoli, so that the airway pressure (P_{aw}) is equal to the alveolar pressure (P_{alv})—that is, 12 cm H_2O. The lung is distended with the sum of pressures that includes P_{alv}, and alveolar outward septal tissue forces (Fo). These pressures are balanced by deflating inward forces that include the pleural pressure (P_{pl}) and the inward tissue recoil forces (Fi). The tissue forces Fi include connective tissue stresses as well as surface tension forces. The alveolar duct wall tension is determined by the Laplace relationship between wall tension (Tw), the radius of curvature (R), and the transmural pressure (P). For a cylinder $Tw = P \times R$, so that for any given transmural pressure, the larger the radius of the airway, the greater the wall tension. The airway pressure distends the alveolar duct wall with 12 cm H_2O pressure, and this is counterbalanced by the adjacent alveolar pressure of 12 cm H_2O. Thus the pressures cancel each other so that the transmural pressure is essentially equal to the alveolar septal tissue distending forces Fo.

There are a number of additional mechanical factors that protect the mature lung from barotrauma. The alveoli and airways are stabilized by lung interdependence (2). Pulmonary interdependence is the physical property of the lung and chest wall which tends to maintain uniform distention throughout the parenchyma during lung volume changes. For example, if a region of the lung is underaerated, forces will be generated at the interface with the neighboring normally aerated region, which will tend to expand the underaerated regions. Lung interdependence does not function well at very low lung volumes, at which the tissue elements are lax (3). A stable chest wall enhances the magnitude of lung interdependence (4). The presence of surfactant in the alveoli and small airways including the small bronchioles is a major factor in stabilizing the small airways and alveoli (1, 5, 6). Because the terminal airways and alveoli have small radii, without a surfactant lining layer they would collapse at end-expiration and would require an opening pressure greater than 25 cm H_2O (7, 8). Surfactant also keeps the airways, interstitium, and alveoli dry (9). Mature airways are less distensible than immature airways, and larger airways are less distensible than smaller airways (10, 11). Surfactant, stiff airway walls, and lung interdependence all help stabilize the small airway wall. In addition, because the airways are anchored distally to the lung parenchyma, with each inspiration the airways not only increase their volume but also undergo lengthening. The distended and lengthened airway is more stable than a collapsed one, just as an inflated balloon resists bending (12). Collateral flow through the pores of Kohn, bronchiole-alveolar channel of Lambert, and interbronchiolar channel of Martin are found in the mature lung and help prevent atelectasis (13, 14). This collateral flow is absent in the immature lung.

Lung Immaturity and Small Airway Barotrauma

Those mechanical properties of the immature lung that make it so susceptible to deformation and rupture during assisted ventilation will now be explored. Figure 5.2 (A) represents an immature lung at end-expiration. A transitional duct which is the precursor of alveolar ducts and respiratory bronchioles is shown connected to the saccules. Because there is no surfactant lining layer, the increased surface tension forces result in fluid being pulled into the interstitium, saccules, and small airways. The saccules and small airways that are not collapsed contain fluid. Due to the small radii of these airways, their wall tension is low. The airway wall, in fact, may be concave because of large surface tension forces acting on the wall at the air-liquid interface. The lax septal tissue in the collapsed or fluid-containing periairway saccules provides almost no outward stress on the small airways. The entire lung volume is low and near residual volume. The connective tissue forces are represented as springs (Fi and Fo in Figure 5.1) and are seen as being relaxed and under little tension. The chest wall is extremely compliant, which permits the pleural pressure to approach atmospheric pressure.

Figure 5.2 (B) shows the terminal unit

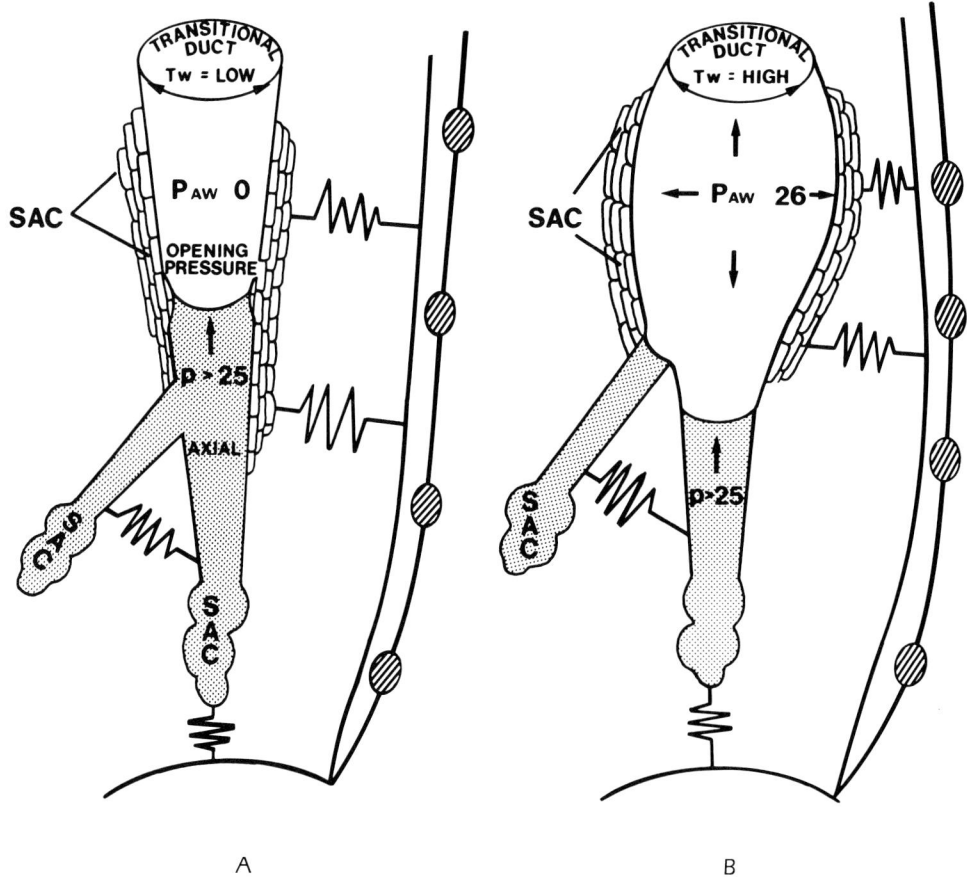

Figure 5.2. (*A*) An immature distal airway at end-expiration. The end-expiratory airway pressure (Paw) equals zero. The saccules (SAC) and airways contain fluid (shaded area). The axial airway is concave at the air-liquid interface, due to the surface tension forces. The periairway saccules (SAC) are collapsed or fluid filled. The lax tissues are represented by relaxed springs. (*B*) Inspiratory airway pressure (Paw) equal to 26 cm H_2O. The distended distal airway has a high wall tension Tw. The liquid front has been pushed peripherally, but the saccules are still not inflated.

when the airway pressure has been increased to 26 cm H_2O. Scarpelli and his colleagues have shown in immature rabbit lungs that the opening pressure required to overcome the surface tension forces and push back the fluid front is approximately 25 cm H_2O (8, 15). The gas-containing proximal portion of the airway dilates as the pressure and volume increase. The volume of the airway and the wall tension increase markedly for the following reasons, all related to the immaturity of the system. As the airway dilates the radius increases, and this increases the wall tension. The immature airway wall is extremely compliant; the saccules surrounding the airway are collapsed and do not provide a counterbalancing force. At low lung volumes the radial tensions in the parenchyma are low, so that the stabilizing effect of mechanical interdependence is also low. Since there is no significant saccule air filling, the airway does not lengthen, which further increases the instability of the airway wall. Thus at this early stage of airway filling and recruitment, there is a risk of overdistending the airway or rupturing it (16). As the airway dilates and increases its radius, it also increases the radius of the air-liquid interface, thereby decreasing the surface tension forces. The liquid front then moves peripherally, first in the axial airways with their larger radii and later into the smaller lateral branches as their radii enlarge. As the saccules fill with air, the saccule pressure rises and eventually counterbalances the airway pressure. The airway volume, radius, and wall tension will then decrease, and the inflated immature lung develops airway stability. The airway structure will then resemble that shown in Figure 5.1 for the mature lung. Mead *et al.* (2) have suggested that if a high transpulmonary pressure is applied to the nonuniformly expanded lung of infants with severe surfactant deficiency, then hemorrhage may occur in the atelectatic regions by virtue of lung interdependent forces. If an immature acinus contains some expanded airways and saccules, then a very large expanding stress could be applied to neighboring collapsed distal airways and saccules during inspiration. This could occur repetitively with each inspiration if parts of an acinus were permitted to collapse during expiration.

The above considerations have dealt with a static system without regard for time. In reality immature infants are ventilated with controlled inspiratory times. The aeration of the small airway is less time dependent—that is, gas has to reach the distal airway, overcome resistive and surface tension forces, recruit and distend airways, and fill saccules, and all this in as short a time as 0.3 seconds at 50–80 times a minute (8).

The implication of this review of respiratory mechanics is that the small, highly compliant airways (bronchioles and transitional ducts) in a surfactant deficient and immature lung are the most likely areas of tissue damage and rupture during inflation.

Small Airway Perturbations and Barotrauma in the Immature Animal Lung

Investigations of the mechanisms of neonatal barotrauma in immature animals have been in agreement that increased surface tension in small airways and alveoli is the seminal predisposing factor. McAdams *et al.* (17) showed that preterm rhesus monkeys receiving positive pressure with either air or oxygen for a period as brief as 5 minutes developed epithelial necrosis or hyaline membranes in alveolar ducts and respiratory bronchioles. Diffuse atelectasis with alveolar duct distention was also a common finding. Schwieler and Robertson (18) in 1976 provided evidence that bronchiolar lesions that characterize the RDS lung may be triggered by abnormal expansion patterns in small surfactant deficient airways and saccules. They also demonstrated that ventilation in rabbits with liquid, a maneuver that lowers surface tension forces, caused far less bronchiolar epithelial necrosis than did gas ventilation. Nilsson *et al.* (19) ventilated surfactant deficient preterm rabbits for 10 minutes shortly after birth with a peak positive airway pressure of 25 cm H_2O at a frequency of 60 breaths per minute. One group of rabbits received surfactant via the trachea before institution of artificial ventilation, and the other group were controls without surfactant. They found bronchiolar epithelial lesions in 90% of the control fetuses, in contrast to only 36% of the surfactant treated animals. Their results indicate that surfactant lined small airways can sustain overventilation and a high intraluminal pressure without significant wall damage. It would appear that the airways walls were stabilized by the surfactant—that is, the intraluminal high airway pressure was counterbalanced by the equally high periairway saccule pressure, so that the bronchioles were not as overdistended or strained as they were in the surfactant deficient controls.

In another study on preterm rabbits, Nilsson et al. showed that treating rabbits with tracheal installation of surfactant was effective in reducing pneumothoraces and small airway lesions, even when given after an initial period of mechanical ventilation (20). Nilsson and his colleagues also demonstrated that preterm rabbits with surfactant deficiency could be treated at birth with artificial surfactant and then supported with high-frequency oscillatory ventilation at relatively low mean airway pressures of 6–8 cm H_2O. These animals showed essentially normal small airways at postmortem examination (21).

Ackerman et al. (22) studied the effects of various modes of mechanical ventilation on the incidence of PIE in preterm baboons. The animals, at birth, were randomly assigned to four groups: 1) intermittent positive pressure ventilation (IPPV) at rates of 30–60 per minute, an inspiratory time of 0.7 to 1.0 seconds with PEEP—these animals did not receive sighs; 2) high-frequency ventilation (HFV) at 10 Hz with one to 12 interposed mechanical sighs per minute; 3) HFV at 10 Hz with manual sighs at a rate of 30 breaths per minute for 5 minutes per hour; 4) HFV at 10 Hz with controlled sighs for 1 minute per hour. All the animals were ventilated for 24 hours or until death. The IPPV-PEEP treated animals that received no sighs did not have PIE and had slightly dilated small airways. The fourth group of animals, with the HFV with controlled sighs for only 1 minute each hour, also showed no PIE and slightly dilated airways. The baboons in group 2 with HFV with 1–12 interposed mechanical sighs per minute had striking distal dilated respiratory bronchioles and alveolar ducts, and all the animals had PIE (Figure 5.3). The PIE was usually contiguous with the respiratory bronchioles or alveolar ducts. In the third group of animals, which had HFV and manual sighs at a rate of 30 breaths per minute for 5 minutes per hour, PIE was found but was less prominent than in those infants that had been mechanically sighed. They, however, also had severe small airway dilatation. The most important deduction from this study on these surfactant deficient baboons is that lung rupture appears to take place in the wall of the small, compliant airways and not the saccules. The authors also concluded that animals that received the most aggressive intermittent sighs during HFV had the most severe dilatation of the small airways and PIE. These animals during ventilation probably had a low alveolar volume and atelectasis, so that the sigh pressures caused large increases in small airway wall tension (Fig. 5.2, B) with frequent rupture (Fig. 5.3).

These animal studies indicate that the small airways in the surfactant deficient lung are the most susceptible to pressure deformation. Also surfactant administration protects the small airway from barotrauma, perhaps by stabilizing the small airway wall by the mechanisms outlined in Figure 5.1.

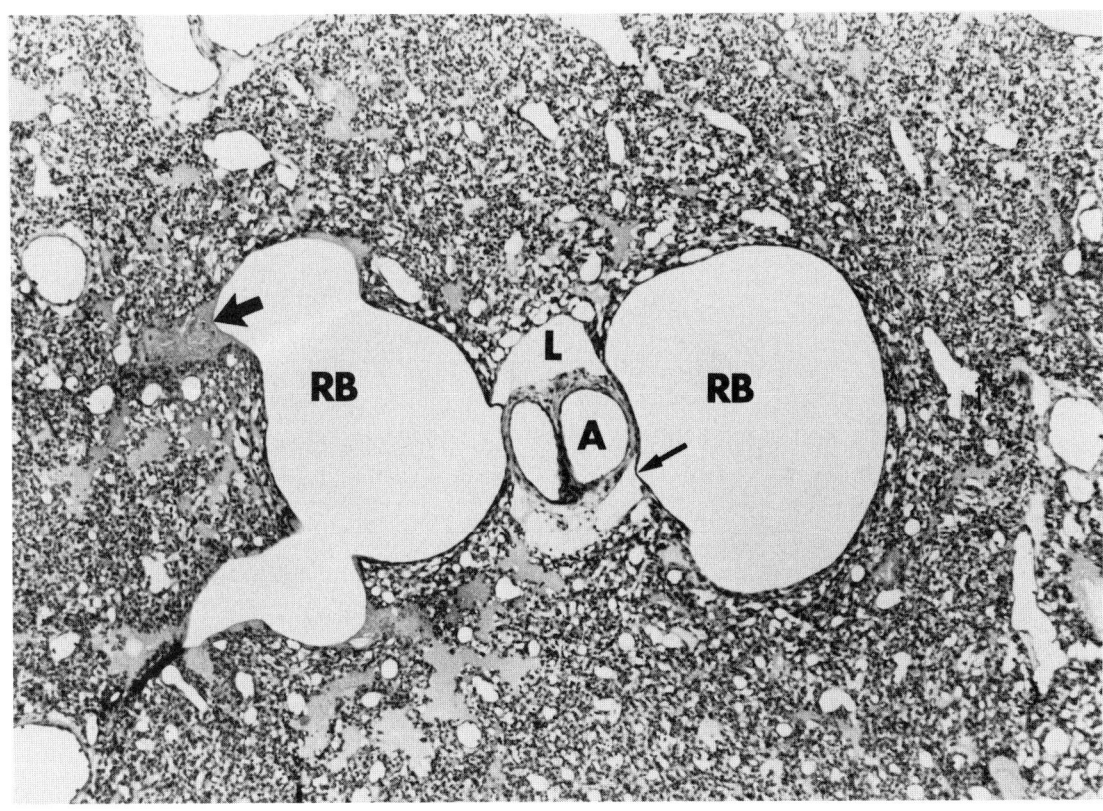

Figure 5.3. Marked dilatation of the respiratory bronchiole (RB) with early extension into an alveolar duct area. Striking atelectasis surrounds the dilated airways. There are hyaline membranes and/or pulmonary edema at both the alveolar duct and saccular levels (thick arrow). The tangentially cut pulmonary artery (A) is surrounded by dilated lymphatics (L). A very thin shelf of tissue separates the engorged lymphatics from the dilated bronchiole (thin arrow). Hematoxylin-eosin; ×37. (Reprinted, with permission, from Ackerman NB Jr, Coalson JJ, Kuehl TJ, et al.. Pulmonary interstitial emphysema in the premature baboon with hyaline membrane disease. This figure has been kindly furnished to us by Dr. Jacqueline J. Coalson. Crit Care Med 1984;12:512.)

The Response of the Alveolus or Saccule with Surfactant to Increased Distention

Preterm infants are more likely to develop diffuse PIE than are full-term infants (23, 24). Indeed full-term infants rarely develop diffuse PIE; their air leak is usually manifested as a pneumomediastinum, pneumothorax, or a large subpleural bleb. An isolated pneumothorax rarely leads to chronic functional changes and is easily treated by the pleural drainage of the gas, whereas diffuse PIE is often followed by chronic pulmonary insufficiency and is very difficult to treat. A general rule can be made that the easily expandable lung is more prone to develop a pneumothorax without diffuse PIE, and the surfactant deficient lung is more likely to develop diffuse PIE without a pneumothorax. This further implies that surfactant, and not gestational age or maturity of the animal, is the critical factor in determining which of the two types of air leak will result following barotrauma (23).

Surrounding the extra-alveolar vessels and airways is an interstitial space, the outer boundary of which is the fascial sheath that extends down from the trachea. Within this interstitial space are lymph vessels and loose connective tissue. The sheath extends farther distally along the vessels than it does along the airways (25). If the small airway ruptures distal to the termination of the fascial sheath, then air will dissect into the interstitium, creating PIE. This is contrasted with the surfactant-containing lung that is prone to develop a pneumomediastinum and pneumothorax without diffuse PIE. This contrast implies that in infants with surfactant the lung rupture is not in the small airways. The site of rupture in the respiratory tree appears to determine the direction of interstitial gas movement. Macklin and Macklin (26) have shown in various mature animal species that lung rupture takes place in overdistended alveoli. For an alveolus to rupture there must be a large pressure gradient across the alveolar wall. In the normal surfactant-containing lung, the pressure in each alveolus is equal, so that no matter how large the applied pressure, each alveolar pressure would counterbalance the pressure in the neighboring alveolus. However, there are sites in the lung parenchyma where alveolar walls do not abut alveolar structures. These nonalveolar structures are the pleura, airways, connective tissue septa, and extra-alveolar arteries and veins.

With positive pressure lung inflation the perivascular (27–29) and peribronchial interstitial space pressures (30–33) become more negative relative to those of the lung interstitium or pleural pressure. This is a result of the pull applied on the perivascular and peribronchial sheath by the expanding alveolar walls. Mead *et al.* (2) have shown that a pressure gradient develops across this sheath during inflation as the sheath fails to follow the expansion of the surrounding parenchyma. Figure 5.4 is a schematic of the forces influencing the pressures in the peribronchial and perivascular spaces. The outward acting airway pressure (P_{aw}) is counterbalanced by the alveolar pressure (P_{alv}). As the alveoli expand with inflation, a stress (Fo) is generated in their walls which pulls on the peribronchial and perivascular sheaths. This generates an airway wall tension (Tw), causing the airway to recoil inward, which results in a negative peribronchial pressure. With a large inflation, if an alveolar wall is anchored against a connective tissue septum, or the sheath surrounding a vessel or airway, then the tissue stresses are favorable to rupture the wall of the alveolus. If the stress generated in that alveolar wall exceeds the opposing force in the sheath or septum by some critical limit, the wall will rupture and air will track into its interstitial space. Caldwell *et al.* (34) have shown that if the chest wall is bound, a maneuver that prevents overdistention of the alveoli, then even high transpulmonary pressures will not cause alveolar rupture. With rupture of alveoli the gas moves preferentially into the lower pressure perivascular or peribronchial spaces and back toward the hilum to form a perihilar bleb or a pneumomediastinum. The trapped gas in the perihilar areas may also rupture to form a pneumothorax. Gas can also move peripherally from the site of the rupture in connective tissue septa and cause subpleural blebs. Occasionally these blebs can rupture to form a pneumothorax (24).

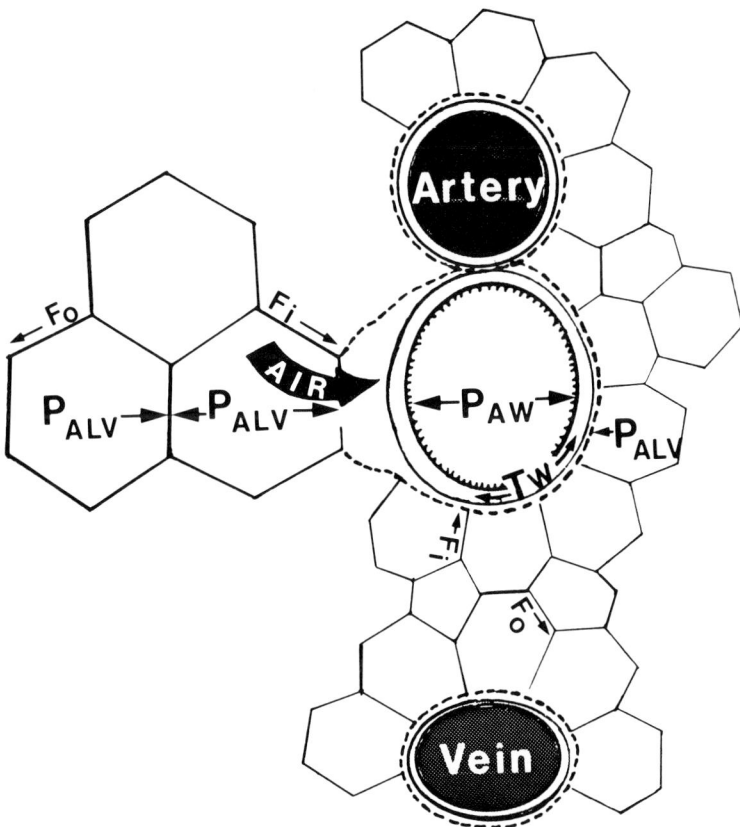

Figure 5.4. Artery, vein, and small airway transversing lung parenchyma. The connective tissue sheath surrounds the airway (dotted line), and it sends a separate sheath over the artery. The vein has its separate sheath. Airway pressure (P_{AW}) equals alveolar pressure (P_{ALV}). Normal alveoli are shown on the right, upper, and lower sides of the schematic. On the left side are overdistended alveoli. The elastic limit of the base of one of the distended alveoli that is attached to the periairway sheath has been exceeded and has ruptured. Gas is shown escaping into the periairway interstitial space.

The conclusion from these observations is that if the alveoli are overdistended and then rupture, the gas is routed generally through tissue planes—that is, in the perivascular or periairway spaces to the hilum—with formation of a pneumomediastinum or pneumothorax. On the other hand, if the small airways are ruptured in surfactant deficient animals, then the gas in the interstitium is trapped, and diffuse PIE occurs. Of course overdistended alveoli in surfactant deficient subjects can also rupture and cause a pneumothorax.

Effects of Pressure Mediated Trauma on Large Airways

The effects of pressure mediated trauma on large airways have become more evident as duration of mechanical ventilation of very small preterm infants has increased. Immature airways have the unique property of being more distensible than mature airways, and the smaller the airway at any level of maturity, the greater the distensibility (10, 11, 35).

Bhutani *et al.* (10) used an *in vitro* animal model and demonstrated a fivefold decrease in specific compliance of the trachea between the 21 day fetal and the adult rabbit. Most of this decline occurred during the fetal period. Following birth at 31 days of gestation, the tracheal compliance continued to decrease at a slower rate until adulthood. Considering that the saccules of immature infants with surfactant deficiency are very stiff and that the airway is very compliant, then the high transmural pressures used during mechanical ventilation can result in substantial increases in anatomic dead space and airway damage.

In another report the same authors investigated the effect of 60 minutes of IPPV or CPAP on compliance, distensibility, and resting volume of excised rabbit tracheas in fetal (21–27 days), term, and adult rabbits (36). They show that the more immature tracheas responded to IPPV and CPAP with a marked decrease in both specific compliance and distensibility (Fig. 5.5). In contrast the resting tracheal volumes were greater in these immature tracheas following mechanical ventilation. The magnitude of these changes from mechanical ventilation decreased as gestation increased, and the changes were not significant in the adult rabbit.

Anatomic maturation of the trachea and large airways is associated with increasing amounts of smooth muscle, collagen, elastin, and cartilage. This anatomic maturation gives structural support to the wall and prevents pressure deformations in the mature upper airway with IPPV (37). The ability of the trachea to withstand the stress and strain of IPPV is therefore less in the immature animal and improves with advancing maturity.

Coburn and Palombini (38) have demonstrated in adult dogs, and Koslo *et al.* (39) in newborn mature lambs, that the greater the tension of the trachealis muscle, the less the tracheal volume will increase for any given pressure increase. This finding has important implications for immature infants on high-pressure IPPV. *In vivo* tracheal smooth muscle tone in the human preterm is yet to be assessed. However, an increase in the tracheal smooth muscle tone would provide a protective mechanism against pressure induced deformation by decreasing the magnitude of the volume change during the respiratory cycle (39).

Bhutani *et al.* (40) have shown that very small preterm infants that have received prolonged mechanical ventilation have significant tracheomegaly when measured 7 days after extubation in comparison with nonventilated controls. This dimensional deformation is thought to be a result of barotrauma on the highly compliant airways of these immature infants. The long-term effects of this deformation remain to be evaluated. Sotomayor *et al.* (41) demonstrated tracheobronchomalacia in five preterm infants who had BPD and had been treated with prolonged mechanical ventilation. These infants demonstrated narrowing of the central airways by as much as 75% or more during expiration. Stocks *et al.* (42) observed an increased airway resistance in preterm infants 4–10 months following mechanical ventilation for RDS. They attributed this increased resistance to retardation of airway growth secondary to damage to the airway walls by mechanical ventilation. The precise pathogenesis and

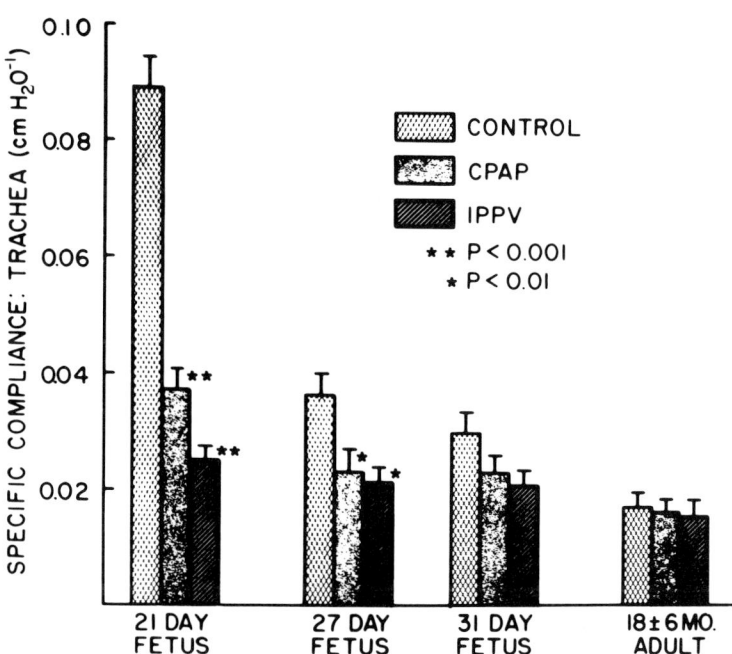

Figure 5.5. Alterations in specific tracheal compliance following mechanical respiratory assistance with IPPV or CPAP. The specific compliance significantly decreased in the immature fetus following IPPV and CPAP. (Reprinted with permission from Bhutani VK, Rubenstein D, Shaffer TH. Pressure-induced deformation in immature airways. Pediatr Res 1981;15:829.)

clinical importance of these large airway functional and structural changes in preterm infants remain to be defined. Nevertheless pressure induced trauma appears to be an important predisposing factor.

Animal Models of Barotrauma and BPD

The incidence of chronic lung disease or BPD is highly correlated with prematurity, surfactant deficiency, prolonged and high-concentration of inspired oxygen, positive pressure ventilation, and diffuse PIE. Any animal model attempting to isolate barotrauma as an etiologic factor in BPD would be required to control these variables. Theoretically this would be possible with extracorporeal membrane oxygenation (ECMO)—that is, with an immature surfactant deficient animal on ECMO, acute airway trauma or diffuse PIE could be produced by high ventilator pressures and volumes. Following this the animal lungs would be ventilated with room air and at low pressures until the lungs healed. This would remove the toxic influence of hyperoxia as the lung heals from barotrauma, and thus establish the relationship of barotrauma to BPD.

The baboon model of BPD as outlined in reports by Escobedo *et al.* (43) and Coalson *et al.* (44) could be utilized in conjunction with ECMO. Their important model of BPD was not able to distinguish the separate influences of oxygen toxicity and barotrauma on the development of BPD for the reasons noted above. Vidyasagar *et al.* (45) have also used this baboon model in the treatment of RDS with exogenous surfactant.

Modes and Patterns of Ventilation Associated with Acute and Chronic Damage to the Human Neonatal Lung

Gruenwald demonstrated at postmortem examination on lungs inflated with air that the small airways of infants with RDS were dilated while the saccules were collapsed (46, 47). He further showed that the expansion of these atelectatic surfactant deficient lungs could easily be achieved with fluid inflation, indicating that increased surface tension forces were the cause of the atelectasis and dilated small airways (48). Taghizadeh and Reynolds also found that the terminal airways in air inflated fixed lungs of infants dying with RDS in the first 5 days of life appeared markedly dilated (49). They concluded that these airways were particularly susceptible to distortion and mechanical damage. From the theoretical analysis, animal investigations, and clinical experience, there is general agreement that the small airway is the site of damage in the surfactant deficient lung. Although lung rupture and PIE are the most obvious clinical findings of barotrauma, it is also clear from animal studies (19) and human material that the small airway can be extensively damaged without an actual rupture of the airway wall. The theoretical analysis above also implies that positive airway pressure mechanical ventilation is not the only means of damaging the small airway walls. If the infant with severe surfactant deficiency (RDS) is capable of generating a large transpulmonary pressure, then the susceptible and unstable small airway walls may be damaged by spontaneous breathing.

Campbell was one of the earliest authors to recognize the increased frequency of PIE in infants with RDS (50). Later investigators demonstrated that PIE was usually associated with prematurity and positive pressure ventilation (23, 24). Also they found that diffuse PIE could occur without a pneumomediastinum or pneumothorax and that the mortality rate with bilateral PIE was very high. The use of the nonspecific term "air leak" for any and all types of lung rupture has made interpretation of the literature difficult. The type of air leak is important since the mortality from a pneumothorax is minimal, whereas that from diffuse PIE is greater than 50% (51, 52). It is generally accepted that PIE and pneumothorax in the preterm infant bear a direct relationship to mechanical ventilation, and furthermore that the method of ventilation is important (53, 54).

Mechanical Ventilatory Techniques and Acute Lung Damage

Reynolds and his coworkers recognized in the early 1970s that mechanical ventilation was associated with acute and chronic lung damage (55). In a series of investigations on various methods of ventilation, they were able to decrease significantly pulmonary barotrauma and its sequelae (55–58). A central problem in mechanically ventilating surfactant deficient infants is the difficulty in achieving good oxygenation without resorting to high ventilator pressures, with their deleterious effects.

PEEP was introduced as a method to improve oxygenation, without elevating peak ventilatory pressures (58, 59). The introduction of CPAP as a mode of neonatal assisted ventilation was potentially a simple and convenient method to eliminate the high ventilator pressures and simultaneously achieve good oxygenation in a safe way (60).

CPAP and PEEP

Our theoretical analysis (Figs. 5.1 and 5.2) implies that all the distal lung units either have surfactant or are surfactant deficient; however, it is evident from bedside observation that RDS can be mild, moderate, or severe, indicating that there are degrees of surfactant deficiency. This nonuniformity of surfactant deficiency has important implications in the cause and prevention of barotrauma. It indicates that there are areas of lung that are normally inflated at all times, others that are atelectatic and surfactant deficient, and others that have a very low volume or are atelectatic but will open and expand relatively easily. Time constants will be unequal across the lung—that is, the atelectatic areas will have short time constants, and the inflated areas will have longer constants.

CPAP is thought to recruit surfactant-containing atelectatic or undervolumed saccules, thereby increasing the lung volume and optimizing oxygenation. An excess of CPAP may also overdistend the normal saccules and decrease compliance, eventually causing lung rupture (61). CPAP is very effective in elevating the PaO_2 (60). An optimum or best CPAP can be found by measuring the esophageal pressure while progressively elevating the CPAP (62–64). There is a sudden increase in the transpulmonary transmission of airway pressure when the optimum CPAP is reached. This optimum pressure appears to be the critical opening pressure of saccules that are atelectatic or undervolumed. At this best CPAP, compliance would be optimized, and further increases of CPAP, would cause overdistention of normal saccules and a decrease in their compliance (61). CPAP at modest levels would not be expected to cause diffuse PIE, but overdistention and pneumothoraces can occur (60, 65).

Intermittent positive pressure ventilation with PEEP achieves the same goal as CPAP—that is, recruitment and increased volume of undervolumed saccules. However, if high peak-inspiratory pressures (PIPs) are used with the PEEP, then there is a risk of overdistending the normal and undervolumed surfactant-containing saccules as well as damaging the small surfactant deficient airways (54). If the applied PEEP is able to keep the airways and saccules patent throughout the respiratory cycles, it will stabilize the small airway walls. Nonuniformity of surfactant-containing saccules explains how diffuse PIE, pneumothorax, pneumomediastinum, and subpleural blebs may all be found in the same lung.

Mean Airway Pressure

The concept of mean airway pressure has been especially useful in understanding the effects of ventilator settings on oxygenation (58, 66, 67). Mean airway pressure is closely related to oxygenation, but there is little available evidence to indicate its usefulness in preventing damage. Herman and Reynolds (58) were able to decrease the peak ventilatory pressures and FiO_2 by increasing the mean airway pressure. They elevated the mean airway pressure by applying PEEP and using a square wave pressure waveform with a high inspiratory to expiratory time ratio (I:E). They also used slow frequencies of 30 cycles per minute. This method of ventilation resulted in a marked decrease in BPD. However, it is difficult to know which of the ventilator changes decreased the long-term damage to the lung.

One can speculate that the collapsed and undervolumed saccules can be recruited by the long inspiration, and the ventilation of areas with varying time constants would be improved. PEEP, by preventing alveolar and airway collapse during expiration (68), would stabilize the small airway walls. However, if the small airways collapsed during expiration, and if the applied pressure was too low to reopen the saccules, then the rapid opening of the airways with the square wave pressure waveform could damage the airway wall. In addition if some airways in an acinus opened and others did not, then lung interdependence forces could cause injury to the walls of the collapsed airways. Taghizadeh and Reynolds have found in some infants that died with RDS, that airway pressures of as much as 60 cm H_2O were required to open some atelectatic areas (49).

Ratner *et al.* (69) modified the ventilatory management instituted by Herman and Reynolds (58) by decreasing the peak inspiratory pressure 30% while maintaining the mean airway pressure constant. This was achieved in 10 infants by increasing the ventilatory frequency from a baseline of 30 breaths per minute to 47. This maneuver maintained the oxygenation, because the mean airway pressure remained constant. It also decreased the PIP and therefore should be less damaging to the small airways.

Ventilatory Rates, Pressure Waveforms, and Tidal Volumes

The slow ventilator rates (<30 breaths per minute) during neonatal ventilation were chosen both for the purpose of decreasing peak pressures and thereby barotrauma and for better oxygenation at a lower pressure (58). In recent years there has been a movement toward faster respiratory frequencies. Boros and Campbell have given convincing evidence that the improvement in oxygenation associated with fast or slow patterns of ventilation was often secondary to changes in the mean airway pressure (67). The changes in mean airway pressure were often produced by changes inadvertently generated by the respirator as the rates increased or decreased. More recently Boros *et al.* tested various infant ventilators and showed that the shape of the pressure waveform and tidal volumes varied with increasing ventilator rates (70). Compliances, lung volumes, tidal volumes, and pressure waveforms are important considerations when assessing any ventilatory strategy to prevent barotrauma, but rarely, if ever, have they been measured in clinical trials.

Ciszek *et al.* (71) demonstrated how the pressure waveform is modified by changing the PEEP and the duration of the positive pressure while maintaining constant the mean airway pressure, peak inspiratory pressure, and the flow rate. Their study also indicated the importance of measuring tidal volume and functional residual capacity (FRC) when assessing ventilator changes. Three of the nine infants they studied became apneic secondary to overdistention of alveoli as the PEEP was decreased and the duration of positive pressure was prolonged while maintaining a constant mean airway pressure. Manginello et al. (72) evaluated infants with RDS, comparing pressure limited ventilation with ventilation regulated by volume in which there was no pressure limit. The rapid rise of the pressure waveform generated by the volume cycled ventilator appeared to be too short to recruit and expand the saccules. Because the prescribed volume was delivered to the lungs, it is clearly possible that significant airway damage was sustained by the infants treated with the volume ventilators.

Bland et al. (73) treated 24 preterm infants with fast ventilator rates of 60–110 per minute, short inspiratory times, and low PIPs and achieved good survival rates and a low incidence of barotrauma and chronic lung disease comparable to achievements in infants treated with slower frequencies. Various ventilators were used during the course of the study, which may have increased the mean airway pressure to levels comparable to those obtained with slower modes of ventilator management (70). In addition the FRC may have been increased by inadvertent PEEP (74–77). However, as discussed by the authors, barotrauma to the small airways may have been minimized by the low tidal volume and low pressures. Those terminal units that had surfactant could be easily opened or expanded by the low applied pressure while the low surfactant airways and units would not open and therefore would not be traumatized.

Heicher et al. (78) carried out a prospective clinical comparison of two methods of mechanical ventilation in 102 neonates with a predominant diagnosis of RDS. In one group slow ventilator rates of 20–40 breaths per minute with a 1 second inspiratory time were used, and in the other group the rate was 60 breaths per minute with a 0.5 second inspiratory time. The main conclusion from the study was a significant decrease in the incidence of pneumothoraces from 35% in the slow rate group to 14% in the fast rate group of infants. The incidences of the types of air leaks in each group were not specifically noted. Chronic lung disease and death occurred in 16.6% of each group. The time on ventilator therapy was also not different in the two groups. The increased incidence of pneumothoraces in the slow rate group suggests that the alveoli were overdistended with the prolonged inspiratory times.

Spahr et al. (79) randomly assigned 69 neonates with RDS on ventilatory therapy to an I:E ratio of either 1:2 or 2:1. Their method of ventilator management generated a square wave similar to that of Reynolds (68). The I:E ratios and the flow rates remained constant throughout the course of mechanical ventilation. The respiratory rates were slow at 20–40 breaths per minute. There were no differences in the mortality, morbidity, or incidence of barotrauma between the two methods of ventilation.

Muscle Relaxants and Mechanical Ventilation

Stark et al. (80) evaluated the effects of muscle paralysis on gas exchange and the incidence of pneumothorax in 35 severely ill infants on mechanical ventilation. One of their concerns was that infants "fighting the ventilator" could superimpose spontaneous respiratory efforts on ventilator inspiratory pressures and thereby generate a transpulmonary pressure large enough to cause lung rupture. They showed that peak transpulmonary pressure was lower after paralysis, and their incidence of pneumothoraces was only 8%. Forty-four percent of their patients improved their oxygenation following the paralysis despite the decreased peak pressure. These results encouraged Pollitzer et al. (81) to study randomly 50 infants with RDS, with one group receiving muscle relaxants during mechanical ventilation and the other no relaxation. The purpose of the study was to see if elimination of spontaneous breathing during mechanical ventilation would decrease the prevalence of barotrauma. Their study showed no reduction in the incidence of pneumothoraces or PIE but did show a significant reduction in the length of time the infants were dependent on added oxygen. They attributed this reduction in oxygen requirement to a decrease in the peak transpulmonary pressure, which resulted in less barotrauma to the terminal airways.

Greenough et al. (82) further studied the patterns of spontaneous respiration of infants on slow mechanical ventilation. Either the infants were totally apneic, or ventilator inflation stimulated one of four distinct respiratory patterns: synchronous breathing, Hering-Breuer reflex, augmented inspiration, or active expiration against ventilator inflation. They consistently observed active expiration against inflation before the development of a pneumothorax. This finding is in contrast to the hypothesis of augmented respiration noted by Stark et al. (80) and Pollitzer et al. (81). Greenough et al. (83) reasoned that by identifying infants on mechanical ventilation with the specific pattern of active expiration against ventilator inflation and then eliminating this pattern with muscle paralysis, a reduction in the incidence of pneumothorax should be achieved. In a randomized study they found 100% incidence of pneumothorax in those infants with the risk pattern who were not paralyzed and only 8% incidence of pneumothorax in those infants who were paralyzed. The study of Stark et al. (80) did show a decrease in the incidence of pneumothoraces with muscle relaxation. In contrast the controlled study of Pollitzer et al. (81) did not demonstrate a decreased incidence of pneumothoraces. The interesting findings of Greenough et al. (83) should be confirmed on a larger number of infants.

There are still many unanswered questions about the optimal method of conventional mechanical ventilation of infants with surfactant deficient lungs. More pulmonary function tests during mechanical ventilation are required, especially measurements of the FRC, tidal volume, and inadvertent PEEP. Rhodes et al. (84) treated all 230 infants with respiratory failure admitted to their nursery over a 2 year period. Ventilator methods were in general similar to those of Herman and Reynolds (58) in that they used long inspiratory times and slow ventilator rates. Their incidence of pneumothorax was 10%, PIE in infants without a pneumothorax was 2%, and BPD was 3.6%. Rhodes et al. (84) achieved very low mean airway and peak-inspiratory pressures by accepting a lower arterial oxygen tension down to 36 mmHg and a pH of 7.21. The carbon dioxide tension was allowed to rise until the pH fell to 7.21. This provocative uncontrolled study indicates that barotrauma of all types can be reduced to very low levels if the lung is slowly ventilated with a long inspiration and no attempt is made to open surfactant deficient airways and saccules.

Surfactant Therapy and Prevention of Barotrauma

It is the absence of surfactant in the small airways and saccules that so markedly enhances the predisposition of the immature lung to barotrauma during conventional ventilation. The availability of exogenous surfactant offers the exciting prospect of simplifying ventilator therapy and decreasing barotrauma, especially diffuse PIE.

Fujiwara et al. in 1980 reported improved gas exchange, decreased oxygen requirements, and decreased peak ventilator pressures in 10 infants with RDS given surfactant endotracheally (85). These infants were studied within 20 hours of birth, and all had severe RDS prior to treatment. None of the infants developed a pneumothorax. A recent randomized prospective clinical study by Hallman et al. (86), using exogenous human surfactant in the treatment of severe RDS, confirmed and extended the findings of Fujiwara et al. (85). Infants were less than 10 hours of age with birth weights less than 1500 g. Infants given surfactant required less oxygen during the first week and had lower mean airway pressures during the first 48 hours. Death or the occurrence of BPD, pneumothorax, and PIE were significantly less in the infants given surfactant. Significant decreases in the mean airway pressure were seen within 1 hour of the surfactant administration. Enhorning et al. (87) gave exogenous surfactant endotracheally to preterm infants of less than 30 weeks' gestation prior to the first breath, with the purpose of preventing the development of RDS. This randomized trial resulted in improved gas exchange during the first 72 hours of life, as well as decreased ventilator pressures and rates. There was a significant decrease in the PIE in the surfactant treated infants but not in the incidence of pneumothorax. There was no difference in the incidence of chronic lung disease. Kwong et al., in a similarly designed study, gave exogenous surfactant to preterm infants prior to the first breath (88). Their results were similar to those of Enhorning et al. (87).

Merritt et al., in a randomized, controlled trial, treated preterm infants at birth with exogenous human surfactant (89). This study differs from that of Enhorning et al. (87) because only infants at very high risk for developing RDS were treated. All had amniotic fluid samples or pharyngeal or tracheal aspirates that revealed an immature phospholipid profile. The control infants also had an immature phospholipid profile but received no surfactant. The surfactant treated group had significantly fewer deaths, fewer cases of BPD, and fewer cases of PIE and pneumothorax.

Exogenous surfactant administration to preterm infants with RDS is a potent means of decreasing mortality and diffuse PIE. However, following exogenous surfactant administration to preterm infants with severe RDS, a rational approach to conventional mechanical ventilation is still required. A patchy distribution of the administered surfactant in the presence of high ventilator settings could lead to small airway damage, as shown in Figure 5.2, or to alveolar overdistention, as shown in Figure 5.4. In addition if some alveolar ducts in an acinus received surfactant and others did not, then large interdependent forces could be applied to the surfactant deficient airways.

High-Frequency Ventilation and the Treatment and Prevention of Barotrauma

This subject is treated in detail in Chapter 21, by Boynton and Frantz. High-frequency ventilation has a unique potential for the prevention of barotrauma. It has also been useful in the treatment of diffuse PIE (90–92), with resolution of the PIE in more than 50% of the infants. It eliminates the large oscillating distending pressures and volumes associated with conventional ventilation that appear to be so damaging to small airway walls. With high-frequency ventilation it is necessary to maintain a constant end-expiratory alveolar volume using PEEP.

Chronic Lung Disease and Barotrauma

The acute harmful effects of PIE with its high mortality rate and subacute effects which require prolongation of assisted ventilation and increased FiO_2 needs are self-evident. There are also obvious chronic sequelae of diffuse PIE. However, the relationship of airway trauma and diffuse PIE to BPD is not well defined. The separation of the influences of hyperoxia from barotrauma in the pathogenesis of BPD is not fully resolved. As discussed above the use of the immature baboon model and ECMO could resolve the problem. Chronic lung disease has been shown to develop in preterm and full-term infants who are not on mechanical ventilators but require prolonged high concentrations of inspired oxygen (93). More subtle airway changes have also been reported following oxygen therapy for RDS in preterm infants who did not receive mechanical ventilation (94). The chronic vascular and pulmonary parenchymal lesions secondary to long-term hyperoxia breathing in mature animals are well known (95, 96). However, these studies do not define the separate influences of diffuse PIE and hyperoxia on the development of BPD in the immature animal. Diffuse PIE appears to be the ultimate barotraumatic challenge to the immature lung. However, as outlined above in our theoretical analysis and animal studies, the repetitive overdistention of the small, immature airway walls with or without rupture may also be chronically damaging. The long-term pulmonary follow-up of infants treated with mechanical ventilation at birth is detailed in Chapters 15 by Tepper and 25 by Heldt.

Stocker and Madewell (97) and others (98) have shown that PIE can persist and cause a chronic lung disease. This condition was termed persistent interstitial pulmonary emphysema (PIPE). Some infants develop a localized form of PIPE with cysts measuring up to 3.0 cm in diameter. There is a more diffuse form of PIPE in which the cysts are predominantly small (<0.3 cm) and can be seen in all the lobes of the lung. This latter form is difficult to differentiate from BPD. Brewer *et al.* (98) suggested that the air or gas in the interstitium may provoke a tissue reaction, causing the gas pockets to be walled off and persist chronically (99). These cystic lesions usually resolve spontaneously over a period of months without treatment. If the lesions are isolated to one lobe and there is respiratory distress and tension occurs with a mediastinal shift, then a lobectomy can be therapeutic.

References

1. Macklem PT, Proctor DF, Hogg JC. The stability of peripheral airways. Respir Physiol 1970;8:191–302.
2. Mead J, Takishima T, Leith D. Stress distribution in lungs: a model of pulmonary elasticity. J Appl Physiol 1970;28:596–608.
3. Greaves IA, Hildebrand TJ, Hoppin FG. Micromechanics of the lung. In: Fishman AP, ed. Handbook of physiology, section 3. The respiratory system, vol. 3. Mechanics of breathing, part 1. Baltimore, Md: American Physiological Society, The Williams & Wilkins Co. 1986, p 217.
4. Sylvester JT, Menkes HA, Stitik F. Lung vol-

ume and interdependence in the pig. J Appl Physiol 1975;38:395–401.
5. Mead J. Mechanical properties of lungs. Physiol Rev 1971;41:281–330.
6. Macklem PT. Airway obstruction and collateral ventilation. Physiol Rev 1971;51:368–436.
7. Scarpelli EM, Humar A, Doyle C, Clutario BC. Functional anatomy and volume-pressure characteristics of immature lungs. Respir Physiol 1981;45:25–41.
8. Kumar A, Clutario BC, Doyle C, Scarpelli EM. Time-dependency and static mechanics of immature airways and saccules. Respir Physiol 1983;51:195–207.
9. Pattle RE. Properties, function, and origin of the alveolar lining layer. Proc Roy Soc Lond 1958;148:217–240.
10. Bhutani VK, Rubenstein SD, Shaffer TH. Pressure-volume relationships of tracheae in fetal, newborn and adult rabbits. Respir Physiol 1981;43:221–231.
11. Martin HB, Proctor DF. Pressure-volume measurements on dog bronchi. J Appl Physiol 1958;13:337–343.
12. Hoppin FG Jr., Hughes JMB, Mead J. Axial forces in the bronchial tree. J Appl Physiol: Respirat Environ Exercise Physiol 1977;42:773–781.
13. Menkes H, Gardiner A, Gamsu G, Lempert J, Macklem PT. Influence of surface forces on collateral ventilation. J Appl Physiol 1971;31:544–549.
14. Menkes HA, Macklem PT. Collateral flow. In: Fishman AP, ed. Handbook of physiology. Section 3. The respiratory system, vol. 3. Mechanics of breathing, part 1. Baltimore, Md: American Physiological Society, The Williams & Wilkins Co. 1986, p 337.
15. Scarpelli EM, Mautone AJ. The surfactant system and pulmonary mechanics. In: Robertson B, Van Golde LMB, Batenburg JJ, eds. Pulmonary surfactant. Amsterdam: Elsevier Science Publishers, 1984.
16. Robertson B. Surface forces in respiratory bronchioles during a first breath-model experiment and some theoretical considerations. Scand J Respir Dis 1976;57:160–162.
17. McAdams AJ, Coen R, Kleinman LL, Tsang R, Sutherland J. The experimental production of hyaline membranes in premature rhesus monkeys. Am J Pathol 1973;70:277–290.
18. Schwieler G, Robertson B. Liquid ventilation in immature newborn rabbits. Biol Neonate 1976;29:343–353.
19. Nilsson R, Grossman G, Robertson B. Pathogenesis of neonatal lung lesions induced by artificial ventilation: evidence against the role of barotrauma. Respiration 1980;4:218–225.
20. Nilsson R, Grossman G, Berggren P, Robertson B. Surfactant treatment in experimental hyaline membrane disease. Eur J Respir Dis 1981;62:441–449.
21. Nilsson R, Berggren P, Curstedt T, Grossman G, Renheim G, Robertson B. Surfactant treatment and ventilation by high frequency oscillation in premature newborn rabbits: effect on survival, lung aeration, and bronchiolar epithelial lesions. Pediatr Res 1985;19:143–147.
22. Ackerman NB Jr., Coalson JJ, Kuehl TJ, et al. Pulmonary interstitial emphysema in the premature baboon with hyaline membrane disease. Crit Care Med 1984;12:512–516.
23. Thibeault DW, Lachman RS, Laul VR, Kwong MS. Pulmonary interstitial emphysema, pneumomediastinum and pneumothorax. Occurrence in the newborn infant. Am J Dis Child 1973;126:611–614.
24. Plenat F, Vert P, Didier F, Andre M. Pulmonary interstitial emphysema. Clin Perinatol 1978;5:351–375.
25. Hayek H Von. The human lung. New York: Hafner, 1960.
26. Macklin MT, Macklin CC. Malignant interstitial emphysema of the lungs and mediastinum as an important occult complication in many respiratory diseases and other conditions: an interpretation of the clinical literature in the light of laboratory experiment. Medicine 1944;23:281–352.
27. Smith JC, Mitzner W. Analysis of pulmonary vascular interdependence in excised dog lobes. J Appl Physiol: Respirat Environ Exercise Physiol 1980;48:450–467.
28. Lai-Fook SJ. A continuum mechanics analysis of pulmonary vascular interdependence in isolated dog lobes. J Appl Physiol: Respirat Environ Exercise Physiol. 1979;46:419–429.
29. Permutt S. Mechanical influences on water

accumulation in the lungs in pulmonary edema. In: Fishman AP, Renkin EM, eds. Pulmonary edema. Bethesda, Md: American Physiological Society, 1979.
30. Inoue H, Inoue C, Hildebrandt J. Vascular and airway pressures, and interstitial edema, affect peribronchial fluid pressure. J Appl Physiol: Respirat Environ Exercise Physiol 1980;48:177–185.
31. Sasaki H, Hoppin FG Jr, Takishma T. Peribronchial pressure in excised dog lungs. J Appl Physiol: Respirat Environ Exercise Physiol 1978;45:858–869.
32. Nakamura M, Luchtel DL, Ikeda Y, et al. Surrounding structures affect pressure-diameter behavior of excised dog bronchi. J Appl Physiol: Respirat Environ Exercise Physiol 1984;57:1632–1639.
33. Lai-Fook SJ, Kallok MJ. Bronchial-arterial interdependence in isolated dog lung. J Appl Physiol: Respirat Environ Exercise Physiol 1982;52:1000–1007.
34. Caldwell EJ, Powell RD, Mullooly JP. Interstitial emphysema: a study of physiologic factors involved in experimental induction of the lesion. Am Rev Respir Dis 1970;102:516–525.
35. Burnard ED, Graftan-Smith P, Picton-Warlow CG, Grauaug A. Pulmonary insufficiency in prematurity. Aust Paediatr J 1965;1:12–38.
36. Bhutani VK, Rubenstein SD, Shaffer TH. Pressure-induced deformation in immature airways. Pediatr Res 1981;15:829–832.
37. Bhutani VK, Shaffer TH. Time-dependent tracheal deformation in fetal, neonatal, and adult rabbits. Pediatr Res 1982;16:830–833.
38. Coburn RF, Palombini B. Time-dependent pressure-volume relationships of the in vivo canine trachea. Respir Physiol 1972;16:282–289.
39. Koslo RJ, Bhutani VK, Shaffer TM. The role of tracheal smooth muscle contraction on neonatal tracheal mechanics. Pediatr Res 1986;20:1216–1220.
40. Bhutani VK, Ritchie WG, Shaffer TH. Acquired tracheomegaly in very preterm neonates. Am J Dis Child 1986;140:449–452.
41. Sotomayor JL, Godinez RI, Borden S, Wilmott RW. Large-airway collapse due to acquired tracheobronchomalacia in infancy. Am J Dis Child 1986;140:367–371.
42. Stocks J, Godfrey S, Reynolds EOR. Airway resistance in infants after various treatments for hyaline membrane disease: special emphasis on prolonged high levels of inspired oxygen. Pediatrics 1978;61:178–183.
43. Escobedo MB, Hillard JL, Smith F, et al. A baboon model of bronchopulmonary dysplasia. I. Clinical features. Exp Mol Pathol 1982;37:323–334.
44. Coalson JJ, Kuehl TJ, Excobedo MS, et al. A baboon model of bronchopulmonary dysplasia. II. Pathologic features. Exp Mol Pathol 1982;37:335–350.
45. Vidyasagar D, Maeta H, Raju TNK, et al. Bovine surfactant (Surfactant TA) therapy in immature baboons with hyaline membrane disease. Pediatrics 1985;75:1132–1142.
46. Gruenwald P. Normal and abnormal expansion of the lungs of newborn infants obtained at autopsy. III. The pattern of aeration as affected by gestational and postnatal age. Anat Rec 1963;146:337–351.
47. Gruenwald P. Normal and abnormal expansion of the lungs of newborn infants obtained at autopsy. II. Opening pressure, maximal volume and stability of expansion. Lab Invest 1963;12:563–576.
48. Gruenwald P. Normal and abnormal expansion of the lungs of newborn infants obtained at autopsy. I. Expansion of the lungs by liquid media. Anat Rec 1961;139:471–479.
49. Taghizadeh A, Reynolds EOR. Pathogenesis of bronchopulmonary dysplasia following hyaline membrane disease. Am J Pathol 1976;82:241–246.
50. Campbell RE. Intrapulmonary interstitial emphysema. A complication of hyaline membrane disease. AJR 1970;110:449–456.
51. Yu VYK, Wong PY, Bajuk B, Szymonowicz. Pulmonary air leak in extremely low birthweight infants. Arch Dis Child 1986;61:239–241.
52. Hart SM, McNair M, Gamsu HR, Price JF. Pulmonary interstitial emphysema in very low birthweight infants. Arch Dis Child 1983;58:612–615.
53. Greenough A, Dixon AK, Roberton NRC. Pul-

monary interstitial emphysema. Arch Dis Child 1984;59:1046–1051.
54. Berg TJ, Pagtakhan RD, Reed MH, Langston C, Chernick N. Bronchopulmonary dysplasia and lung rupture in hyaline membrane disease. Influence of continuous distending pressure. Pediatrics 1975;55:51–54.
55. Hawker JM, Reynolds EOR, Taghizadeh A. Pulmonary surface tension and pathological changes in infants dying after respirator treatment for severe hyaline membrane disease. Lancet 1967;2:75–77.
56. Reynolds EOR, Taghizadeh A. Improved prognosis of infants mechanically ventilated for hyaline membrane disease. Arch Dis Child 1974;49:505–515.
57. Reynolds EOR. Effects of alterations in mechanical ventilator settings on pulmonary gas exchange in hyaline membrane disease. Arch Dis Child 1971;46:152–159.
58. Herman S, Reynolds EOR. Methods for improving oxygenation in infants mechanically ventilated for severe hyaline membrane disease. Arch Dis Child 1973;48:612–616.
59. Llewellyn MA, Swyer PR. Assisted and controlled ventilation in the newborn period: effect on oxygenation. Br J Anaesth 1971;43:926–932.
60. Gregory GA, Kitterman JA, Phibbs RH, et al. Treatment of the idiopathic respiratory distress syndrome with continuous positive airway pressure. N Engl J Med 1971;284:1333–1378.
61. Suter PM, Fairley HB, Isenberg MD. Optimum end-expiratory airway pressure in patients with acute pulmonary failure. N Engl J Med 1975;292:284–289.
62. Tanswell AK, Clubb RA, Smith BT, Boston RW. Individualised continuous distending pressure applied within 6 hours of delivery in infants with respiratory distress syndrome. Arch Dis Child 1980;55:33–39.
63. Bonta BW, Uauy R, Warshaw JB, Motoyama EK. Determination of optimal continuous positive airway pressure for the treatment of IRDS by measurement of esophageal pressure. J Pediatr 1977;91:449–454.
64. Landers S, Hansen TN, Corbet AJS, Stevener MJ, Rudolph AJ. Optimal constant positive airway pressure assessed by arterial alveolar difference for CO_2 in hyaline membrane disease. Pediatr Res 1986;20:884–889.
65. Rhodes PG, Hall RT. Continuous positive airway pressure delivered by face mask in infants with the idiopathic respiratory distress syndrome: a controlled study. Pediatrics 1973;52:17–21.
66. Boros SJ, Matalon SV, Ewald R, Leonard AS, Hung CE. The effect of independent variations in inspiratory-expiratory ratio and end expiratory pressure during mechanical ventilation in hyaline membrane disease: the significance of mean airway pressure. J Pediatr 1977;91:794–798.
67. Boros SJ, Campbell K. A comparison of the effects of high frequency—low tidal volume and low frequency–high tidal volume mechanical ventilation. J Pediatr 1980;97:108–112.
68. Reynolds EOR. Pressure wave form and ventilator settings for mechanical ventilation in severe hyaline membrane disease. Intern Anesth Clin 1974;12:259–277.
69. Ratner I, Hernandez J, Accuroso F. Low peak pressure inspiratory pressures for ventilation of infants with hyaline membrane disease. J Pediatr 1982;100:802–804.
70. Boros SJ, Bing DR, Mammel MC, et al. Using conventional infant ventilators at unconventional rates. Pediatrics 1984;74:487–492.
71. Ciszek TA, Modanlou HD, Owings D, et al. Mean airway pressure—significance during mechanical ventilation of neonates. J Pediatr 1981;99:121–126.
72. Manginello FP, Grassi AE, Schechner S, Krauss AN, Auld PAM. Evaluation of methods of assisted ventilation in hyaline membrane disease. Arch Dis Child 1978;53:878–881.
73. Bland RD, Kim MH, Light MJ, et al. High frequency mechanical ventilation in severe hyaline membrane disease: an alternative therapy? Crit Care Med 1980;8:275–280.
74. Weigl J. The infant lung: a case against high respiratory rates in controlled neonatal ventilation. Respir Therapy 1973;3:57–62.
75. Donahue LA, Thibeault DW. Alveolar gas trapping and ventilator therapy in infants. Respir Therapy 1979;9:47–51.

76. Cartwright DW, Willis MM, Gregory GA. Functional residual capacity and lung mechanics at different levels of mechanical ventilation. Crit Care Med 1984;12:422–427.
77. Simbruner G. Inadvertent positive end-expiratory pressure in mechanically ventilated newborn infants: detection and effect on lung mechanics and gas exchange. J Pediatr 1986;108:589–595.
78. Heicher DA, Kasting DS, Richards JR. Prospective clinical comparison of two methods for mechanical ventilation of neonates: rapid rate and short inspiratory time versus slow rate and long inspiratory time. J Pediatr 1981;98:957–761.
79. Spahr RC, Klein AM, Brown DR, et al. Hyaline membrane disease. A controlled study of inspiratory to expiratory ratio. Am J Dis Child 1980;134:373–376.
80. Stark AR, Bascom R, Frantz ID. Muscle relaxation in mechanically ventilated infants. J Pediatr 1979;94:439–444.
81. Pollitzer MJ, Reynolds EOR, Shaw DG, Thomas RM. Pancuronium during mechanical ventilation speeds recovery of lungs of infants with hyaline membrane disease. Lancet 1981;1:346–348.
82. Greenough A, Morley CJ, David JA. Interaction of spontaneous respiration with artificial ventilation in preterm babies. J Pediatr 1983;103:769–773.
83. Greenough A, Wood S, Morley CJ, Davis JA. Pancuronium prevents pneumothoraces in ventilated premature babies who actively expire against positive pressure ventilation. Lancet 1983;1:1–4.
84. Rhodes PG, Graves GR, Patel DM, Campbell SB, Blumenthal BI. Minimizing pneumothorax and bronchopulmonary dysplasia in ventilated infants with hyaline membrane disease. J Pediatr 1983;103:634–637.
85. Fujiwara T, Maeta H, Chida S, Watabe Y, Abe T. Artificial surfactant therapy in hyaline membrane diseases. Lancet 1980;1:55–59.
86. Hallman M, Merritt TA, Jarvenpaa A, et al. Exogenous human surfactant for treatment of severe respiratory distress syndrome: a randomized prospective clinical trial. J Pediatr 1985;106:963–969.
87. Enhorning G, Shennan A, Possmayer F, Dunn M, Chen CP, Milligan J. Prevention of neonatal respiratory distress syndrome by tracheal instillation of surfactant: a randomized clinical trial. Pediatrics 1985;76:145–153.
88. Kwong MS, Egan EA, Notter RH, Shapiro DL. Double-blind clinical trial of calf lung surfactant extract for the prevention of hyaline membrane disease in extremely premature infants. Pediatrics 1985;76:585–592.
89. Merritt TA, Hallman M, Bloom BT, et al. Prophylactic treatment of very premature infants with human surfactant. N Engl J Med 1986;315:785–790.
90. Boynton BR, Mannino FL, Davis RF, Kopotic RJ, Friederichsen G. Combined high-frequency oscillatory ventilation and intermittent mandatory ventilation in critically ill neonates. J Pediatr 1984;105:297–302.
91. Boros SJ, Mammel MC, Coleman JM, et al. Neonatal high-frequency jet ventilation: four years' experience. Pediatrics 1985;75:657–663.
92. Frantz ID III, Werthammer J, Start AR. High-frequency ventilation in premature infants with lung disease: adequate gas exchange at low tracheal pressure. Pediatrics 1983;71:483–488.
93. Thibeault DW, Grossman H, Hagstrom HWC, Auld PA. Radiologic findings in the lungs of premature infants. J Pediatr 1969;74:1–10.
94. Coates AL, Desmond K, Willis D, Nogrady MB. Oxygen therapy and long-term pulmonary outcome of respiratory distress syndrome in newborns. Am J Dis Child 1982;136:892–895.
95. Ludwin SK, Northway WH Jr, Bensch KG. Oxygen toxicity in the newborn. Necrotizing bronchiolitis in mice exposed to 100 per cent oxygen. Lab Invest 1974;31:425–435.
96. Bonikos DS, Bensch KG, Northway WH Jr. Oxygen toxicity in the newborn Am J Pathol 1976;85:623–650.
97. Stocker TJ, Madewell JE. Persistent interstitial pulmonary emphysema: another complication of the respiratory distress syndrome. Pediatrics 1977;59:847–857.
98. Brewer LL, Moskowitz PS, Carrington CB, Bensch KG. Pneumatosis pulmonalis, a com-

plication of the idiopathic respiratory distress syndrome. Am J Pathol 1979;95:171–190.
99. Wright AW. The local effect of the injection of gases into the subcutaneous tissues. Am J Pathol 1930;6:87–124.

Comments

Bruce R. Boynton

A great deal has been learned about the mechanisms of barotrauma in immature lungs. However, as the authors point out, we still do not understand how barotrauma interacts with the toxic effects of oxygen metabolites and proteases to cause BPD. Moreover our increased understanding of barotrauma has not, as yet, enabled us to prevent lung injury. It is now clear that high-frequency ventilation does not prevent pneumothoraces, pulmonary interstitial emphysema, or BPD completely, although it may reduce their incidence. Barotrauma continues to be a frequent complication of conventional mechanical ventilation, partly because we do not know which combinations of ventilator settings are least injurious. However, there is cause for optimism. Exogenous surfactant treatment of infants with RDS shows great promise for reducing lung injury. Combining high-frequency ventilation with surfactant administration may facilitate the uniform distribution of phospholipids and thereby enhance their beneficial effects.

6

Development of Antioxidant Systems

JONATHAN R. WISPE AND ROBERT J. ROBERTS

Introduction

At birth the fetus is required to rapidly adapt biochemically and physiologically to extrauterine existence. With birth and the onset of respiration, there is a sudden increase in the concentration of oxygen in the lung. The replacement of fetal lung fluid with air results in a fivefold increase in oxygen tension in the lung. This increase is substantially greater in premature infants who require oxygen therapy. This increased oxygen tension is associated with the potential for oxygen induced tissue injury. The exact mechanisms of oxygen injury are unknown. In 1954 Gerschman and Gilbert proposed that the damaging effects of oxygen could be due to the formation of oxygen radicals (1). Several oxidative pathways have been implicated in the genesis of oxygen induced tissue injury. The free radical theory of oxygen toxicity states that increased oxygen concentrations in aerobic cells cause the formation of reactive oxygen metabolites (2, 3). These metabolites are generated by metabolic processes in which oxygen is incompletely reduced. A summary of the biochemical pathways involved in the formation of reactive oxygen metabolites is presented in Figure 6.1 along with the enzymatic and nonenzymatic systems that are believed to protect the cell from these reactive metabolites.

Several authors have compared the evolutionary changes that resulted from a progressively aerobic environment with the adaptations that a newborn baby must make at birth (5). Coincident with increasing atmospheric oxygen, there was an increase in the number of organisms dependent upon aerobic metabolism. As described by Haugaard, survival in an aerobic environment requires efficient protective antioxidant systems (6). In one sense the newborn infant is recapitulating this evolutionary process. At birth the newborn is suddenly exposed to increased oxygen and must have functioning antioxidant protective systems. In premature infants who require hyperoxic therapy, these systems must be able to compensate for even greater oxidative stresses. Antioxidant systems are an important homeostatic mechanism for adaptation to environmental oxygen content whether evolutionarily or developmentally.

The objective of this chapter is to review available information about the development of enzymatic and nonenzymatic systems. In considering the role of antioxidant protection in the genesis of bronchopulmonary dysplasia, it is important to understand the normal development of antioxidant systems and also the ability of these systems to respond to an oxidant challenge.

Enzymatic Antioxidant Protective Systems

Table 6.1 lists the various enzymatic antioxidants and the reactive metabolites that are the substrates for each enzyme. The action of these enzymes is to decrease the toxicity of the substrate.

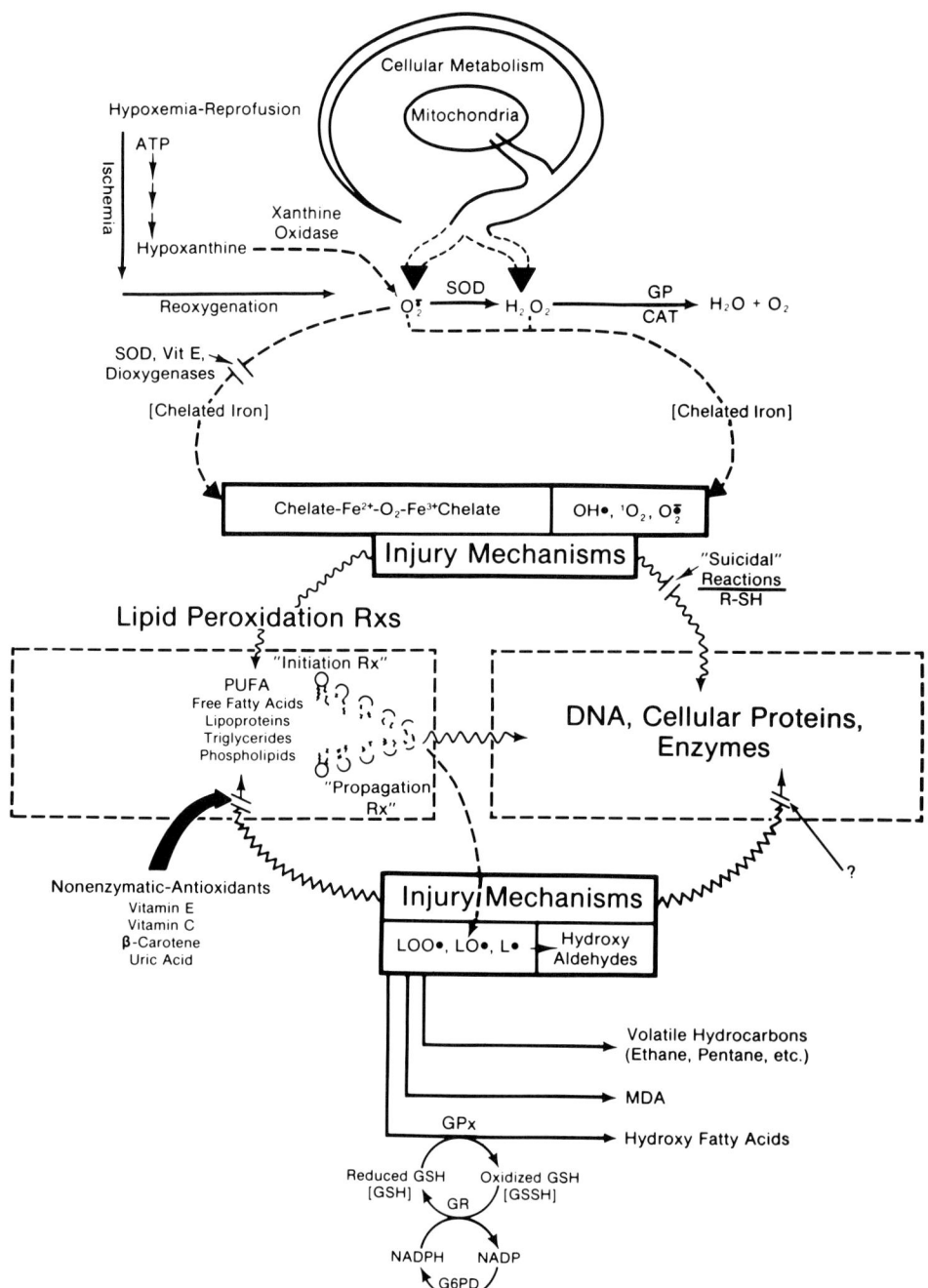

Figure 6.1. Schematic representation of the source and generation of free radicals and reactive intermediates, and the enzymatic and nonenzymatic protective systems available to the cell. Additional details are provided in the text. Adapted from Roberts, 1984 (4).

Table 6.1 Antioxidant Systems ("Protectants") in the Developing Lung

"Protectant"	Toxic Substrate
Enzymatic	
Superoxide dismutase (SOD)	O_2^-
Catalase	H_2O_2
Glutathione peroxidase	H_2O_2, LOOH
Indoleamine 2,3-dioxy genase	O_2^-
Glutathione S-transferases	LOOH
Nonenzymatic	
Vitamin E (α-tocopherol)	LOO·, $^1O_2$, O_2^-, OH·
Vitamin C	LOO·, LO·, $^1O_2$, O_2^-, OH·
β-Carotene	$^1O_2$
R-SH, Unsaturated lipids; amino acids	"Suicidal binding" of various toxic species
Glutathione	H_2O_2, LOO·, hydroxy aldehydes
Uric acid	$^1O_2$, O_2^-, OH·

The major endogenous protective systems along with the proposed reactive or toxic species against which they act are listed. The list of protectants and toxic substrates is not intended to be comprehensive and does not reflect the controversies about their biologic significance or relevance.

Superoxide Dismutase

Superoxide Dismutase (SOD) is a key protective enzyme because it catalyzes the reduction of superoxide anion (O_2^-). Superoxide dismutase is actually a family of metalloproteins that efficiently catalyze the dismutation of the superoxide radical to hydrogen peroxide and oxygen:

$$2O_2^- + 2H^+ \xrightarrow{SOD} H_2O_2 + O_2$$

Eukaryotic cells contain two SOD enzymes: CuZnSOD and MnSOD. The CuZnSOD enzymes contain two identical subunits with a combined molecular weight of 32,000 daltons. The MnSOD enzyme is composed of four identical 21,500 dalton subunits. Although differences exist among animal species and in different tissues, CuZnSOD is located primarily in the cytosol whereas MnSOD is located in the soluble matrix of mitochondria. The major SOD in the extracellular space in mammals is a tetrameric, slightly hydrophobic glycoprotein with a molecular weight of approximately 135,000, which contains four copper and possibly four zinc atoms (7). The physiologic significance of extracellular SOD is unclear.

SOD can also indirectly affect the production of hydroxyl radical (OH·), a very reactive and potentially damaging oxygen metabolite. Superoxide anion participates in an iron catalyzed reduction with hydrogen peroxide to produce hydroxyl radical (Haber-Weiss and Fenton reactions):

$$Fe^{3+} + O_2^- \rightarrow Fe^{2+} + O_2$$
$$Fe^{2+} + H_2O_2 \rightarrow Fe^{3+} + OH^- + OH·$$

Therefore SOD mediated decreases in superoxide anion could decrease FE^{+3} reduction. Conversely SOD could accelerate OH· production by increasing the amount of hydrogen peroxide present, particularly if conditions of excess superoxide anion existed. Under circumstances of excess O_2^-, removal of hydrogen peroxide by catalase and/or the glutathione system would prevent hydroxyl radical production (see following discussions).

SOD activity has been quantitated in fetal lung and lung from animals of various ages.

Although there are species differences, there is a progressive increase in SOD activity during late gestation which continues after birth (8, 9, 10). The increase in SOD activity during fetal life is developmentally regulated and parallels the maturation of other pulmonary systems, such as the surfactant system (11, 12, 13). Tanswell and Freeman (13) examined the contribution of CuZnSOD and MnSOD to total SOD activity at various ages in rats. They observed that the relative contributions of the various isoenzymes vary according to the denominator used to normalize activity. When compared on the basis of SOD activity per unit lung weight, the majority of the lung SOD activity in the fetus is due to MnSOD. At birth MnSOD and CuZnSOD contribute equally to total lung SOD activity. When levels of SOD activity are normalized to DNA content, Tanswell and Freeman found that most of the developmental increase in SOD activity is due to increased CuZnSOD activity. Because mitochondrial mass per cell increases during lung development, it may be more appropriate, when comparing data from lung tissue obtained from different age groups, to relate SOD activity to a mitochondrial enzyme; for example, cytochrome oxidase. When increases in SOD activity are normalized to cytochrome oxidase activity, the developmental patterns of MnSOD and CuZnSOD are comparable. In adults CuZnSOD activity accounts for the majority of lung SOD activity. Marklund (7) has recently described a third form of SOD, extracellular SOD. There are no published data available on extracellular SOD activity in the fetus or newborn. In adult lungs extracellular SOD activity is equal to MnSOD activity.

The most intriguing question about the developmental changes in SOD activity is what factors regulate these changes. One possible explanation for the increase in antioxidant activity is that it is a response to increased production of superoxide anion. Such substrate regulation is known to occur in other enzyme systems. Warshaw *et al.* demonstrated increased activity of the enzymes responsible for glucose and fatty acid utilization as the availability of these substrates increased (14). With this dependence on oxidative metabolism, more oxygen is utilized by mitochondria. Associated with this utilization of oxygen is the increased potential for mitochondrial generation of superoxide anion (15). Therefore the mechanism driving maturation of SOD activity during fetal life and early postnatal life may be increased substrate availability. However, other factors are certainly involved, including hormonal and metabolic influences. Dexamethasone administration increased SOD activity (16) and hypothyroid lamb fetuses had decreased SOD activity (17). Since SOD activity is known to be inhibited by H_2O_2, changes in SOD activity in the first few days after birth (10) may be explained by significant changes in quantity of available toxic substrate (O_2^-, H_2O_2, $OH\cdot$, etc.). It is crucial to develop a better understanding of regulatory mechanisms if there is to be any hope of manipulating antioxidant activity in newborn infants.

The role of antioxidant enzymes, including SOD, in facilitating adaptation to, or tolerance of, hyperoxia is of great interest and controversy. Increased activity of these protective enzymes could be vital in protecting against oxygen injury (8). As shown in Table 6.2 the response of pulmonary SOD activity to oxygen exposure differs between newborns and adults in most animal species. In most newborn animals SOD activity increases after oxygen exposure. In adult ani-

Table 6.2 Protective Enzyme Activity in the Lung: Developmental Changes and Adaptation to Hyperoxic Exposure

Enzyme	Developmental Changes*	Response to Oxygen†
SOD	Fetus < newborn < adult	Newborn–increase Adult–variable
Catalase	Fetus < newborn > adult	Newborn–increase Adult–variable
Glutathione peroxidase	Fetus < newborn newborn > or < adult	Newborn–increase Adult–no change or decrease

*Relative enzyme activity at various ages compared on a per unit weight, DNA, or protein basis. Animal species studied include rat, rabbit, mouse, guinea pig, hamster.

†Response to oxygen differs among species (10, 18) and with concentration and duration of oxygen exposure (19).

mals oxygen effects vary with dose and length of oxygen exposure. There are also differences in the protective effects of increased SOD activity. In adult animals there is a strong correlation between the capacity for SOD to increase and the resistance to oxygen induced lung injury and lethality. In newborn animals there is a positive association between the length of survival in hyperoxia and the ability to increase lung SOD activity (18). However, despite increased pulmonary SOD activity in newborn animals, microscopic lung injury still occurs and further lung growth and maturation is inhibited (19, 20). Interpretations of quantitative changes in lung SOD activity in oxygen exposed newborn animals are complicated by changes in commonly used denominators, total protein, DNA content, or lung weight.

In adult rats gradual increases in oxygen concentration induce an adaptation that allows these animals to survive when they are subsequently exposed to ordinarily lethal 100% oxygen. This adaptation is associated with increased activity of all pulmonary antioxidant enzymes, including SOD. Some animal species, for example adult mice or guinea pigs, cannot be "preadapted" to survival in 100% oxygen by pre-exposure to lower oxygen concentrations. The molecular basis of the differences in preadaptability among different species is unknown.

Catalase

Catalase consists of four protein subunits, each of which contains a heme group bound to its active site. Catalase can be found in most aerobic cells, although the activity varies considerably between different tissues and even in different regions of the same tissue. Catalase activity is believed to be located primarily in the peroxisomes.

Catalase catalyzes the reactions:

$$2 H_2O_2 \rightarrow 2 H_2O + O_2$$

Although H_2O_2 is potentially damaging itself, it has greater injury potential because it serves as a precursor for more reactive radicals, including the hydroxyl radical. (See previous discussion of the Haber-Weiss and Fenton reactions.) Most eukaryotic cells have two enzyme systems to metabolize H_2O_2: catalase and glutathione peroxidase. These two enzymes have very different affinities for H_2O_2, and each may be important in different situations. Glutathione peroxidase has greater affinity for H_2O_2 and probably serves as the primary catalytic enzyme during low rates of H_2O_2 production. However, when H_2O_2 concentrations are high, catalase has a greater capacity for H_2O_2. This dual antioxidant system allows for greater participation of catalase during periods of increased cellular H_2O_2 production. If the cells were solely dependent upon glutathione peroxidase in situations of high oxidant stress, there would be the potential for depletion of reduced glutathione (GSH) and/or glutathione disulfide (GSSG) accumulation. GSH availability is important for many cellular processes, and depletion of GSH stores causes cellular dysfunction. Therefore the relative function of catalase or glutathione peroxidases depends on intracellular location of the enzyme in relation to the site of H_2O_2 production, and on the rate of H_2O_2 production. There are also metabolic regulatory influences on catalase. Superoxide anion (O_2^-) inhibits catalase, and H_2O_2 inhibits SOD. These interactions, and the differences in substrate affinity, imply a complex regulatory relationship between these two major cellular antioxidant systems.

Catalase is developmentally regulated, with differences in activity between fetal, newborn, and adult lung tissue. Catalase activity in the lung increases during gestation and for the first few days after birth (10, 11, 12, 13). The activity of catalase in adult lung is reported to be less than in the newborn lung in most species. Gerdin *et al.* speculated that the increase in catalase activity after birth may be secondary to increased tissue levels of H_2O_2 (12). The *in vitro* generation of H_2O_2 by isolated lung mitochondria is proportional to oxygen tension (15). If the same relationship exists *in vivo*, then the increase in pulmonary oxygen exposure associated with birth would lead to increased H_2O_2 production and a substrate induction of catalase.

There are a few reports on the effect of hyperoxic exposure on lung catalase activity. Newborn rats and rabbits exposed to hyperoxia showed an increase in lung catalase activity whereas the mouse, hamster, and guinea pig newborns failed to show a significant change (11, 18). Studies of newborn rats, in which oxygen concentration and duration of exposure were varied, demonstrated little change in lung catalase activity unless the rats were exposed to 95% oxygen for 5 days. The explanation for these results is not clear. During exposure to hyperoxia hydrogen peroxide formation should be increased, and catalase would be expected to play a more important antioxidant role. Conversely glutathione peroxidase would be expected to be the major factor in normoxic conditions with low concentrations of hydrogen peroxide present (12).

Glutathione System

The glutathione system consists of glutathione, glutathione peroxidase, and glutathione reductase. Glutathione peroxidase is a soluble protein consisting of four uniform subunits. Each subunit contains a single selenium atom. The molecular weight of the functional tetrameric protein is about 85,000 daltons. Glutathione peroxidase activity is located primarily in the cytosol and mitochondrial matrix. Glutathione peroxidase converts hydrogen peroxide to water and molecular oxygen. As described above, this process indirectly decreases the production of hydroxyl radicals. Glutathione peroxidase also catalyzes the conversion of lipid peroxides (LOOH) to nontoxic hydroxy fatty acids (Figure 6.1). GSH provides the reducing equivalents necessary for removal of hydrogen peroxide and lipid peroxides. Lipid peroxides, resulting from peroxidation of polyunsaturated fatty acids, can cause tissue injury. The term glutathione peroxidase is best reserved for the selenoprotein that catalyzes the reduction of both hydrogen peroxide and lipid peroxides.

It is important for cellular integrity that glutathione depletion and/or glutathione disulfide accumulation be avoided. Under conditions of high oxidant stress, glutathione status is preserved partially by increased catalase activity and partially by the action of glutathione reductase. Glutathione reductase reduces GSSG and keeps the ratio of GSH to GSSG high. The reaction requires NADPH:

$$GSSG + NADPH + H^+ \rightarrow 2\ GSH + NADP^+$$

The NADPH required is supplied mainly by the pentose phosphate pathway through the action of glucose-6-phosphate dehydrogenase.

Several investigators have studied the developmental pattern of the glutathione system. Glutathione peroxidase activity increasing during fetal life in all species examined (10, 11, 12, 13, 21). As with SOD, there is an apparent decrease in glutathione peroxidase activity in the first few days after birth (10). Activity of glutathione peroxidase in adult animals is greater or less than in newborns depending upon the species investigated. In contrast total glutathione (both GSH and GSSG) is unchanged or decreased during fetal life, declines shortly after birth, and then increases to adult levels equal to or slightly above those in the newborn. Glutathione reductase activity follows the pattern of total glutathione.

Newborn rats placed in hyperoxia at birth have a rapid increase in glutathione peroxidase activity (18). Again the response to hyperoxia is concentration and time dependent (19). There are species differences, however, particularly with respect to the response of the adult lung to hyperoxic exposure (18). In newborn rats glutathione content increases rapidly in the lung in response to hyperoxic exposure (21). The changes in GSH are believed to relate to an increase in *de novo* synthesis in the lung of GSH as well as to maintenance of the high GSH/GSSG ratio through the concerted activities of glutathione reductase and G-6-PDH. The nature of the stimulus responsible for increased glutathione peroxidase activity and glutathione levels in response to hyperoxic therapy is unclear. Hormonal regulation appears unlikely on the basis of studies by Warshaw *et al.* (21). Lung explants from human fetal lung or from fetal rats showed increased total and reduced glutathione when cultured in 95% oxygen, 5% CO_2. These results suggest an intrinsic lung response to oxygen rather than external regulatory influences.

Glutathione S-transferases

Glutathione S-transferases are included in the family of protective enzymes because they help in the conjugation of potentially toxic substances including xenobiotics and lipid hydroperoxides to reduced glutathione (GSH). Glutathione S-transferase also detoxify some damaging metabolites by "suicidal binding" reactions. In this process cellular damage is prevented at the expense of destruction of the transferases. These non-selenium-containing enzymes do not reduce hydrogen peroxide and are therefore distinct in their spectrum of activity from selenium dependent glutathione peroxidase activity. Glutathione S-transferase activity is located mainly in the cytosol along with small amounts in the mitochondria.

There are no reports dealing with the developmental aspects of glutathione S-transferase activity in the lung. Oxygen exposure of adult rats has been shown to increase lung glutathione S-transferase activity (22). There are no similar reports in newborns.

Nonenzymatic Antioxidant Protective Systems

There are a number of nonenzymatic antioxidant defenses present in cells (Table 6.1). The relative contribution of the nonenzymatic protectants to cellular defenses against oxygen-induced lung injury has not been fully explored. The developmental features of these nonenzymatic protectants in the lung have also not been systematically examined. The following sections summarize the available information relative to the developmental aspects of the nonenzymatic protectants in the lung and their role as modifiers of oxygen-induced lung injury.

Vitamin E

Vitamin E (α-tocopherol) is the most thoroughly investigated and best understood of the nonenzymatic antioxidants. α-Tocopherol's ability to prevent or modulate oxygen-induced lung injury has been investigated in several laboratories. α-Tocopherol is a lipid soluble antioxidant that is intimately integrated into membrane lipids, where it provides antioxidant activity by hydrogen donation to lipid peroxy radicals:

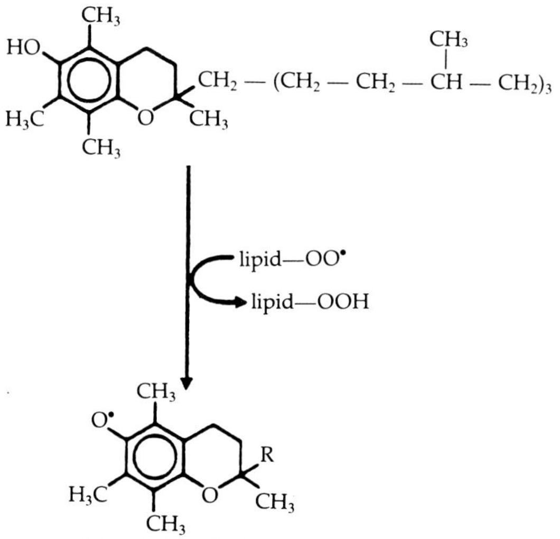

The membrane antioxidant function of vitamin E is facilitated by the physiochemical interaction between the phytyl side chain of α-tocopherol and the polyunsaturated fatty acids in membrane phospholipids. α-Tocopherol is found in highest concentrations in subcellular membranes of nuclei, mitochondria, and microsomes. Although vitamin E is believed to interact primarily with lipid peroxy radicals (LOO·), it has also been shown in nonbiologic systems to react with singlet oxygen, superoxide radical, and hydroxyl radical (Table 6.1). γ-Tocopherol is the other commonly occurring natural form of vitamin E. Although it is less active biologically (10% to 30% of the antioxidant activity of α-tocopherol), the major portion of total dietary vitamin E intake may be γ-tocopherol. The most common synthetic form of vitamin E is

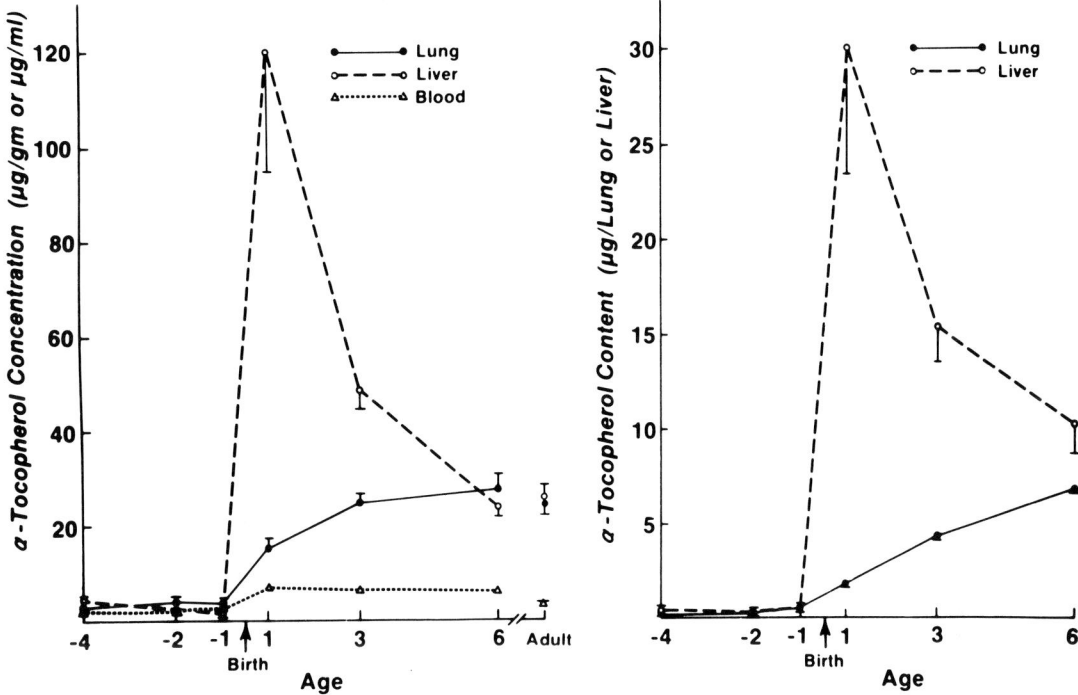

Figure. 6.2. α-Tocopherol concentrations in tissues from experimental rats in late fetal, early neonatal, and adult periods. Values are means ±SE. Adapted from Bucher and Roberts, 1981 (23).

α-tocopherol acetate, an ester form of vitamin E that has no antioxidant activity because the important phenolic hydrogen is replaced with acetate. α-Tocopheryl acetate is the most prevalent form of vitamin E in infant enteral nutrition products and enteral or parenteral vitamin preparations.

There is very little change in the total body tocopherol concentration or in lung tocopherol concentration during fetal life. Figure 6.2 represents the changes in α-tocopherol concentration in tissues from experimental animals. Liver α-tocopherol concentrations increase dramatically within the first days of life and then decline to those of the adult. Lung α-tocopherol concentration increases gradually after birth, reaching a value similar to that seen in adults by one week. As is clearly shown in Figure 6.2, blood concentrations of alpha-tocopherol do not accurately reflect these dynamic changes occurring in tocopherol concentration in other tissues. In general plasma tocopherol concentrations in newborns are about 50% lower than in adults. The pattern of α-tocopherol changes in the liver suggest that this organ is a storage depot, releasing α-tocopherol to other tissues during the early phases of maturation.

Several studies have convincingly demonstrated that changes in tissue α-tocopherol levels after birth result from dietary intake of α-tocopherol (23). There is no increase in tissue α-tocopherol levels if α-tocopherol intake is denied. Furthermore tissue α-toco-

Table 6.3 α-Tocopherol Concentration of Lung Tissue from Infants and Children

Group	No. Patients	Birth Weight (g)	Age at Death	Est. Total α-Tocopherol Intake (mg)*	Lung α-Tocopherol Concentrations (μg/g)*†
Infants‡					
Normoxia	2	380–1880	0–3 hr	None	2.7 (2.4–3.0)
Hyperoxia	5	1230–2700	24–36 hr	None	2.5 (1.9–3.5)
Normoxia	2	780–1050	9–1 mo	22 (5–39)§	8.2 (5.9–10.5)
Hyperoxia	2	1000–1230	5–7 d	1.4 (0.7–20)	5.7 (4.2–7.2)
Children	3	—	6 mo–2 yr	Normal diet	14.3 (3.7–33.2)

*α-Tocopherol intake and lung concentrations represent means in the number of patients indicated, with the range of values shown in parentheses.
†Infant received 5 mg α-tocopherol intravenously and 34 mg by mouth; all other α-tocopherol treated infants received intravenous administration.
‡Lung α-tocopherol concentrations are given for four groups of infants (including term and prematures). Inclusion in a particular group was based on estimated total α-tocopherol intake, age at death, and exposure to hyperoxia (arbitrarily defined as exposure to $FiO_2 > 0.6$ for at least 24 hr).
§Comparison of mean lung α-tocopherol concentrations in α-tocopherol treated (7.0 ± 1.3) and nontreated infants (2.6 ± 0.2) revealed significantly elevated lung concentrations in the treated group, Student's t-test < .01. From Bucher and Roberts, 1981 (23).

pherol levels at birth in term and premature infants are similar; the apparent "low" serum tocopherol concentrations in premature infants are probably due to inadequate nutritional intake including inadequate vitamin E. Typical enteral and parenteral nutritional programs given to premature infants in the first few days of life have low alpha-tocopherol content (23, 24, 25). Table 6.3 illustrates the alpha-tocopherol concentration of lung tissue from infants and children. The close relationship between total α-tocopherol intake and lung α-tocopherol concentrations is obvious.

The role of lipid peroxidation in the injury process arising from hyperoxic exposure remains unresolved. In vitamin E deficient adult animals, administration of α-tocopherol reduced oxygen induced lung injury (23). These data suggest that lipid peroxidation is involved in oxygen injury and that adequate tissue α-tocopherol levels are required for antioxidant defense. In vitamin E sufficient newborn animals, pharmacologic doses of α-tocopherol fail to modify the hyperoxic effects on lung growth and maturation (26). However, α-tocopherol does appear to be effective in preventing the oxygen induced changes in lung compliance, possibly by decreasing the oxygen-induced decrease in surfactant lipids (27). Pharmacologic doses of vitamin E also decreased parameters of lipid peroxidation in newborn rabbits, including newborn rabbits given parenteral infusions of lipid emulsion preparations (28).

Exposure to hyperoxia does not change α-tocopherol concentrations in lung (26). The proposed antioxidant mechanism of α-tocopherol involves H^+ donation to the lipid radicals, with subsequent conversion of α-tocopherol to α-tocopherol quinone. Therefore if lipid peroxidation plays a prominent role in oxygen injury, some decrease in tissue α-tocopherol concentration might be anticipated. However, α-tocopherol may be regenerated from its oxidized metabolites including α-tocopherol quinone:

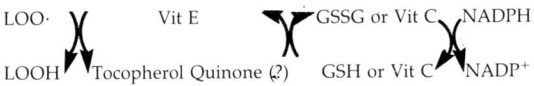

Vitamin C

Vitamin C or ascorbic acid is a water soluble vitamin required *in vivo* as a cofactor for a number of enzymes. Its most prominent chemical activity is to act as a reducing agent (electron donor), as exemplified by its ability to reduce Fe^{3+} to Fe^{2+}. Ascorbate reacts rapidly with superoxide anion and even more rapidly with hydroxyl radical. It also scavenges singlet oxygen. This scavenging activity of ascorbate has led to the conjecture that ascorbate may well assist in protecting cells against oxygen derived toxic species in biologic systems.

Ascorbic acid has been proposed to act in antioxidant synergy with vitamin E. In this model vitamin E acts as the primary antioxidant, and ascorbic acid regenerates oxidized vitamin E (see reactions in vitamin E discussion). In the lung ascorbate appears to accumulate in extracellular spaces including the fluid lining the alveoli. Intracellular ascorbate concentrations in several lung cells are reported to be in the millimolar range, which is significantly greater than the concentrations of 50 micromoles or less reported for other tissues and fluids (29).

Paradoxically ascorbate reduction of Fe^{3+} ions to Fe^{2+} ions in the presence of hydrogen peroxide can stimulate hydroxyl radical formation by the Fenton reaction. The overall impact of ascorbate on free radical production may depend on relative concentrations of ascorbate and iron. In nonbiologic systems low concentrations of ascorbate, with a given concentration of iron (Fe^{3+}), stimulate peroxidation, probably by reducing Fe^{3+} to Fe^{2+}. High concentrations of ascorbate, relative to iron, inhibit peroxidation, possibly by reducing lipid peroxy radicals directly to hydroperoxides (30).

Tissue ascorbic acid content in humans depends on nutritional intake. Ascorbic acid levels during fetal rat development are largely unchanged during the late stages of gestation (31). Exposure of adult animals to elevated oxygen concentrations causes a decrease in the ascorbic acid content of the lungs (29). There is no information available on the influence of oxygen on newborn lung ascorbate levels.

Miscellaneous Nonenzymatic Protectants

β-Carotene is an efficient quencher of singlet oxygen and oxygen centered radicals (32). β-Carotene has been shown to possess a dual action: decreasing the formation of singlet oxygen *in vivo* and removing singlet oxygen which is formed. β-Carotene also reacts directly with peroxy and alkoxy radicals and interferes with the chain reaction of lipid peroxidation (*e.g.*, propagation). Thus β-carotene may be an effective agent for protecting cells against a variety of processes that can lead to cellular damage by several different and distinct free radical mechanisms.

The binding of singlet oxygen, hydroxyl radical, and lipid peroxidation products to cellular constituents including sulfhydryl-containing amino acids, glutathione, and polyunsaturated fatty acids has been demonstrated in various experimental systems (29). This "suicidal binding" may protect the cells if the loss of the protecting substance is not critical to cell homeostasis and the products formed are not toxic.

Uric acid may act as a scavenger of singlet oxygen, superoxide anion, and hydroxyl radical (33). The high reactivity between uric acid and these toxic species as well as the high concentration of uric acid in biologic fluids suggests an important role for uric acid in oxidant and radical induced cellular injury. Uric acid has also been shown to inhibit Fenton-type reactions by complex formations between uric acid and iron, thus inhibiting iron dependent peroxidation of lipids.

Summary

Bronchopulmonary dysplasia (BPD) occurs frequently in premature infants, especially in those infants that require respiratory support with hyperoxia. The reasons for the apparent predisposition to develop BPD may include susceptibility to oxygen injury. The relationship between oxygen radical production and tissue antioxidant capabilities could have major implications regarding susceptibility to oxygen injury. Therefore it is crucial to understand the normal developmental changes in lung antioxidants as well as the influence of hyperoxic therapy on lung antioxidants. In the aggregate there appears to be a late gestational rise in the specific activity of pulmonary antioxidant enzymes including superoxide dismutase, catalase, and glutathione peroxidase. The late fetal maturation of antioxidant activity may be viewed as an important step in preparation for air breathing (*e.g.*, relative hyperoxic exposure).

The premature infant who requires oxygen therapy has several risk factors for oxygen injury. Because of the hyperoxia there is a greater potential for oxygen radical generation. Because of the prematurity enzymatic antioxidant activity may be insufficient to deal with the increased radical generation associated with hyperoxic therapy. Nonenzymatic antioxidant activity may also be inadequate if nutritional factors, including α-tocopherol, β-carotene, and ascorbic acid, are not provided as part of the management of the sick infant. Pulmonary oxygen injury in premature infants aggravates an already precarious situation of pulmonary insufficiency resulting from immaturity of the lung. Therapeutic hyperoxia may cause further damage to the lung by disrupting important normal maturational events in the lung including structural, physiologic, and biochemical processes.

References

1. Gerschman R, Gilbert DL, Nye SW. Oxygen poisoning and x-irradiation: a mechanism in common. Science 1954;119:623–626.
2. Freeman BA, Crapo JD. Biology of disease: free radicals and tissue injury. Lab Invest 1982;47:412–426.
3. Fridovich I. The biology of oxygen radicals. Science 1978;201:875–880.
4. Roberts RJ. Pulmonary oxygen toxicity in the premature and full term infant: its relationship to the development and pathogenesis of RDS and of its complications. In: Stern L, ed. Hyaline membrane disease: pathogenesis and pathophysiology. Chapter 9. Orlando, Fla: Grune and Stratton, 1984, pp 211–232.
5. Frank L, Massaro D. Oxygen toxicity. Am J Med 1980;69:117–126.
6. Haugaard N. Cellular mechanisms of oxygen toxicity. Physiol Rev 1968;48:311–373.
7. Marklund SL. Extracellular superoxide dismu-

tase in human tissues and human cell lines. J Clin Invest 1984;74:1398–1403.
8. Frank L, Autor AP, Roberts RJ. Oxygen therapy and hyaline membrane disease: the effect of hyperoxia on pulmonary superoxide dismutase activity and the mediating role of plasma or serum. J Pediatr 1977;90:105–110.
9. Roberts RJ. Employment of pulmonary superoxide dismutase, catalase, and glutathione peroxidase activity as criteria for assessing suitable animal models for studies of bronchopulmonary dysplasia. J Pediatr 1979;95:904–909.
10. Yam J, Frank L, Roberts RJ. Age-related development of pulmonary antioxidant enzymes in the rat. Proc Soc Exp Biol Med 1978;157:293–296.
11. Frank L, Groseclose EE. Preparation for birth into an O_2-rich environment: the antioxidant enzymes in the developing rabbit lung. Pediatr Res 1984;18:240–244.
12. Gerdin E, Tyden O, Eriksson UJ. The development of antioxidant enzymatic defense in the perinatal rat lung: activities of superoxide dismutase, glutathione peroxidase and catalase. Pediatr Res 1985;19:687–691.
13. Tanswell AK, Freeman BA. Pulmonary antioxidant enzyme maturation in the fetal and neonatal rat. I. Developmental profiles. Pediatr Res 1984;18:584–587.
14. Warshaw JB, Terry ML, Ranis MB. Metabolic adaption in developing lung. Pediatr Res 1980;14:296–299.
15. Turrens JF, Freeman BA, Levitt JG, Crapo JD. The effect of hyperoxia on superoxide production by lung sub-mitochondrial particles. Arch Biochem Biophys 1982;217:401–410.
16. Frank L, Lewis PL, Sosenko IRS. Dexamethasone stimulation of fetal rat lung antioxidant enzyme activity in parallel with surfactant stimulation. Pediatrics 1985;75:569–574.
17. Erenberg A, Frank L, Roberts RJ, Rhodes ML. Pulmonary superoxide dismutase activity in the euthyroid and hypothyroid ovine fetus. Pediatr Res 1982;16:570–572.
18. Frank L, Bucher JR, Roberts RJ. Oxygen toxicity in neonatal and adult animals of various species. J Appl Physiol: Respirat Environ Exercise Physiol 1978;45:699–704.
19. Bucher JR, Roberts RJ. The development of the newborn rat lung in hyperoxia: a dose-response study of lung growth, maturation, and changes in antioxidant enzyme activities. Pediatr Res 1981;15:999–1008.
20. Yam J, Roberts RJ. Oxygen-induced lung injury in the newborn piglet. Early Hum Dev 1980;4:411–424.
21. Warshaw JB, Wilson CW III, Saito K, Prough RA. The response of glutathione and antioxidant enzymes to hyperoxia in developing lung. Pediatr Res 1985;19:819–823.
22. Jenkinson SG, Lawrence RA, Burk RF, Gregory PE. Non-selenium-dependent glutathione peroxidase activity in rat lung: association with lung glutathione S-transferase activity and the effects of hyperoxia. Toxicol Appl Pharmacol 1983;68:399–404.
23. Bucher JR, Roberts RJ. α-Tocopherol (vitamin E) content of lung, liver, and blood in the newborn rat and human infant: influence of hyperoxia. J Pediatr 1981;98:806–811.
24. Wright SW, Filer LJ, Mason KE. Vitamin E blood levels in premature and full term infants. Pediatrics 1951;7:386–393.
25. Bell EF, Filer LJ. The role of vitamin E in the nutrition of the premature infants. Am J Clin Nutr 1981;34:414–422.
26. Bucher JR, Roberts RJ. Effects of α-tocopherol treatment on newborn rat lung development and injury in hyperoxia. Pediatr Pharmacol 1982;2:1–9.
27. Ward JA, Roberts RJ. Vitamin E inhibition of the effects of hyperoxia on the pulmonary surfactant system of the newborn rabbit. Pediatr Res 1984;18:329–334.
28. Wispe JR, Knight M, Roberts RJ. Lipid peroxidation in newborn rabbits: effects of oxygen, lipid emulsions and vitamin E. Pediatr Res 1986;20:505–510.
29. Halliwell B, Gutteridge JMC. Free radicals in biology and medicine. New York: Oxford University Press, 1985, pp 100–105.
30. Aust SD, Svingen BA. The role of iron in enzymatic lipid peroxidation. In: Payor WA, ed. Free radicals in biology, vol 5. New York: Academic Press, 1982, pp 1–28.
31. Kratzing CC, Kelly JD. Tissue levels of ascorbic acid during rat gestation. Int J Vit Nutr Res 1982;52:326–332.

32. Krinsky NI, Deneke SM. Interaction of oxygen and oxy-radicals with carotenoids. J Natl Cancer Inst 1982;69:205–210.
33. Hochstein P, Hatch L, Sevanian A. Uric acid: function and determination. In: Packer L, ed. Methods in enzymology, vol 105. Orlando, Fla: Academic Press, 1984, pp 162–166.

Comments

William H. Northway, Jr.

Understanding the factors that stimulate or limit the response of the immature antioxidant systems of the lung to supplemental oxygen exposure at various stages of development is a major part of developing a strategy for reducing oxygen injury in the very small premature infant. This strategy would include prenatal and postnatal stimulation of the lung antioxidant system and exogenous treatment with antioxidants as well as efforts to limit further the concentration and duration of supplemental oxygen usage. Significant increases in our knowledge of the free radical theory of oxygen toxicity and the antioxidant system in the lung have roughly paralleled the recognition and development of interest in BPD and the adult respiratory distress syndrome.

7

Interactions in the Immature Lung: Protease–Antiprotease Mechanism of Lung Injury

T. ALLEN MERRITT AND MIKKO HALLMAN

Introduction

Since the earliest descriptions of lung pathology in preterm infants dying with radiographic evidence of bronchopulmonary dyplasia (1), profound alterations of lung interstitial connective tissue, with fibrosis and thickening of the endothelial basement membrane and alveolar epithelia, altered or denuded ciliary epithelia, and vascular smooth muscle hyperplasia, have been described (2–5). The correlation of these pathologic findings, especially interstitial fibrosis and radiologic features at a month or more of age is quite high: (r = 0.72) (6). Although the pathogenesis of bronchopulmonary dysplasia (BPD) can be inferred neither from these radiographic features nor from autopsy results, the role of a variety of agents or insults (oxidant injury, barotrauma, air dissection, pulmonary edema, lung immaturity, and nutritional deficiencies) have been the focus of investigations since the National Heart, Lung, and Blood Institute's Workshop on Bronchopulmonary Dysplasia, the proceedings of which were published in 1979 (7).

Neonatologists presently are unable to determine whether in a given infant the resolution of severe respiratory distress syndrome (RDS) will be manifested by recovery of near normal lung function and a normal or near normal chest radiograph, or may rather be associated with characteristic radiographic features of BPD. These infants demonstrate increased airway resistance and decreased lung volume associated with epithelial metaplasia of the bronchioles, interstitial and peribronchial smooth muscle proliferation, alveolar inflammation, and interstitial fibrosis with lobular distention by emphysematous foci. Despite intensive clinical studies and limited preventive strategies, it remains unclear whether interacting factors including a familial predisposition—(especially among families with reactive airway disease (8)—)or immaturity of host defenses to oxidant induced pulmonary injury or dysfunctional antiprotease mechanisms result in BPD. This chapter focuses on the protease–antiprotease interactions in the neonates and their function in alterations of lung connective tissue in BPD. The protease–antiprotease imbalance supports the role of oxidant induced lung injury in the pathogenesis of BPD, and the role(s) of the oxidant and antiprotease activities in mechanisms on lung remodeling.

Lung Injury in the Newborn

The mechanisms that result in neonatal lung injury occur simultaneously during efforts to maintain normoxemia with elevated inspiratory oxygen concentrations and positive mean airway pressures in order to distend the atelectatic lung (Figure 7.1). These efforts to sustain both oxygenation and ventilation are necessary until adequate surfactant synthesis and secretion can maintain lung stability or until respiratory control mechanisms develop more fully and spontaneous breathing achieves normal gas exchange. Inadequate surfactant quantity and composition (9) in RDS affected infants is associated with high alveolar-capillary permeability following air breathing. Therefore proteinaceous filtrates leak into the air spaces, disrupting the surfactant and inhibiting to various degrees the surface activity (10, 11). This high-permeability alveolar edema further decreases compliance and gas exchange, making continued ventilatory support and supplemental oxygen mandatory. Further increases in lung water result both from increased lung blood flow through the left-to-right ductal shunt (12) and from low-pressure pulmonary edema secondary to endothelial junction "immaturity" (13). Filtration pressure of the pulmonary circulation is higher than normal and higher yet during episodes of hypoxia. Plasma protein osmotic pressure is low (14), and excessive fluid intake (frequently used clinically in metabolic resuscitation and to meet ongoing metabolic demands) often not only worsens the clinical state, but also is associated with the occurrence of BPD (15). Because the airway spaces are low in surfactant and have increased water and other serum components, the transpulmonary pressure must be large for adequate gas exchange. The distending pressures used in assisted ventilation may produce leaks (16) in the epithelial junctions and reduce interstitial pressure around extra-alveolar vessels, thus contributing to edema formation (17). These factors are at least "additive" in further diminishing lung compliance, resulting in scattered foci of atelectasis and dilated bronchioli alveolar ducts—frequently denuded of normal ciliated epithelium by mechanical ventilation (18). The damaged epithelia become metaplastic (19, 20) with abnormal nuclear repair seen on cytologic examination. These alterations result in functional changes in both water and chloride homeostasis of the airway cells (21). Loss of chloride-secreting cells and alteration in water transport across the trachea promote mucus secretion by increasing the number of globlet cells (22). This increased mucus production can result in airway obstruction, atelectasis, or a predisposition to airway infection.

Besides the striking changes in the cellular elements of fluids obtained from the airway, these secretions contain higher concentrations of glycolipids, especially lactosyl ceramide, normally present only in trace amounts. These glycolipids may result from an excessive shedding of plasma membrane components from the lining cells and are capable of disrupting the surfactant aggregate and inhibiting the surface activity. According to current concepts lactosyl ceramide appears to be a biochemical marker of advanced lung injury in preterm infants, likely to result in BPD (M. Hallman, unpublished results). Positive pressure ventilation may result in epithelial necrosis within 30 minutes of initiation of ventilation (23). The shear forces of the ventilation "fluid wave" not only distend and possibly disrupt the epithelial lining of respiratory bronchioles and basement membrane, but also result in pulmonary air leaks from the distal airways into the pulmonary lymphatics and perivascular space (24)—noted radiographically as pulmonary interstitial emphysema. There exists a

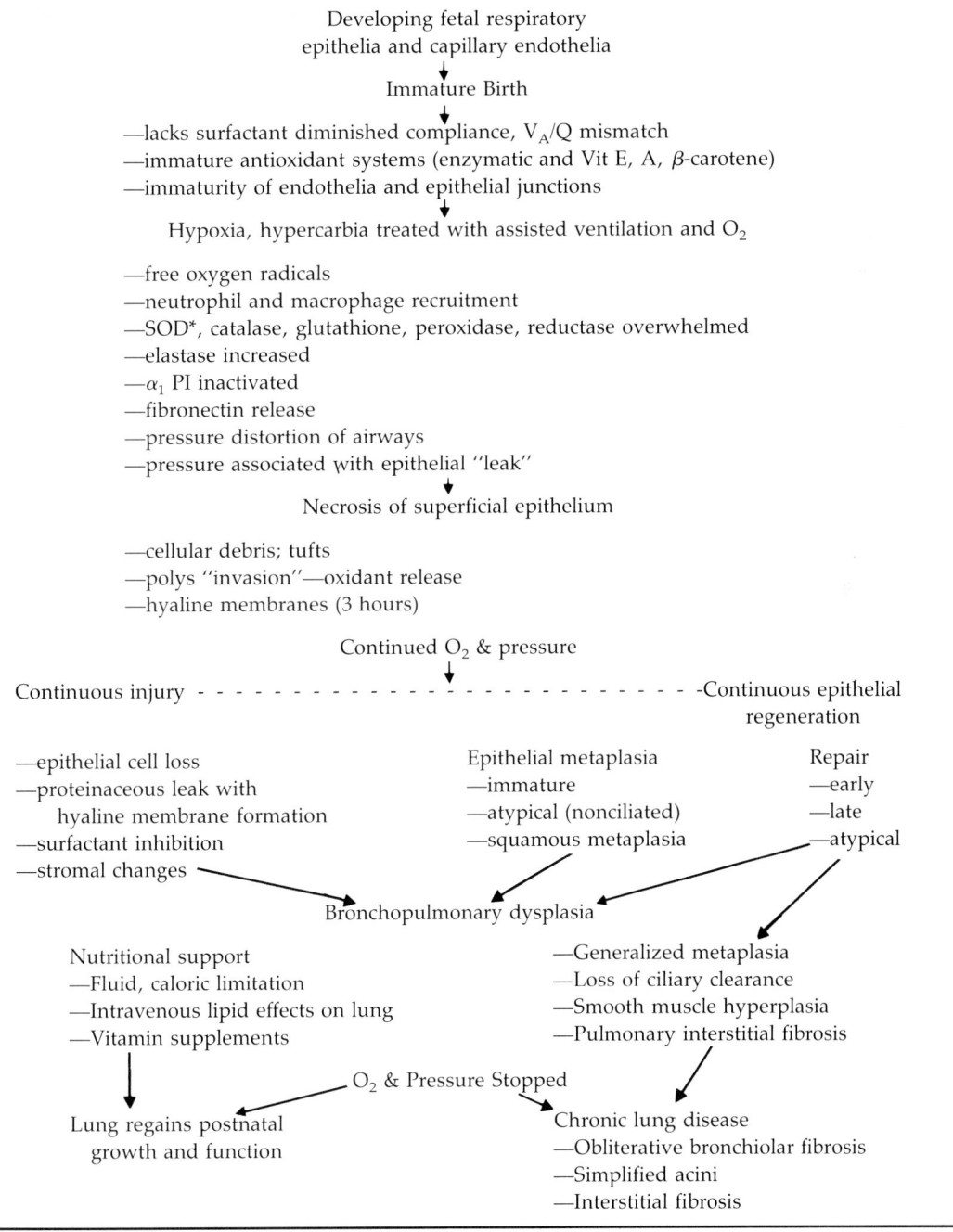

*SOD system = superoxide dismutase enzyme system

Figure 7.1. Pathophysiologic response to respiratory therapy and the development of BPD.

strong epidemiologic association between pulmonary interstitial emphysema and the eventual diagnosis of BPD (25). This association suggests that airway disruption and the resulting need for elevated mean airway pressures and prolonged oxygen exposure are due both to intrinsic properties of the immature airway and to the mechanical injury of ventilation. The mere presence of an endotracheal tube can cause direct mechanical damage to the underlying tracheal epithelium. Furthermore frequent suctioning of the endotracheal tube as a part of "pulmonary toilet" may lead to mechanical trauma and damage to the bronchial epithelium and be associated with granuloma formation in major bronchi, leading to selective overdistention or atelectasis of distal lung units (26). Furthermore the humidification of inspired gas may also influence mucociliary function and transport. Oxygen itself has been shown to impair ciliary motility in a dose dependent fashion (22). When these airway lining cells are replaced by squamous metaplasia or dysplastic cells with impaired ciliary movement, functional clearance of pulmonary secretions is undoubtedly limited.

Thus multiple, simultaneous events must be considered as interacting etiologic factors in the development of BPD. These include mechanical stresses on the immature lung, lung inflammation with alterations in cell ciliary and clearance functions, and water flux across the epithelial and endothelial membranes. Convincing evidence documents the elaboration of both extracellular and intracellular oxidants and proteolytic enzymes by inflammatory cells. In addition to supplemented inspired oxygen, these conditions have been demonstrated in neonatal animals to result in fibrosis of lung tissue.

Lung Injury in Adult Respiratory Distress Syndrome

Sudden respiratory failure with diffuse lung involvement, known as adult respiratory distress syndrome (ARDS), may occur among children or adults who sustain systemic or pulmonary insults. Although a variety of insults including sepsis, aspiration, circulatory collapse, inhaled toxins, emboli, and metabolic, neurologic, or hematologic disorders precede ARDS, the resulting severe lung injuries have strikingly similar features (27, 28). The pathogenesis involves an increase in capillary permeability (29, 30), abnormalities of the surfactant system, diminished lung compliance (31) and glycolipid accumulation in the bronchoalveolar space (32, 33). Although they differ in their primary initiating events, there are many similarities between ARDS and severe RDS resulting in BPD. Although there are differences in the temporal courses of ARDS and the development of chronic lung disease in neonates, similarities in the protease–antiprotease patterns in lung effluent during these diseases have been demonstrated (34, 35). These observations regarding elaboration of protelytic enzymes in ARDS and BPD have permitted a better appreciation of mechanisms that result in structural lung damage.

Changes in the Protease–Antiprotease System in Lung Injury

The antiprotease system is designed to protect the alveolar-capillary unit from autolytic proteolysis. Lung fibroblasts, fibrillar collagen (primarily types I and III), elastin fibers, the ground substance (laminin in the epithelial cells and endothelial basal laminae; fibronectin in the interstitium and on the surface of collagen bundles) can be degraded by proteases. In addition contractile cells with extensive cytoplasmic projections (comprised of actin and myosin fibrils) on the epithelial basal lamina and smooth muscle cells can be degraded when proteases are not inactivated by endogenous proteins. Interspersed among these fibrils and basement membranes are migratory cells including monocytes, macrophages, and mast cells. These cells respond to, and participate in, the enzymatic changes accompanying lung injury. The initial description of airway fluids in infants with BPD revealed an increase in inflammatory cells (36). Furthermore studies by Merritt et al. found that neutrophilic elastase was elevated in airway lavage of infants with RDS developing BPD and often preceding radiographic evidence for the disorder. Infants requiring endotracheal intubation but an $FiO_2 < 0.4$ for primarily nonpulmonary disease served as comparison infants. They did not demonstrate a predominance of inflammatory cells in tracheal aspirates, even when ventilated for weeks. Infants with radiographically confirmed BPD had detectable elastase activity in lung effluent obtained during pulmonary toilet (37). Injury to lung connective tissues, primarily elastin and collagen, takes place when there is an imbalance between the elaboration of proteases and the capacity of inhibitory proteins, primarily α_1-globulins. The presence of free elastase activity in the airway secretions of neonates undergoing mechanical ventilation may therefore be a hallmark of lung injury. Analysis of bronchoalveolar lavage fluid of individuals with ARDS by Lee and associates (34) and McGuire et al. (35) identified altered α_1-protease inhibitor activity (α_1PI) and free neutrophilic elastase during the course of the illness. Furthermore studies by Gadek et al. have demonstrated that α_1PI is the predominant inhibitor of neutrophil elastase in the gas exchange regions of the lungs in adult humans (38). Unlike adults, preterm infants have low levels of serum proteins including the antiproteases. Evans and coworkers (39) described low serum trypsin inhibitory protein in cord blood of infants developing RDS. Similar findings by others (40–42) most likely reflected the generalized hypoproteinemia described by Bland (43) in preterm infants with RDS. In none of these studies was the total α_1PI activity evaluated. Recently Rosenfeld et al. (44) measured trypsin inhibitory capacity (a measure of α_1PI functional capacity) in cord sera and found that infants with the most severe RDS also had the lowest trypsin inhibitory capacity on the first day after birth and that low inhibitory capacities on the first day generally predicted development of BPD several days or weeks later.

Although several serum antiproteases in addition to α_1PI exist (including α_2-macroglobulin, α_1-antichymotrypsin, antithrombin III, α_2-antiplasmin inhibitor, and C_1 esterase inhibitor), only α_1PI has been extensively studied in preterm infants. Andrew and coworkers (45) evaluated levels of several plasma protease inhibitors in well and sick preterm and term neonates. Infants (preterm and term) with disseminated intravascular coagulopathies had depressed level of α_2-macroglobulin, α_2-antiprotease, antithrombin III, and C_1 esterase activities. Ill infants at 1 week of age had depressed α_2-antiprotease and α_2-macroglobulin globulin, whereas α_1PI increased some 28% over levels at birth, similar to acute phase proteins. Kueppers and Offord (46) found, however, that by 30 postnatal days there was an approximately 30% decrease in absolute levels for the genotypes

PiM, M$_2$, and PiMS isotypes. It is critical to distinguish between "active" protease inhibitor and that which is bound or complexed to protease (*i.e.*, elastase). The latter can be measured immunologically but not functionally. Bruce and coworkers (47) reported the inactivation of α_1PI in infants exposed to oxygen concentrations ≥ 0.4, documenting the importance of determining functionally active levels of the antiproteases, as well as their total quantity.

Connective Tissue in Bronchopulmonary Dysplasia

Up to 6% of the fetal or neonatal lung parenchyma is elastin, and up to 85% of the connective tissue mass is collagen (48), of which types I and III (fibrillar collagen) are predominant (49). The lungs of infants with pulmonary fibrosis associated with BPD (29 weeks of gestation) have a higher collagen type I/III ratio than somewhat older (34 weeks' gestation) control infants dying of other causes. This excess of type I collagen relative to type III collagen is also found in adults succumbing to ARDS (50, 51). Shoemaker and coworkers reported on a preterm infant with RDS who developed severe BPD (52). By 147 days of ventilator therapy with high inspiratory oxygen, the collagen type I/III ratio was higher than 4 (normal I/III ratio = 1.6). No differences have yet been reported in lung collagen type V/III ratios in infants dying of BPD. These findings are consistent with an increase in the number of fibroblasts and quantities of fibroblast products (*i.e.*, type I collagen) during the acute phase of lung injury. The accumulation of type I collagen within the alveolar wall most likely results from a shift in the relative proportions of parenchymal cells to alveolar cells. Fibroblastic proliferation is seen histochemically (Masson trichrome staining) in the alveolar walls (fibrosis) and within the interstitial matrix. This proliferation leads to production of type I collagen (80% to 90% of the collagen produced by fibroblasts is type I) (53–55). Unfortunately the mechanism inducing production of collagen by fibroblasts is incompletely understood, although a macrophage derived growth factor for fibroblasts (18,000 dalton protein that induces fibronectin primed fibroblasts to release a fibroblastic growth factor) has been suggested by Bitterman and coworkers (56).

Alveolar macrophages also are thought to modulate the accumulation and replication of interstitial fibroblasts. Alveolar macrophages in adults with interstitial lung diseases release increased amounts of fibronectin (57), an adhesive glycoprotein that is chemotactic for fibroblasts (58). Fibronectin appears to "fix" fibroblasts to the interstitial matrix (59, 60, 61) and provides them with one of the "inducers" of fibroblastic proliferation. Ratios of fibronectin to albumin in tracheal effluent are increased over the second to third week after birth and are coincident with the decreased plasma levels in preterm infants with BPD (62).

These findings are suggestive of similar reports of enhanced pulmonary vascular permeability associated with plasma fibronectin deficiency during sepsis. However, macrophage derived fibronectin (63) may also be reflected in these measurements. Preliminary results in our laboratory have demonstrated specific cellular fibronectin in tracheal effluent from infants with BPD. Fibronectin undergoes proteolytic degradation and the peptide fragments have been found to retain fibroblastic and monocyte chemotactic properties (64, 65).

The recruitment of fibroblasts to areas of lung injury (and enhanced permeability) may be an important mechanism in interstitial and alveolar fibrosis, or alternatively increased fibronectin levels may stimulate phagocytosis by alveolar macrophages of cellular debris resulting from lung injury and inflammation (66). Fibronectin in lung secretions is of cellular origin (presumably macrophage derived) and an ultrafiltrate of serum. In lung effluent fibronectin may promote the clearance of cellular debris and connective tissue fragments (61). Yoder et al. (67) reported that plasma fibronectin levels are decreased in newborn cord blood and the low levels correlate with the degree of prematurity. Our laboratory evaluated plasma fibronectin levels in tracheal effluent in infants recovering from RDS and in infants developing BPD. Compared with preterm infants recovering from RDS, infants with BPD had a twofold elevation in fibronectin expressed per milligram of albumin. Recently Gerdes and coworkers reported a reduction in plasma fibronectin during the first 3 weeks after birth compared with infants with uncomplicated RDS (62). Efforts to determine the origin of pulmonary effluent fibronectin (cellular or plasma) are under way. Furthermore the possible role of fibronectin in the pathogenesis of BPD associated fibrosis remains to be determined.

Inflammation as a Cause of Lung Damage

Evidence of neutrophilic influx into the air spaces of neonatal animals, and in human neonates with RDS is well documented (Figure 7.2) (68, 69). Ogden et al. (70) found neutrophilic influx into airway secretions by 48 to 96 hours after birth in RDS infants, but

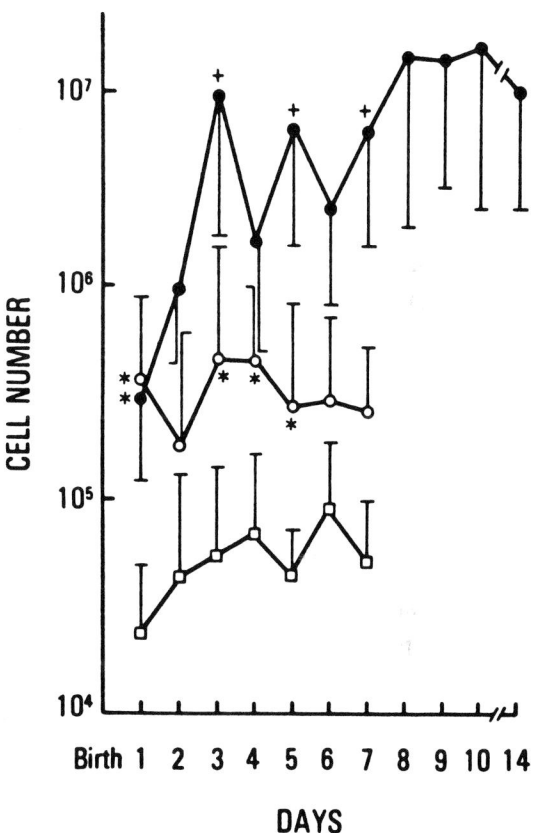

Figure 7.2. Tracheal aspirate inflammatory cell in 3 groups of preterm infants. Preterm infants intubated for non-pulmonary disorders (□) who never demonstrated radiographic evidence of BPD. Infants with RDS (○) had higher inflammatory cell number than comparison infants, but were significantly lower than infants destined to develop BPD (●). Infants in the latter group developed radiographic BPD at 21–30 days after birth. (Reprinted with permission from Rockefeller Press, From Merritt TA, Cochrane CG, Holcomb K, et al. J Clin Invest 1983;72:656–662).

cell numbers returned to levels found in control infants by the end of the first week (Figure 7.3). Infants later developing BPD had similar increases in inflammatory cell numbers, but the polymorphonuclear neu-

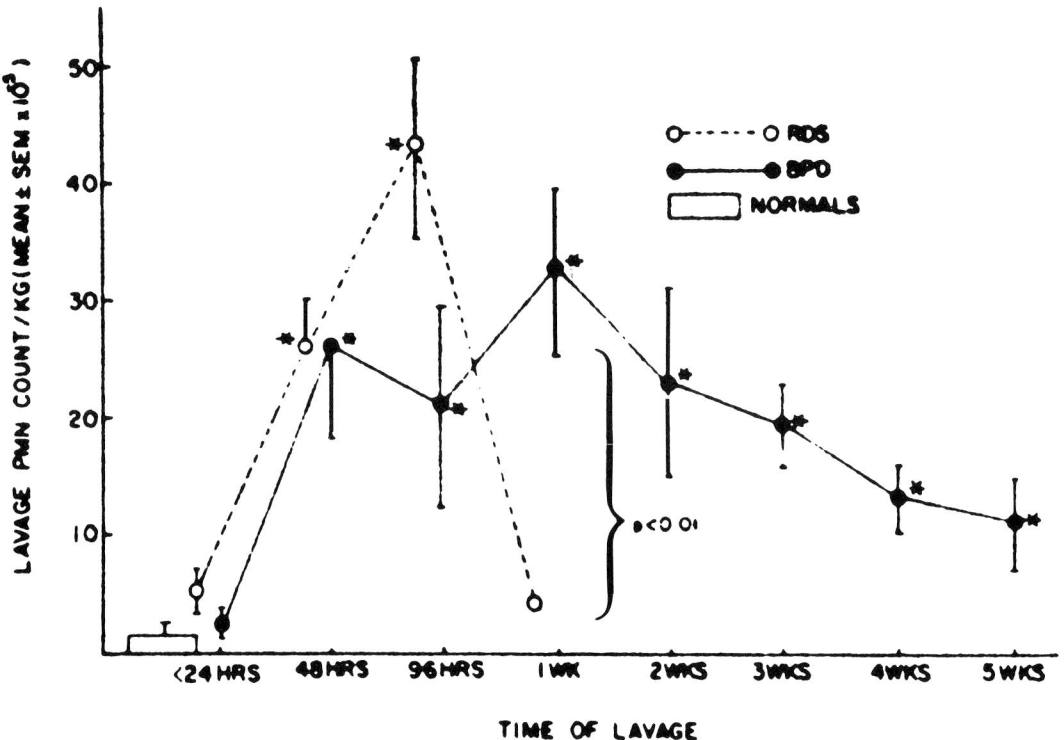

Figure 7.3. Neonatal lung lavage polymorphonuclear cell count throughout the course of RDS and BPD compared to normal infants. (Reprinted, with permission of the American Lung Association, From Ogden B, Murphy S, Saunders G, Pathak D, Johnson J. Neonatal lung neutrophils and elastase/proteinase inhibitor imbalance. Am Rev Resp Dis 1984;130:817–821).

trophilic leukocyte (PMN) counts remained elevated for the entire 5 week study period.

Our laboratory (37) reported that during the first week infants with RDS had a similar elevation in total inflammatory cells (PMNs plus alveolar macrophages), but that infants destined to develop BPD had a 20-fold increase in cell numbers compared with RDS infants with uneventful recoveries. This magnitude of increase was unassociated with concurrent lung infection. As we described and as Ogden et al. (70) confirmed, there is a persistent increase in inflammatory cell populations in airway secretions throughout the course of ventilation and for up to 6 weeks after initiation of assisted ventilation. Although alveolar macrophages and monocytes were early predominant inflammatory cells, PMNs represented more than 90% of the airway cells after day 7. By 2 weeks macrophages became more prominent in airway secretions, and continued to be in significant populations throughout the period of oxygen treatment; however, neutrophils are seen in abundance in the airways around the organizing hyaline membranes.

Human neutrophils produce a potent serine protease. This enzyme contains a serine residue at position 195 of the primary amino acid sequence which contributes a nucleophilic hydroxyl group to attack carbonyl carbons of target peptide bonds. The enzyme has several isoenzyme forms and is active in neutral pH. With a molecular weight of 33,000 daltons, it is stored in the promyelocyte cytoplasmic azurophilic granules (71). Each neutrophil has approximately 0.5 to 3 picograms of elastase (72, 73). This protease is discharged into tissues when neutrophils encounter objects to be phagocytized or after cell death. Upon secretion, hydrolysis of connective tissue matrix results, with degradation of tissue protein and glycoprotein in connective tissue ground substance. Collagen types III and IV are also structural targets of serine elastases; and fibronectin, a cellular adhesion molecule critical in basement membranes, is enzymatically cleaved by this enzyme (74). In addition to connective tissue architectural components, many plasma proteins can be hydrolyzed by neutrophil elastase, including immunoglobulins, fibrinogen, and complement proteins (75). Indeed proteolytic degradation may be one of several methods whereby the hyaline membranes are broken down. Although some of the effects of proteolytic digestion by elastase may be beneficial (e.g., clearing the necrotic hyaline membranes), the over-riding impact of unremitting proteolytic activity can be viewed as harmful.

Other inflammatory cell types including monocytes and macrophages also contain elastase. Monocytic elastase has been shown to digest elastin, fibronectin, and serum amyloid. Macrophage elastase is secreted directly into the extracellular milieu and is thought to be a calcium ion dependent enzyme (76). Degradation of lung connective tissue by macrophages appears to involve elastase and plasminogen activator. Plasminogen activator converts plasminogen to plasmin in exudative fluids and can facilitate elastinolysis (77). Human alveolar macrophages also contain cathepsin B (78), which has been shown in adults to be responsible for alveolar macrophage elastinolytic activity. While macrophage, calcium dependent elastase activity has been identified in neonatal pulmonary effluent, thus far the predominant protease identified has been neutrophilic elastase (Figure 7.4). We previously reported that infants with RDS developing BPD had elevated (sixfold) elastase levels during the first week of life compared with RDS infants not developing chronic lung disease. These elevations persisted for 2 to 3 weeks after birth and antedated radiographic appearance of BPD. Ogden et al. reported a nearly identical pattern using a different method of elastase analysis (70). The observation of Bruce et al. (79) is consistent with these findings. She reported that infants exposed to F_iO_2 concentrations > 0.4 for 3 to 4 days required greater amounts of $\alpha_1 PI$ added to a standardized measure porcine pancreatic elastase activity (to measure the elastase inhibition) to achieve a 15% inhibition of elastase than infants exposed up to 9 days at $FiO2 \leq 0.4$.

In order to determine whether the elastolytic activity altered connective tissue components, Bruce et al. quantitated by amino acid analysis the elastin degradation products (desmosines) excreted in the urine of 14 premature male infants during the first 3 weeks of life. Eight infants exposed to $FiO2 \leq 0.4$ were compared with six infants ventilated with $FiO2 > 0.6$. By the end of the first week of life, urine desmosine excretion was significantly greater in the infants who later developed BPD than in the infants exposed to lower FiO2. Elevated desmosine excretion

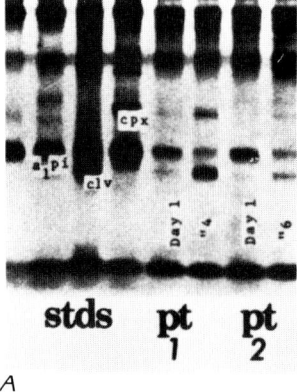

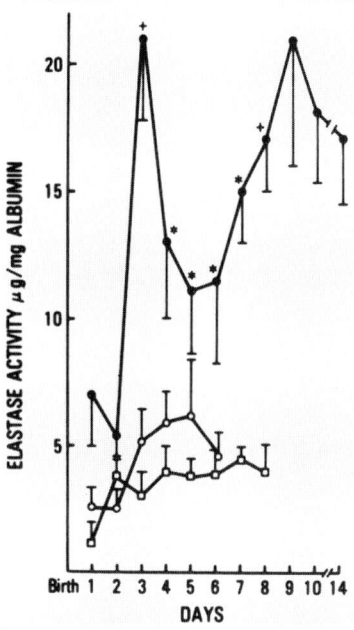

Figure 7.4. (*A*) Polyacrylamide gel electrophorises in 2 infants with BPD. On day 1 α, proteinase inhibitor shows only slight elastase complexing (cpx) and no cleavage (clv). By days 4 or 6, respectively, elastase-complexing of α, proteinase inhibitor and oxidative cleavage of this protein is evident.

Figure 7.4. (*B*) Elastase activity in tracheal aspirates (per mg albumin) from infants cited in Figure 7.2. (Reprinted with permission from Rockefeller Press, From Merritt TA, Cochrane CG, Holcomb K. et al. J Clin Invest 1983;72:656–662).

persisted for up to 9 days, but decreased thereafter, suggesting impaired elastin synthesis or turnover, perhaps related to nutritional deficiencies (80).

These findings document that proteolytic enzymes released by inflammatory cells in the lungs may play a pivotal role in the development of lung epithelial injury and connective tissue remodeling in the developing lung exposed to supplemental oxygen and mechanical ventilation. Indeed Jefferies *et al.* recently observed rapid pulmonary clearance of diethylenetriaminepentacetate (DTPA) labeled aerosols into the lungs of neonates with RDS developing BPD in a time course parallel to lung effluent protease activity (81). This observation suggests that proteolytic degradation of basement membrane and intercellular junctions are influencing fluid and gaseous exchange within the lung.

Several independent studies have provided complementary data demonstrating that elaboration of leukocytic proteases is coupled with low levels of antiprotease activities in preterm infants with respiratory distress who subsequently develop chronic lung disease. Although neutrophils may not be essential for oxidant induced lung injury (82), their universal abundance in pulmonary secretions of ventilated, oxygen treated infants strongly suggests their role in oxidant release on activation during the respiratory burst, and the release of proteolytic enzymes when degradation occurs. Importantly these biochemical measures precede the classical radiologic findings of BPD. Thus therapies designed to prevent or ameliorate BPD may require institution prior to, or soon after, the elaboration of free elastase or other proteases into the air spaces and before structural alteration of lung connective tissue and basement membrane structures ensues. Furthermore these measurements may provide useful indices of reduced or enhanced lung injury when employing new therapies. Although classical α_1PI deficiency is not found disproportionately among infants developing BPD, immature synthesis and increased inactivation or oxidation of this protein occurs in infants developing BPD. Whether antioxidant therapy, either as exogenous superoxide dismutase or catalase, or nutritional supplementation with α-tocopherol or retinol, will maintain pulmonary effluent antiprotease activity by reducing oxidant production or protect the retinol connective tissues from these proteolytic enzymes is under investigation. Other therapies using exogenous antioxidants including superoxide dismutase, catalase, or combinations of antioxidants are being evaluated in clinical trials. Recently Gerdes confirmed that dexamethasone treatment for BPD is associated with a 45% decrease in elastase levels (expressed as elastase/$2\alpha_1$PI) (83). Recent developments focused on restoring circulating antiprotease in PiZZ α_1-antiprotease deficient adults have been encouraging (84). Both a blood derived product and a deglycosylated form obtained by recombinant DNA technology have been used in pilot studies in deficient adults to restore levels in PiMA adults and maintain inhibitor balance in fluid obtained by bronchoalveolar lavage. Should these investigations show efficacious restoration of antiprotease activity and safety, clinical trials in neonates at high risk for developing BPD will be warranted. As cited in Chapter 22, by Rosenfeld and Concepcion, clinical trials using a variety of antioxidants and enzymes critical to the reduction of oxygen toxicity, with quenching of superoxide anion or $^-$OH are currently under way. One hopes that in the near future combination antioxidant therapy and enhanced antiprotease activity can ameliorate the outcome of oxidant induced lung injury in newborn infants.

References

1. Northway WH Jr, Rosan RC, Porter DY. Pulmonary disease following respirator therapy of hyaline membrane disease: bronchopulmonary dysplasia. N Engl J Med 1967;276:357–361.
2. Rosan RC. Hyaline membrane disease and related spectrum of neonatal pneumopathies. In: Rosenberg HS, Bolande RP, eds. Perspectives in pediatric pathology, vol 2. Chicago: Year Book Medical Publishers, 1975, pp 15–60.
3. Taghizadeh A, Reynolds EOR. Pathogenesis of bronchopulmonary dysplasia following hyaline membrane disease. Am J Pathol 1976;82:241–252.
4. Bonikos DS, Bensch KG, Northway WH Jr, Edwards DK. Bronchopulmonary dysplasia: the pulmonary pathologic sequel of necrotizing broncholitis and pulmonary fibrosis. Hum Pathol 1976;7:643–651.
5. Reid L. Bronchopulmonary dysplasia: pathology. J Pediatr 1976;95:836–841.
6. Edwards DK, Colby TV, Northway WH Jr. Radiologic-pathologic correlation in bronchopulmonary dysplasia. J Pediatr 1979;95:836–838.
7. National Heart, Lung, and Blood Institute. Workshop on Bronchopulmonary Dysplasia. J Pediatr 1979;85:815–920.
8. Nickerson BG, Taussig LM. Family history of asthma in infants with bronchopulmonary dysplasia. Pediatrics 1980;65:1140–1144.
9. James DK, Chiswick ML, Harkes A, Williams M, Hallworth J. Nonspecificity of surfactant deficiency in neonatal respiratory disorders. Parit Med J 1984;288:1635–1638.
10. Ikegami M, Jobe A, Jacobs H, Lam R. A protein from airways of premature lambs that inhibits surfactant function. J Appl Physiol 1984;57:1134–1142.
11. Seeger W, Stohr G, Wolf H, Neuhoff H. Alteration of surfactant function due to protein leakage: special interaction with fibrin monomer. J Appl Physiol 1985;58:326–338.

12. Bland R. Edema formation in the newborn lung. Clin Perinatol 1982;9:593–601.
13. Bland RD. Dynamics of pulmonary water before and after birth. Acta Pediatr Scand (suppl) 1983;305:12–20.
14. Bland RD. Cord-blood total protein level as a screening and for idiopathic respiratory distress syndrome. N Engl J Med 1972;287:9–13.
15. Brown ER, Stark A, Sosenko I, Lawson EE, Avery ME. Bronchopulmonary dysplasia: possible relationship to pulmonary edema. J Pediatr 1978;92:982.
16. Jobe A, Ikegami M, Jacobs H. Permeability of preterm lamb lungs to protein and the effect of surfactant on that permeability. J Appl Physiol: Respirat Environ Exercise Physiol 1983;55:169–176.
17. Inoue H, Inoue C, Hildebrandt J. Vascular and airway pressures and interstitial edema affect peribronchial fluid pressure. J Appl Physiol 1980;48:177–181.
18. Nilsson R, Grossman G, Robertson B. Lung surfactant and the pathogenesis of neonatal bronchiolar lesions induced by artificial ventilation. Pediatr Res 1978;12:249–254.
19. Merritt TA, Stuard ID, Puccia J, et al. Newborn tracheal aspirate cytology: classification during respiratory distress syndrome and bronchopulmonary dysplasia. J Pediatr 1981;98:949–954.
20. Doshi N, Kanbour A, Fujikura J, Klionsky B. Tracheal aspiration in neonates with respiratory distress: histopathologic correlation. Acta Cytol 1982;26:15–19.
21. Warner A. Clinical aspects of mucociliary transport. Am Rev Dis 1977;116:73–125.
22. Boat TF. Studies of oxygen toxicity in cultured human neonatal respiratory epithelium. J Pediatr 1979;95:916–918.
23. Nilssen R. Lung compliance and lung morphology following artificial ventilation in the premature and fullterm rabbit neonate. Scand J Respir Dis 1979;60:206–210.
24. Wood BP, Anderson VM, Mauk JE, Merritt TA. Pulmonary lymphatic air: locating "pulmonary interstitial emphysema" of the premature infant. AJR 1982;138:809–814.
25. Berg TJ, Pajtkhan RD, Reed MH, Langston C, Chernick V. Bronchopulmonary dysplasia and lung rupture in hyaline membrane disease and influence of continuous distending pressure. Pediatrics 1975;55:51–54.
26. Miller KE, Edwards DK, Hilton S, Collins D, Lynch F, Williams R. Acquired lobar emphysema in premature infants with bronchopulmonary dysplasia: an iatrogenic disease? Radiology 1981;138:589–591.
27. Petty TL, Ashbaugh DG. The adult respiratory distress syndrome: clinical features, factors influencing prognosis and principles of management. Chest 1971;60:233–239.
28. Ashbaugh DG, Bigelow DB, Petty TL, Levine BE. Acute respiratory distress syndrome in adults. Lancet 1967;2:319–339.
29. Rinaldo JE, Rogers RM. Adult respiratory distress syndrome: changed concepts of lung injury and repair. N Engl J Med 1982;306:900–909.
30. Bone RC. Adult respiratory distress syndrome. Clin Chest Med 1982;3:1–215.
31. Thorgeirsson G, Robertson AL. The vascular endothelium—pathobiologic significance: a review. Am J Pathol 1978;93:808–838.
32. Hallman M, Spragg R, Harrell J, Moser K, Gluck L. Evidence of lung surfactant abnormality in respiratory failure: study of bronchoalveolar lavage phospholipids, surface activity, phospholipase activity, and plasma myoinositol. J Clin Invest 1982;70:673–683.
33. Rauvala H, Hallman M. Glycolipid accumulation in bronchoalveolar space in adult respiratory distress syndrome. J Lipid Res 1984;25:1257–1262.
34. Lee CT, Fein A, Lippman M, Holtzman H, Kimbel P, Weinbaum G. Elastolytic activity in pulmonary lavage fluid from patients with adult respiratory distress syndrome. N Engl J Med 1981;304:192–196.
35. McGuire W, Spragg R, Cohen A, Cochrane C. Studies on the pathogenesis of adult respiratory distress syndrome. J Clin Invest 1982;69:543–553.
36. Merritt TA. Oxygen exposure in the newborn guinea pig lung lavage cell populations, chemotactic, and elastase response: a possible relationship to neonatal bronchopulmonary dysplasia. Pediatr Res 1982;16:798–805.
37. Merritt TA, Cochrane CG, Holcomb K. et al.

Elastase and alpha-1-proteinase activity in tracheal aspirates: inflammation in the pathogenesis of bronchopulmonary dysplasia. J Clin Invest 1983;72:656–662.

38. Gadek JE, Fells GA, Zimmerman RL, Rennard SI. Antielastases of the human alveolar structures: implications for the protease–antiprotease theory of emphysema. J Clin Invest 1981;68:889–898.

39. Evans HE, Keller S, Mandl I. Serum trypsin inhibitory capacity and the idiopathic respiratory distress syndrome. J Pediatr 1972;81:588–595.

40. El-Bardeesy MW, Johnson AM. Serum proteinase inhibitors in infants with hyaline disease. J Pediatr 1972;81:579–583.

41. Mathis RK, Freier E, Hunt C, Krivit W, Sharp H. Alpha-1-antitrypsin in respiratory distress syndrome. N Engl J Med 1973;288:59–63.

42. Singer AD, Thibeault D, Hobel C, Heiner D. Alpha-1-antitrypsin in amniotic fluid and cord blood of preterm infants with respiratory distress syndrome. J Pediatr 1976;88:87–92.

43. Bland RD. Cord blood total protein level as a screening aid for the idiopathic respiratory distress syndrome. N Engl J Med 1972;287:9–13.

44. Rosenfeld W, Concepcion L, Evans H, Jhaveri R, Brunst V. Alpha-1-antitrypsin (AAT) activity in development of bronchopulmonary dysplasia. Pediatr Res 1984;18:403A.

45. Andrew M, Massicotte-Nolan P, Karpaatkin M. Plasma protease inhibitors in premature infants: influence of gestational age, postnatal age, and health status. Proc Exp Biol Med 1983;173:495–500.

46. Kueppers F, Offord KP. Alpha-1-antitrypsin in health neonates. J Lab Clin Med 1979;94:475–480.

47. Bruce MC, Boat TF, Martin RJ, Dearborn D, Fanaroff A. Inactivation of alpha proteinase inhibitor in infants exposed to high concentrations of oxygen. Am Rev Respir Dis 1981;123:166.

48. Keeley FW, Fagan DG, Webster SI. Quantity and character of elastin in developing human lung parenchymal tissues of normal infants and infants with respiratory distress syndrome. J Lab Clin Med 1977;90:981–989.

49. Hance A, Crystal RG. The connective tissue of lung. Am Rev Respir Dis 1975;112:657.

50. Zapol WM, Trelsted RL, Coffey JW, Tsai L, Salvador RA. Pulmonary fibrosis in severe acute respiratory failure. Am Rev Respir Dis 1979;119:547.

51. Last JA, Siefkin AD, Reiser KM. Type I collagen is increased in lungs of patients with adult respiratory distress syndrome. 1983;38:364.

52. Shoemaker CT, Reiser KM, Goetzman B, Last J. Elevated ratios of type I/III collagen in the lungs of chronically ventilated neonates with respiratory distress. Pediatr Res 1984;18:1176–1180.

53. Rennard SI, Ferrans VJ, Bradley KH, Crystal RG. Lung connective tissue. In: Witschi H, ed. Mechanisms in respiratory toxicology, vol 2. Boca Raton, Fla: CRC Reviews, 1982, pp 115–153.

54. Hance AJ, Crystal RG. The connective tissue of lung. Am Rev Respir Dis 1975;112:657–711.

55. Hance AJ, Bradley K, Crystal RG. Lung collagen heterogeneity: synthesis of type I and type III collagen by rabbit and human lung cells in culture. J Clin Invest 1976;57:102–111.

56. Bitterman PB, Rennard SI, Adelberg S, Crystal RG. Role of fibronectin as growth factor for fibroblasts. J Cell Biol 1983;97:1925–1932.

57. Bitterman PB, Rennard SI, Adelberg S, Crystal RG. Role of fibronectin as a growth factor for fibroblasts. J Cell Biol 1983;97:1925–1932.

58. Yamada KM, Olden K. Fibronectin-adhesive glycoproteins of cell surface and blood. Nature 1978;275:1979–1981.

59. Niehaus GD, Schumacker PT, Saba TM. Influence of opsonic fibronectin deficiency on lung fluid balance during bacterial sepsis. J Appl Physiol 1980;49:693–697.

60. Rennard SI, Crystal RG. Fibronectin in human bronchopulmonary lavage fluid: elevation in patients with interstitial lung disease. J Clin Invest 1981;69:113–117.

61. Saba TM, Jaffe E. Plasma fibronectin (opsonic glycoprotein): its synthesis by vascular endothelial cells and role in cardiopulmonary integrity after trauma as related to reticuloendothelial function. Am J Med 1980;68:577–581.

62. Gerdes JS, Yoder M, Douglas S, Paul M, Harris M, Polin R. Tracheal lavage and plasma

fibronectin: relationship to respiratory distress syndrome and development of bronchopulmonary dysplasia. J Pediatr 1986;108:601–606.
63. Rennard SI, Hunninghake GW, Bitterman PB, Crystal RG. Production of fibronectin by the human alveolar macrophage: mechanism for the recruitment of fibroblasts to sites of injury in interstitial lung diseases. Proc Nat Acad Sci USA 1981;78:7147-7149.
64. Czop JK, Kadish JL, Austen K. Augmentation of human monocyte opsonin independent phagocytosis by fragments of human plasma fibronectin. Proc Nat Acad Sci USA 1981;78: 3649–3651.
65. Norris DA, Clark RAF, Swigard LM, Huff JC, Weston WL, Howell SE. Fibronectin fragments are chemotactic for human peripheral blood monocytes. J Immunol 1982;129:1612–1614.
66. Villiger B. Function of pulmonary alveolar macrophage fibronectin. Curr Probl Clin Biochem 1983;13:190–192.
67. Yoder MC, Douglas SD, Gerdes JS, Kline J, Polin RA. Plasma fibronectin in healthy newborn infants, respiratory distress syndrome, and perinatal asphyxia. J Pediatr 1983;102:777–779.
68. Delemos R, Wolfsdorf J, Hachman R. Lung injury from oxygen in lambs. Anesthesiology 1969;30:609–618.
69. Frank L, Bucher JR, Roberts RJ. Oxygen toxicity in neonatal and adult animals of various species. J Appl Physiol 1978;45:699–704.
70. Ogden B, Murphy S, Saunders G, Pathak D, Johnson J. Neonatal lung neutrophils and elastase/proteinase inhibitor imbalance. Am Rev Respir Dis 1984;130:817–821.
71. Ohlsson K, Olsson I. The neutral proteases of human granulocytes: isolation and partial characterization of granulocyte elastase. Eur J Biochem 1974;42:519–527.
72. Weissman G, Smolen JE, Korchak HME. Release of inflammatory mediators from stimulated neutrophils. N Engl J Med 1980;303:27–34.
73. Sklar L, McNeil V, Jesaitis A, Pointer RG, Cochrane C. A continuous spectroscopic analysis of the kinetics of elastase secretion by neutrophils. J Biol Chem 1982;257:5471–5475.

74. McDonald JA, Kelly DG. Degradation of fibronectin by human leukocyte elastase: release of biologically active fragments. J Biol Chem 1980;225:8848–8858.
75. Havemann K, Gramse M. Physiology and pathophysiology of neutral proteinases of human granulocytes. Adv Exp Med 1984;167:1–20.
76. Lavi G, Zucker-Franklin D, Franklin EC. Elastase-type proteases on the surface of human blood monocytes: possible role in amyloid formation. J Immunol 1980;125:175–180.
77. Werb Z, Banda MJ, Jones PA. Degradation of connective tissue matrices by macrophages. I. Proteolysis of elastin, glycoproteins, and collagen by proteinases isolated from macrophages. J Exp Med 1980;150:1527–1536.
78. Orlowski M, Orlowski J, Lesser M, Kilburn KH. Proteolytic enzymes in bronchopulmonary lavage fluids: cathespin B like activity and prolylendopeptidase. J Lab Clin Med 1981;97:467–476.
79. Bruce M, Boat T, Martin R, Dearborn D, Fanaroff A. Proteinase inhibitors and inhibitor inactivation in neonatal airway secretions. Chest 1982;81(suppl):445–455.
80. Bruce MC, Wedig E, Jentoft N, Martin RJ, Cheng PW, Boat TF, Fanaroff A. Altered urinary excretion of elastin cross-links in premature infants who develop bronchopulmonary dysplasia. Am Rev Respir Dis 1985;131:568–572.
81. Jefferies AL, Coates G, O'Brodovich H. Pulmonary epithelial permeability in hyaline membrane disease. N Engl J Med 1984;811: 1075–1080.
82. Raj JH, Hazinski TA, Bland RD. Oxygen-induced lung microvascular injury in neutropenic rabbits and lambs. J Appl Physiol: Respirat Environ Exercise Physiol 1985;58:920–927.
83. Gerdes JS, Harris M, Dworanczyk R, Polin R. Effect of dexamethasone and intercurrent infection on tracheal lavage elastase and alpha-1-proteinase inhibitor in bronchopulmonary dysplasia. Pediatr Res 1986;20:429A.
84. Wewers MD, Casolaro MA, Sellers S. et al. Replacement therapy for alpha$_1$-antitrypsin deficiency associated with emphysema. N Engl J Med 1987;316:1053–1061.

8

Alterations in Surfactant Composition

MICHAEL OBLADEN

Introduction

Two decades of extensive research on pulmonary surfactant have not resulted in the coining of a generally accepted definition for this unique biologic material, and some controversy still exists concerning its biochemical composition and physical structure. The classic function of surfactant is lowering of surface tension at the air-water interphase, which counteracts the tendency for alveolar collapse during expiration. Other important functions are adsorption from the subphase, formation of a highly organized film, respreading, promotion of capillary filling and mucociliary clearance, prevention of pulmonary edema, and prevention of mucus adhesion to the airways.

The major compound responsible for the surface tension lowering potential is phosphatidylcholine, which is mainly esterified with palmitic acid; the properties and metabolism of this substance have been extensively studied. The enormous mobility rendering different physical status to the film during inspiration and expiration is achieved by negatively charged, partly unsaturated "minor" phospholipids, mainly phosphatidylglycerol (in mature surfactant) or phosphatidylinositol (in preterm infants). Hallman and Gluck have shown that phosphatidylglycerol is absent in the surfactant of infants with respiratory distress syndrome (1). Specific surfactant apoproteins (34,000 daltons) seem to enhance spreading in the presence of calcium ion, while the lower molecular proteins (9,000 and 18,000) promote rapid adsorption and lower surface tensions of phospholipids.

In vivo surfactant exists in different physical and chemical forms and accumulates in at least three different pools: storage in the lamellar bodies within the type II cells; newly secreted material forming tubular myelin in the subphase; and functionally active material forming a film with monolayer characteristics at the air-water interphase.

In clinical studies different materials have been investigated, especially amniotic fluid, tracheal aspirates, and bronchoalveolar lavage. As demonstrated by film balance analysis, these fluids contain surface active material but they are not surfactant. Isolation and purification can be achieved by pelleting and density gradient centrifugation of bronchoalveolar lavage. Studies of tracheal aspirates, the only material obtainable from ventilated infants, however, do not allow extensive purification due to lack of quantity. Therefore metabolic studies cannot be performed with this material. Cells in tracheal aspirates have been analyzed by Merritt et al. (2), who found an increase in neutrophils and in elastase of neutrophil origin in infants who later developed bronchopulmonary dysplasia (BPD). The phospholipid profile of neonatal tracheal aspirates is well known and has been characterized by several groups (3, 4, 5, 6) in order to study the course of respiratory distress syndrome (RDS). It seemed justified, therefore, to look for the phospholipid profile

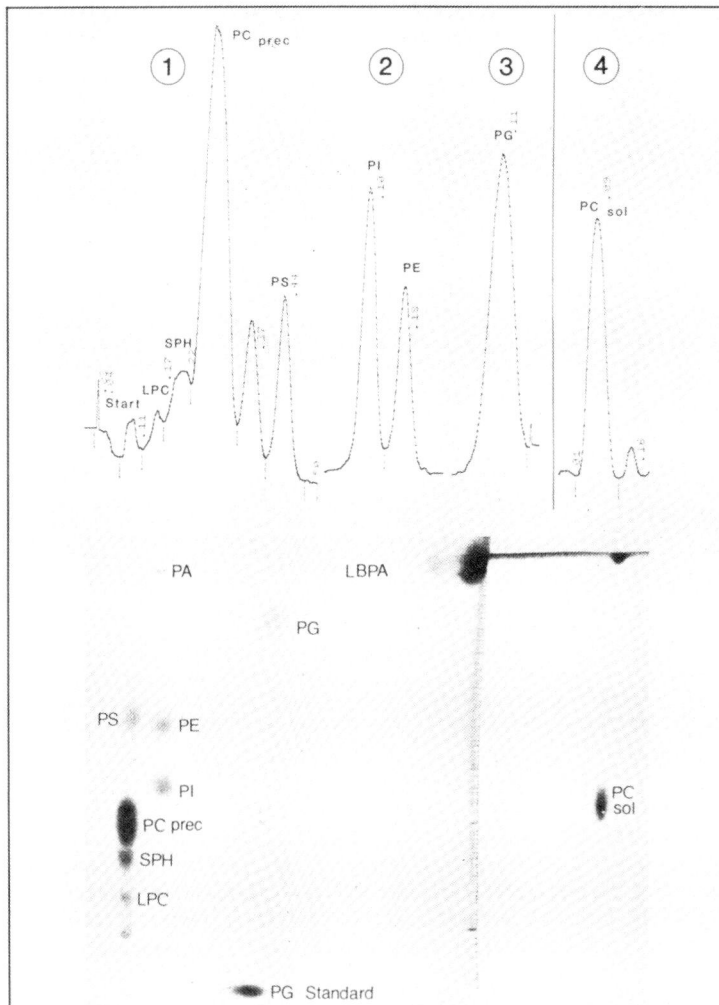

Figure 8.1. Tracheal aspirate phospholipid profile of a term neonate without pulmonary problems at birth. (*Bottom*) Two-dimensional thin layer chromatogram. (*Top*) Four scans of the same chromatogram as obtained by reflectance densitometry. Lecithin/sphingomyelin ratio 4.8; phosphatidylinositol/phosphatidylserine ratio 1.5, phosphatidylglycerol present, acetone precipitable lecithin 73% of total phosphatidylcholine. LPC = lysophosphatidylcholine; SPH = sphingomyelin; PC prec = acetone precipitable phosphatidylcholine; PI = phosphatidylinositol; PS = phosphatidylserine; PE = phosphatidylethanolamine; PA = phosphatidic acid; PG = phosphatidylglycerol; LBPA = lyso-bis-phosphatidic acid; PC sol = acetone soluble phosphatidylcholine.

in tracheal aspirates of infants with BPD beyond the neonatal period.

Materials and Methods

Tracheal aspirates of artificially ventilated infants were collected when therapeutic suctioning of the tracheal tube was required. After instillation of 0.5 to 1.0 ml of 0.15 M sodium chloride solution into the tube, the material was sampled into a type 478 collecting trap (Unoplast, Hundested, Denmark). Usually three subsequent suctionings were pooled and frozen at $-18°$ C. Phospholipid analysis was performed using the "lung profile" technique described by Kulovich et al. (7). Cellular debris was removed by 5 minutes of centrifugation at $750 \times$ g. Lipids were extracted according to Folch et al. (8), acetone precipitation was performed according to

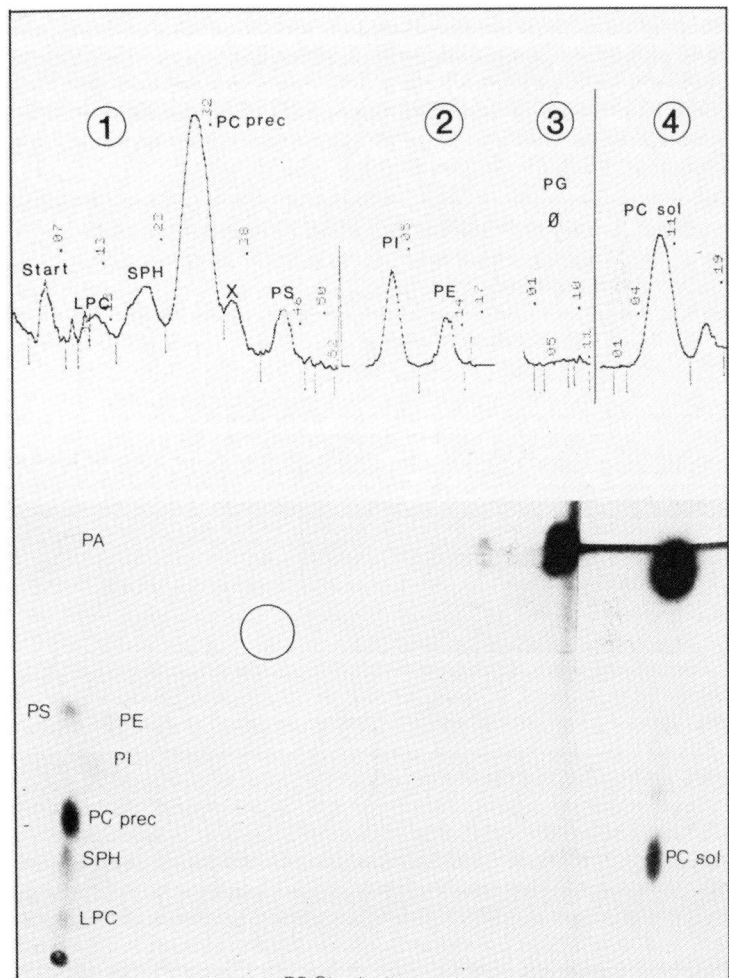

Figure 8.2. Tracheal aspirate phospholipid profile of an infant with Stage IV bronchopulmonary dysplasia requiring artificial ventilation with an FiO$_2$ of 1.0 at the age of 3 months. (*Bottom*) Two-dimensional thin layer chromatogram. (*Top*) Four scans of the same chromatogram as obtained by computer corrected reflectance densitometry. Lecithin/sphingomyelin ratio 3.7; phosphatidylinositol/phosphatidylserine ratio 0.9; phosphatidylglycerol still absent (circle), acetone precipitable lecithin 67% of total phosphatidylcholine. See Figure 8.1 for abbreviations.

Gluck et al. (9), and acetone soluble fractions and precipitable fractions were processed separately. Separation of phospholipids was achieved with two-dimensional thin layer chromatography according to Body and Gray (10) on silica gel H plates coated with a 200 μm layer prepared with 5% ammonium sulfate. Phospholipids were visualized by charring at 290° C. The chromatograms were evaluated by reflectance densitometry (Desaga Quick scan, Heidelberg, FRG); correction for baseline drift and incomplete peak separation was achieved with a computerized chromatography integrator (Spectra Physics 4100, Santa Clara, CA), as previously described (11).

Patients and Ventilator Management

Infants suffering from RDS were ventilated with time cycled, pressure limited ventilators (Bourns BP 200, Stephan monitor respirator) at rates of 50 to 60 min^{-1} and (an inspiratory-

Table 8.1. Tracheal Aspirate Phospholipid Patterns in Artificially Ventilated Human Infants

Infants	No.	Gest. Age (wk)	L/S	PI/PS	PG (+/−)	PC prec (%)
Term neonates without pulmonary problems	24	40.0 ± 1.5	4.88 ± 2.45	1.59 ± 1.09	24/0	46
Accelerated preterm infants without RDS	21	31.7 ± 3.5	4.65 ± 2.04	2.82 ± 1.10	17/4	42
RDS, day 1	26	31.8 ± 3.5	1.51 ± 0.41	0.93 ± 0.61	0/26	34
RDS, day 5	28	31.8 ± 2.9	4.89 ± 3.55	3.52 ± 2.08	2/26	44
BPD, day 18	20	27.9 ± 1.8	6.68 ± 4.59	3.52 ± 2.74	3/17	59
BPD, 3 mo	10	27.7 ± 2.0	8.21 ± 4.86	1.64 ± 0.87	4/6	67

L/S = ratio of lecithin to sphingomyelin; PI/PS = ratio of phosphatidylinositol to phosphatidylserine; PG = phosphatidylglycerol (+/− = PG present/PG absent); PC prec = acetone precipitable phosphatidylcholine, ratios represent mean ± SD; RDS = respiratory distress syndrome; BPD = bronchopulmonary dysplasia.

to-expiratory) ratio of 1:1 to 1:2. Initially peak inspiratory pressure was set to 20–25 cm H_2O. During recovery peak pressure was gradually reduced to 12 cm H_2O. Thereafter rates were reduced to intermittent mandatory ventilation or to continuous positive airway pressure. When BPD was suspected prolonged inspiration was avoided. BPD was diagnosed in infants requiring ventilator support or oxygen longer than 28 days (12) and showing typical radiologic evidence of BPD (13, 14). The following analysis is restricted to infants with birth weight below 1500 g and BPD Stages III or IV, according to the description of Northway et al. (15).

Results

A "normal" tracheal aspirate phospholipid profile obtained from a term neonate without pulmonary disease is shown in Figure 8.1. All surfactant phospholipids are present including phosphatidylglycerol and phosphatidylinositol. Figure 8.2 shows the tracheal aspirate phospholipid profile of a 3 month old preterm boy with severe BPD. At the time of analysis the infant is 2 weeks post-term. The aspirate's phospholipid content is lower than in the term neonate, phosphatidylcholine (PC) is normal, but phosphatidylinositol (PI) is low, and phosphatidylglycerol (PG) is still absent.

Typical lung profiles are shown in Table 8.1. At term the ratio of lecithin to sphingomyelin is usually above 2.0, PI is relatively low, and PG is present (this phospholipid usually appears after 35 weeks' gestation). Following chronic perinatal stress such as prolonged rupture of membranes, tocolytic treatment, or amniotic infection, some premature infants do not develop RDS because of "accelerated" lung maturation. In their tracheal effluent PI is increased, and often PG is present despite prematurity. Infants with RDS are characterized by decreased L/S ratio and total absence of PG. During the recovery phase of RDS a dramatic increase in PI occurs, but PG usually remains absent until 35 weeks' gestation. In infants with BPD the phospholipid lung profile may vary consider-

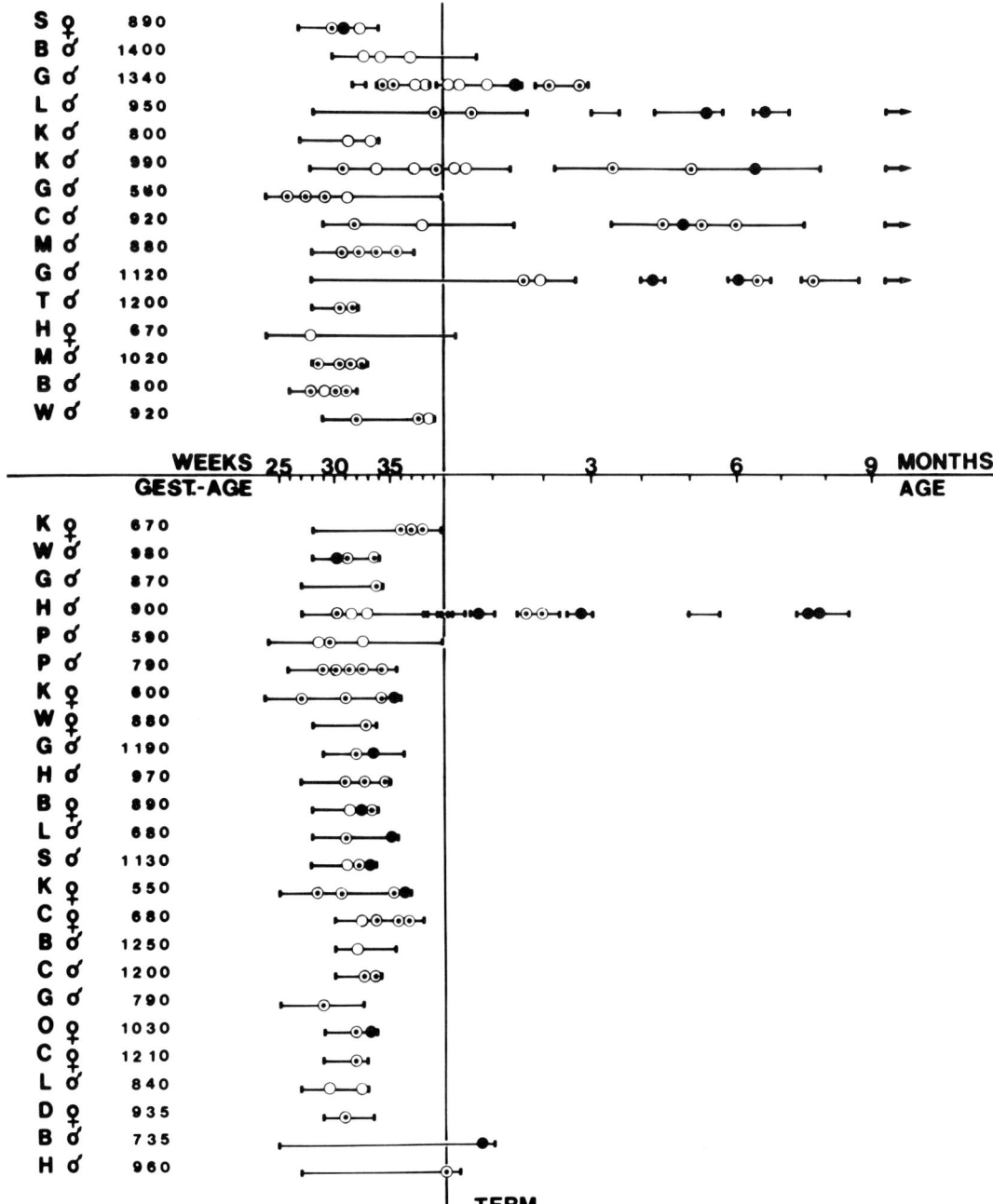

Figure 8.3. Birth weight (g), sex, duration of artificial ventilation (bars), and tracheal aspirate phospholipid patterns in 39 infants with bronchopulmonary dysplasia studied beyond 14 days of age. All infants ventilated since birth and plotted according to gestational age. Open circles: no phospholipids detectable in tracheal aspirate. Closed circles: all phospholipids including phosphatidylglycerol detectable in tracheal aspirate. Dotted circles: phosphatidylcholine and phosphatidylinositol, but not phosphatidylglycerol, detectable in tracheal aspirate. (*Top*) 15 infants with lethal course. (*Bottom*) 24 infants surviving BPD. In phases of clinical deterioration phosphatidylglycerol may disappear.

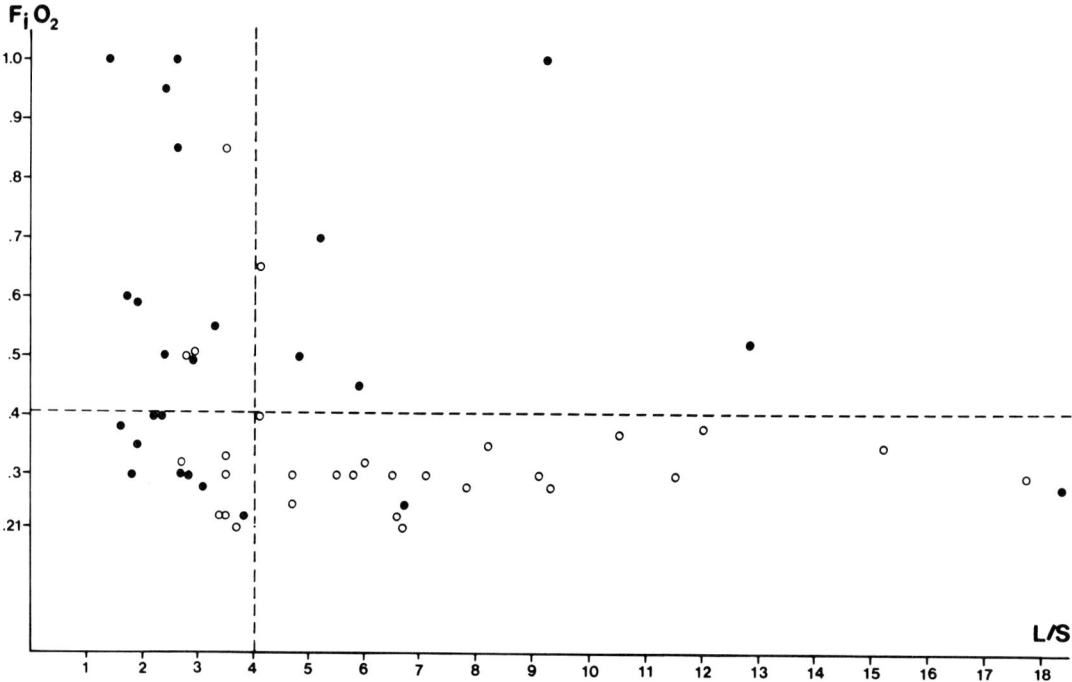

Figure 8.4. Tracheal aspirate lecithin/sphingomyelin ratio (L/S) compared with oxygen requirement (FiO$_2$). Measurements from infants with bronchopulmonary dysplasia, artificially ventilated longer than 28 days after birth. Both first and last samples are given for each infant. Closed circles: data from infants who later expired. Open circles: data from infants who later survived.

ably: usually the L/S ratio and the PI/PS ratio are high, and PG is absent even after term. The amount of acetone precipitable PC is higher than in the other groups.

In 156 very low birth weight infants admitted for RDS, serial tracheal aspirate analyses were performed. Stage III and IV BPD was diagnosed in 39 infants with prolonged (more than 28 days) respiratory insufficiency and typical x-ray findings. Of these infants fifteen died and 24 survived. Of the 39 BPD infants, 28 were male, as were 13 of the 15 infants who died. Figure 8.3 depicts duration of artificial ventilation and results of 128 tracheal aspirate analyses performed in these infants at the age of more than 2 weeks, when RDS was no longer present and BPD was suspected (mean age at first suspicion = 16 days). In many infants with BPD, tracheal aspirates remained free of PG for a prolonged period. In some infants who had to return to artificial ventilation, this phospholipid had disappeared again, even if formerly present. In infants with lethal course of BPD (upper part of graph), PG appeared several months later than in infants surviving BPD.

Figure 8.4 compares the ratio of lecithin to sphingomyelin with the need for oxygen. No linear correlation was found, but infants with FiO$_2$ above 0.4 usually had an L/S ratio below 4.0. An L/S ratio below 2.5 was found in nonsurvivors only.

ALTERATIONS IN SURFACTANT COMPOSITION

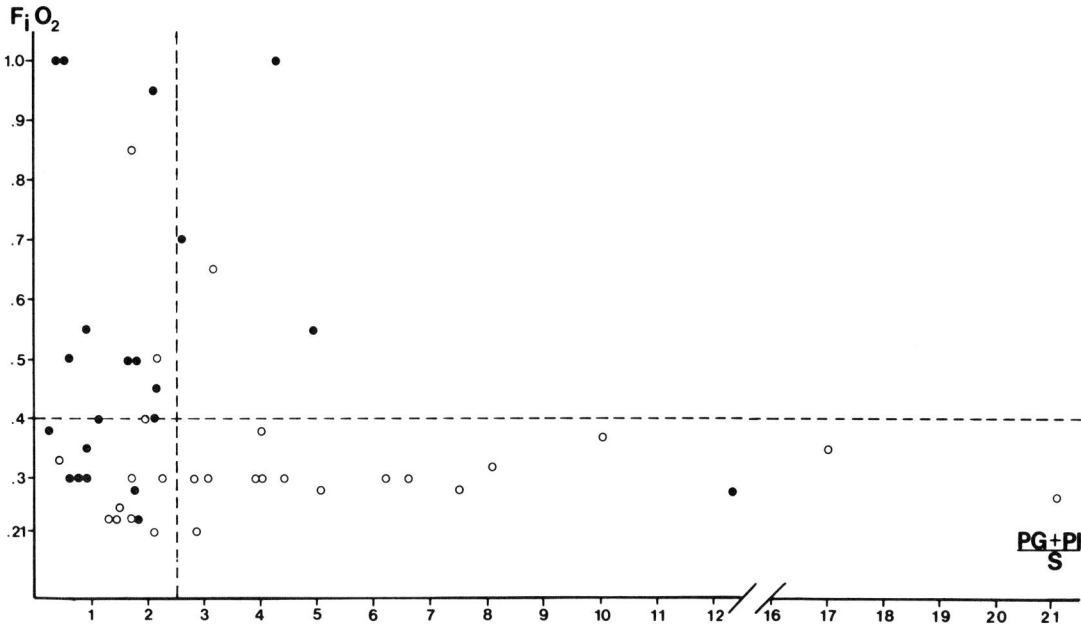

Figure 8.5. Tracheal aspirate ratio of phosphatidylglycerol plus phosphatidylinositol to sphingomyelin (PG+PI/S) compared with oxygen requirement (FiO$_2$). Measurements from infants with bronchopulmonary dysplasia, artificially ventilated longer than 28 days after birth. Both first and last samples are given for each infant. Closed circles: data from infants who later expired. Open circles: data from infants who survived.

Figure 8.5 shows the same type of correlation between oxygen need and the minor phospholipids, with PI and PG cumulated. Presence or absence of PI and PG allowed the discrimination of survivors and nonsurvivors of BPD ($p < .01$). In half of the infants with lethal BPD (Fig. 9.4), *no* phospholipids could be detected in tracheal aspirates around term.

Discussion

The data presented here suggest a persisting inadequacy of the surfactant system in BPD. The usual recovery phase of RDS, increase of phosphatidylinositol and appearance of phosphatidylglycerol (5), does not occur or may be delayed for several months. The abnormalities in phospholipid composition differ somewhat from those characteristic for RDS, as phosphatidylcholine is usually present and is diminished only in terminal stages of BPD. These findings do not allow us to ascribe a causative role in the pathogenenesis of BPD to surfactant deficiency, as this may well be secondary to the proliferative changes leading to diminished type II cells (15, 16). However, surfactant pathology may help to explain several pathophysiologic mechanisms present in BPD. Surfactant has several biologic functions other than lowering of surface tension during expiration, which is the main characteristic of a mixed film containing saturated phosphatidylcholine (Figure 8.6). Increased surface ten-

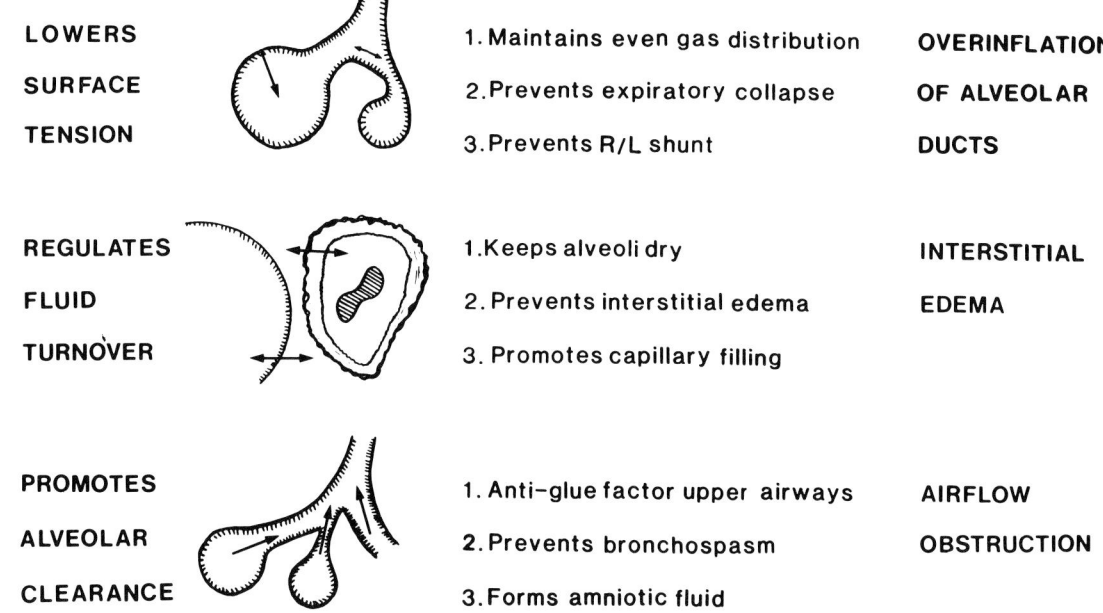

Figure 8.6. Basic surfactant functions and possible contribution of persisting surfactant inadequacy to specific features of bronchopulmonary dysplasia.

sion promotes closure of alveoli and dilates alveolar ducts during artificial ventilation, which may contribute to the early cyst formation in BPD (17).

Pressures at the air-water interphase cannot be evaluated independent of pressures in capillaries and interstitial fluid. The pressure equilibration causes considerable movement of the surfactant layer within the alveoli. This mechanism normally leads to a fluid transfer from capillaries to alveolar surface, and from alveolar surface to lymphatic vessels, which has been termed "alveolar wash mechanism" by Guyton et al. (18). An increased transvascular pressure gradient will promote edema (19). As recently demonstrated by Jefferies et al. (20), the lung of neonates with RDS is abnormally permeable to small solutes, and this increased permeability persists in infants with BPD.

Surfactant is not only present in the alveoli but also covers bronchioli and upper airways, promoting mucociliary clearance (21) and exerting an anti-glue effect within the airways. Persisting inadequacy of the surfactant layer may lead to adhesion of mucus and may promote airway obstruction, a feature regularly present in BPD. Bronchial hyperreactivity has been described in survivors of the disorder (22) and may be enhanced by increased mucus adhesion.

In infants who had died from sudden infant death syndrome, Morley et al. (23) found levels of surfactant phospholipids to be diminished in comparison with those in infants who died from other causes. If surfactant inadequacy persists for many months, or if surfactant disintegrates in BPD patients during lower airway infections, this finding may explain the increased incidence of sudden infant death syndrome in infants with BPD (24).

Oxygen toxicity to the lungs of preterm infants with RDS, was suspected as early as 1835 by Jörg (25). Free oxygen radicals seem to play a role in producing chronic lung injury following neonatal RDS. Several studies have shown that oxygen intermediates can damage the surfactant system and do interfere with phospholipid metabolism (26, 27).

The analysis of tracheal aspirates gives valuable insights to the still incompletely understood pathogenetic pathways in BPD. It may help to evaluate new forms of treatment such as high-frequency oscillatory ventilation (28, 29, 30) or corticosteroids (31, 32), and to establish a reliable prognosis in infants suffering from this often fatal disorder.

References

1. Hallman M, Gluck L. Phosphatidylglycerol in lung surfactant. III. Possible modifier of surfactant fuction. J Lipid Res 1976;17:257–262.
2. Merritt TA, Stuard ID, Puccia J, et al. Newborn tracheal aspirate cytology: classification during respiratory distress syndrome and bronchopulmonary dysplasia. J Pediatr 1981;98:949–956.
3. Blumenfeld ThA, Driscoll JM, James LS. Lecithin/sphingomyelin ratios in tracheal and pharyngeal aspirates in respiratory distress syndrome. J Pediatr 1974;85:403.
4. Motoyama EK, Namba Y, Rooney SA. Phosphatidylcholine content and fatty acid composition of tracheal and gastric liquids from premature and fullterm newborn infants. Clin Chim Acta 1976;70:449–454.
5. Obladen M. Factors influencing surfactant composition in the newborn infant. Eur J Pediatr 1978;128(3):129–143.
6. Shelley SA, Kovacevic M, Paciga J, Balis JU. Sequential changes of surfactant phosphatidylcholine in hyaline-membrane disease of the newborn. N Engl J Med 1979;300:112–116.
7. Kulovich MV, Hallman M, Gluck L. The lung profile. I. Normal pregnancy. Am J Obstet Gynecol 1979;133:57.
8. Folch J, Lees M, Stanley GHS. A simple method for the isolation and purification of total lipids from animal tissue. J Biol Chem 1957;226:497.
9. Gluck L, Kulovich MV, Borer RC. Estimates of fetal lung maturity. Clin Perinatol 1974;1:125.
10. Body DR, Gray GM. The isolation and characterisation of phosphatidyl-glycerol and a structural isomer from pig lung. Chem Phys Lipids 1967;1:254–263.
11. Stevens P, Thiemann U, Obladen M. Computer-corrected neonatal lung profile. In: Herzog H, ed. Progress in respiration research. Volume 18. Basel: S Karger, 1984, pp 230–234.
12. Bancalari E, Abdenour GF, Feller R, Gannon J. Bronchopulmonary dysplasia: clinical presentation. J Pediatr 1979;95:819–823.
13. Edwards DK, Colby TV, Northway WH Jr. Radiographic-pathologic correlation in bronchopulmonary dysplasia. J Pediatr 1979;95:834–836.
14. Opperman HC, Wille L, Bleyl U, Obladen M. Bronchopulmonary dysplasia in premature infants. A radiological and pathological correlation. Pediatr Radiol 1977;5:137–141.
15. Northway WH Jr, Rosan RC, Porter DY. Pulmonary disease following respirator therapy of hyaline-membrane disease. N Engl J Med 1967;276:357–368.
16. Bonikos DS, Bensch KG, Northway WH Jr, Edwards DK. Bronchopulmonary dysplasia: the pulmonary pathologic sequel of necrotizing bronchiolitis and pulmonary fibrosis. Hum Pathol 1976;7:643–666.
17. Taghizadeh A, Reynolds EOR. Pathogenesis of bronchopulmonary dysplasia following hyaline membrane disease. Am J Pathol 1976;82:241–258.
18. Guyton AC, Moffatt DS, Adair T. Role of surface tension in trans-epithelial movement of fluid. In: Robertson B, von Golde LMG, Batenburg JJ, eds. Pulmonary surfactant. Amsterdam: Elsevier, 1984, pp 171–185.

19. Beck KC, Lai-Fook SJ. Alveolar liquid pressure in excised edematous dog lung with increased static recoil. J Appl Physiol 1983;55:1277–1283.
20. Jefferies AL, Coates G, O'Brodovich H. Pulmonary epithelial permeability in hyaline-membrane disease. N Engl J Med 1984;311:1075–1080.
21. Morgenroth K, Balz J. Morphological features of the interaction between mucus and surfactant on the bronchial mucosa. Respiration 1985;47:225–231.
22. Smyth JA, Tabachnik E, Duncan WJ, Reilly BJ, Levinson H. Pulmonary function and bronchial hyperreactivity in long-term survivors of bronchopulmonary dysplasia. Pediatrics 1981;68:336–340.
23. Morley CJ, Brown BD, Hill CM, Barson AJ. Surfactant abnormalities in babies dying from sudden infant death syndrome. Lancet 1982;1:1320–1323.
24. Werthammer J, Brown ER, Neff RK, Taeusch HW Jr. Sudden infant death syndrome in infants with bronchopulmonary dysplasia. Pediatrics 1982;69:301–304.
25. Jörg E. Die foetuslunge im geborenen kinde. Grimma, 1835.
26. Gross NJ, Smith DM. Impaired surfactant phospholipid metabolism in hyperoxic mouse lungs. J Appl Physiol: Respirat Environ Exercise Physiol 1981;51(5):1198–1203.
27. Ward JA, Roberts RJ. Effect of hyperoxia on phosphatidylcholine synthesis, secretion, uptake and stability in the newborn rabbit lung. Biochim Biophys Acta 1984;796:42–50.
28. Ennema JJ, Reijngoud D-J, Egberts J, Mook PH, Wildevuur CRH. High-frequency oscillation affects surfactant phospholipid metabolism in rabbits. Respir Physiol 1984;58:29–39.
29. Truog WE, Standaert TA, Murphy J, Palmer S, Woodrum DE, Hodson WA. Effect of high-frequency oscillation on gas exchange and pulmonary phospholipids in experimental hyaline membrane disease. Am Rev Respir Dis 1983;127:585–589.
30. Frantz ID, Werthammer J, Stark AR. High-frequency ventilation in premature infants with lung disease: adequate gas exchange at low tracheal pressure. Pediatrics 1983;71:483–488.
31. Mammel MC, Green TP, Johnson DE, Thompson TR. Controlled trial of dexamthasone therapy in infants with bronchopulmonary dysplasia. Lancet 1983;2:1356–1357.
32. Avery GB, Fletcher AB, Kaplan M, Brudno DS. Controlled trial of dexamethasone in respirator-dependent infants with bronchopulmonary dysplasia. Pediatrics 1985;75:106–111.

Comments

T. Allen Merritt

Those factors that initate the development of BPD are also harmful to preterm infants recovering from RDS associated with surfactant deficiency. Indeed a circular pathogenesis of RDS → early BPD → delayed surfactant recovery → chronic BPD can be envisioned and is supported by the data of Obladen. Precisely how ongoing lung injury by oxidants, barotrauma, and suboptimal nutrition during acute RDS results in alterations in surfactant quantity and composition (absence of phosphatidylglycerol for weeks or months and lower total surfactant phospholipids in pulmonary effluent during recovery from BPD) or in function within the terminal airways and alveoli is incompletely understood.

One goal of surfactant therapy is to replenish functional surfactant to enable the restoration of surface forces that will maintain alveolar expansion at end-expiration. This approach has tentatively proved successful in reducing BPD. Further efforts at nutritional modification (see Chapter 20) will undoubtedly prove a method to enhance synthesis and release of "mature" surfactant.

Little is known about the effects of chronic diuretic therapy on the surfactant system. Several beta-agonists and even theophylline are known to enhance surfactant synthesis in a variety of animal models. Prenatal glucocorticoid therapy for acceleration of pulmonary maturity has had limited success in reducing the occurrence of RDS, and it remains an attractive hypothesis that postnatal dexamethasone treatment may not only attentuate the inflammatory response to ongoing injury but also stimulate surfactant production.

In an era of surfactant treatment for RDS, one hopes that clinicians will have fewer cases of BPD, but the role of surfactant supplementation in infants with BPD remains to be explored.

9

Pulmonary Edema in Respiratory Distress Syndrome and Bronchopulmonary Dysplasia

HUGH M. O'BRODOVICH AND GEOFFREY COATES

Introduction

Bronchopulmonary dysplasia (BPD) is a chronic lung disease that develops all too frequently in very premature infants who have suffered acute lung injury in the first days or weeks of life (1). In order to increase the consistency of the diagnostic criteria and avoid relatively milder and transient forms of neonatal lung disease, in general BPD is not diagnosed until 28 days of life. The mechanisms responsible for the development of BPD, however, have likely been operative since, or perhaps even before, the birth of the infant. Therefore to understand the evolutionary process leading to BPD, attention must be focused on the early days and weeks of life. There is ever-increasing evidence that infants with BPD suffer appreciable lung injury during the early weeks of life, which results in pulmonary inflammation and edema. The purpose of this chapter is to discuss the potential mechanisms for the edema formation and inflammatory response that occur in these critically ill infants.

In 1967 Northway and coworkers (2) reported that BPD occurred in infants with severe respiratory distress syndrome (RDS) and that the evolution of chronic lung disease was steady and relentless. It has since become clear that very low birth weight infants can develop chronic lung disease without much radiographic evidence of pulmonary parenchymal disease, or even when ventilatory assistance is provided because of apnea (1). Although the latter is becoming an increasing problem with the increasing survival rate of babies weighing less than 750 grams at birth, this chapter focuses on the more typical evolutionary pathway to BPD—namely, acute pulmonary parenchymal lung disease (RDS) in the first week of life—and its progression to BPD.

Evidence of Pulmonary Edema

The lungs at the time of birth are completely filled with fluid. Fortunately the protein concentration of fetal lung liquid is extremely low (30 mg/100 mL). This negligible protein concentration enables the alveolar liquid to move rapidly out of the air space (3) and in large part explains the rapid fall in lung water content following birth observed in healthy newborn rabbits (4), lambs (5), and humans (6, 7) (Fig. 9.1). The mode of delivery can influence lung water content: even when a fetal animal has normal mature lungs, caesarean section delivery can result in an increase in the gravimetric lung water content for at least the first day of life (4). The human clinical correlate of this inadequate clearance of normal lung water at birth is transient tachypnea of the newborn. It could therefore be anticipated that

EFFECT OF GESTATIONAL AGE, POSTNATAL AGE AND RESPIRATORY DISTRESS ON INFANT LUNG WATER CONTENT

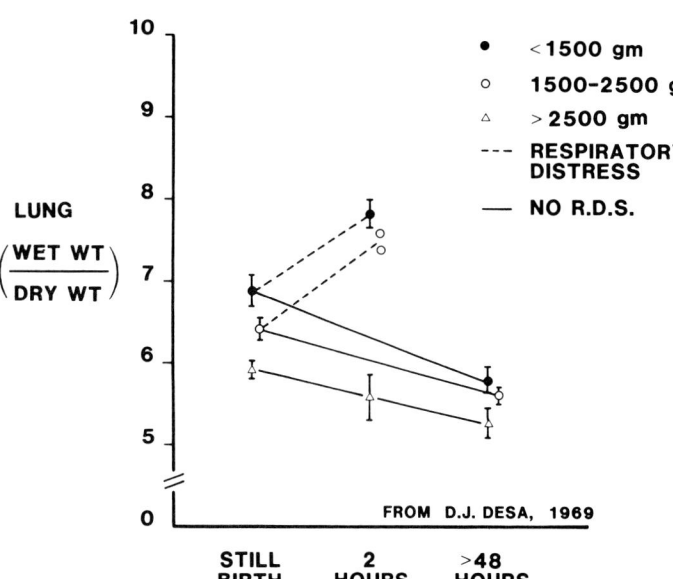

Figure 9.1. Effect of birth weight, postnatal age, and clinical respiratory distress on postmortem lung water content, calculated from the data of deSa (6, 7). Regardless of birth weight infants who develop respiratory distress increase their lung water content rather than showing the usual postpartum decline. (Reprinted, with permission, from H. M. O'Brodovich. Pulmonary edema in unresolved neonatal acute lung injury. In: Farrell PM, Taussig LM, eds. Bronchpulmonary dysplasia and related chronic respiratory disorders, Report of the 90th Ross Conference on Pediatric Research. Columbus, Ohio: Ross Laboratories, 1986, p 69.)

caesarean section delivery of infants at risk for RDS would further increase the excess fluid burden on their lungs.

Neonatal pulmonary parenchymal disease could alter lung water content by impairing the clearance of fetal lung liquid. The protein concentration of pulmonary edema fluid, although lower in high-pressure pulmonary edema than it is in increased permeability pulmonary edema, is substantially greater than the protein concentration in fetal lung liquid. Therefore the presence of edema from either of these mechanisms will delay the clearance of excess lung water because of the intra-alveolar protein. Matthay *et al.* have shown that protein, once in the air space, is cleared extremely slowly (1%/hr), and that this intra-alveolar protein slows fluid clearance by its osmotic properties (8). It could therefore be anticipated that pulmonary edema occurring in the first day of life will be slow to resolve, especially when alveolar capillary permeability and protein leakage are increased, as is the case in RDS (see below).

Pulmonary edema is an invariable component of RDS in newborn infants (6, 7, 9). deSa has provided gravimetric evidence that preterm human neonates who develop respiratory distress demonstrate increasing lung water content instead of the normal postnatal decline toward adult values (6, 7) (Fig. 8.1). This finding of increased lung water content has been confirmed in studies of prematurely born primates with RDS in which lung water measurements could be more carefully controlled (10). Lung water content has not been measured in BPD, but the postmortem examinations of human infants who were developing BPD have edematous interstitial spaces and distended lymphatics (11, 12) (Fig. 9.2). There is marked pulmonary edema in RDS, and the hyaline membranes signify that this edema fluid is protein-rich. Therefore, on the basis of our knowledge of alveolar fluid clearance (see above), it is likely that lung water content is increased in BPD.

Mechanisms of Edema Formation in HMD and BPD

There is a normal continuous net outward movement of water and solute from fluid-exchanging vessels (microvasculature) into the pulmonary interstitium. This fluid is then cleared by the lymphatics or reabsorbed by the downstream pulmonary or bronchial vasculature. When the efflux of fluid from the microvasculature exceeds the capacity of the lung's clearance mechanisms, fluid will accumulate, and by definition pulmonary edema is present. When this excess lung fluid remains within the interstitial space, it has minimal effect on lung function; however, when the reservoirs for storing excess fluid (predominantly the bronchovascular sheaths) are overwhelmed, then fluid spills into the terminal lung units with deleterious effects on pulmonary hemodynamics and gas exchange (12a).

The pressures involved in transvascular fluid exchange were described by Starling in the nineteenth century. Subsequent investigators expanded upon his basic observations and developed the equation that bears Starling's name and describes fluid movement across a semipermeable membrane.

$$\dot{Q} = K_f (P_{mv} - P_{pmv}) - K_f \cdot \sigma(\pi_{mv} - \pi_{pmv})$$

Where $\dot{Q}$ is the net flow rate of fluid across the membrane, K_f is the filtration coefficient and represents the membrane surface area available for fluid exchange and permeability of that membrane to fluid, P_{mv} and P_{pmv} are the hydrostatic pressures inside and outside (perimicrovascular) the microvessel, π_{mv} and π_{pmv} are the protein osmotic pressures inside and outside the microvessels, while σ is the reflection coefficient and describes the ability of the membrane to restrict transvascular protein movement. The equation is easier to understand in conceptual terms—that is, the amount of fluid leaving a vessel is affected by the net transvascular hydrostatic pressure gradient ($P_{mv} - P_{pmv}$), the net transvascular protein osmotic pressure gradient ($\pi_{mv} - \pi_{pmv}$), the amount of perfused microvascular surface area (part of the K_f term), and the permeability of the microvessels to fluid (K_f) and protein (σ). To aid in the understanding of mechanisms involved in the production of pulmonary edema in RDS and presumably in BPD, the next portion of the chapter discusses each of the components of the Starling equation in relationship to the pathophysiologic characteristics of these pulmonary disorders.

Intravascular Forces

Two opposing forces within the microvessel influence transvascular water and solute movement: the intravascular hydrostatic pressure promotes outward movement of fluid whereas the intravascular protein osmotic pressure retains fluid within the vessel

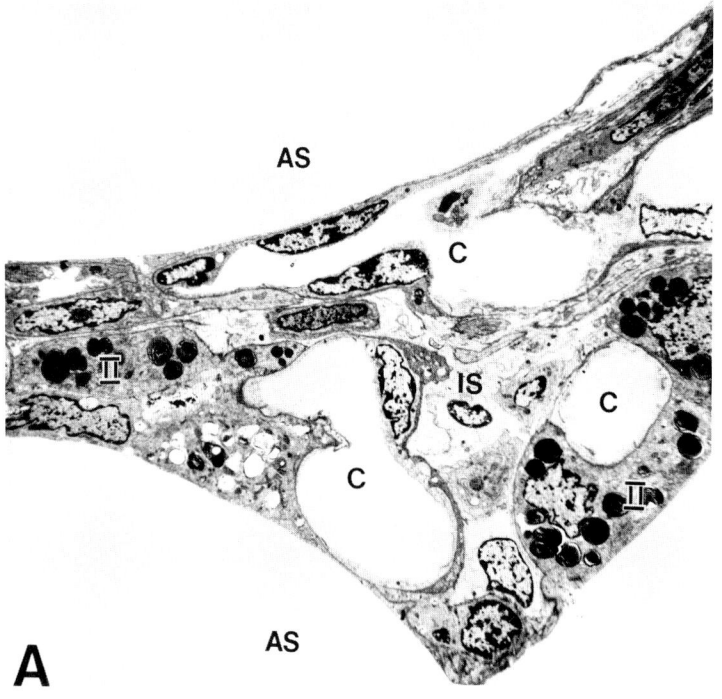
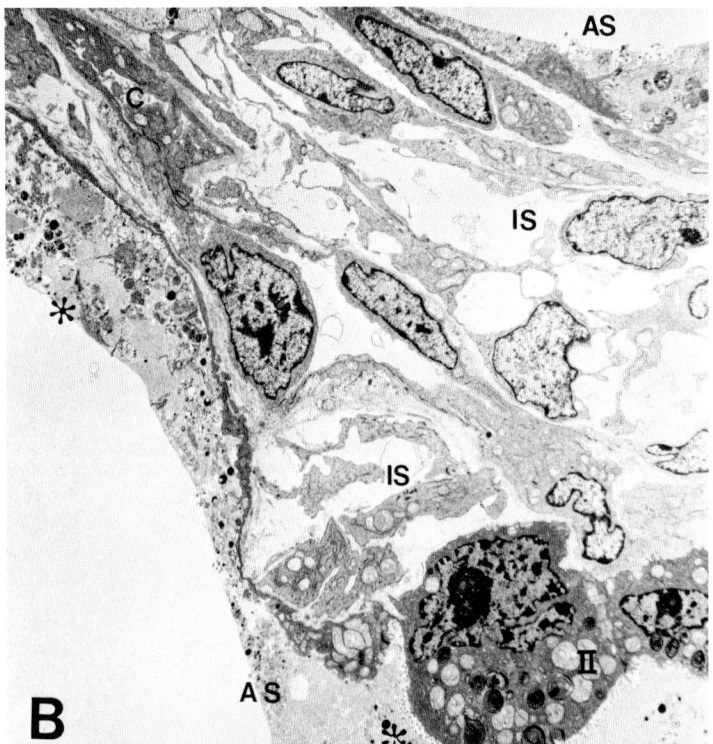

Figure 9.2. (*A*) Specimen from a premature baboon (75% gestation) ventilated for 11 days with oxygen only as needed shows several capillaries (C), a few cells within the interstitium (IS) and types I and II epithelial cells (II). (*B*) Specimen from a premature baboon ventilated for 11 days with 100% oxygen has a markedly widened interstitium (IS), which shows edema and increased cells. Only one capillary (C) is evident. Cellular debris and edema are evident over the epithelium (*). AS = alveolar space. Uranyl acetate and lead citrate; ×2000 and ×2300, respectively. (Electronmicrographs courtesy of J. J. Coalson, Ph.D., San Antonio, Tex.)

and promotes reabsorption of fluid from the interstitium back into the microvessel.

The intravascular hydrostatic pressure within the pulmonary microvasculature is not known precisely, especially when the lung is diseased. It must be greater than left atrial pressure and less than pulmonary arterial pressure, the actual valve being influenced by the magnitude and distribution of resistances upstream and downstream from the lung's fluid-exchanging vessels (microvasculature). Changes in left atrial pressure can significantly affect pulmonary microvascular pressure and lung water content. Left atrial pressure, however, is normal in RDS (13) and established BPD (14), as it is in the adult respiratory distress syndrome (ARDS). Pulmonary arterial pressure is elevated in both RDS (13) and BPD (14), but it is uncertain how much of this pressure is "seen" by microvasculature. In other words if the pulmonary arterial resistance is high and located predominantly or exclusively upstream from the microvasculature, the pulmonary hypertension in these disorders will have no effect on lung water or solute movement. This is unlikely, however, as extra-alveolar vessels can leak water and solute in response to pressure. Further support for the speculation that an elevated pulmonary arterial pressure can, to some degree, be seen by the microcirculation comes from experiments in 1 week old lambs. Lambs of this age normally have an elevated pulmonary arterial pressure and have a greater transvascular filtration of fluid per unit lung mass than adult animals do (15). Similarly, newborn lambs (16), in contrast to adult sheep (17), increase lung lymph flow in response to hypoxia. Hypoxia must increase the intravascular pressure within fluid-exchanging vessels to increase lung water and solute movement in newborn lambs. This might result from either vasoconstriction of vessels downstream from fluid-exchanging vessels, or an intense vasoconstriction of some vessels with an associated overperfusion of other vessels (18). Therefore in RDS and BPD it is possible that the intravascular hydrostatic pressure within the microvasculature is increased to some degree because of the elevated pulmonary arterial pressures that occur in these diseases.

The microvasculature impairs the movement of protein across its walls and acts as a semipermeable membrane. The plasma protein therefore creates an osmotic pressure, which helps retain fluid within the vascular space, or promotes reabsorption from the pulmonary interstitium. This osmotic pressure of the intravascular protein plays an important role in limiting the amount of fluid leaving the vascular space. Markarian *et al.* (19) first recognized that infants with RDS had lower plasma total protein concentration than control infants. It was subsequently observed (20) that total protein concentration was directly related to maturity, thus leaving the more premature infants at a higher risk of pulmonary edema. This is emphasized by direct measurements of plasma colloid osmotic pressure. Normal adults have a colloid osmotic pressure of approximately 25 mmHg whereas healthy premature infants can have values as low as 12 mmHg (21).

Extravascular Forces

The perimicrovascular hydrostatic and protein osmotic pressures are the pertinent extravascular (interstitial) forces involved in lung water and solute exchange. It was the lack of appreciation of these forces that led earlier workers to conclude incorrectly that there was no net fluid movement out of the pulmonary microvascular bed. They had calculated that in the adult the *intra*vascular oncotic pressure was −25 mmHg, the intravascular hydrostatic pressure was only 10 to 20 mmHg, and therefore there should be a net inward force. It is now appreciated that even within the normal lung there are significant extravascular forces promoting egress of fluid from the vascular space. These forces are magnified in acute lung disease.

Controversy still exists as to what the interstitial fluid pressure is within the lung. Good data exist which suggest that it varies with both the anatomic site (bronchovascular sheaths are more negative than perialveolar areas) and degree of total and regional lung inflation (phenomena of interdependence of the lung). Most investigators now agree that in normal lungs the pressure in the bronchovascular sheaths is negative relative to atmospheric pressure and that the interstitial pressure within the mid portion of the alveolar septum is close to, or equal to, zero. The presence of surfactant within the alveolus plays an important role in minimizing lung water and solute movement by reducing the pressure drop across the curved alveolar air-liquid interface, thus presumably minimizing the negativity of the interstitial hydrostatic pressure.

The importance of surfactant in lung water and solute movement is illustrated by the work of several investigators. If surface tension is experimentally increased in previously normal adult lungs, marked pulmonary edema ensues (22, 23). Presumably the initial increase in lung water content arises, in large part, from the increased negativity of the interstitial hydrostatic pressure sucking fluid out of the vascular space. When surfactant is inactivated (24), or immature surfactant deficient lungs (25) are studied, direct micropuncture measurements demonstrate a significant fall in alveolar liquid and presumably in perimicrovascular interstitial fluid pressures. Experiments in dogs have suggested that surfactant inactivation results in an increased flow of protein-poor lymph consistent with a hydrostatic type of pulmonary edema (26). It is likely, however, that if the increase in surface active forces is persistent and great, then the alveolar capillary membrane is damaged and the permeability to water and solutes increases (see below).

Increased surface tension induced increases in alveolar-capillary permeability allow plasma protein to enter the distal lung unit. This results in lung dysfunction, formation of the hyaline membrane, and importantly inactivation of any surfactant that is present. Ikegami *et al.* (27) have isolated and purified a specific plasma protein that is an especially potent surfactant inhibitor. They have isolated this protein from the lungs of premature lambs (27), human neonates with RDS (28), and adults with ARDS (29). The latter may explain in part the findings of Hallman *et al.* (30), who demonstrated marked surfactant abnormalities in adults with ARDS. As illustrated in Figure 9.3, the flow of this and other proteins (31) into the distal lung unit sets up a vicious circle promoting further lung dysfunction, surfactant inactivation, and edema production. For a more detailed description of alterations in surfactant see Chapter 8, by Obladen.

There is a significant amount of protein in the perimicrovascular space. The exact concentration of the protein is unknown, but if it is comparable to lung lymph, it is approximately 60% of the plasma concentration. Therefore in the normal adult human the perimicrovascular protein would generate an osmotic pressure of approximately −15 mmHg. Note that the absolute value is comparable to the intravascular hydrostatic pres-

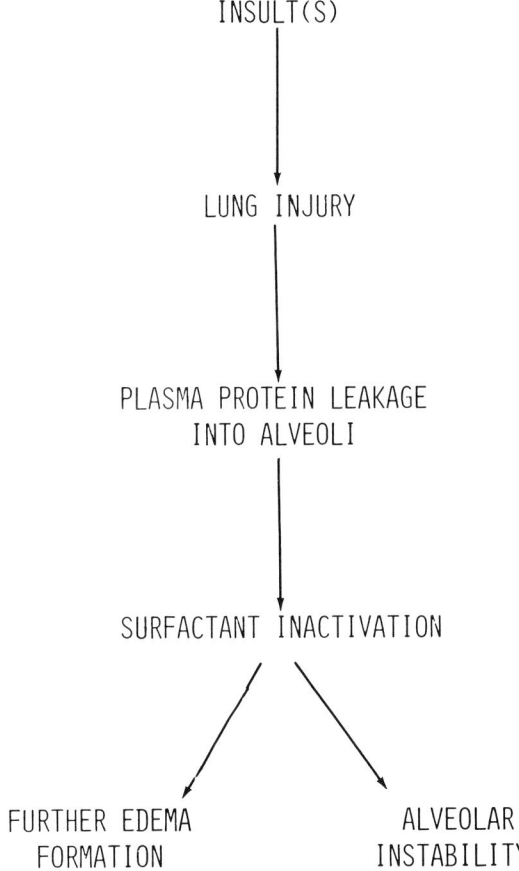

Figure 9.3. Hypothesis to explain the continuing lung dysfunction in disorders characterized by pulmonary edema and decreased pulmonary compliance. Although the initiating insults leading to the development of RDS and ARDS are different, the effects on the remaining or subsequently synthesized surfactant are comparable.

sure, and together they would result in an estimated force of 30 mmHg promoting fluid movement out of vessels. When this 30 mmHg pressure is compared with the 25 mmHg osmotic pressure from the intravascular protein, it is apparent that there is a net force promoting the movement of fluid out of the microvasculture into the lung's interstitium. Although premature infants have lower total protein concentrations than adults, the interstitial protein will still have a significant effect on lung fluid movement.

Pulmonary Permeability to Water and Solutes

Pulmonary permeability, or in other words the ease with which water and solutes pass through the alveolar-capillary membrane, plays a critical role in lung water balance. Before one can discuss the permeability of the lungs in RDS and BPD, it is important to know whether the permeability of the healthy infant lung to solutes is comparable to that of the adult lung. There is only one report of data from premature infants. That study demonstrated that premature infants who have recovered from RDS or who had respiratory insufficiency due to high-pressure pulmonary edema (32; O'Brodovich and Coates, unpublished observations) had normal pulmonary *epithelial* permeability to the small hydrophilic compound ^{99m}technetium diethylenetriaminepentacetate (^{99m}Tc-DTPA, molecular weight 492).

Endothelial permeability to water and solutes has been assessed in fetal and newborn animals. Humphrey *et al.* (33) demonstrated that fetal lambs had a higher flow rate of water and protein from their lung lymphatics than adult sheep did. The interpretation of these early experiments is difficult in view of the subsequent discoveries that there was significant systemic contamination of the presumed pulmonary lymph and that acute anesthesia and surgery had deleterious effects on lung lymph flow. Bland and McMillan (15) subsequently used a chronic lung lymph fistula preparation that enabled the collection of nearly pure lung lymph. They confirmed the earlier observations that 1 week old lambs have a higher rate of transvascular filtration of fluid per unit lung mass than adult sheep do. Their experiments, however, provided data that demonstrated that the endothelial permeability of newborn lungs to protein is similar to that of adult lungs, and therefore the increased lung lymph flow must have resulted from an increase in the net transvascular pressure gradient and/or the relatively great amount of perfused microvascular bed. Subsequent investigations by Bland et al. (5) demonstrated that the lamb fetus in utero near term and during birth has normal lung vascular permeability to protein. Their conclusions are supported by the work of Brigham et al. (34). Using a different technique they demonstrated that the pulmonary permeability to small hydrophilic solutes is similar in lambs and sheep.

Epithelial permeability to small solutes has been assessed in great detail by Olver et al. (35) in fetal sheep with gestational ages ranging from 69 to 147 days (term = 147 days). They demonstrated that the fetal lung epithelium is extremely restrictive to the movement of small solutes, even at the earliest gestation studied. Utilizing a different technique our laboratory (32) has demonstrated that epithelial permeability to ^{99m}Tc-DTPA is comparable in newborn and adult pigs and sheep.

Hyaline membrane disease is characterized by severe lung injury, and several lines of evidence suggest that pulmonary permeability to solutes is increased in this lung disease. Lambs who were delivered prematurely developed an HMD-like lung disease and had increased bidirectional flux of protein across the alveolar-capillary membrane (36). In human infants with established RDS there is widespread pulmonary edema in the face of normal left atrial pressures (7, 8, 13). The hyaline membrane, although a nonspecific finding in itself, is formed from a coagulum of plasma derived protein. This suggests that the normal barrier to protein has been damaged. Finally there is histologic evidence of extensive damage to the alveoli and terminal airway in RDS (7, 8, 11).

Jefferies et al. (32) have provided the first data regarding pulmonary permeability to solutes in infants with RDS. It was observed that the pulmonary epithelial clearance of inhaled and deposited ^{99m}Tc-DTPA was abnormally fast and comparable to that observed in adults with ARDS (38), or in animals with experimentally induced increased pulmonary permeability (37). In uncomplicated RDS this assessment of permeability returned to normal prior to extubation during the first week of life. These original observations have been extended, and thus far 28 patients with RDS have been studied on 48 occasions (unpublished observations). In all but two patients RDS was characterized by a biphasic clearance curve for ^{99m}Tc-DTPA, with a very fast initial clearance phase representing a population of damaged lung units. Seven premature infants who were receiving assisted ventilation for reasons other than RDS were also studied. Only one patient, who had severe meconium aspiration, had an abnormal pulmonary clearance of ^{99m}Tc-DTPA, a finding not unexpected given the pathophysiologic characteristics of that disorder. Several infants also underwent sequential studies as they progressed from RDS to BPD. These infants had abnormally fast clearances that persisted for 7–20 days. Their lung clearances returned to normal once their lung disease stabilized, even though they required continued ventilatory support. Therefore rapid epithelial clearance of ^{99m}Tc-DTPA is seen in severe lung injury, the most common form in the neonatal period being RDS. The clearance can remain rapid during the initial few weeks of life but can then normalize as before BPD is subsequently diagnosed at 28 days of age.

The site of increased pulmonary epithelial permeability and rapid clearance of ^{99m}Tc-DTPA to the lung is uncertain. Our laboratory has utilized a submicron-size aerosol to deliver the ^{99m}Tc-DTPA to the lung, and experiments in newborn piglets with normal and abnormal lungs have demonstrated that approximately three-fourths of the aerosol is deposited distal to ciliated airways—that is, the terminal lung units (39). Since many alveoli in HMD are airless and fluid filled, it is unlikely that our measurements are assessing these air spaces; however, we could be assessing partly damaged alveoli. Our preferred explanation is that we are detecting the markedly distended and disrupted alveolar ducts that are characteristic of RDS. After the initial weeks of life, the distended ducts are able to undergo some epithelial repair, and clearance of ^{99m}Tc-DTPA returns to normal. This speculation is supported by further experiments that show marked increases in small solute clearance when excessively large lung volumes are reached (40, 41).

The etiology of the increased alveolar-capillary permeability to solutes in disorders characterized by increased surface tension is unknown. It is possible that surfactant itself modulates pulmonary epithelial permeability. A more likely explanation is that the increased surface tension at the alveolar air-liquid interface results in mechanically induced alterations in lung shape or lung damage. Weibel (42) has discussed the effects of increased surface tension on the distal lung unit—namely, to promote alveolar collapse and concomitant alveolar duct overdistention. Similar alveolar duct overdistention is seen when simple mechanical stresses are applied to the lung (43). This alveolar duct overdistention could lead to epithelial injury and exudation of plasma into the distal lung unit. An alternative (or additional) explanation is that surfactant functions as an antiglue to prevent an excessively strong adherence of the distal terminal bronchioles. Thus if surfactant is deficient or inhibited, the rhythmic inflation and deflation of the lung would rip the epithelium in this region. These speculations are supported by the observation that the alveolar duct is the site of hyaline membrane formation (7, 8), and when immature rabbits receive assisted ventilation, characteristic bronchiolar epithelial lesions are seen (44).

Perfused Microvascular Surface Area

The lung has an enormous pulmonary vascular surface area. In the normal adult human morphometric measurements have shown the capillaries to have a potential surface area of 126 m^2 and a potential volume of 213 mL (45). In the resting adult only a fraction of this surface area is perfused and is participating in lung water and fluid movement. The potential capillary surface area has not been quantified in the premature infant, but it is likely that it is similar in proportion to body size.

The amount of perfused microvascular surface area will influence the amount of fluid leaving the vascular space since there is a continuous net outward flow of fluid from the microvascular bed into the lung interstitium. A newborn infant can be subjected to significant changes in pulmonary blood flow and amount of perfused microvascular surface area. This is best illustrated by the infant who is born with an atrial septal defect, has a pulmonary blood flow that is two to three times normal, yet has normal pulmonary arterial pressures. Recruitment and/or distention of the vascular bed with a concomitant increase in perfused microvascular bed must have occurred. More relevant to the present discussion is the presence of a patent ductus arteriosus (PDA) in the premature infant with HMD. In spite of elevated pulmonary artery pressures, there are both direct hemodynamic evidence (13) and echocardiographic evidence (46) that the vast majority of infants have significant left-to-right shunting across the PDA. The clinical evolution from HMD to BPD is frequently characterized by a PDA along with persistent ventilator dependence and clinical deterioration.

Our laboratory has been investigating the effect of this increased pulmonary blood flow on lung water and solute movement in lungs that have normal or increased permeability to water and solutes. To address this question both a sensitive index of lung water and solute movement and a reproducible method of increasing pulmonary blood flow were required. The experiments used sheep with a chronic lung lymph fistula who exercised on a treadmill. Lung lymph flow has been demonstrated to be a sensitive indicator of pulmonary transvascular fluid exchange. Exercise yields a reproducible increase in cardiac output with a concomitant increase in the carbon monoxide uptake by the lung, the latter indicating a recruitment of gas-exchanging vessels within the lung.

The principal observation from our initial experiments (47) was that under either normoxic or hypoxic conditions, exercise induced increases in cardiac output were associated with proportional increases in lung lymph flow. The increase in lymph flow was due principally to a recruitment of pulmonary microvascular bed (Fig. 9.4). In critically ill infants cardiac output, and hence pulmonary blood flow, is frequently augmented by use of vasoactive agents; therefore it was important to determine whether all methods of increasing cardiac output would have similar effects on lung water and solute movement. Isoproterenol was infused into sheep at rest to increase cardiac output to a level similar to that observed in the exercise experiments. In contrast to exercise isoproterenol induced increases in cardiac output did not increase lung lymph flow.

The likely explanation for these observations is that exercise induced increases in cardiac output recruit previously unperfused vascular bed whereas isoproterenol induced increases in cardiac output recruit previously unperfused vascular bed whereas isoproterenol induced increases in cardiac output merely dilated already perfused pulmonary vessels and thus had little effect on lymph flow (48). Therefore it appears that the mechanism responsible for the increase in pulmonary blood flow can influence the response of the pulmonary microvascular bed. If shunting left to right through a PDA is analogous to an experimentally induced arteriovenous shunt or an atrial septal defect (49), then the effect on lung water and solute exchange would be comparable to exercise—namely, a one-to-one increase in lymph flow for increase in pulmonary blood flow.

Infants with RDS have lungs with increased pulmonary permeability to water and solutes. To study the effect of increased pulmonary blood flow on lung water and solute exchange in abnormally permeable lungs, additional experiments have been performed. Similarly prepared sheep underwent

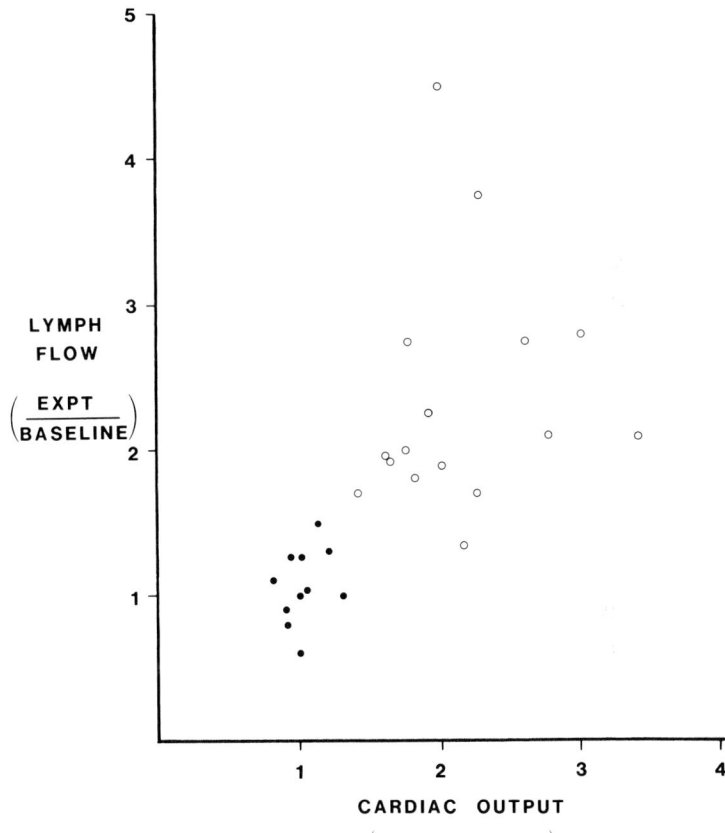

Figure 9.4. Lung lymph flow during (○) and immediately following (●) exercise in chronically instrumented unanesthetized sheep. Exercise induced increases in cardiac output resulted from a 1:1 increase in lung lymph flow. Data from O'Brodovich and Coates, 1986 (48).

intravenous infusions of air microemboli to produce a stable and prolonged increase in lung vascular permeability and were then exercised on a treadmill to increase cardiac output. In these experiments lung lymph flow increased on a three-to-one basis relative to the increase in cardiac output (50). This indicates that when there is increased lung vascular permeability, an increase in pulmonary blood flow produces large increases in lung water and solute movement.

Two potential explanations exist for the above observations. The increase in cardiac output may have recruited damaged pulmonary microvascular bed. Alternatively the marked increase in lymph flow may have resulted from small undetectable increases in pulmonary microvascular pressures, since changes of only 5 mmHg in pulmonary capillary wedge pressures can further increase lung water content in abnormally permeable lungs (51). During acute RDS there may be vascular decruitment in view of the profound lung injury. Under these conditions the presence of left-to-right shunting would be even more important, as this blood flow would add to the relative overperfusion of the vessels that remain patent.

Lung Inflammation and Injury

As discussed above the physiologic characteristics of the premature infant's cardiopulmonary system and the consequences of surfactant deficiency provide several mechanisms for the pulmonary edema that characterizes RDS. There is relatively less knowledge regarding the mechanisms of continuing lung injury in infants who do not demonstrate a normal resolution of their RDS and progress on to BPD. Indeed there is little evidence to suggest that surfactant *deficiency* is the cause of continuing lung dysfunction. Recent investigations have focused attention on inflammation within the lung as an important marker and potential mechanism for the evolutionary steps from RDS to BPD.

Leukocytes had been identified within the lungs of infants dying from BPD (1); however, the significance of this finding was unknown. Merritt and coworkers sequentially studied premature infants and identified a group of infants who developed BPD. They observed neutrophils and macrophages in the tracheal secretions of these infants, but not in those of infants with uncomplicated RDS, during the latter part of the first week of life. These infants did not have clinical evidence of active infection (52). Subsequent studies by the same group demonstrated that the infants who went on to develop BPD also had elevated levels of neutrophil derived elastase and reduced elastase inhibitor capacity in their airway secretions (53).

Reports by other investigators have provided supportive evidence of neutrophil influx and elastase–protease inhibitor imbalance in infants who developed BPD (54, 55). The imbalance between neutrophil elastase and its major inhibitors likely results from both increased release of enzyme and diminished inhibitor availability. Andrew *et al.* (56) have demonstrated that the plasma concentrations of protease inhibitors decrease with decreasing gestational age (for a more detailed description of protease–antiprotease interaction in BPD see Chapter 7, by Merritt and Hallman).

The inflammatory response within the lung is not limited to the neutrophil. Irving *et al.* (57) have demonstrated that as infants fail to recover spontaneously from HMD and begin their evolutionary process to BPD, their tracheal fluids have increased numbers of activated macrophages that are secreting large amounts of cytokines (presumably interleukin-1) that modulate fibroblast function.

Lung inflammation, and specifically neutrophil activation, is believed on the basis of experiments in animals to play an important pathogenic role in disorders characterized by increased pulmonary permeability (58). Preliminary data have shown that one form of experimentally produced surfactant deficiency and hyaline membrane formation is leukocyte dependent (59). There are many mechanisms that could be involved in the intrapulmonary sequestration and activation of neutrophils. One such mechanism is activation of the complement cascade, with generation of the leukocyte chemotactic factors. Our laboratory has measured the systemic arterial plasma concentrations of complement degradation products in eight infants with HMD during the first weeks of life. The levels of C_{3a} des Arg and D_{4a} des Arg were not elevated, and importantly the concentration of the potent leukocyte chemoattractant C_{5a} des Arg remained below detectable levels (<10 ng/mL). It should, however, not be assumed that this is not an important mechanism for activation of leukocytes in HMD, since sampling of arterial blood may be too insensitive to detect intrapulmonary complement activation. Further studies are required to answer this question.

The above observations indicate that there is an association between indices of lung inflammation and the development of BPD. Although it seems logical to assume that inflammation plays a pathogenic role, it may be just an association rather than a direct cause and effect relationship. Caution is needed in interpreting the observations made, but certainly this is a promising area for further investigation.

Treatment Related Mechanisms of Edema Formation

Infants with acute RDS and BPD are critically ill and require complex and invasive care. This necessary supportive care, however, can also be associated with deleterious effects. There must be appreciation of these potential negative effects as each intervention is taken.

Oxygen is the most important medication required by infants with RDS and BPD. Prolonged inhalation of high concentrations of oxygen can damage the lung in multiple ways including an increase in pulmonary endothelial permeability (60) and epithelial permeability (61) to solutes. Wilson et al. (62) have demonstrated that the inhalation of 80% oxygen will impair lung growth and will have a deleterious effect on the remodeling of the pulmonary vascular bed. There are data to suggest that premature infants are less able to mount a defence against an oxidant stress. Positive pressure ventilation may also contribute to the lung injury by mechanically damaging the lung. These issues are discussed in more detail in a previous review on BPD (1) and in Chapters 5 by Thibeault and Lang and 6 by Wispe and Roberts.

Intravenous infusions are necessary to maintain fluid, electrolyte, and nutritional balance. There is the potential, however, for these to have a deleterious effect on lung water and solute movement. Intravascular hydrostatic pressure could increase and intravascular protein osmotic pressure decrease with the infusion of crystalloid solutions. As demonstrated by Prewitt et al. (51), a change of only 5 mmHg pressure can significantly affect lung water content when pulmonary vascular permeability is increased. Similarly an increase in cardiac output, if associated with an increase in perfused microvascular surface area, would increase lung water and solute movement (see previous discussion). Finally, intravenous infusions of lipid at rates used in clinical situations have been associated with an increase in pulmonary arterial pressures and vascular resistance (63). This could both increase the amount of right-to-left shunting if there is a sufficient increase in resistance and increase lung water and solute movement if a portion of the elevated pulmonary arterial pressure was transmitted to the pulmonary microvascular bed.

Significance of Pulmonary Edema in RDS and BPD

The occurrence of pulmonary edema in premature infants has dramatic effects on cardiorespiratory function. In contrast to the adult, the infant who has pulmonary overperfusion and interstitial pulmonary edema has significant increases in peripheral airway resistance and impaired gas exchange (64). When alveolar flooding occurs gas exchange is worsened because of the resultant intrapulmonary shunt and increase in pulmonary vascular resistance, which will promote right-to-left shunting through fetal vascular channels. The flooding of the alveoli with protein-containing fluid will inactivate any surfactant present, worsen pulmonary function, and promote further edema production as previously discussed. Interstitial or alveolar edema will stimulate juxtacapillary receptors and increase the respiratory rate with a resultant increase in the work of breathing and the total oxygen demand. Unresolved inflammation and edema promote fibrosis both in animals (65) and in humans (66, 67).

Summary

Pulmonary edema is invariably associated with RDS, the most important precursor of BPD. The edema results both from an increase in the transvascular pressure gradient and from an increase in pulmonary permeability to water and solutes. The increased lung water content and inflammation have both acute and long-term implications for long structure and function.

References

1. O'Brodovich HM, Mellins RB. State of the art. Bronchopulmonary dysplasia: unresolved neonatal acute lung injury. Am Rev Respir Dis 1985;132:694–709.
2. Northway WH Jr, Rosan RC, Porter DY. Pulmonary disease following respirator therapy of hyaline-membrane disease. N Engl J Med 1967;276:357–368.
3. Matthay MA, Landolt CC, Staub NC. Differential liquid and protein clearance from the alveoli of anesthetized sheep. J Appl Physiol 1982;53:96–104.
4. Bland RD, McMillan DD, Bressack MA, Dong L. Clearance of liquid from lungs of newborn rabbits. J Appl Physiol 1980;49:171–177.
5. Bland RD, Hansen TN, Haberkern CM, et al. Lung fluid balance in lambs before and after birth. J Appl Physiol 1982;53:992–1004.
6. deSa DJ. The pathogenesis of the respiratory distress syndrome of the newly born. Ph.D. thesis, Oxford University, 1967.
7. deSa DJ. Pulmonary fluid content in infants with respiratory distress. J Pathol 1969;97:469–479.
8. Matthay MA, Berthiaume Y, Staub NC. Long term clearance of liquid and protein from the lungs of anesthetized sheep. J Appl Physiol 1985;59:928–934.
9. Lauweryns JM. Hyaline membrane disease: pathological study of 55 infants. Arch Dis Child 1965;40:618–625.
10. Truog WE, Standaert TA, Murphy JH, Woodrum DE, Hodson WA. Effects of prolonged high frequency oscillatory ventilation in premature primates with experimental hyaline membrane disease. Am Rev Respir Dis 1984;130:76–80.
11. Taghizadeh A, Reynold EOR. Pathogenesis of bronchopulmonary displasia following hyaline membrane disease. Am J Pathol 1976;82:241–258.
12. Rosen RC. Hyaline membrane disease and a related spectrum of neonatal pneumopathies. Perspect Pediatr Pathol 1975;2:15–60.
12a. Staub NC. Pathogenesis of pulmonary edema. Am Rev Respir Dis 1974;109:358–372.
13. Rudolph AM, Drorbaugh JE, Auld PAM, et al. Studies on the circulation in the neonatal period: the circulation in the respiratory distress syndrome. Pediatrics 1961;27:551–566.
14. Berman W Jr, Yabek SM, Dillon T, Burstein R, Corlew S. Evaluation of infants with bronchopulmonary dysplasia using cardiac catheterization. Pediatrics 1982;70:708–712.
15. Bland RD, McMillan DD. Lung fluid dynamics in awake newborn lambs. J Clin Invest 1977;60:1107–1115.
16. Bressack MA, Bland RD. Alveolar hypoxia increases lung fluid filtration in unanesthetized newborn lambs. Circ Res 1980;46:111–116.
17. Bland RD, Demling RH, Selinger SL, Staub NC. Effects of alveolar hypoxia on lung fluid and protein transport in unanesthetized sheep. Circ Res 1977;40:269–274.
18. Hansen TN, LeBlanc AL, Gest AL. Hypoxia and angiotensin II infusion redistribute lung

blood flow in lambs. J Appl Physiol 1985;58: 812–818.
19. Markarian M, Jackson JJ, Bannon AE. Serial serum total protein values in premature infants with and without respiratory distress syndrome. J Pediatr 1966;69:1046–1053.
20. Bland RD. Cord-blood total protein level as a screening aid for the idiopathic respiratory distress syndrome. N Engl J Med 1972;287: 9–13.
21. Ekblad H, Kero P, Korvenranta H, Erkkola R, Valimaki I. Colloid osmotic pressure of umbilical cord plasma in healthy and sick newborn infants. Pediatrics 1985;75:764–769.
22. Albert RK, Lakshminarayan S, Hildebrandt J, Kirk W, Butler J. Increased surface tension favors pulmonary edema formation in anesthetized dogs' lungs. J Clin Invest 1979;63: 1015–1018.
23. Nieman GF, Bredenberg CE. High surface tension pulmonary edema induced by detergent aerosol. J Appl Physiol 1985;58:129–136.
24. Beck NC, Lai-Fook SJ. Alveolar liquid pressures in excised edematous dog lung with increased static recoil. J Appl Physiol 55: 1277–1283.
25. Raj JU. Alveolar liquid pressure measured by micropuncture in isolated lungs of mature and immature fetal rabbits. J Clin Invest 1987;79: 1579–1588.
26. Bredenberg CE, Nieman GF, Paskanik AM, Hart AKE. Microvascular permeability in high surface tension pulmonary edema. J Appl Physiol 1986;60:253–259.
27. Ikegami M, Jobe A, Jacobs H, Lam R. A protein from airways of premature lambs that inhibits surfactant function. J Appl Physiol 1984;57:1134–1142.
28. Ikegami M, Jacobs H, Jobe A. Surfactant function in respiratory distress syndrome. J Pediatr 1983;102:443–447.
29. Ikegami M, Kaneda M, Nozaki M. Adult respiratory distress syndrome surfactant inhibition. J Jpn Med Soc Biol Interface 1985;16: 43–50.
30. Hallman M, Spragg R, Harrell JH, Moser KM, Gluck L. Evidence of lung surfactant anormality in respiratory failure. J Clin Invest 1982;70: 673–683.
31. Seeger W, Stohr G, Wolf HRD, Neuhof H. Alteration of surfactant function due to protein leakage: special interaction with fibrin monomer. J Appl Physiol 1985;58:326–338.
32. Jefferies AL, Coates G, O'Brodovich HM. Pulmonary epithelial permeability in hyaline membrane disease. N Engl J Med 1984;311: 1075–1080.
33. Humphrey PW, Normand ICS, Reynolds EOR, Strang CB. Pulmonary lymph flow and the uptake of liquid from the lungs of the lamb at the start of breathing. J Physiol 1967;193: 1–29.
34. Brigham KL, Sundell H, Harris TR, Catterton Z, Kovar I, Stahlman M. Lung water and vascular permeability in sheep. Newborns compared with adults. Circ Res 1977;42: 851–855.
35. Olver RE, Schneeberger EE, Walters DV. Epithelial solute permeability, ion transport and tight junction morphology in the developing lung of the fetal lamb. J Physiol 1981;315: 395–412.
36. Jobe A, Ikegami M, Jacobs H, Jones S, Conaway D. Permeability of premature lamb lungs to protein and the effect of surfactant on that permeability. J Appl Physiol 1983;55:169–176.
37. Jefferies AL, Coates G, Webber CE, O'Brodovich HM. Measurement of pulmonary clearance of radioaerosol using a portable sodium iodide probe. J Appl Physiol 1984;57: 1908–1912.
38. Mason GR, Effros RM, Uzler JM. Small solute clearance from the lungs of patients with cardiogenic and non-cardiogenic pulmonary edema. Chest 1985;88:327–334.
39. Kay JD, Coates G, O'Brodovich H. Pulmonary deposition sites of an inhaled radiolabelled submicronic aerosol Pediatr Res 1986;20: 1297–1300.
40. Egan EA. Lung inflation, lung solute permeability and alveolar edema. J Appl Physiol 1982;53:121–125.
41. O'Brodovich H, Coates G, Marrin M. Effect of increased inspiratory resistance and PEEP on pulmonary clearance of ^{99m}Tc-DTPA. J Appl Physiol 1986;60:1461–1465.
42. Weibel ER. The pathway for oxygen. Cam-

bridge: Harvard University Press, 1985, pp 317–325.
43. Robertson CH, Hall DL, Hogg JC. A description of lung distortion due to localized pleural stress. J Appl Physiol 1973;34:344–350.
44. Nilsson R, Grossman G, Robertson B. Lung surfactant and the pathogenesis of neonatal bronchiolar lesions induced by artificial ventilation. Pediatr Res 1978;12:249–255.
45. Burri PH. Handbook of physiology: the respiratory system, section 3, vol 1. Fishman AP, ed. Bethesda, Md: American Physiological Society, 1985, pp 1–47.
46. Dudell GG, Gersony WM. Patent ductus arteriosus in neonates with severe respiratory disease. J Pediatr 1984;104:915–920.
47. Coates G, O'Brodovich H, Jefferies AL, Gray GW. Effects of exercise on lung lymph flow in sheep and goats during normoxia and hypoxia. J Clin Invest 1984;74:133–141.
48. O'Brodovich H, Coates G. Effect of isoproterenol or exercise on pulmonary lymph flow and hemodynamics. J Appl Physiol 1986;60:38–44.
49. Grover RF, Wagner WW, McMurtry IF, Reeves JT. Handbook of Physiology, section 2, vol 3. Shepherd JT, Abboud FM, eds. Bethesda, Md: American Physiological Society, 1983, pp 103–136.
50. O'Brodovich H, Coates G. Effect of exercise on lung lymph flow in unanesthetized sheep with increased pulmonary vascular permeability. Am Rev Respir Dis 1986;134;862–866.
51. Prewitt RM, McCarthy J, Wood LDH. Treatment of acute low pressure pulmonary edema in dogs: relative effects of hydrostatic and oncotic pressure, nitroprusside, and positive and expiratory pressure. J Clin Invest 1981;67:409–418.
52. Merritt TA, Stuard IK, Puccia J, et al. Newborn tracheal aspirate cytology: classification during respiratory distress syndrome and bronchopulmonary dysplasia. J Pediatr 1981;98:949–956.
53. Merritt TA, Cochrane CG, Holcomb K, et al. Elastase and α_1-proteinase inhibitor activity in tracheal aspirates during respiratory distress syndrome. Role of inflammation in the pathogenesis of bronchopulmonary displasia. J Clin Invest 1983;72:656–666.
54. Ogden BE, Murphy SA, Sauners GC, Pathak D, Johnson JD. Neonatal lung neutrophils and elastase/protease inhibitor imbalance. Am Rev Respir Dis 1984;130:817–821.
55. Bruce MC, Wedig KE, Jentoft N, et al. Altered excretion of elastin cross-links in premature infants who develop bronchopulmonary dysplasia. Am Rev Respir Dis 1985;131:568–572.
56. Andrew M, Massicotte-Nolan PM, Karpatkin M. Plasma protease inhibitors in premature infants: influence of gestational age, postnatal age, and health status. Proc Soc Exp Biol Med 1983;173:495–500.
57. Irving LB, Jordana M, O'Brodovich H, Gauldie J. Alveolar macrophage activation in bronchopulmonary dysplasia (abstr). Am Rev Respir Dis 1986;133:A207.
58. Brigham KL, Meyrick B. Interaction of granulocytes with the lungs. Circ Res 1984;54:623–635.
59. Kawano T, Mori S, Cybulsky M, Burger R, Ballin A, Cutz E, Bryan C: Effect of granulocyte depletion in a ventilated surfactant-depleted lung. J Appl Physiol 1987;62:27–33.
60. Hansen TN, Hazinski TA, Bland RD. Vitamin E does not prevent oxygen-induced lung injury in newborn lambs. Pediatr Res 1982;16:583–587.
61. Davis WB, Rennard SI, Bitterman PB, Crystal RG. Pulmonary oxygen toxicity. Early reversible changes in human alveolar structures induced by hyperoxia. N Engl J Med 1983;309:878–883.
62. Wilson WL, Mullen M, Olley PM, Rabinovitch M. Hyperoxia-induced pulmonary vascular and lung abnormalities in young rats and potential for recovery. Pediatr Res 1985;19:1059–1067.
63. McKeen CR, Brigham KL, Bowers RE, Harris TR. Pulmonary vascular effects of fat emulsion infusion in unanesthetized sheep. J Clin Invest 1978;61:1291–1297.
64. Hordof AJ, Mellins RB, Gersony WM, Steeg CN. Reversibility of chronic obstructive lung disease in infants following repair of ventricular septal defect. J Pediatr 1977;90:187–191.
65. Meyer EC. Acute and chronic clearance of lung fluids, proteins, and cells. In: Staub NC,

ed. Lung water and solute exchange. New York: Marcel Dekker, 1978, pp 277–321.
66. Crystal RG, Bitterman PB, Rennard SI, Hance AJ, Keogh BA. Interstitial lung diseases of unknown cause. I. Disorders characterized by chronic inflammation of the lower respiratory tract. N Engl J Med 1984;310:154–166.
67. Zapol WM, Trelstad RL, Coffey JW, Tsai I, Salvador RA. Pulmonary fibrosis in severe acute respiratory failure. Am Rev Respir Dis 1979;119:547–554.

Acknowledgments

This work was supported by grants-in-aid from the Heart and Stroke Foundation of Ontario and the Medical Research Council of Canada. Dr. O'Brodovich is a scholar of the Canadian Heart Foundation.

Comments

Bruce R. Boynton

The experimental findings reviewed here have important implications for the use of exogenous surfactant (see Chapter 20 by Merritt and Hallman). Even a short period of positive pressure ventilation may damage the respiratory epithelium and permit protein entry into the air spaces with consequent inactivation of surfactant. This implies that administration of surfactant may be more effective in the delivery room than when RDS is fully established. Further research is needed to assess the effect of exogenous surfactant on pulmonary edema. By facilitating alveolar expansion, surfactant may decrease overdistention and epithelial damage to the terminal airways. Reduction in surface tension may also reduce fluid leak by decreasing alveolar-capillary permeability. On the other hand increasing lung volume after surfactant treatment may decrease pulmonary vascular resistance and increase left-to-right shunting through the PDA. This increase in pulmonary blood flow might promote edema by increasing pulmonary capillary blood volume and hydrostatic pressure.

10

Bronchopulmonary Dysplasia: Can the Laboratory Duplicate Factors That Influence Its Pathogenesis and Evolution?

JACQUELINE J. COALSON

The descriptive term bronchopulmonary dysplasia (BPD) was coined by Northway, Rosan, and Porter (1) in 1967 to describe a clinical syndrome in infants with respiratory distress syndrome (RDS) who received prolonged respiratory assistance and developed chronic pulmonary changes. Premature infants with severe respiratory distress treated 24 hours or more with supplemental oxygen and intermittent positive pressure ventilation (IPPV) were categorized into four stages with Stage IV (the most severe) seen in infants who had been treated with 80% to 100% oxygen and IPPV.

The pathologic features of the four stages were also detailed. Stage I was seen in infants 2 to 3 days of age who had classical acute respiratory distress syndrome. A patchy loss of ciliated cells and sites of metaplasia and necrosis of the bronchiolar mucosa were present along with the typical findings of hyaline membranes, hyperemia, and atelectasis.

Stage II was seen in infants 4 to 10 days of age and was noted to be the period of regeneration. Necrosis and regeneration of alveolar epithelium, persistent hyaline membranes, and emphysematous coalescence of alveoli were the pathologic findings. Airway changes included patchy bronchiolar necrosis with overlying hyaline membranes and sites of squamous metaplasia.

Stage III was seen in infants 10 to 20 days of age and was called the period of transition to chronic disease. Fewer hyaline membranes were present, but alveolar epithelium still showed regenerative activity. Widespread bronchial and bronchiolar mucosal metaplasia was evident. Spherical circumscribed groups of emphysematous alveoli with surrounding atelectatic alveoli were described. Alcin blue staining of the interstitial tissues, first noted in Stage II, was more prominent, and an increase in interseptal collagen was seen.

Stage IV was seen in infants older than 1 month and was called the period of chronic disease. At autopsy circumscribed areas of emphysematous alveoli in which bronchioles showed peribronchiolar smooth muscle hypertrophy alternated with areas of atelectasis that showed normal bronchioles. Increased connective tissue deposition and pulmonary hypertensive vascular changes were present.

These histopathologic features were expanded by Rosan (2) to include changes in the bronchial and bronchiolar mucosae, the pulmonary interstitium, the lymphatics, and the inflation pattern. Bonikos et al. (3) further adapted and refined Rosan's criteria and developed a detailed grading system of mild, moderate, severe, and very severe for the histopathologic changes. Additional pathologic studies have further detailed many of these described lesions. Anderson et al. (4–6) evaluated the fibroproliferative obliterative bronchitis and bronchiolitis and noted that the cystic emphysematous lesions resulted from marked ectasia of bronchioles. They suggested that the partial obliteration of airways could result in bronchiolar ectasia, or that cyst formation occurred in neighboring bronchioles when bronchioles underwent complete obliteration. Taghizadeh and Reynolds (7) and Sobonya and coworkers (8) have noted that small airway bronchiolar lesions are seen more frequently in sites of residual atelectasis. The histopathologic features of BPD described above would comprise the "gold standard" pathologic criteria desired in an animal model.

Of the multiple factors that have been suggested to cause BPD, pulmonary immaturity, oxygen exposure, which elicits cellular damage via free radicals, and barotrauma induced by mechanical ventilation continue to be prime considerations. These etiologic possibilities were appreciated by the participants at the National Institutes of Health Workshop on Bronchopulmonary Dysplasia in 1979 who recommended that animal models of BPD be developed (9). Criteria suggested for an animal model of BPD included 1) pathology similar to, if not indistinguishable from, human BPD, 2) viability following premature delivery by caesarean section, 3) susceptibility to RDS, 4) sufficient size to permit appropriate physiologic and biochemical studies of the lungs, 5) availability of timed gestation, 6) littermates, species specific normal data, or appropriate control animals for comparison, and 7) availability of resources needed to maintain and study the animals. Some of these criteria have been difficult to achieve in very small species such as mice, rats, and rabbits, but the newborn mice models of oxygen poisoning described by Northway and his group in a series of papers (10–12) do show a necrotizing bronchiolitis and a distal connective tissue response. However, as most cases of BPD occur in premature infants with RDS, more effort has been directed to studies in larger animals.

Robertson has reviewed the experimental models of RDS, including naturally occurring RDS, RDS induced by artificial techniques, and RDS that occurs in premature animals with deficient surfactant (13). Spontaneous RDS occurs in the foal, puppy, and calf, and in piglets with the "barker syndrome." The clinicopathologic features of RDS have been especially well characterized in the foal and the barker piglet, but these species have not been studied further for development of BPD.

Several animals, including the sheep, rhesus monkey, pigtail monkey, baboon, and rabbit, have been delivered prematurely and maintained with mechanical ventilation and oxygen therapy. With the exception of the baboon, none of these animals has been maintained successfully for a prolonged period, and BPD Stages II through IV have not been characterized.

The premature lamb has proved to be an excellent model of RDS and has been studied extensively (14; reviewed in 13). However, most studies reflect data that have been obtained within a few hours of delivery, and only rarely have 48 hour endpoints been examined (15). This species to date has not been manipulated successfully to yield a BPD model.

Several investigators have studied RDS in

the rhesus and pigtail monkeys. McAdams and coworkers (16) theorized that premature rhesus monkeys delivered at 60% gestation aspirated gastric fluid, which either caused necrosis of the bronchiolar epithelium or sensitized it to oxygen. Following delivery the animals were ventilated with hand-operated positive pressure and 60% to 70% oxygen for 0 to 120 minutes, which resulted in hyaline membranes within alveolar ducts and respiratory bronchioles by 5 minutes of age.

Cutz and coworkers (17) evaluated the effects of intratracheally instilled surfactant in rhesus monkeys delivered by caesarean section at about 70% of gestation. One group of animals received surfactant, whereas a control group was ventilated with IPPV and oxygen as needed. All animals were studied for 6 hours. Bronchiolar epithelial necrosis, aspiration of amniotic fluid cells, and hyaline membranes were quantitatively more numerous in the control IPPV group than in the surfactant treated group.

Hodson and coworkers (18–20) have characterized RDS in the *Macaca nemestrina* monkey in several 2 to 6 hour studies. In later studies, these workers examined the effects of high-frequency oscillatory ventilation on RDS in this species in 7 and 24 hour studies (21, 22).

In the baboon model of RDS/BPD, animals are delivered prematurely by caesarean section at 140 days ± 2 days (total gestation 180 days (1) (23, 24). Over 95% of the premature animals will develop RDS. Delivered animals that do not breathe do not show hyaline membranes.

The evolution of RDS in the baboon has been characterized and is very similar to that of the human. At 2 hours animals show hyaline membranes at the respiratory bronchiolar level, saccular atelectasis, and inflation primarily of the more compliant airways (24). Unlike the human lung, the baboon lung has very short terminal bronchioles, if any, but has multiple orders of respiratory bronchioles. By 24 hours of age animals treated with IPPV and appropriate oxygen have striking dilation lesions at the bronchiolar level when perfusion-fixed at a known airway pressure (25). Hyaline membranes are evident at the respiratory bronchiolar and alveolar duct levels and occasionally within the partially expanded saccules. The bronchiolar epithelium shows severe thinning and focal loss of epithelial continuity. By 96 hours, if premature baboons are maintained on appropriate oxygen and any type of ventilatory mode, lungs show sparse hyaline membranes and good inflation to the saccular level (26). The only residual sites of atelectasis consistently seen in these premature baboons are in alveoli or saccules directly adjoining the larger airways and in occasional focal subpleural sites.

Using IPPV ventilation and 100% oxygen Stage III histopathologic changes have been induced in the premature baboon in a period of 11 to 17 days (24). As compared with the premature baboons maintained on appropriate oxygen and mechanical ventilation for 96 hours, the animals treated with 100% oxygen and mechanical ventilation show persistent airway and saccular disease at 4 days (27). Degenerative epithelial airway changes, atelectasis, foci of extravasated red blood cells and pulmonary edema, and hyaline membrane formation are seen (Fig. 10.1) The distribution of the hyaline membrane is not that seen in typical RDS; the membranes are primarily at the alveolar duct and saccular levels and are associated with the edema and extravasated red blood cells. The pattern is similar to that seen in the adult counterpart of exu-

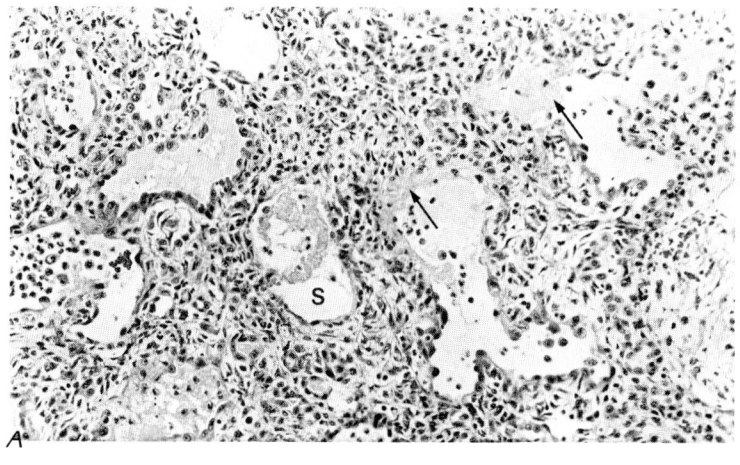

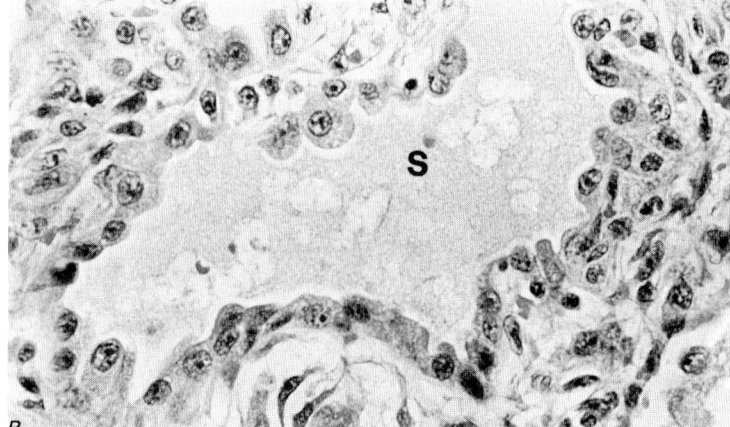

Figure 10.1. (*A*) The saccules (S) contain edema, hyaline membranes (arrow), and scattered PMNs and alveolar macrophages. The saccular walls are thickened and are lined by hyperplastic type 2 cells. (*B*) A higher magnification details the saccular wall's interstitium and hyperplastic type 2 cells. S-saccules. Hematoxylin-eosin; ×150 in *A*, ×560 in *B*.

dative diffuse alveolar damage (DAD) described below.

After treatment with 9 to 11 days of 100% oxygen and mechanical ventilation, alternating sites of atelectasis and overinflation (Fig. 10.2), striking metaplastic/hyperplastic epithelial lesions in the larger airways (Fig. 10.3), and at the respiratory bronchiolar and alveolar duct levels (Figs. 10.4 and 10.5), peribronchial and peribronchiolar fibrosis (Fig. 10.6), and interstitial edema and early connective tissue deposition in the saccules are seen (Fig. 10.7). The hyperplastic/metaplastic small airway changes invariably are found in the areas of atelectasis and are less severe in the better expanded portions of the lung. The epithelium of the saccules at the 140 day window normally shows an abundance of type 2 epithelial cells. However, the type 2 cells in the BPD induced lesions show an increase in number and variation in size during this repair phase. Some of these re-

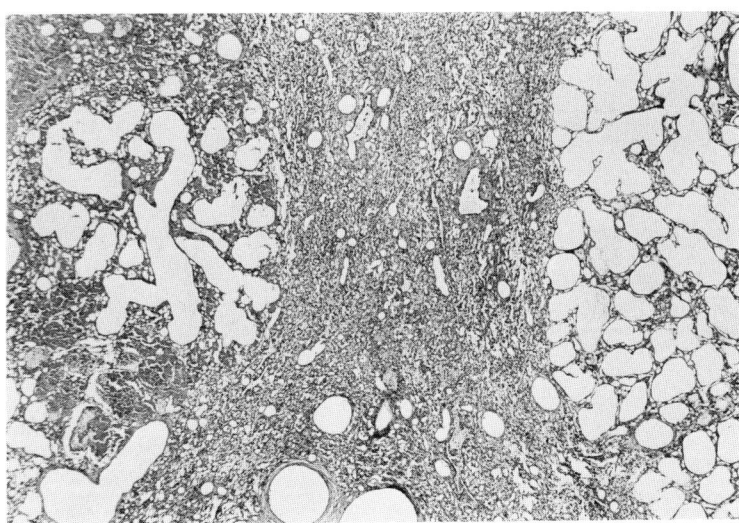

Figure 10.2. Pattern of alternating atelectasis and overinflation is depicted. Hematoxylin-eosin; ×38.

parative responses of the immature lung overlap with features of reparative diffuse alveolar damage in the adult lung.

DAD is a descriptive term that reflects a consistent, though nonspecific sequence of findings in the lung following acute injury by a variety of agents. It can be separated into exudative and reparative (proliferative) phases (28). The exudative phase of 1 to 6 days includes pulmonary edema, hyaline membranes, alveolar wall edema, and microatelectasis (28–38). There is hyaline membrane formation at the respiratory bronchiolar and alveolar levels (30–32, 36) and particularly at the alveolar level (31, 32, 38). Fibrin strands are within the damaged alveolar wall and free within the alveolar space, frequently forming a major component of the hyaline membrane. Polymorphonuclear leukocytes (PMNs) are seen in the edematous alveolar walls and alveolar spaces within 24 to 36 hours following injury. The edema of DAD has been characterized as protein-rich fluid resulting from increased permeability rather than increased hydrostatic pressure (39–41).

Six days after lung injury in the adult with *adult respiratory distress syndrome* (ARDS), the reparative phase of DAD has usually begun and is characterized by hyperplasia of epithelial type 2 cells and interstitial mononuclear inflammatory infiltrate, and the "rounding up" of hyaline membranes either by mural application or by encirclement with alveolar macrophages. Increased numbers of fibroblasts are in thickened alveolar walls and in organizing alveolar exudates. Residual fibrin is invariably found in these lesions with prominent fibroplasia (31, 36, 42). The reparative phase lasts about 2 weeks and is followed either by widespread fibrosis or by resolution of the lesion (38, 43).

Although BPD and adult DAD have some histologic characteristics in common, there are significant differences. Newborns of many species have rare, if any, pores of Kohn (44). They are not found in humans until 10 months of age, after which time they slowly

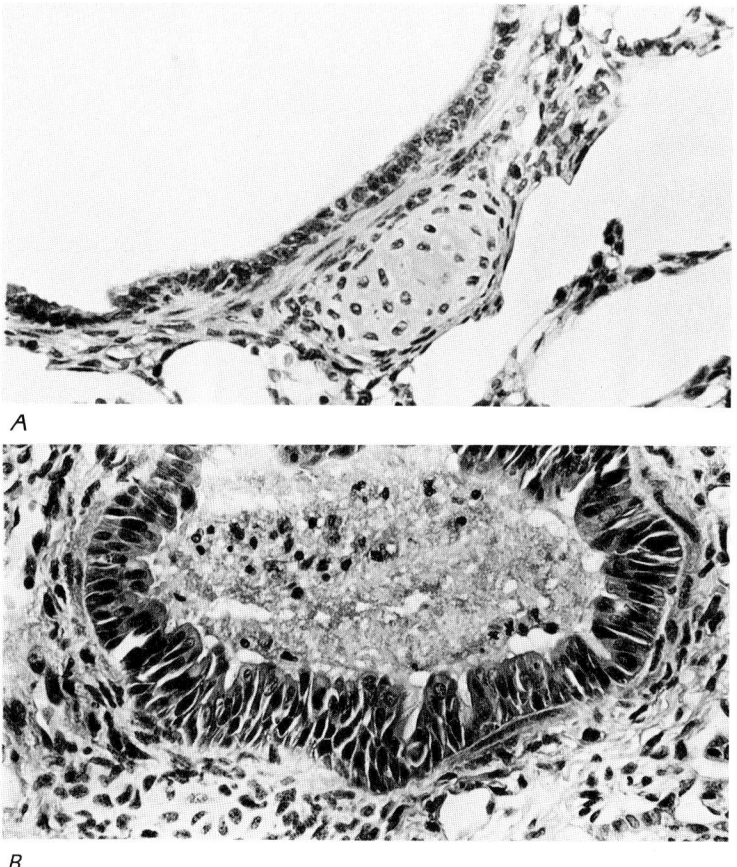

Figure 10.3. (*A*) Normal bronchial epithelium. (*B*) Hyperplastic epithelium of the bronchus from a baboon with BPD. Hematoxylin-eosin; ×380.

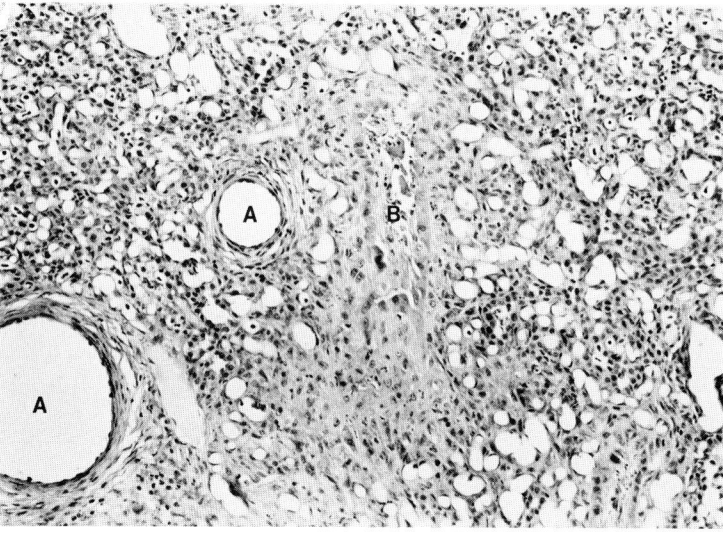

Figure 10.4. The small bronchiole (B) show reparative squamous epithelium. A-pulmonary artery. Hematoxylin-eosin; ×150.

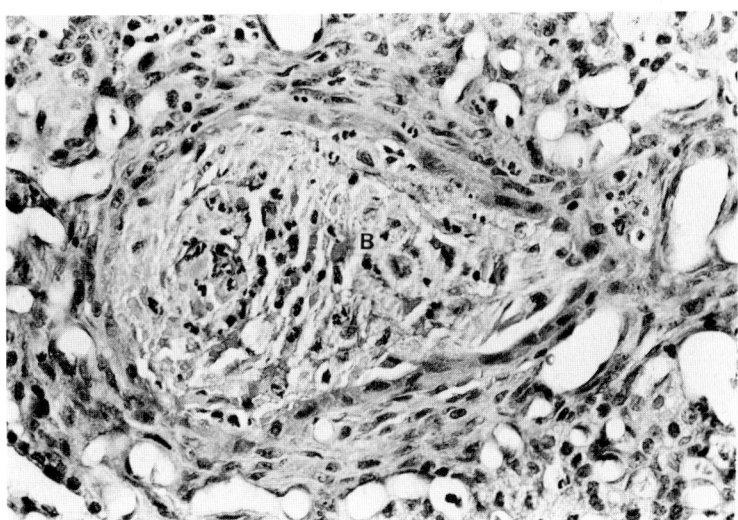

Figure 10.5. Higher magnification of a small bronchiole (B) which is plugged with necrotic cellular debris. Hematoxylin-eosin; ×380.

increase in number into adulthood. The adult lung has pores of Kohn, and bronchiolar-bronchiolar and bronchiolar-alveolar collateral channels. The lack of adequate collateral ventilation in infant lungs, combined with a deficiency of surfactant, produces an atelectasis pattern that is more confluent and uniform than that seen in the adult, which is predominantly a diffuse but focal reduction in the size of alveolar spaces.

The atelectasis pattern in the premature infant may also be aggravated by positive pressure ventilation. Reynolds described a maldistribution of intrapulmonary air in in-

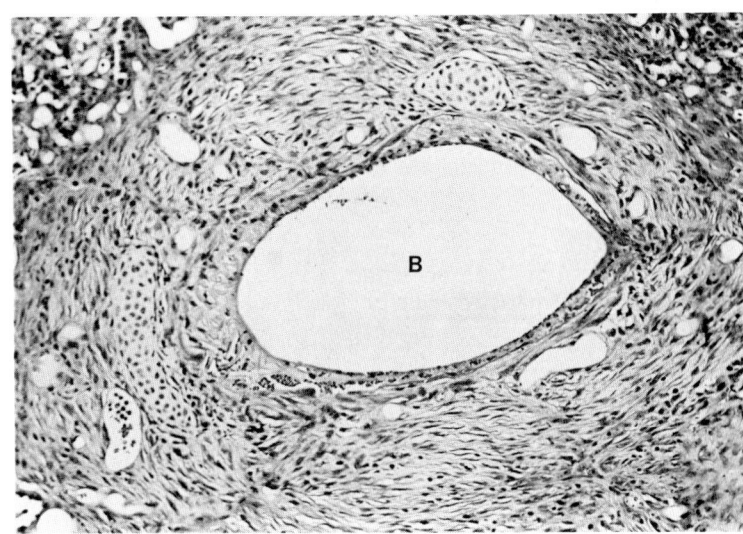

Figure 10.6. Striking peribronchial fibrosis is evident. The bronchus (B) is lined by reparative simple squamous epithelium. Hematoxylin-eosin; ×150.

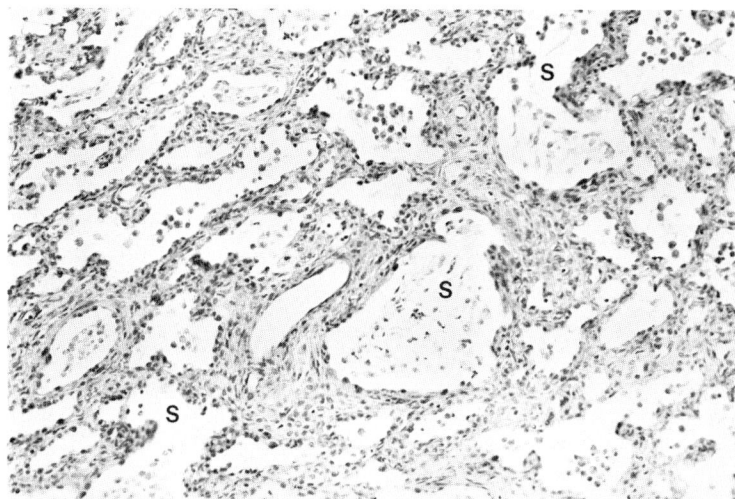

Figure 10.7. Saccular wall interstitial fibrosis and saccular space (S) size variation are seen. The saccules contain scattered cells. Hematoxylin-eosin; ×150.

fants with RDS (7). In the premature baboon with RDS ventilated for 24 hours with positive pressure ventilation and positive end-expiratory pressure (PPV/PEEP), the majority of the air is located in overdilated, distorted airway with poor saccular aeration (25). Baboons ventilated with high-frequency oscillatory ventilation (HFOV) have more rapid saccular recruitment manifested physiologically by a rapid rise in the arterial-alveolar ratio and pathologically by more uniform aeration and less airway dilation. The use of HFOV in an 11 day baboon study has clearly resulted in a significantly lower incidence of interstitial pulmonary emphysema when compared with conventional positive pressure ventilation (25, 45). These results support the use of high-frequency ventilation in the ventilatory management of infants with RDS.

Bronchiolar epithelial responses in adult DAD are not well described in the literature, but are evident if sought in lungs from patients dying of ARDS with diffuse alveolar damage at autopsy (46). In the recent report of BPD in adults with ARDS who required high PEEP pressures and oxygen during life (47), cystic structures, probably derived from dilated alveolar ducts, with surrounding fibrotic alveolar parenchyma were seen. Obstructive airway epithelial changes were not mentioned.

The small size of airways in infants would make them more susceptible to obstruction secondary to marked epithelial proliferative responses to injury. It is our thought that the dilation lesion of the fetal compliant airway results from barotrauma induced by positive pressure ventilation. This airway lesion has been appreciated by a number of investigators including Hochheim (48), Taghizadeh and Reynolds (7), and Nilsson *et al*. (49, 50). High oxygen levels probably act as a significant additive injurant to both the injured airway and the more distal noncompliant parenchymal unit.

Several investigators have reported increases in cell numbers (PMNs and alveolar macrophages), elastase–proteinase activities, and protein levels in BPD and oxygen toxicity

(51–53). This "alveolitis" has not been as well characterized in the BPD literature as in the adult DAD literature. Scant numbers of PMNs can be found in experimentally induced BPD in the baboon, but are not evident histologically until 6 days and longer (27). Alveolar macrophages are not present in the 140 day premature baboon, but are recruited into the saccules as the BPD lesions evolve (27). The role of oxygen in the recruitment of white blood cells from the vascular stream into the saccules through release of chemotactic factors, its role in the deactivation of the antiprotease defense mechanisms, and its role in inducing toxic changes in alveolar macrophages need to be further studied for their possible effects in the evolution of infant BPD.

The role of bronchopulmonary infection in the course and outcome of BPD has not been prospectively studied in either animal models or humans. It is generally recognized by clinicians that infection is commonly seen in infants hospitalized with BPD. Evidence of infection has been consistently noted in the published pathologic studies of infants who have died with BPD (54, 55). A review of the autopsies performed on infants with BPD during 1980–1984 yielded 30 at Medical Center Hospital in San Antonio, of whom 20 had confirmed evidence of infection. This may be an underestimate of the presence of infection in that there was not a systematic approach to determine by microbiologic culture either its presence or absence in these infants. In this patient population *Pseudomonas aeruginosa* was the most frequently cultured organism, which differed from the pre-1980 autopsied BPD infants in which *Klebsiella, Serratia,* and occasional *E. coli* organisms were more prevalent.

Newborns are known to develop their bacterial flora within the first week of life (56–59). However, aberrations in colonization patterns following antibiotic treatment and intubation and the propensity for the intubated premature infant to aspirate have been documented (60–66). Infection, which frequently ensues following these occurrences, has been noted to be an important determinant of morbidity and mortality in the neonatal intensive care unit (67).

The effects of a superimposed nosocomial pneumonia on the ongoing exudative–reparative processes in the BPD injured lung are not known. In the adult counterpart of ARDS, there are two clinical reports that suggest an association between lung infection and the occurrence of lung fibrosis (68, 69). The premature infant is certainly at great risk if infection occurs; there is an impairment of PMN bactericidal activity in the preterm infant (70), the lungs' normal upper respiratory antimicrobial defenses are bypassed via intubation and ventilation, and the newborn is born with lower levels of antioxidants (51). Alveolar macrophages are also sparse in number, increasing the susceptibility of the premature to infection (71).

The outcomes of patients who survive their BPD episode continue to be examined by various workers. It is suspected that the striking and severe connective tissue alterations seen in BPD will produce adverse effects on lung maturation, and this is supported by one case report (8). Sobonya and his colleagues performed morphometric analyses on the lungs and heart of a male infant who had died at 33 months of age with BPD resulting from prematurity, RDS, and its subsequent treatment. They found that the alveolar internal surface area was only one-third to one-half that expected for age matched controls, while the number of alveoli was only one-eighth to one-sixth of the normal number found in age matched controls. Of interest, minimal airway abnormalities were noted. When these workers compared the data from this BPD child with control data from children of the same height or weight, the number of alveoli was still found to be markedly reduced, being less than that of a full-term newborn.

There has been a recent resurgence of interest in postnatal lung development (72, 73). Although it has been studied in a number of laboratory animals, few definitive studies have been done in human infants and fetuses. A number of established concepts are now being questioned, and intrauterine and postnatal lung growth standards are being redefined. At one time preacinar airways were thought to increase in number during lung growth after birth (74), but later work implied that they may be complete at birth (75). The preacinar airways are formed by the 16th week of gestation, so following birth they do not increase in number, but they increase in both length and diameter, in parallel with the increase in body size. The significant increases of lung volume and weight from birth to adulthood occur predominantly as a result of growth within the acinar portion of the lung. Tracheal diameter increases directly with the increase in chest circumference. Studies examining relative rates of growth of intrapulmonary airways (proximal *vs.* distal) have yielded conflicting data. The work of Hogg *et al.* showed that the airways of children under 5 years of age were disproportionately narrow beyond the 18th airway generation, suggesting a retarded rate. They conjectured that conduction of peripheral airways was low in the first year of life but increased markedly at about 4 to 5 years of age (76). Studies of acinar development have shown that respiratory bronchioles are present by 19 weeks of gestation, and alveolar ducts by 28 weeks (77). Acinar development continues postnatally; the large increase in the number of respiratory bronchioles in the postnatal period has generally been accounted for by alveolization of bronchioles.

However, probably the areas of most disagreement relate to the number and extent of multiplication of alveoli in the neonatal period and early childhood (78–80), and the time alveolar multiplication ceases (78, 81–84). Workers over the years have felt that new alveoli continue to be formed to at least 8 years of age (78, 83, 84). However, Thurlbeck has noted that there is an increase in total alveolar number to 2 years of age in boys and to 4 years of age in girls, suggesting that the majority of alveoli are present by the age of 2 years and that no significant alveolar multiplication occurs subsequently (72). Langston and workers have also noted that in infants there is not a striking increase in alveolar number at 1 to 4 weeks following birth, suggesting that birth and air breathing, in and of themselves, do not stimulate alveolar development (73). This challenges the earlier work of Reid and Simon, who assumed that ventilation of peripheral lung units was important for the development of alveoli (85).

In those human infants with RDS who developed BPD, bronchiolar reactivity, increased small airway resistance, and abnormal blood gas levels have been identified during the first year following recovery and in survivors of 7 to 9 years of age (86–89). Kattan, in several reports, has examined long-term sequelae of various respiratory illnesses in infancy and childhood and has noted that several entities, including tracheaesophageal fistula, bronchiolitis, adenoviral infection, hydrocarbon pneumonitis, and croup, can result in long-term residual abnormalities in lung function and especially airway function (90, 91). Tepper and his colleagues have recently demonstrated that the small airway functional deficit seen in children with BPD is comparable to that seen in children with bronchiolitis and cystic fibrosis (personal communication). The finding that these respiratory illnesses can result in long-term residual abnormalities in lung function would support the hypothesis generated by several epidemiologic studies that childhood respiratory problems can be important risk factors for the development of chronic lung disease in adulthood. There are multiple epidemiologic studies in the British literature which show reduced flow rates in children and adults who have had childhood respiratory diseases (92–95). Burrows and his co-workers have demonstrated that patients with childhood respiratory disorders have lower levels of FEV_1 and that the rate of decline in FEV_1 with age is more rapid than that found in normal children (96). When smoking is considered the rate of decline is even more dramatically aggravated.

The human infant with BPD will probably be shown to stratify into several outcome categories, similar to what has been noted in adult ARDS patients. However, there is a unique feature in the infant lung which adds a new dimension; the infant has to accomplish his program of continued lung growth and development, a program which can be seriously disrupted by an injury that requires extensive repair and remodeling. This uniqueness of the infant lung may set the infant apart from ARDS adult survivors, most of whom can be expected to regain normal pulmonary function within 6 months (97–100). A recent report of children who survived ARDS supports this suspicion (101). Nine ARDS survivors, studied 0.9 to 4.2 years after the acute illness, had abnormal lung function including ventilation inequalities and hypoxemia. The authors suggested that a pediatric-age patient possibly is more susceptible to the primary insult or the respiratory treatment than the adult ARDS patient.

The use of a nonhuman primate as a BPD model has many valuable attributes—namely, an established knowledge of the anatomy of the lung, including morphometric data, similar cardiopulmonary physiology, appropriate size for intensive care monitoring, and comparable pathology of RDS/BPD. Their use for elucidating the pathogenesis, determining what factors may influence the course, and determining the long-term complications of perinatal injury will contribute greatly to the understanding, and ultimately the prevention, of RDS/BPD in the newborn.

Acknowledgments

The author thanks her colleagues (R. deLemos and T. Kuehl) and staff (E. Rominger, S. Hadick, L. Buchanan, and G. Canales) for their valuable contributions. Special thanks to G. Wolfe for superb secretarial assistance and E. Rominger for photographic support are extended.

References

1. Northway WH Jr, Rosan RC, Porter DY. Pulmonary disease following respirator therapy of hyaline-membrane disease. N Engl J Med 1967;276:357.
2. Rosan RC. Hyaline membrane disease and a related spectrum of pneumonopathies. In: Rosenberg HS, ed. Perspectives in pediatric pathology, vol 2. Chicago: Year Book Publishers, 1975, p 15.
3. Bonikos DS, Bensch KG, Northway WH Jr, et al. Bronchopulmonary dysplasia: the pulmonary pathologic sequel of necrotizing bronchiolitis and pulmonary fibrosis. Hum Pathol 1976;7:643.
4. Anderson WR, Strickland MB. Pulmonary complications of oxygen therapy in the neonate: postmortem study of bronchopulmonary dysplasia with emphasis on fibroproliferative obliterative bronchitis and bronchiolitis. Arch Pathol 1971;91:506.
5. Anderson WR, Strickland MB, Tsai SH, et al. Light microscopic and ultrastructural study of the adverse effects of oxygen therapy on the neonate lung. Am J Pathol 1973;73:327.
6. Anderson WR, Engel RR. Cardiopulmonary sequelae of reparative stages of bronchopulmonary dysplasia. Arch Pathol Lab Med 1983;107:603.
7. Taghizadeh A, Reynolds EOR. Pathogenesis of bronchopulmonary dysplasia following hyaline membrane disease. Am J Pathol 1976; 82:241.
8. Sobonya RE, Logvinoff MM, Taussig LM, et al. Morphometric analysis of the lung in prolonged bronchopulmonary dysplasia. Pediatr Res 1982;16:969.
9. Northway WH Jr, Brown E, Bancalari E, et al. Workshop on Bronchopulmonary Dysplasia. J Pediatr 1979;95:815.
10. Ludwin SK, Northway WH Jr, Bensch KG. Oxygen toxicity in the newborn: necrotizing bronchiolitis in mice exposed to 100 percent oxygen. Lab Invest 1974;31:425.
11. Bonikos DS, Bensch KG, Northway WH Jr. Oxygen toxicity in the newborn: the effect of chronic continuous 100 percent oxygen exposure on the lungs of newborn mice. Am J Pathol 1976;85:623.
12. Pappas CTE, Obara H, Bensch KG, Northway WH Jr. Effect of prolonged exposure to 80% oxygen on the lung of the newborn mouse. Lab Invest 1983;48:735.
13. Robertson B. Review of experimental hyaline membrane disease. Diagn Histopathol 1981; 4:49.
14. Stahlman M, LeQuire VS, Young WC, Merill RE, Birmingham RT, Payne GA. Pathophysiology of respiratory distress in newborn lambs. Am J Dis Child 1964;108:375.
15. Jobe A, Ikegami M, Glatz T, Yoshida Y, Diakomanolis E, Padbury J. Saturated phosphatidylcholine secretion and the effect of natural surfactant on premature and term lambs. Exp Lung Res 1983;4:259.
16. McAdams AJ, Coen R, Kleinman LI, et al. The experimental production of hyaline membranes in premature rhesus monkeys. Am J Pathol 1973;70:277.
17. Cutz E, Enhorning G, Robertson B, et al. Hyaline membrane disease: effect of surfactant prophylaxis on lung morphology in premature primates. Am J Pathol 1978;92:581.
18. Prueitt JL, Palmer S, Standaert TA, et al. Lung development in the fetal primate Macaca nemestrina. III. HMD. Pediatr Res 1979;13:654.
19. Hodson WA, Luchtel DL, Murphy JH, et al. Hyaline membrane disease: does sequential alveolar collapse occur? In: Stern L, Oh W, Friis-Hansen B, eds. Intensive care in the newborn, vol 2. New York: Masson Publishing, 1978, p 51.
20. Kessler, DL, Truog WE, Murphy JH, et al. Experimental hyaline membrane disease in the premature monkey: effects of antenatal dexamethasone. Am Rev Respir Dis 1982;126: 62.
21. Truog WE, Standaert TA, Murphy J, et al. Effect of high-frequency oscillation on gas exchange and pulmonary phospholipids in experimental hyaline membrane disease. Am Rev Respir Dis 1983;127:585.
22. Truog WE, Standaert TA, Murphy JH, et al. Effects of prolonged high-frequency oscilla-

tory ventilation in premature primates with experimental hyaline membrane disease. Am Rev Respir Dis 1984;130:76.
23. Escobedo MB, Hilliard JL, Smith F, et al. A baboon model of bronchopulmonary dysplasia. I. Clinical features. Exp Mol Pathol 1982;37:323.
24. Coalson JJ, Kuehl TJ, Escobedo MB, et al. A baboon model of bronchopulmonary dysplasia. II. Pathologic features. Exp Mol Pathol 1982;37:335.
25. deLemos RA, Coalson JJ, Null DM, Jr, et al. Ventilatory management of infant baboons with hyaline membrane disease: the use of high frequency ventilation. Ped Res 1987;21:594–602.
26. Bell RE, Kuehl TJ, Coalson JJ, et al. High-frequency ventilation compared to conventional positive-pressure ventilation in the treatment of hyaline membrane disease in primates. Crit Care Med 1984;12:764.
27. Coalson JJ, Kuehl TJ, deLemos RA. Bronchopulmonary dysplasia in the baboon: the role of diffuse alveolar damage in its pathogenesis, submitted.
28. Orell SR. Lung pathology in respiratory distress following shock in the adult. Acta Pathol Microbiol Scand 1971;79:65.
29. Katzenstein AA, Bloor CM, Leibow AA. Diffuse alveolar damage—the role of oxygen, shock and related factors. A review. Am J Pathol 1976;85:210.
30. Ashbaugh DG, Bigelow DB, Petty TL, et al. Acute respiratory distress in adults. Lancet 1967;2:319.
31. Nash G, Blennerhassett JB, Pontoppidan II. Pulmonary lesions associated with oxygen therapy and artificial ventilation. N Engl J Med 1968;276:368.
32. Soloway HB, Castillo Y, Martin AM. Adult hyaline membrane disease: relationship to oxygen therapy. Ann Surg 1968;168:937.
33. Weston JT, Liebow AA, Dixon MG, et al. Untoward effects of exogenous inhalants on the lung. J Forensic Sci 1972;17:199.
34. Bachofen M, Weibel ER. Alterations of the gas exchange apparatus in adult respiratory insufficiency associated with septicemia. Am Rev Respir Dis 1977;116:589.
35. Lamy M, Fallat RJ, Koeniger E, et al. Pathologic features and mechanisms of hypoxemia in adult respiratory distress syndrome. Am Rev Respir Dis 1976;114:267.
36. Nash G, Foley FD, Langlinais PC. Pulmonary interstitial edema and hyaline membranes in adult burn patients. Hum Pathol 1974;5:149.
37. Teplitz C. The core pathobiology and integrated medical science of adult acute respiratory insufficiency. Surg Clin North Am 1976;56:1091.
38. Pratt PC, Vollmer RT, Shelburne JD, et al. Pulmonary morphology in a multihospital collaborative extracorporeal membrane oxygenation project. I. Light microscopy. Am J Pathol 1979;95:191.
39. Anderson RR, Holliday RL, Driedger AA, et al. Documentation of pulmonary capillary permeability in the adult respiratory distress syndrome accompanying human sepsis. Am Rev Respir Dis 1979;119:869.
40. Carlson RW, Schaeffer RC Jr, Michaels SG, et al. Pulmonary edema fluid: spectrum of features in 37 patients. Circulation 1979;60:1161.
41. Sibbald WJ, Anderson RR, Holliday RL. Pathogenesis of pulmonary edema associated with the adult respiratory distress syndrome. Can Med Assoc J 1979;120:445.
42. Porte A, Stoeckel ME, Mantz JM, et al. Acute interstitial pulmonary fibrosis: comparative light and electron microscopic study of 19 cases—pathogenic and therapeutic implications. Intensive Care Med 1978;4:181.
43. Zapol WM, Trelstad RL, Coffey JW, et al. Pulmonary fibrosis in severe acute respiratory failure. Am Rev Respir Dis 1979;119:547.
44. Loosli CG. Interalveolar communications in normal and pathologic mammalian lungs. Arch Pathol 1937;24:743.
45. deLemos RA, Coalson JJ, Gerstmann DR, et al. Oxygen toxicity in the premature baboon with hyaline membrane disease. Am Rev Respir Dis 1987;136:677–682.
46. Coalson JJ. Pathophysiologic features of respiratory distress in the infant and adult. In Shoemaker WC, Thompson WL, Holbrook

PR, eds. The textbook of critical care. Section 5, Cardiovasculor. Chapter 50. Philadelphia: W.B. Saunders Co., 1984, p 344.
47. Churg A, Golden J, Fligiel S, Hogg JC. Bronchopulmonary dysplasia in the adult. Am Rev Respir Dis 1983;127:117.
48. Hochheim K. Ueber einige befunde in den lungen von neugborenen und die beziehung derselben zur aspiration von fruchtwasser. (Arb. a.d. pathol. Inst. zu Gottingen. Festschrift fur Orth. Berlin (1903). Zentralbl Pathol 1903;14:537.
49. Nilsson R, Grossman G, Robertson B. Pathogenesis of neonatal lung lesions induced by artificial ventilation: evidence against the role of barotrauma. Respiration 1980;40:218.
50. Nilsson R, Grossman G, Robertson B. Bronchiolar epithelial lesions induced in the premature rabbit neonate by short periods of artificial ventilation. Acta Path Microbiol Scand Sect A 1980; 88:359.
51. McCarthy K, Bhogal M, Nardi M, and Hart D. Pathogenic factors in bronchopulmonary dysplasia. Pediatr Res 1984;18:483.
52. Merritt TA. Oxygen exposure in the newborn guinea pig lung lavage cell populations, chemotactic and elastase response: a possible relationship to neonatal bronchopulmonary dysplasia. Pediatr Res 1982;16:798.
53. Ogden BE, Murphy SA, Saunders GC, Pathak D, Johnson JD. Neonatal lung neutrophils and elastase/proteinase inhibitor imbalance. Am Rev Respir Dis 1984;130:817.
54. Vapaavuori EK, Krohn K. Intensive care of small premature infants. II. Postmorten findings. Acta Paediatr Scand 1971;60:49.
55. Shankaran S, Szego E, Eizert D, Siegel P. Severe bronchopulmonary dysplasia—predictors of survival and outcome. Chest 1984;86: 607.
56. Smith JW, Bloomfield AL. The development of the aerobic bacterial flora of the throat in newborn babies. J Pediatr 1950;36:51.
57. McAllister TA, Givan J, Black A, Turner MJ, Kerr MM, Hutchinson JH. The natural history of bacterial colonization of the newborn in a maternity hospital. I. Scot Med J 1974;19: 119.
58. Long SS, Swenson RM. Development of anaerobic fecal flora in healthy newborn infants. J Pediatr 1977;91:298.
59. Rotimi VO, Duerden BI. The development of the bacterial flora in normal neonates. J Med Microbiol 1981;14:51.
60. Eisenach KD, Reber RM, Eitzman DV, Baer H. Nosocomial infections due to kanamycin-resistant, [R]-factor carrying enteric organisms in an intensive care nursery. Pediatrics 1972;50:395.
61. Harris H, Wirtschafter D, Cassady G. Endotracheal intubation and its relationship to bacterial colonization and systemic infection of newborn infants. Pediatrics 1976;56:816.
62. Goldmann DA, Leclair J, Macone A. Bacterial colonization of neonates admitted to an intensive care environment. J Pediatr 1978;93: 288.
63. Brook I, Martin WJ. Bacterial colonization in intubated newborns. Respiration 1980;40: 323.
64. Sprunt K, Leidy G, Redman W. Abnormal colonization of neonates in an intensive care unit: means of identifying neonates at risk of infection. Pediatr Res 1978;12:998.
65. Borderon JC, Gold F, Laugier J. Enterobacteria of the neonate—normal colonization and antibiotic-induced selection. Biol Neonate 1981;39:1.
66. Goodwin SR, Graves SA, Haberkern CM. Aspiration in intubated premature infants. Pediatrics 1985;75:85.
67. LaGamma EF, Drusin LM, Mackles AW, Machalek S, Auld PAM. Neonatal infections—an important determinant of late NICU mortality in infants less than 1,000g at birth. Am J Dis Child 1983;137:838.
68. Lamy M, Fallat RJ, Koeniger E, et al. Pathologic features and mechanisms of hypoxemia in adult respiratory distress syndrome. Am Rev Respir Dis 1976;114:267.
69. Ashbaugh DC, Petty RL. Sepsis complicating the acute respiratory distress syndrome. Surg Gynecol Obstet 1972;135:865.
70. Chirico G, Marconi M, De Amici M, et al. Deficiency of neutrophil bactericidal activity

in term and preterm infants—a longitudinal study. Biol Neonate 1985;47:125.
71. Alenghat E, Esterly JR. Alveolar macrophages in perinatal infants. Pediatrics 1984; 74:221.
72. Thurlbeck WM. Postnatal human lung growth. Thorax 1982;37:564.
73. Langston C, Kida K, Reed M, Thurlbeck WM. Human lung growth in late gestation and in the neonate. Am Rev Respir Dis 1984;129:607.
74. Broman I. Uber die ureaschen der asymmetrie der lungen und der herzlage bei den saugetieren. Anat Anz 1924;57:95.
75. Bucher U, Reid L. Development of the intrasegmental bronchial tree: the pattern of branching and development of cartilage at various stages of intrauterine life. Thorax 1961;16:207.
76. Hogg JC, Williams J, Richardson JB, Macklem PT, Thurlbeck EM. Age as a factor in the distribution of lower-airway conductance and in the pathologic anatomy of obstructive lung disease. N Engl J Med 1970;282:1283.
77. Hislop A, Reid L. Development of the acinus in the human lung. Thorax 1974;29:90.
78. Dunnill MS. Postnatal growth of the lung. Thorax 1962;17:329.
79. Angus GE, Thurlbeck WM. Number of alveoli in the human lung. J Appl Physiol 1972;32:483.
80. Davis G, Reid L. Growth of alveoli and pulmonary arteries in childhood. Thorax 1970; 25:669.
81. Hieronymi G. Veranderungen der lungenstruktur in verschiedenen liebensaltern. Verh Dtsch Ges Pathol 1960;44:129.
82. Hietronymi G. Uber den durch das alter bedingten formwandel menschlicher lungen. Ergeb Allerg Path Anat 1961;41:1.
83. Wilson HG. Postnatal development of the lung. Am J Anat 1928;41:97.
84. Emery JL, Mithal A. The number of alveoli in the terminal respiratory unit of man during late intrauterine life and childhood. Arch Dis Child 1960;35:544.
85. Reid L, Simon G. The role of alveolar hypoplasia in some types of emphysema. Br J Dis Chest 1964;58:158.
86. Bryan MH, Hardie MJ, Reilly BJ, Swyer PR. Pulmonary function studies during the first year of life in infants recovering from the respiratory distress syndrome. Pediatrics 1973;52:169.
87. Stocks J. Godfrey S, Reynolds EOR. Airway resistance in infants after various treatments for hyaline membrane disease: special emphasis on prolonged high levels of inspired oxygen. Pediatrics 1978;61:178.
88. Smyth JA, Tabachnik E, Duncan WJ, Reilly BJ, Levison H. Pulmonary function and bronchial hyperreactivity in long-term survivors of bronchopulmonary dysplasia. Pediatrics 1981;68:336.
89. Johnson JD, Malachowski NC, Grobstein R, Welsh D, Daily WJR, Sunshine P. Prognosis of children surviving with the aid of mechanical ventilation in the newborn period. J Pediatr 1974; 84:272.
90. Kattan M, Keens TG, Lapierre J-G, Levison H, Bryan AC, Reilly BJ. Pulmonary function abnormalities in symptom-free children after bronchiolitis. Pediatrics 1977;59:683.
91. Kattan M. Long-term sequelae of respiratory illness in infancy and childhood. Pediatr Clin N Am 1979;26:525.
92. Colley JRT, Douglas JWB, Reid DD. Respiratory disease in young adults: influence of early childhood lower respiratory tract illness, social class, air pollution and smoking. Br Med J 1973;3:195.
93. Holland WW, Halil T, Bennett AE, et al. Factors influencing the onset of chronic respiratory disease. Br Med J 1969;2:205.
94. Leeder Sr, Corkhill RT, Wysocki MJ, et al. Influence of personal and family factors on ventilatory function in children. Br J Prev Soc Med 1976;30:219.
95. Lunn JE, Knowelden J, Handyside AJ. Patterns of respiratory illness in Sheffield infant schoolchildren. Br J Prev Soc Med 1967;21:7.
96. Burrows B, Krudson RJ, Lebowitz MD. The relationship of childhood respiratory illness to adult obstructive airway disease. Am Rev Respir Dis 1977;115:751.

97. Elliott CG, Morris AH, Cengiz M. Pulmonary function and exercise gas exchange in survivors of adult respiratory distress syndrome. Am Rev Respir Dis 1981;123:492.
98. Lakshminarayan S, Stanford RE, Petty TL. Prognosis after recovery from adult respiratory distress syndrome. Am Rev Respir Dis 1976;113:7.
99. Rotman HH, Lavelle H, Duncheff DG, et al. Long-term physiologic consequences of the adult respiratory distress syndrome. Chest 1977;72:190.
100. Yahav J, Lieberman P, Molho M. Pulmonary function following the adult respiratory distress syndrome. Chest 1978;74:247.
101. Fanconi S, Kraemer R, Weber J, Tschaeppler H, Pfenninger J. Long-term sequelae in children surviving adult respiratory distress syndrome. J Pediatr 1985;106:218.

Comments

William H. Northway, Jr.

Since the incidence of BPD has shifted to become very high in infants with a birth weight of less than 1000 grams, a major challenge for an animal model is to duplicate this marked degree of prematurity and still survive. The factors that may have caused BPD in more mature babies, high concentration of oxygen and high peak pressures, have been reduced, but lower concentrations of oxygen and lower pressures may be just as injurious to the very immature lung.

III

Clinical Manifestations and Management of Bronchopulmonary Dysplasia

11

Clinical Presentation of Bronchopulmonary Dysplasia

T. ALLEN MERRITT AND BRUCE R. BOYNTON

Bronchopulmonary dysplasia (BPD) arises in the clinical setting as a gradually emerging chronic lung disease superimposed upon acute lung injury. Herein lies the problem of BPD diagnosis. Emerging BPD and acute lung injury often present many of the same symptoms including oxygen dependency, CO_2 retention, tachypnea, and labored respirations. For this reason it is usually impossible during the early stages of lung injury to distinguish the contributions of BPD to illness from those of acute lung injury. Only when the acute phase of illness has subsided can we diagnose BPD with certainty and, in retrospect, attribute the prolongation of clinical symptoms to emerging BPD.

In the vast majority of cases, BPD begins with the birth of a preterm infant. There are no other specific prenatal or intrapartum complications associated with later development of BPD, although infants with HLA-A2 antigen (1) or family history of reactive airway disease (2) may be at increased risk. In addition to a high incidence of surfactant deficient RDS (the acute lung disease most closely associated with development of BPD), preterm infants have immaturity of the lung airways, parenchyma, and antioxidant enzyme systems that may predispose them to lung injury from pressure or oxidant stresses.

Although ventilatory assistance for meconium aspiration, pneumonia, and apnea have all been linked to the development of BPD, its most frequent precursor is respiratory distress syndrome (RDS). Typically the infant is in distress from the time of birth, with tachypnea, expiratory grunting, and subcostal retractions. Infants with RDS usually require a fraction of inspired oxygen (FiO_2) greater than 0.6 to maintain an arterial oxygen tension greater than 50 torr and need assisted ventilation with continuous distending pressure. A frequent, and often unrecognized, accompaniment of RDS is systemic-to-pulmonary shunting of blood through a patent ductus arteriosus. The combination of surfactant insufficiency, pulmonary interstitial edema, and parenchymal immaturity produces a noncompliant and poorly aerated lung that exchanges gas poorly, thereby necessitating the use of elevated FiO_2 and high inspiratory pressures. In immature infants this therapy frequently produces pulmonary interstitial emphysema, a disease that complicates management and greatly increases the risk of BPD (3). The substantially lower activity of pulmonary antioxidants found in fetal and newborn rabbits, rats, and hamsters probably also exists in human preterm infants (4). Thus inflammatory cell mediated oxidants and high molecular oxygen concentrations can lead to lipid peroxidation, oxidation of sulfhydryl-containing enzymes, and inhibition of protein, nucleotide, and fatty acid biosynthesis. Cellular injury coupled with barotrauma sets the stage for that subtle transformation from acute lung injury to chronic BPD.

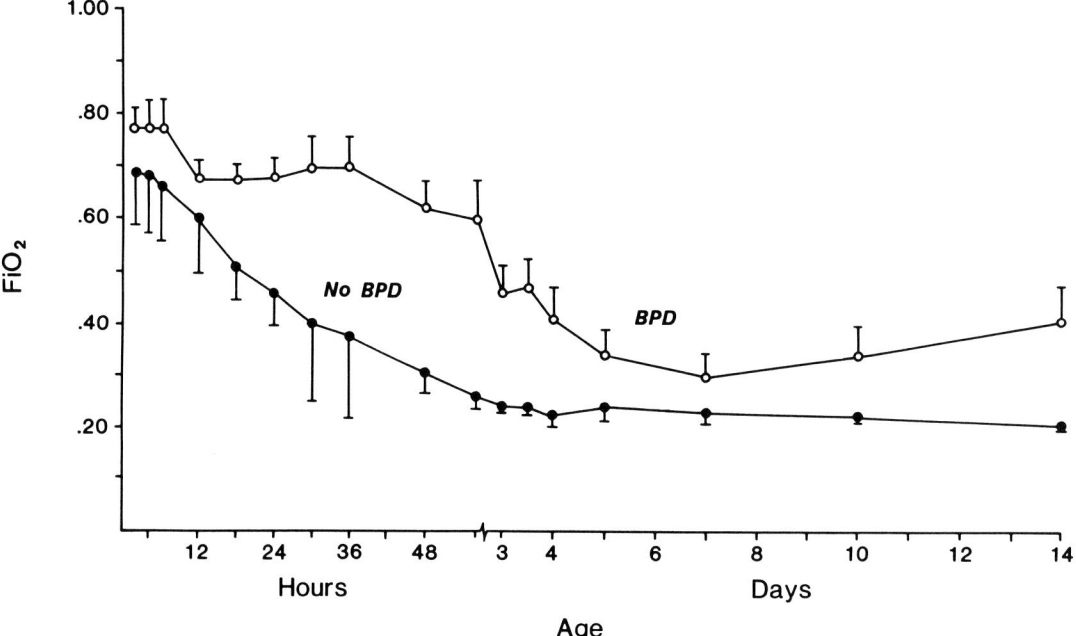

A

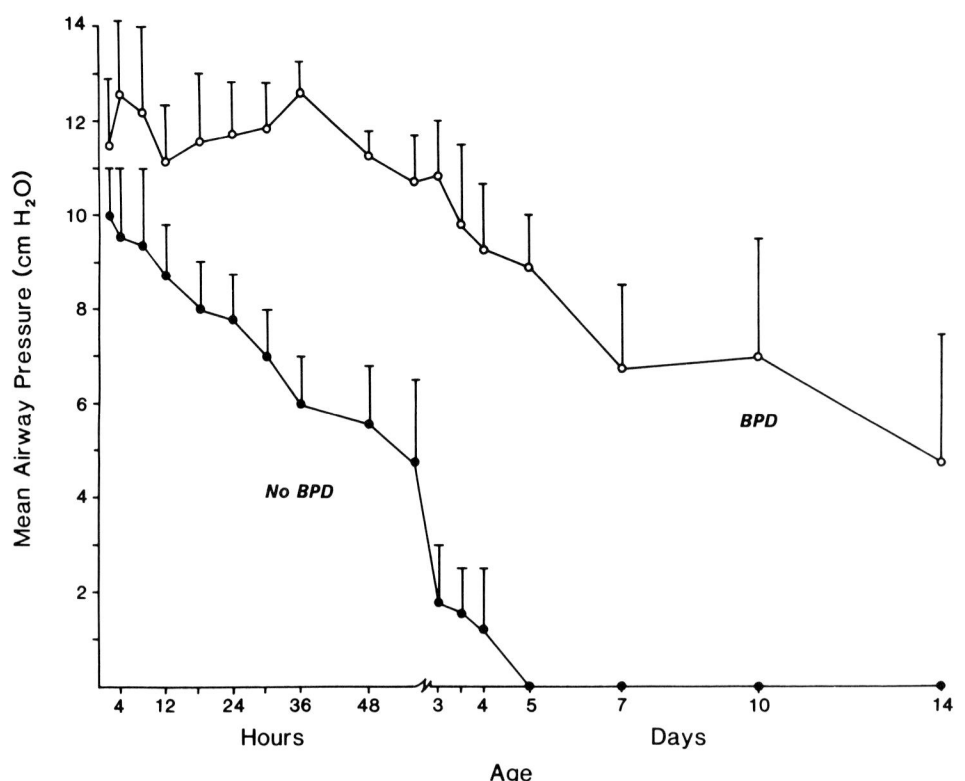

B

CLINICAL PRESENTATION OF BPD

The first sign of incipient BPD is usually a prolongation of the clinical course of RDS. Whereas most infants with RDS recover by 1 to 2 weeks of age, infants who are developing BPD continue to require supplemental oxygen and may be resistant to weaning from the ventilator. This is illustrated in Figure 11.1, which shows FiO_2 and mean airway pressure requirements of two groups of infants with RDS. One group went on to develop BPD, and the other recovered without sequelae. Obladen described the natural course of surfactant maturation among very low birth weight infants with RDS (5). By 7 to 10 days of life, lung stability was sufficient to permit at least an initial extubation, even in the absence of phosphatidylglycerol. Jacob et al. plotted the ventilatory course of infants with RDS of varying weight with or without a complicating patent ductus arteriosus and defined added duration of ventilation and supplemental oxygen exposure in these groups of infants (6).

Although opinions abound, there is little solid evidence to implicate a particular type of ventilator or method of ventilation in the pathogenesis of BPD. Neither Boros and Orgill (7) nor Toce et al. (8) were able to implicate any specific ventilator or ventilatory pattern (slow rate vs. rapid rate). There are anecdotal reports that BPD is rare in infants ventilated only by negative pressure ventilators (9). Heicher et al. (10) found no difference in the incidence of BPD between infants ventilated at a rate of 60 breaths a minute (0.5 second inspiration) and those ventilated at 20 to 40 breaths a minute (1.0 second inspiration). Rhodes et al. (11) and Boynton et al. (12) reported a low incidence of BPD in infants who were ventilated under a program that permitted lower values of PO_2 and higher values of PCO_2 than are usually considered acceptable. Although these reports are encouraging, they have yet to be verified by prospective clinical trial.

The neonatologist must strongly suspect BPD if an infant continues to require assisted ventilation and/or supplemental oxygen beyond 2 weeks after birth. However, the diagnosis of BPD should never be assumed, and other explanations for the infant's failure to wean from the ventilator must be sought. During the physical examination the clinician should pay special attention to respiratory frequency and the quality and distribution of breath sounds. In BPD breath sounds are often diminished in the peripheral lung fields, with bronchial sounds heard in synchrony with the inspiratory cycle of the ventilator. Expiration may produce wheezy, turbulent sounds or squeaks or explosive crackles (also heard in inspiration). These auscultatory findings frequently are not modified by pulmonary toilet, chest percussion, or airway suctioning. Rhonchi or gurgling sounds in the large airways can be auscultated over both anterior and posterior lung fields. The uniform, fine, crisp sounds of air entry are obscured by "junky" chest sounds. Unfortunately the stethoscope provides little information that is useful in determining either the onset or the severity of BPD. Never-

---

Figure 11.1. A & B: The F_iO_2 and mean airway pressures are plotted by age in hours or days from 15 infants between 750–1500 grams born at New England Center in 1986 who were diagnosed as bronchopulmonary dysplasia (○) compared to 15 infants not developing bronchopulmonary dysplasia (●). Each point represents the mean ± 1 standard deviation.

theless listening to breath sounds is a useful exercise in determining the response to various therapies such as inhaled agents. Thus the clinical presentation and physical examination are of little use in differentiating the infant developing BPD from the infant recovering from RDS.

Once the radiographic manifestations of BPD have appeared, the clinical signs are more distinctive. Whether still receiving assisted ventilation or able to be supported with supplemental oxygen alone, the infant with BPD will have elevated airways resistance associated with intercostal and subcostal retractions, tachypnea, and prolongation of the expiratory phase of breathing. During the second or third month of life, these infants will have frequent episodes of tachypnea during any exertion but especially during feeding, bowel movements, and procedures that cause pain or stress such as placement of intravenous needles and physical therapy.

Infants with BPD have wide oscillations in blood gas tensions whether measured by intermittent arterial or capillary puncture or by more contemporary methods such as transcutaneous measurement or pulse oximetry. Arterial PCO_2 ($PaCO_2$) values usually fluctuate between 60 and 80 torr. Frequent adjustment of FiO_2 may be required to maintain PaO_2 above 50 torr. It is essential to understand that during the recovery phase of BPD gas exchange is activity dependent (a reflection of oxygen consumption) and that the need for supplemental oxygen and other therapies such as diuretics, bronchodilators, and anti-inflammatory agents depends upon the demands placed on oxygen consumption and CO_2 elimination.

The 1979 Workshop on Bronchopulmonary Dysplasia concluded that the term BPD "should be used to describe the disease which is associated with intensive therapy for respiratory difficulty in newborn infant and which leads to chronic lung disease characterized by hypoxia, hypercarbia, and oxygen dependence with an associated chest radiograph showing hyperexpansion and focal hyperlucency alternating with strands of opacification" (13). In these recommendations no specific clinical signs were designated as indicative of BPD. Bancalari and coworkers provided a clinical description of "chronic respiratory disease characterized by tachypnea, intercostal and subcostal retractions, and rales on auscultation, all persisting for longer than 28 days" (14). Stahlman pointed out the major problems of hypercarbia, enhanced susceptibility to pulmonary infection, and the concomitant problems with nutrition and growth failure (15). At this conference there was only limited discussion of rickets, nephrolithiasis, nutritional deficiencies, cor pulmonale, and the psychosocial issues involved in this chronic disease.

Since that workshop there have been attempts at developing clinical and combined clinical and radiographic scoring systems. Toce *et al.* performed serial clinical assessments of infants with and without BPD (8). In these studies (see Chapter 23, Table 23.1) observations of respiratory patterns were averaged over several days and retractions were scored as previously described by Silverman and Anderson (16). This study failed to evaluate prospectively and objectively the infants' auscultatory findings. Retrospective and subjective assessment of chest sounds did not improve the predictive nature of the scoring. In other words no clinical sign or laboratory test was pathognomonic of BPD.

Important conclusions from this study were that it is preferable to wait 14 or more days after birth to make a clinical diagnosis of

BPD, and if examination at 21 days of age does not reveal signs of respiratory distress, the infant does not have BPD. If there are signs of tachypnea, dyspnea on exertion, hypercarbia (>46 torr), a need for supplemental oxygen, and insufficient weight gain, then further clinical and radiographic studies should be undertaken. The possibility of persistent patent ductus arteriosus or other causes of heart failure and pneumonia must always be considered. Coupled with the evidence provided by serial chest radiographs, this approach fulfills the desire of many neonatologists for uniform diagnositic criteria. However, the clinical scoring system of Toce *et al.* (8) has a number of problems. BPD in 600 g, 24 week gestation infants may be dramatically different from the disease seen in 1600 g, 32 week gestation infants. This scoring system does not account for heterogenous patterns of recovery from RDS, including systemic-to-pulmonary shunting through the patent ductus arteriosus, pulmonary infections, and immaturity of respiratory control, necessitating supplemental oxygen or assisted ventilation for extended periods. Furthermore, the radiographic score does not exclude Mikity-Wilson syndrome or interstitial pneumonitis due to a variety of infectious processes. Indeed recovery from RDS complicated by pneumonia (viral, bacterial, or fungal) may produce a chest radiograph not unlike BPD. Thus, while BPD scoring systems have sought to assess objectively the clinical and radiographic criteria upon which a diagnosis can be based, the National Heart, Lung, and Blood Institute publication, *Pediatric Respiratory Disorders*, stressed that the "lack of an appropriate, widely accepted definition" for BPD continues to be a major problem and questioned whether the diagnosis could be made at a specific point in time (17).

How will new therapies for RDS affect the clinical presentation of BPD? The efficacy of high-frequency oscillatory ventilation (HFOV) in the prevention of BPD is under investigation in a national collaborative trial. Thus far it seems clear that BPD does occur in neonates treated only with HFOV, but whether or not the use of this technique will reduce the incidence or severity of the disease is not known. Several centers are studying the use of high-frequency jet ventilation in infants, but little information is available about its effect on the clinical presentation of BPD. Therapy with exogenous surfactant accelerates the resolution of the reticulogranular infiltrates of RDS and improves oxygenation but does not appreciably alter the clinical findings on the first 1–2 days of life. A perihilar fluffiness has been described in a few infants treated with human surfactant (18), but this should not be confused with early BPD. The use of exogenous surfactant in extremely premature infants with surfactant insufficiency does appear to decrease the incidence of BPD (19). Whether the clinical presentation of BPD or its severity will be affected is as yet unknown.

Further investigation of the clinical manifestations of BPD must focus on a uniform definition of what constitutes a case, the heterogeneity of response to pulmonary injury in infants of different gestational ages, and the influence of new, and ever-changing therapies. Refinements in care and new therapies may also alter the clinical severity, age at "firm" diagnosis, and radiographic presentation of BPD.

The clinician must be aware of those variables associated with increased risk of BPD, objectively assess the infant, confirm radiographic changes, and evaluate other confirmatory data such as tracheal aspirate cytology and studies of pulmonary mechanics before assuming that chronic lung disease is BPD.

References

1. Clark DA, Pincus LG, Oliphant M, Hubbell C, Oates RP, Davey FR. HLA-A2 and chronic lung disease in neonates. J Am Med Assoc 1982;248:1868–1869.
2. Nickerson BG, Taussig LM. Family history of asthma in infants with bronchopulmonary dysplasia. Pediatrics 1980;65:1140–1144.
3. Moylan FMB, Walker AM, Krammer SS, Todres ID, Shannon DC. Alveolar rupture as an independent predictor of bronchopulmonary dysplasia. Crit Care Med 1978;6:10–13.
4. Frank L, Sosenko I. Prenatal development of lung antioxidant enzymes in four species. J Pediatr 1978;110:106–110.
5. Obladen M. Factors influencing surfactant composition in the newborn infant. Eur J Pediatr 1978;128:129–143.
6. Jacob J, Gluck L, DiSessa T, et al. The contribution of PDA in the neonate with severe RDS. J Pediatr 1980;96:79–87.
7. Boros S, Orgill A. Mortality and morbidity associated with pressure-and volume-limited infant ventilators. Am J Dis Child 1978;32:865–869.
8. Toce S, Farrell P, Leavitt L, Samuels D, Edwards D. Clinical and roetgenographic scoring systems for assessing bronchopulmonary dysplasia. Am J Dis Child 1984;138:581–585.
9. Stern L. The role of respirators in the etiology and pathogenesis of bronchopulmonary dysplasia. J Pediatr 1979;867–869.
10. Heicher DA, Kasting DS, Richards JR. Prospective clinical comparison of two methods for mechanical ventilation of neonates: rapid rate and short inspiratory time versus slow rate and long inspiratory time. J Pediatr 1981;98:957–961.
11. Rhodes PG, Graves GR, Patel DM, Campbell SB, Blumenthal BL. Minimizing pneumothorax and bronchopulmonary dysplasia in ventilated infants with hyaline membrane disease. J Pediatr 1983;103:634.
12. Boynton BR, Mannino FL, Randel RC, Merritt TA, Coen RW, Edwards D, Gluck L. Minimizing bronchopulmonary dyplasia in VLBW infants (letter). J Pediatr 1984;104:962.
13. National Heart, Lung, and Blood Institute. Workshop on Bronchopulmonary Dyplasia. J Pediatr 1979;85:920.
14. Bancalari E, Abdenour G, Feller R, Gannon J. Bronchopulmonary dysplasia: clinical presentation. J Pediatr 1979;85:819–823.
15. Stahlman M. Clinical description of bronchopulmonary dysplasia J Pediatr 1979;85:829–834.
16. Silverman W, Anderson D. A controlled clinical trial of effects of water mist on obstructive respiratory signs, death rate and necropsy findings among premature infants. Pediatrics 1956;17:1–10.
17. Division of Lung Disease, National Heart, Lung, and Blood Institute. Pediatric respiratory disorders. NIH Publication No. 86-2107, pp 51–55.
18. Edwards D, Hilton S, Merritt T, Hallman M, Mannino F, Boynton B. Respiratory distress syndrome treated with human surfactant: radiographic findings. Radiology 1985;157:329–334.
19. Merritt T, Hallman M, Bloom B, et al. Prophylactic treatment of very premature infants with human surfactant. N Engl J Med 1986;315:785–790.

12

The Radiology of Bronchopulmonary Dysplasia and Its Complications

DAVID K. EDWARDS III

Introduction

Bronchopulmonary dysplasia was initially described, named, and abbreviated (BPD) by a group under the direction of a diagnostic radiologist (1). In the years since Dr. Northway's initial description in 1967, radiology has maintained a crucial role in the diagnosis and surveillance of BPD. Indeed the formal definition of the disease proposed by a National Institutes of Health workshop includes chest radiographic abnormalities as a *sine qua non* of BPD: ". . . chronic lung disease characterized by hypoxia, hypercarbia, and oxygen dependence with an associated chest radiograph showing hyperexpansion, and focal hyperlucency alternating with strands of opacification" (2). This radiographic description is an oversimplification, but the importance of radiology in the study and clinical management of BPD is beyond dispute.

Despite this importance, relatively little has been published about the purely radiologic aspects of BPD. Some of this informational paucity may be ascribed to the adequacy and elegance of the initial radiographic description of the disease (3). Nonetheless few radiologists who deal with active neonatal intensive care nurseries would deny that the radiographic character of BPD has been changing since its initial description, and that the radiographic manifestations of the disease are more complex, varied, and occasionally confusing than originally recognized.

Additionally BPD generally occurs in the complex physical and physiologic environment of a preterm infant in a neonatal intensive care unit, an infant who is subjected to a wide variety of therapeutic maneuvers, the overall effects of which are often poorly understood. These effects on premature, developing organisms can be surprising. For example, until recently cholelithiasis in children was limited largely to those suffering from hemolytic diseases; yet infants with BPD occasionally develop gallstones. Infants with BPD are also subject to nephrocalcinosis, multiple fractures, airway granulomas, and other conditions whose diagnosis is usually radiographic. Thus the radiology of BPD patients is not limited to the lung parenchyma.

This chapter attempts to survey the important radiographic abnormalities that may be expected in the clinical setting of BPD. The most important of these, of course, are pulmonary, but several extrathoracic associations of BPD are discussed as well. It must be recalled that prematurity itself is associated with numerous pathologic conditions that may coincide with BPD (4). Because of space limitations, diseases of prematurity that do not appear closely related to BPD (*e.g.*, intracranial hemorrhage and necrotizing enterocolitis) are not discussed, although they certainly may be important in individual patients with BPD.

Two caveats are in order. First, the radiology of BPD and the radiology of neonates in general are areas in which there are numerous "unknowns"; many phenomena that are fairly commonly seen have not been scrutinized and clarified by formal, rigorous study or pathologic confirmation. For this reason assertions in this chapter that are not graced by bibliographic citation are the subjective, unsubstantiated clinical impressions of the author, whose experience is extensive but by no means exhaustive. I apologize for the errors that time will doubtless reveal.

Second, classical "plain film" radiology, upon which most of the radiology of neonates is based, is a crude instrument. The shadow-pictures of many diseases resemble those of many other diseases, even to the most expert eyes. The reason for this is not only the crudity of the instrumentation, but also the limited number of ways a human body can respond to the diseases that beset it. Thus there are relatively few findings that are absolutely pathognomonic in radiology, and a common expression of this defect is the radiographic differential diagnosis, which is emphasized in this chapter. As I often tell my neonatologist friends, there is absolutely no way I can diagnose BPD confidently on a single chest film, and I can diagnose it only with a variable (but higher) level of certainty after examining all prior films and learning the clinical history. Radiology in BPD is a powerful tool, but like all tools it is best used with full understanding of its limitations.

The Radiographic Progression of Bronchopulmonary Dysplasia

General

It was recognized early that the radiographic appearance of BPD within a given patient varied as a function of time (1). Instead of appearing full-blown, or appearing in a mild version and becoming more severe, the disease changed in its radiographic manifestations through a succession of fairly distinct appearances, each of which was generally more diagnostically specific than its predecessor. Experience has shown, first, that this succession of appearances varies widely in its timing and radiographic specificity from patient to patient, and second, that the radiographic progression of BPD is not as predictably stereotyped as initially thought.

Obviously the radiographic environment from which BPD arises is that of the underlying chest disease. In the great majority of cases the underlying chest disease is respiratory distress syndrome (RDS, or pulmonary surfactant deficiency, used here interchangeably with "hyaline membrane disease"), upon which the major emphasis of this discussion is placed. It is, however, well recognized that BPD arises from other conditions as well, including very small preterm infants without RDS (5–9), meconium aspiration syndrome (10), other conditions causing aspiration pneumonitis (11–13), sepsis with pneumonia (14), left-to-right shunt from the patent ductus arteriosus (7), large extracardiac left-to-right shunt from an arteriovenous malformation (15), congenital heart disease (13, 16), neonatal tetanus (17), a congenital muscular disorder (18), and Wilson-Mikity syndrome (12). Even adults may acquire a condition that strongly resembles, and may in fact be, BPD (19, 20). Indeed the final, chronic appearance of BPD seems to be an end-point that may be reached by a variety of pathways from an underlying substrate of almost any condition that necessitates extensive respiratory support.

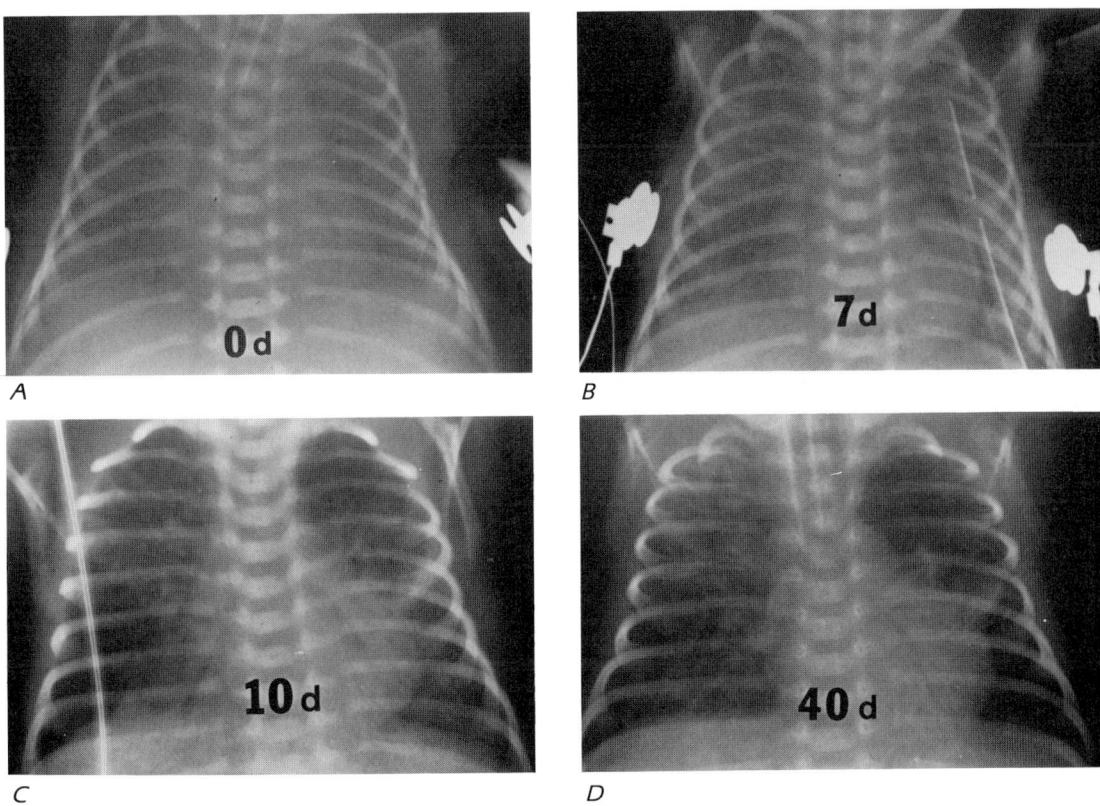

Figure 12.1. Four stages of developing BPD, with patient's age in days indicated. (A) Stage I is identical to uncomplicated RDS. (B) Stage II, a period of parenchymal opacification, was not notable in this patient; the left chest tube reflects PDA ligation. (C) Stage III, mildly bubbly lungs, with a prominent interstitial pattern. (D) Stage IV BPD, or chronic lung disease.

The Development of Bronchopulmonary Dysplasia in the Setting of Respiratory Distress Syndrome

Progression in Four Stages in the Setting of Respiratory Distress Syndrome

As initially described by Northway and associates (1, 3), BPD arose in the setting of RDS through a series of four stages that were both radiographically (Fig. 12.1) and pathologically fairly distinct:

Stage I: Radiographically indistinguishable from uncomplicated RDS, but with distinctive pathologic changes involving considerable mucosal necrosis (1 to 3 days of age).

Stage II: Marked radiopacity of the lungs, pathologically involving necrosis and repair of alveolar epithelium, with exuberant exudate into the airway lumen (4 to 10 days of age).

Stage III: Clearing of the radiopacity into a cystic, bubbly pattern, pathologically marked by widespread mucosal metaplasia and alveolar coalescence alternating with regions of alveolar emphysema (10 to 20 days of age).

Stage IV: Defined by the presence of chronic abnormalities beyond 1 month of age. The radiograph typically shows hyperexpansion, streaks of abnormal density, and areas of emphysema, with variable cardiomegaly (1 month and beyond).

Stage I BPD is radiographically indistinguishable from the underlying RDS. Furthermore the radiographic appearance of RDS itself may be simulated by other diseases; these are listed in Table 12.1. Ideally all of these conditions could be distinguished from RDS because RDS is the only one that is typically *underinflated;* RDS is an atelectatic disease. However, underinflation can be masked when the infant is radiographed while being treated with mechanical ventilation, as most such infants are, and in this setting patients with definite RDS are sometimes unequivocally hyperinflated rather than normally inflated or underinflated.

Of the entities in Table 12.1 the most treacherous is diffuse pneumonitis, especially that caused by the group B *Streptococcus* (21–23). Diffuse pneumonitis should be suspected when "RDS" is seen in a large infant, especially one who is not an infant of a diabetic mother. The presence of a pleural effusion should be sought; effusion is common in diffuse pneumonitis, but seldom seen in uncomplicated RDS (24, 25). Of course RDS and pneumonitis can coexist (26, 27).

Simple retained fetal lung fluid, if radiographed early when the excessive fluid is largely alveolar, can present with a reticulogranular pattern suggesting RDS (28). However, such patients are commonly hyperinflated, and small pleural effusions are common. The distinctive and rapid clearing, during which the excessive fluid tends to become largely interstitial before vanishing

Table 12.1. Radiographic Differential Diagnosis of Respiratory Distress Syndrome and Stage I Bronchopulmonary Dysplasia

1. Diffuse pneumonia accompanying sepsis (group B *Streptococcus* and several other organisms)
2. Retained fetal lung fluid ("transient tachypnea of the newborn"), in early hours when the excessive fluid is largely alveolar
3. Pulmonary edema, especially secondary to intracranial hemorrhage
4. Very small premature infant with accelerated lung maturity and normal or borderline surfactant status
5. Pulmonary hemorrhage
6. Occasionally, pulmonary venous congestion (prototype is total anomalous pulmonary venous connection with obstruction)

within about 72 hours, is retrospectively quite helpful in distinguishing this condition from RDS, which seldom clears rapidly.

Pulmonary edema for any cause can also sometimes simulate RDS. In a small premature infant, pulmonary edema can result from intracranial hemorrhage and from left-to-right shunting through the patent ductus arteriosus (PDA). Pulmonary hemorrhage simulates pulmonary edema and sometimes RDS (29); it generally clears rapidly (within 24 hours) if the bleeding stops. The causes of severe pulmonary venous congestion that can cause RDS's "ground glass" appearance are usually clinically obvious from the associated profound cyanosis that is refractory to elevated inspired oxygen (30). The chest radiographs of very small premature infants who have etiologies of respiratory insufficiency other than RDS are discussed separately below.

Similarly Stage II BPD may be simulated by a variety of other causes of pulmonary parenchymal opacity (the so-called "whiteout") in the setting of RDS; indeed such other causes are probably more common than Stage II BPD. Some of these other phenomena are listed in Table 12.2. Respiratory distress syndrome can definitely worsen radiographically during the first 1 to 2 days of life, presumably because of exhaustion of endogenous surfactant; this occurrence can cause increased parenchymal radiopacity in the absence of any other disease process.

Probably a more commonly seen cause of "whiteout" that generally occurs with about the same timing as Stage II BPD is pulmonary edema from significant left-to-right shunting through the PDA. Indeed the clinical course during Stage II BPD is often dominated by the PDA; as pulmonary vascular resistance falls in the first days of life, the lungs may be flooded by fluid, causing a sustained need for high oxygen and ventilator pressures and necessitating treatment by diuretics, indomethacin, or surgical ligation (31). Other radiographic findings accompanying PDA, such as enlarged "shunt" vessels in the perihilar regions and cardiomegaly, may help to distinguish shunting from Stage II BPD. If these are masked by the extensive edema, the echocardiographic visualization of the ductus and ductal flow (32), assessment of left atrial size (33), or aortography (34) are diagnostically more useful than the radiograph.

Conditions causing a radiographic picture of pulmonary edema, and sometimes producing a "whiteout" include simple iatrogenic fluid overload, pulmonary edema from intracranial hemorrhage, the so-called "weaning effect," and pulmonary hemorrhage. Iatrogenic fluid overload is frequent; in small, preterm infants, fluid balance can shift considerably in response to remarkably small volume changes. Pulmonary edema following intracranial hemorrhage may be considered when such hemorrhage is diagnosed ultrasonographically. Pulmonary hemorrhage occasionally occurs in the setting of diffuse hemorrhagic disease, but is frequently primary in the lung or secondary to a necrotizing pneumonitis.

Table 12.2. Radiographic Differential Diagnosis of Stage II Bronchopulmonary Dysplasia ("Whiteout" in RDS)

1. Worsening RDS (first 1 to 2 days only)
2. Congestive heart failure, usually secondary to patent ductus arteriosus
3. Iatrogenic fluid overload
4. Pulmonary edema secondary to intracranial hemorrhage
5. "Weaning effect" following extubation or decrease in ventilator pressure
6. Pulmonary hemorrhage
7. Superimposed pneumonitis
8. Massive aspiration
9. Expiratory examination
10. Underpenetrated examination

The "weaning effect" is a curious radiographic phenomenon that fairly commonly follows endotracheal extubation or large decreases in ventilator pressure. The lungs undergo a transient period of radiopacity, although the patient generally remains clinically stable or even improved. This phenomenon occurs fairly frequently, and seems to be a more common cause of parenchymal opacity than Stage II BPD, in the setting of RDS (35).

Massive pneumonitis (bacterial or viral) can produce diffuse opacity (26), although a patchy appearance is more common. The same is true of massive aspiration, which in a supine infant tends to involve the upper lobes preferentially. Although it can occur, aspiration is relatively uncommon when an endotracheal tube is in place.

Another condition that may be suspected when a radiographic "whiteout" occurs, especially when the patient has not decompensated clinically, is a hypoventilatory examination. As little as one interspace difference in ventilation in the setting of RDS can make a great difference in the opacity of the lungs. If a hypoventilatory examination (or one that is badly underpenetrated) is suspected, the examination should be repeated.

The clearing of the "whiteout" of Stage II BPD into a bubbly appearance is strongly suggestive of Stage III disease. Indeed it is at this point that one may first suspect that the previous period of radiopacity represented Stage II BPD.

The appearance of Stage III BPD heralds the onset of chronic lung disease. The radiographic distinction between Stage III and Stage IV BPD is not clear-cut; recall that Stage IV BPD is defined chronologically, not radiographically. The prototypic transition between these two stages is the gradual change of the fairly homogeneous bubbles of Stage III disease to a more irregular alternation of heterogeneous regions of emphysema with strands of abnormal density that represent fibrosis and/or atelectasis. However, many patients do not undergo this transition; instead the Stage III bubbly appearance may persist with little change for weeks to months. The definition of Stage IV chronologically is useful, however, because it is at about a month of life that one can usually distinguish clearly between infants who have BPD and those who do not (31).

Insidious Progression in the Setting of Respiratory Distress Syndrome

It is widely agreed that the stepwise radiographic progression of BPD through the four stereotyped stages is presently not commonly seen (16, 18, 35–41). Specifically a period of dense parenchymal opacification in the first week of life is relatively uncommon (35, 38), and when it occurs it is usually found to represent some process other than Stage II BPD (Table 12.2). Similarly the distinct bubbly appearance of Stage III developing from the setting of radiopacity is also uncommon. It is quite difficult to find a single, contemporary patient whose radiographs typify all four stages of BPD.

It is nevertheless true that in the past these four stages were seen with regularity; when my colleagues and I examined and extended through 1973 the original series of Northway *et al.* (1), most patients demonstrated a clear-cut, stepwise transition (42). The question arises as to when this pattern became uncommon; my impression is that it occurred during the period when important changes in ventilatory techniques were made, specifically the use of continuous positive airway pressure. During this period the spectrum of radiographic changes seen in chronic or Stage IV BPD appeared to shift toward a picture of milder disease.

In my experience and that of others, the most common contemporary onset and progression of BPD in the setting of RDS are gradual and insidious, without specific early radiographic landmarks (16, 38). In patients with uncomplicated RDS who develop BPD, a faint, lacy pattern that is predominantly interstitial appears, which is usually noted at 20 to 30 days of life. An example of this progression is shown in Figure 12.2. Occasionally this pattern appears after a period of hazy-appearing lungs, which could represent a delayed or attenuated Stage II BPD or some other process.

In patients whose initial course is complicated with air leaks, PDA shunting, superimposed pneumonia, atelectasis, and the myr-

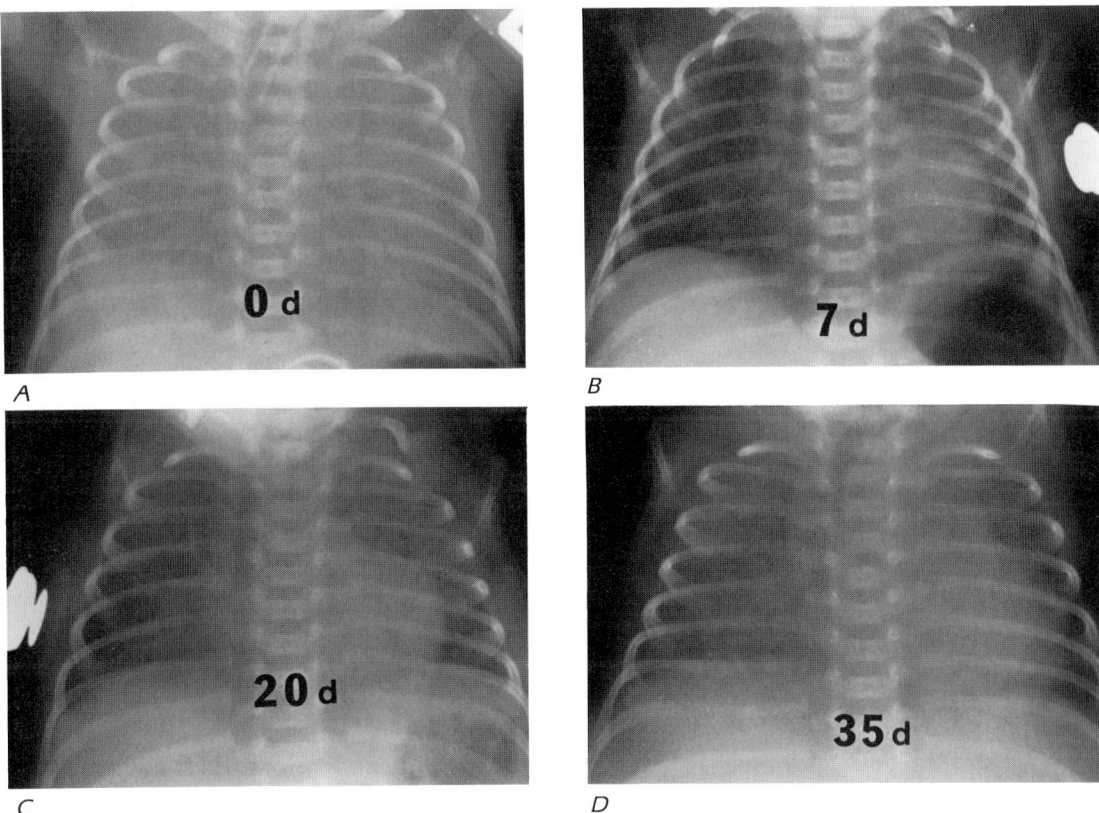

Figure 12.2. Insidious development of BPD; patient's age in days is noted. (A) Initial film shows moderately severe RDS. (B) Much of the granularity has cleared; prominent central vessels suggest a PDA. (C) A faint, lacy infiltrate obscures the central vessels. (D) Lungs are diffusely involved with a hazy process that clinically represented mild to moderate BPD.

iad other difficulties to which RDS patients are subject, BPD commonly becomes manifest as a diffuse interstitial pattern that persists after the various other pulmonary problems have subsided. In such patients the four stages of BPD may have occurred, but their appearance was masked by the more compelling acute abnormalities.

Some such patients, instead of subsiding into chronic interstitial changes after their acute phases, exhibit a prolonged period of considerable pulmonary opacity before the interstitial pattern becomes apparent. Commonly in these patients there are scattered radiographs—often following diuretic therapy—that offer tantalizing glimpses of a pattern of parenchymal irregularity developing beneath the overall opacity. When the opacity finally clears irregular lungs of moderate to severe BPD are seen. Perhaps this period of opacity is a lengthy, delayed, and severe version of Stage II disease, or perhaps merely leaky capillaries secondary to oxygen damage, or an infantile version of adult respiratory distress syndrome. The exact nature of the abnormality is uncertain, but I have learned to associated this appearance with chronic BPD.

The interstitial pattern that develops in these cases may remain stable, regress, or worsen radiographically during the ensuring weeks. In any case clinically most of these patients have BPD, and the lesion is generally confirmed if the patients come to autopsy. The behavior of chronic BPD is a separate subject, discussed below.

Progression in the Setting of Pulmonary Interstitial Emphysema

The incidence of BPD appears to be considerably higher in infants who develop "air leaks" (episodes of airway rupture leading to collections of intrathoracic extra-alveolar gas) than in infants who are spared this complication (43, 44). Moylan and associates (45) estimate that the relative odds of developing BPD are increased by a factor of 39 if air leak occurs. The reason for this is uncertain, but there are two plausible explanations. The first is a speculated direct effect, by which interstitial ectopic gas sets up an inflammatory, scarring response in the pulmonary interstitium. The second is that the ectopic gas, by occupying a significant intrathoracic volume, reduces the area available for gas exchange, leading to the necessity of increased respiratory support and hence increased iatrogenic damage to the lungs by the conventionally stipulated mechanisms of oxygenation and ventila-

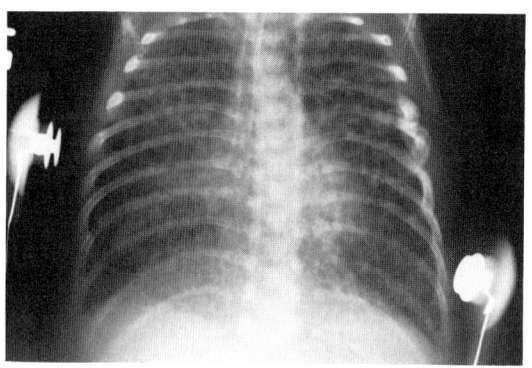

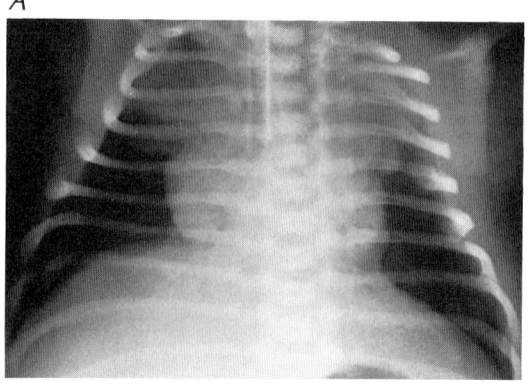

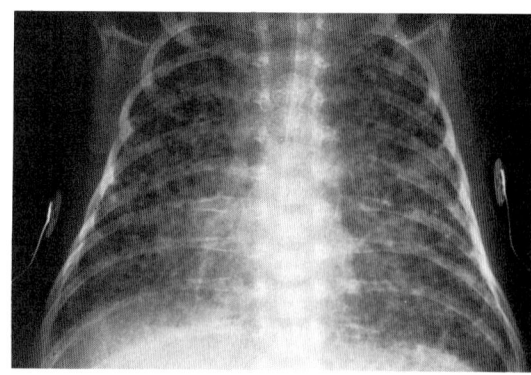

Figure 12.3. BPD developing in the setting of pulmonary interstitial emphysema (PIE). (*A*) Two month old infant with clinical BPD; at 3 days of age, diffuse PIE developed in the setting of RDS, and the radiographs since that time remained essentially unchanged. (*B*) Infant with pulmonary hypoplasia secondary to oligohydramnios, with bilateral pneumothoraces on the day of birth. Diffuse PIE ensued and persisted, radiographically unchanged; at 2 months (*C*) patient clinically has chronic BPD.

tion (46). Whatever the mechanism it is clear that air leaks increase the likelihood of BPD.

One aspect of this phenomenon is a distinct progression of BPD (or what *may* be BPD) that is radiographically even more confusing than the insidious appearance described above. The typical patient with this progression—who generally, but not invariably, has underlying RDS—develops bilateral pulmonary interstitial emphysema, which is commonly diffuse and relatively mild. Instead of resolving, however, the pulmonary interstitial emphysema persists for days and then weeks, changing little in its radiographic appearance (Fig. 12.3). As time passes the neonatologist and radiologist begin to wonder if in fact the infant may have BPD; certainly the process on any individual film resembles BPD, and the clinical picture suggests BPD as well.

On the other hand chronic interstitial emphysema has been described (47–49), although the cases reported have had involvement of only a single lobe or lung. Furthermore such localized collections tend to resolve, given enough time (50), whereas the bilateral cases described here do not. Certainly the affected infants have chronic lung disease, and the disease resembles BPD clinically and radiographically, but the progression causes uncertainty about the true diagnosis. To date I know of no such patients who have come to autopsy.

The Development of Bronchopulmonary Dysplasia in Settings Other Than That of Respiratory Distress Syndrome

Premature Infants with Accelerated Lung Maturity

At the University of California at San Diego Newborn Intensive Care Nursery, the second most common setting in which BPD occurs is in a somewhat confusing group of infants of very low gestation and birth weight (1500 g or less) who "ought" to have RDS because of their prematurity, but who are spared RDS for reasons that are not altogether clear; a plausible theory is that one or another intrauterine stress (or maternal steroid therapy) has accelerated the maturity of their pulmonary surfactant system (5). Such infants are born with relatively normal lungs, at least in terms of pulmonary compliance and gas exchange.

These infants are not themselves unduly confusing; they form a cohort at least as coherent as that composed of RDS patients. The confusion arises from nomenclature: nobody seems quite sure what to call them. When such infants require assisted ventilation because of apnea, they are referred to as having "apnea of prematurity" (8), "apnoea repetens of immaturity" (51), "repeating apnoea" (52), "pulmonary insufficiency of prematurity" (9), and like terms. "Chronic pulmonary insufficiency of prematurity" seems to be a related condition (53).

The first radiographic description of these infants used the term "immature lung syndrome" (54), which we abbreviated as "immature lung" in a later study (5). This proved not to be a popular name for this condition (55), possibly because the lungs seem to be the most mature things about these infants, biochemically at least, despite the fact that such lungs seen at autopsy are morphologically immature.

Currently we call the condition of a low birth weight (1500 g or less) infant who does not have RDS a PALM baby, which is an acronym for premature with accelerated lung maturity. RDS is defined biochemically as the absence of phosphatidylglycerol in lung effluent (56).

The chest radiographic findings in PALM infants include normal inflation, a mild granularity or an interstitial "wet" appearance, an absence of abnormal air bronchograms, and generally a small thymic shadow; the latter presumably reflects intrauterine stress. The most important cardiorespiratory difficulties encountered by PALM infants are significant left-to-right shunting through the PDA, and apnea. A few PALM infants who are mistakenly diagnosed as having RDS and subjected to excessive ventilator pressures may develop air leaks. In PALM infants who require prolonged ventilatory assistance for any of these difficulties, radiographic changes suggesting BPD may occur, as well as clinically significant BPD in a few (5).

The radiographic progression of BPD in PALM infants does not evolve through the four stages described in the setting of RDS (1). Instead, like the insidious progression in RDS, faint interstitial markings appear at about 15 to 20 days. Often these first become perceptible after the pulmonary abnormalities reflecting ductal shunting resolve. The interstitial markings become chronic, and generally disappear slowly after a few weeks to months in infants who no longer require respiratory assistance. In a few infants who require very prolonged respiratory assistance, the changes may become progressively severe until the radiograph suggests frank Stage IV BPD as seen in RDS (Fig. 12.4). Generally, however, the radiographic severity of BPD is substantially less in PALM infants than in RDS survivors.

Infants with Meconium Aspiration Syndrome, Severe Pneumonia, Persisting Fetal Circulation, or Pulmonary Hypoplasia

BPD has been noted to follow meconium aspiration syndrome (10), severe neonatal pneumonia (14), persisting neonatal pulmonary hypertension ("persisting fetal circulation") (57), and pulmonary hypoplasia (Fig. 12.3). Despite the seeming diversity of these conditions, the progression of BPD appears radiographically similar in all of them. Perhaps the reason for this is that the diversity may be more apparent than real; both meconium aspiration syndrome and severe pneumonia may be accompanied by neonatal pulmonary arterial hypertension—the so-called "secondary" form of persisting pulmonary hypertension (58)—and hypoplastic lungs also appear to demonstrate elevated arterial pressures, so that affected patients clinically simulate those with persisting fetal circulation (59). A common denominator may be pulmonary arterial hypertension, which clinically demands high oxygen tension and strenuous ventilatory efforts to maintain oxygenation (60).

Patients with the "primary" type of persisting pulmonary hypertension generally have clear to slightly hyperlucent lungs radiographically, whereas patients with the "secondary" type generally demonstrate the findings of the underlying disease, which is most commonly meconium aspiration syndrome or severe pneumonia. Patients with pulmonary hypoplasia also have clear, small lungs, but very frequently there are air leaks, usually pneumothorax (59).

Infants with these conditions who progress to chronic lung disease commonly develop relative parenchymal opacity for a period that begins after 1 to 3 days of vigorous respiratory support. This opacity, which may be superimposed on the initial abnormalities, is a diffuse, granular "infiltrate" with abnormal air bronchograms; the appearance is most suggestive of RDS. Interestingly phospholipid analysis of patients with "primary" persisting pulmonary hypertension reveals low levels of surfactant comparable with lev-

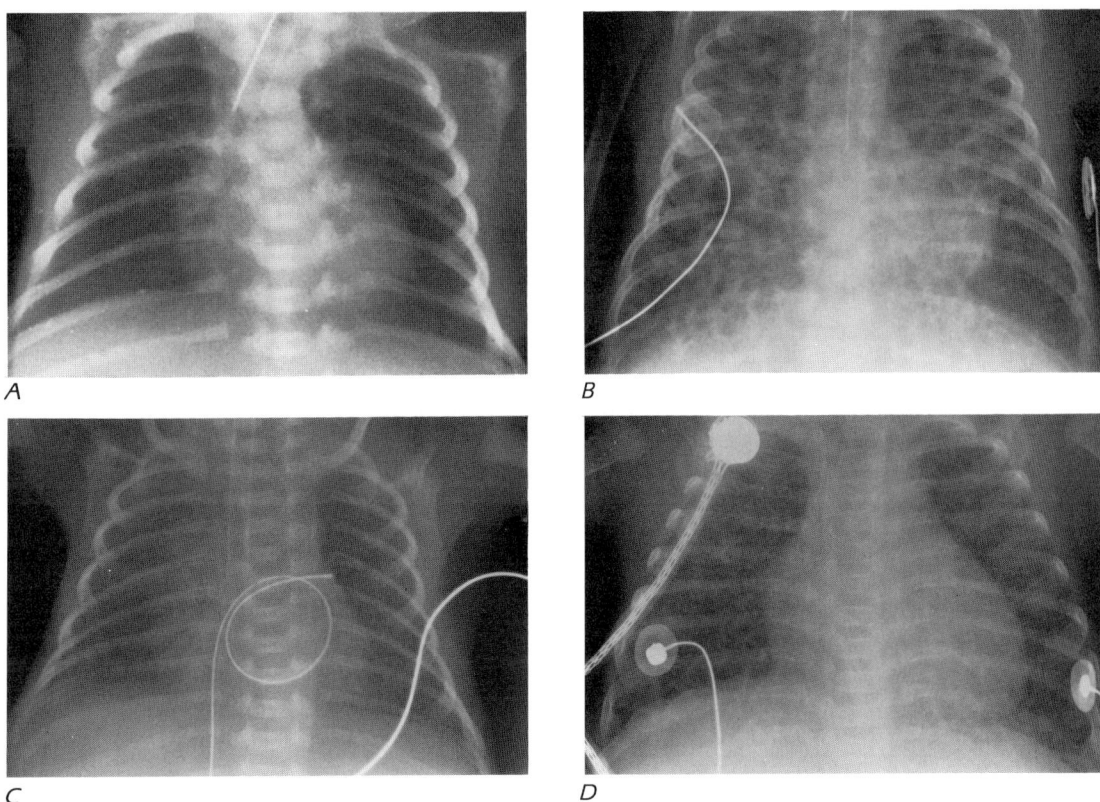

Figure 12.4. BPD developing in the setting of immaturity without RDS or other lung disease ("PALM" infants). (*A*) Premature infant on the day of birth with very little lung disease and normal surfactant, ventilated for apnea. (*B*) Same infant at 1 month of age, with severe chronic BPD. (*C*) Another premature infant on the day of birth with mild granularity and normal surfactant, also ventilated for apnea (an intravenous line has crossed the foreamen ovale and is coiled in the left atrium). (*D*) Same infant at 4 months, with mild chronic BPD.

els seen in RDS (61). The history of extensive ventilation and oxygenation followed by an RDS appearance is quite suggestive of adult respiratory distress syndrome (ARDS), which is described in children (62, 63); in this setting one could expect a BPD-like picture to develop.

The pattern of global opacity may be accentuated by overlying thickened thoracic soft tissues reflecting anasarca, secondary to pancuronium bromide paralysis. Clearing of the RDS pattern usually occurs over 1 to 2 weeks, after which a chronic interstitial pattern appears. While this appearance is long-lived, and probably represents mild BPD, it seldom is as extensive as Stage IV BPD seen following RDS, and is usually not associated with significant medical compromise (57). That these residua are relatively benign is somewhat surprising considering the extensive ventilatory support to which such infants are subjected; possibly the fact that most are full-term rather than premature infants is at least partly protective.

The Early Radiographic Diagnosis of Bronchopulmonary Dysplasia

In recent years there have been numerous efforts to identify therapeutic agents such as antioxidants that might prevent, ameliorate, or halt the course of BPD. Of these the most successful to date seems to be the administration of steroids to infants already diagnosed as having BPD (64), but long-term efficacy and safety of these have not been established. Certainly steroids are not innocuous drugs; increased incidence of infection is but one of several potential hazards (65). It would clearly be preferable to halt the progression of BPD before the stage of chronic disease is reached.

It is thus desirable to identify as early in their clinical courses as possible which of the infants at risk are developing BPD and which are not, to permit the testing and application of interventional maneuvers. Radiologic assistance in early identification is frequently sought in this setting.

The pathologic lesions of early BPD are often seen as early as the first several hours of life (66), and in many cases the disease seems to be established in the first days of life (67). Unfortunately, as indicated in the discussion above, distinctive radiologic changes suggesting BPD do not appear for a matter of days to weeks. The radiograph is thus a very poor instrument in monitoring the early phases of BPD; by the time the radiograph is unequivocal, it may be too late for successful intervention (68). At present the early stages of BPD in living infants would appear to be best assessed by cytologic and biochemical analysis of tracheal effluent (69–71).

This does not, however, suggest that the radiologist should not attempt to diagnose BPD as early as possible in a patient's course, if for no other reason than to permit prognosis. In a patient *with an appropriate clinical and radiographic history* (and this cannot be emphasized too strongly!), early radiographic indicators of BPD include those discussed below.

1. Clearing of a period of parenchymal opacity into a bubbly pattern or a pattern of notably disarrayed aeration suggests the transition of Stage II to Stage III BPD. This finding, while currently fairly uncommon, is reasonably reliable diagnostically.

2. Appearance of a diffuse, generally homogeneous pattern that is essentially interstitial suggests BPD. However, chronicity is a hallmark of BPD; such interstitial markings cannot reliably be ascribed to BPD until the pattern is seen to be long-lived rather than evanescent. The longer the pattern persists, the more confidently the diagnosis of BPD can be made. Thus the diagnosis of BPD in this setting is necessarily retrospective by days to weeks, depending on the level of confidence desired.

3. Occasionally patients during the healing phase of RDS display a prolonged period of pulmonary opacity or near opacity, as described previously; such patients frequently prove to have BPD, although it is difficult to establish its earliest appearance. When the degree of opacity wanes, which it may do in response to diuretics, an irregular pattern of aeration may be seen; generally this ultimately proves to represent moderate to severe BPD, and when it is seen the diagnosis of BPD should be strongly entertained.

Speaking very generally and empirically, I am reluctant to attempt diagnosing BPD radiographically (in the prospective setting, at least) before 2 weeks of age. Further delays in prospective diagnosis result from the necessary chronicity of the condition. Interstitial patterns that on a single film can confusingly simulate the interstitial pattern of BPD are not uncommon. For example, simple fluid overload can sometimes seemingly flood the interstitium rather than the more conventional alveolar filling, presenting a radiograph that simulates BPD except that the findings are transient (16). Similarly left-to-right shunting through the PDA can produce a transient picture of bubbly lungs that suggests BPD or Wilson-Mikity syndrome (72).

The radiologist who attempts to diagnose BPD early in its course—or even late in its course—should use great circumspection. The radiographic appearance of BPD in its late as well as early stages is quite varied and may be mimicked by a number of different conditions. These are discussed in a subsequent section.

Radiographic-Pathologic Correlation in Bronchopulmonary Dysplasia

The chest radiograph reveals, at best, gross pathology. Yet to some extent the radiograph's value may be estimated by the degree to which it predicts the microscopic as well as the gross pathology of the lung. This is particularly important in BPD, because lung biopsy of affected infants is rare and the radiograph is an important modality in the diagnosis and surveillance of the disease.

Three studies have compared the radiographic staging with the pathologic staging of BPD (18, 73, 74); the cumulative results of these studies are presented in Table 12.3. These data indicate radiograph-pathologic agreement in staging in only 72 of 181 cases (40%). In 94 of these cases (52%) the radiographic staging lagged behind the pathologic staging; in only

Table 12.3. Radiographic-Pathologic Correlation in Bronchopulmonary Dysplasia

Radiographic Stage	Pathologic Stage			
	I	II	III	IV
0	1			
I	22	40	11	4
I to II	3	2	2	
II	1	13	12	8
II to III			3	1
III		7	13	13
IV			1	24

Summary of autopsy data from 181 patients. From Oppermann et al., 1977 (18); Edwards et al., 1979 (73); and Kwok-Liu et al., 1980 (74).

15 cases (8%) was the radiographic stage higher than the pathologic stage. This radiographic "lag" has also been noted in living patients whose tracheal aspirate cytology has been examined for changes suggesting BPD (69).

These data, of course, are of greatest relevance in those patients in whom the stepwise progression of BPD through four stages occurs; the pathologic situation when the radiographic changes of BPD appear insidiously or in some other manner is uncertain. Nevertheless, the tendency for the chest film abnormalities to underestimate the pathologic progression of BPD should be borne in mind when interpreting films of patients at risk for BPD.

Chronic or Stage IV Bronchopulmonary Dysplasia

The Typical Radiographic Appearances of Chronic Bronchopulmonary Dysplasia

Because of the great and confusing variability of the radiographic appearances encountered

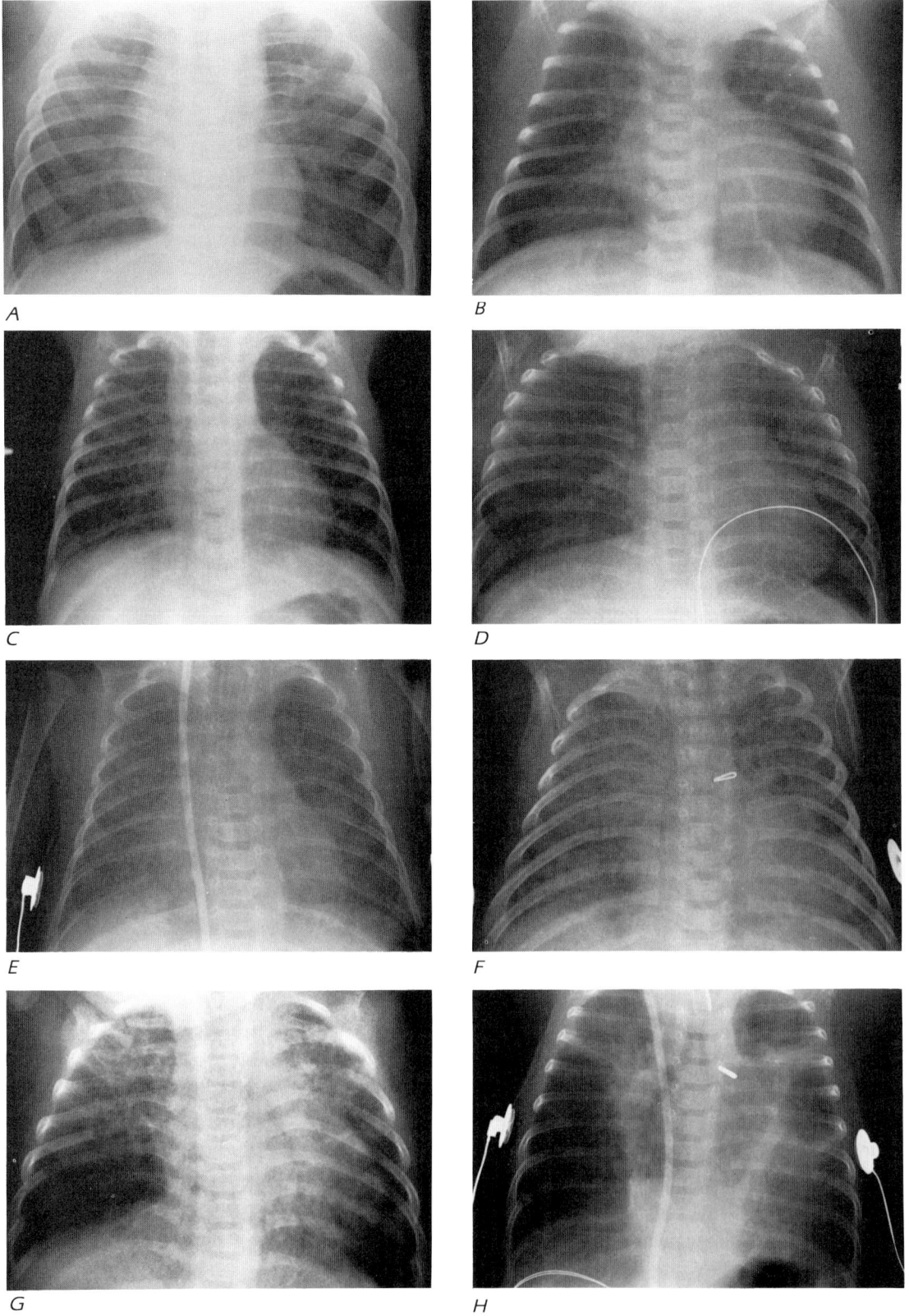

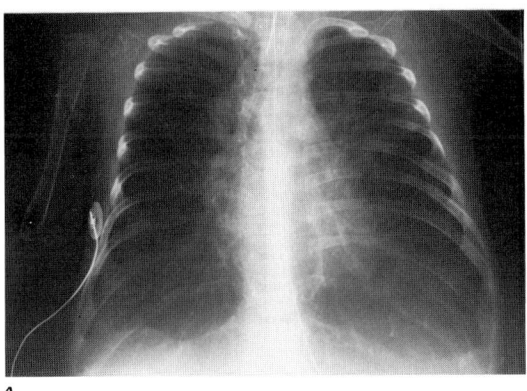 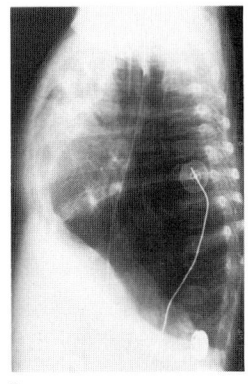

Figure 12.6. Radiographically (and clinically) very severe chronic or Stage IV BPD: 4 month old patient in frontal (A) and lateral (B) views. Lateral view reveals inverted hemidiaphragms.

in developing BPD, and because the chronicity of BPD is probably its most important clinical feature at present, the appearance of chronic or Stage IV BPD is of considerable interest and importance. Indeed in common neonatal parlance "BPD" is taken to mean chronic disease, the condition that persists after the infant has survived the acute and immediately life-threatening phases of his neonatal course. In other words BPD is generally considered more of an endpoint than a process. Thus in conventional jargon a "BPD-er" is a patient with persisting radiographic abnormalities and oxygen requirement after a variable period of postnatal time, usually 2 weeks to a month or longer. It is with such patients that this section is concerned.

Just as the radiographic appearance of BPD during its development is extremely variable, so is the appearance of the chronic lung disease that results. I prefer to consider this variable appearance as reflecting an essentially continuous spectrum from mild to-severe (Fig. 12.5) rather than differing forms of the disease, although others find it prognostically profitable to distinguish the severe, emphysematous form of BPD from its milder appearances (41).

Severe BPD, which is the "classical" picture of chronic disease initially described by Northway and associates (1), is radiographically dramatic (Fig. 12.6). The chest shows hyperinflation that is often profound. The lungs, while globally involved, reveal an inhomogeneous pattern of sharply delineated abnormal densities (presumably reflecting atelectasis and/or fibrosis) alternating with bulky, hyperlucent areas of emphysema. Cardiomegaly that is sometimes marked, often with right ventricular hypertrophy, is

---

Figure 12.5. Chronic BPD, in approximate order of subjective radiographic severity. (A) 8 months of age; (B) 2 months; (C) 3 months; (D) 4 months; (E) 2 months; (F) 3 months; (G) 3 months; (H) 2 months. The patient shown in H and possibly that shown in G, might be considered to have a different kind of BPD ("Type II") by the criteria of Heneghan et al. (41).

variably present and occasionally masked by hyperinflation. The extensive lung disease suggested radiographically is usually, but not invariably, reflected by clinically severe pulmonary insufficiency (41).

At the other end of the spectrum are those patients whose films reveal nothing more than mild interstitial accentuation; many of these patients have no clinical abnormalities at all (75), and it is questionable whether they may properly be said to have "BPD."

More distinctive pulmonary abnormalities may be seen in patients with mild to moderate BPD. The resultant radiographic picture seems to be more frequently encountered at present than are the exuberant abnormalities associated with severe, or classical Stage IV, BPD (16, 38, 41). This more contemporary picture involves a level of inflation that is normal to mildly hyperinflated. Instead of coarse infiltrates alternating with hyperlucencies, the lungs are relatively homogeneously involved, with each portion of lung looking much like every other portion. The abnormal densities tend to be fine, lacy, and ill defined, obscuring vascular markings and extending to or near the lung periphery. Possibly these densities represent summation shadows of the septal fibrosis that is common in infants who die with long-standing BPD (76). More severe cases show a more prominent alteration of the opacities with small areas of relative hyperlucency.

The important hallmarks of chronic BPD radiographically are as follows:

1. *Chronicity:* Although several evanescent phenomena, such as focal atelectasis, heart failure, superimposed pneumonia, and the like, continue to be seen in chronic BPD patients, the abnormal radiographic background changes little with time. This chronicity is an important diagnostic feature of BPD.

2. *Interstitial prominence:* The parenchymal abnormalities appear to involve primarily the pulmonary interstitium, the peribronchial regions, and airways, rather than the alveoli; the radiographic abnormalities are thus primarily interstitial in character, so fine line shadows predominate over nodular shadows.

3. *Global abnormalities:* Allowing that emphysema appears somewhat more marked at the bases in BPD, the disease is usually a global process, involving all parts of both lungs symmetrically. Focal disease, with only one lung or lobe involved, is unlikely to represent BPD.

4. *Inflation normal to increased:* If BPD affects aeration, it does so by causing hyperinflation, not underaeration. This, of course, is not the case when transient phenomena such as mucus plug or more long-lived phenomena such as cardiomegaly produce focal atelectasis. The basic process is emphysematous.

5. *BPD is not a congenital disorder:* The process is not noted at birth, but rather almost always develops in the setting of another, underlying neonatal lung disease that is treated with respiratory assistance.

6. *Gradual onset:* Whether or not four distinct phases of BPD are observed, the disease's radiographic onset tends to be gradual rather than abrupt.

An additional feature is that uncomplicated BPD is not associated with pleural effusion or with marked pleural thickening, although pleural thickening may be seen following long-term therapy with a chest tube.

Table 12.4. Radiographic Differential Diagnosis of Stage III-IV Bronchopulmonary Dysplasia

Usually occur in a clinical setting different from BPD:
1. Recurrent pneumonia with scarring (gastroesophageal reflux, H-type tracheoesophageal fistula, immune deficiency, etc.)
2. Cystic fibrosis
3. Idiopathic pulmonary fibrosis
4. "Cardiogenic asthma" (chronic hyperexpansion and scarring usually from an acyanotic left-to-right shunt [VSD or PDA] or cardiomyopathy)

Often occur in a clinical setting comparable to that of BPD:
1. Pulmonary interstitial emphysema
2. Perinatally acquired viral pneumonitis, particularly cytomegalovirus
3. Wilson-Mikity syndrome
4. Patent ductus arteriosus (uncommon appearance)
5. Overhydration (uncommon appearance)
6. Following surfactant administration

Similarly adenopathy should suggest another or a superimposed process.

Radiographic Differential Diagnosis of Chronic Bronchopulmonary Dysplasia

General

Unfortunately none of the preceding hallmarks of BPD, either alone or in combination, is radiographically pathognomonic. Table 12.4 lists other important conditions that can simulate the radiographic findings in chronic BPD. Other conditions (which are not listed) exist for which the radiographic findings on a single film could simulate BPD in an informational vacuum. For example, the streaky densities of congenital pulmonary lymphangectasia could simulate the abnormalities of BPD, but the changes are present at birth, whereas BPD is not.

Other conditions that do develop over time can also produce radiographs that simulate BPD, but generally these do not cause diagnostic confusion. Recurrent pneumonias with scarring can cause overinflated, scarred lungs that can suggest BPD; these may be seen in numerous conditions, such as gastroesophageal reflux with aspiration, H-type tracheoesophageal fistula, severe asthma, and a variety of immunodeficiency states. Similarly cystic fibrosis in its early phases often produces mild emphysema and increased interstitial markings. Idiopathic pulmonary fibrosis (Hamman-Rich syndrome) seems to present rarely, if at all, in newborns (77), although it has been described in the setting of Wilson-Mikity syndrome (78). Large left-to-right shunts sometimes cause emphysematous effects on the lungs (79) that can suggest BPD. While such diseases can or could occur in the clinical setting of a neonatal intensive care unit, they usually do not, and the distinctive clinical history of BPD patients usually ensures correct diagnosis.

The most difficult entities to distinguish radiographically from BPD are those that develop at some time following delivery, in the clinical setting of a neonatal nursery. Occasionally these conditions present vexing diagnostic problems, some of which admit no ready solution. These are discussed individually below.

Pulmonary Interstitial Emphysema

The process of pulmonary interstitial emphysema (PIE) presents no diagnostic difficulties when it is focal in a lobe or a lung, and only temporary difficulty when it is diffuse but transient; however, it can create a diagnostic dilemma when it is both diffuse and long-lived. Two helpful diagnostic features are that the onset of appearance of PIE is usually early (commonly in the first week of life) and it usually appears rapidly, unlike the gradual development of BPD. The abnormal lucencies of PIE may appear between one day and the next; the development seldom takes more than 2 to 3 days. Furthermore PIE commonly begins focally, often in an upper lobe, before spreading globally, and it is often associated with other air leaks such as pneumothorax and pneumomediastinum.

Frequently the usual appearance of PIE can be distinguished from BPD by close examination of the abnormal lucencies encountered (80). The lucencies of PIE tend to be of similar size, nodular or "wormy," and meandering in a radiating fashion from the hilus, whereas the lucencies of BPD are usually rounded and variable in size, with larger "bubbles" at the lung bases (80). Sometimes, however, the bubbles of PIE can become bullous and rounded, simulating BPD; furthermore PIE is sometimes associated with subpleural blebs of ectopic gas (81) that may be more suggestive of BPD than of PIE. Fortunately these latter gas collections, unlike those of BPD, are usually confined to a focal region; however, like BPD, these can be quite long-lived (48–50).

The differential diagnostic difficulties in this setting are confounded by the fact that PIE and other intrathoracic air leaks are strongly associated with the ultimate development of BPD (41, 43–46). When BPD develops insidiously in the setting of diffuse PIE, as discussed earlier, it is extremely difficult to recognize when the abnormalities on the film no longer represent stable PIE but instead reflect BPD; the question is perhaps no more than academic.

Viral Infection

Perinatally acquired viral pneumonia, especially that caused by cytomegalovirus (CMV), can be reflected radiographically by a very long-lived pneumonitis that can convincingly simulate BPD of mild to severe degree (68, 82). Furthermore CMV is a frequent pathogen in the intensive care nursery setting, and patients in this setting are at distinct risk for colonization and infection (83). In patients with no underlying lung disease, the appearance of CMV pneumonitis can be confused with Wilson-Mikity syndrome, but should not be mistaken for BPD because of the patient's lack of antecedent oxygenation and ventilation.

However, it seems clear that CMV pneumonitis can also affect preterm infants with RDS and perhaps other underlying respiratory diseases. In such patients radiographic diagnosis can be extremely confusing (Fig. 12.7). We have recently examined a series of newborn infants who were treated for RDS and from whom CMV was subsequently cultured. In comparison with matched controls, the incidence of radiographic "BPD" was strikingly and significantly higher in the infected infants (84). Patients who secrete CMV relatively early in their course have an increased incidence of "BPD" compared with infants who excrete virus late in their course (85). One infant has been described whose BPD worsened after infection with CMV (86). Furthermore at autopsy the lungs of some infants with "BPD" have been found to contain cytomegalic inclusions (87).

In such patients, when the underlying RDS evolves into a pattern suggesting BPD, it is virtually impossible radiographically to determine whether the chronic abnormality seen reflects BPD or the infection or a combination of both. It is evident that the possible contribution of viral infection to the development of BPD deserves closer scrutiny.

Wilson-Mikity Syndrome

The entity that has been most commonly confused with BPD is the (much rarer) Wilson-Mikity syndrome (88). It is freely admitted at the outset that the radiographs in this syndrome can exactly simulate those of BPD (Fig. 12.8), and that infants affected with Wilson-Mikity syndrome can exhibit chronic pulmonary insufficiency that also resembles that of chronic BPD. However, at this point the similarity ends; both the early clinical courses and the pathologic findings in Wilson-Mikity syndrome (88) and BPD (1, 66) differ markedly. It has been pointed out that it is incorrect to "lump" these diseases (89); it is certainly incorrect to consider them synonymously, as has occasionally been done (90).

Typically a patient with Wilson-Mikity syndrome begins his clinical course with prematurity and not much else; radiographically his lungs may be clear or show the findings of a PALM infant (5, 78). Then, in a few hours to days, findings of respiratory insufficiency are noted, and the chest radiograph shows a diffuse, bubbly pattern. This pattern, which is often quite suggestive of BPD, becomes chronic. The onset is relatively abrupt compared with that of BPD, and much earlier than conventionally seen with BPD, and of course there is no or minimal antecedent oxygenation and assisted ventilation. The distinction is thus readily made on clinical grounds.

The etiology of Wilson-Mikity syndrome is unknown. The last several patients I have

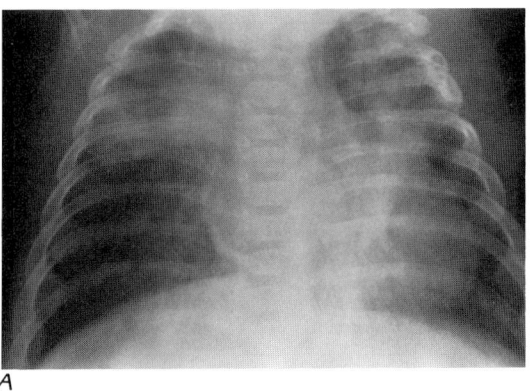
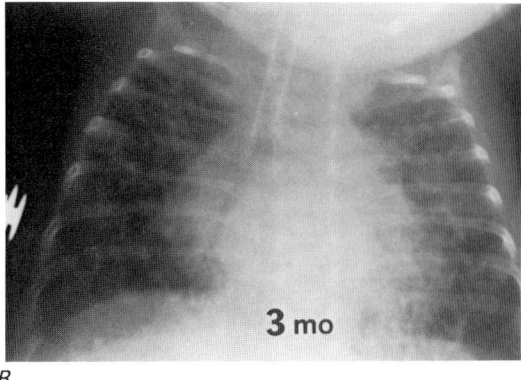

A B

Figure 12.7. Chronic cytomegaloviral infection and/or BPD. Two patients (A, 1 month; B, 3 months) who were ventilated for RDS and from whom endotracheal cytomegalovirus was cultured on multiple occasions while chronic lung disease developed.

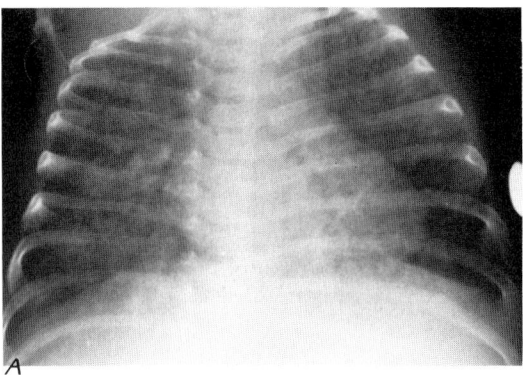
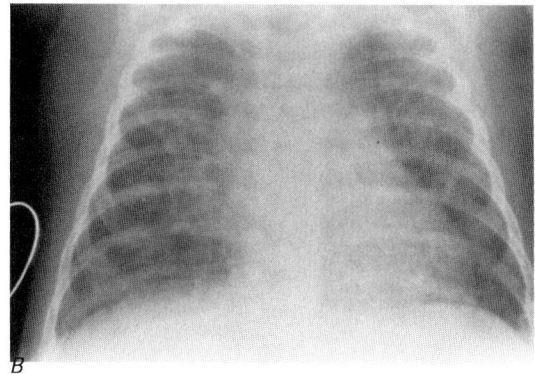

Figure 12.8. Two patients with presumed Wilson-Mikity syndrome, both 2 months old; both patients were encountered in past years when viral cultures were not commonly done, and the clinical and radiographic courses suggested Wilson-Mikity syndrome.

seen who demonstrated typical radiographic and clinical courses of Wilson-Mikity syndrome have all proved, after a few or many cultures, to contain CMV in their tracheal aspirates (Fig. 12.9). Chlamydial pneumonia has also been described as simulating Wilson-Mikity syndrome (91). Pathologically the pulmonary inflammatory cells seen in Wilson-Mikity syndrome (78, 88) suggest an infectious etiology. Perhaps occasional cases of Wilson-Mikity syndrome exist that are not examples of occult pneumonitis, but I suspect these are uncommon.

Patent Ductus Arteriosus and Fluid Overload

The typical radiographic findings in PDA are engorged perihilar vessels, diffuse but largely central pulmonary edema, and often cardiomegaly (33). In unusual cases, however, the radiograph may show hyperinflation and shadows that suggest cystic lucencies and hence BPD or Wilson-Mikity syndrome (72). One feature that distinguishes this manifestation of PDA from BPD is that the PDA manifestations usually occur earlier in the patient's clinical course than expected for BPD. Additionally the cystic appearance of a PDA is transient, lasting only a few days before being replaced by the more usual appearance of ductal shunting (72).

Fairly frequently simple overhydration exhibits a picture showing mild hyperinflation and diffusely increased interstitial markings instead of the more usual pulmonary edema pattern (16). These findings can appear at virtually any time in a patient's course, and in the correct time setting can suggest mild BPD, but the onset is usually abrupt. Unlike the findings in BPD, the interstitial pattern can disappear within a day following fluid restriction. This phenomenon can be unsettling to observe in a patient at risk for BPD, but it is not chronic, and time unmasks the true diagnosis.

Following Surfactant Therapy

We have observed in infants with RDS treated with human surfactant that a small number (3 of 18) developed a transient interstitial pattern on their radiographs that ap-

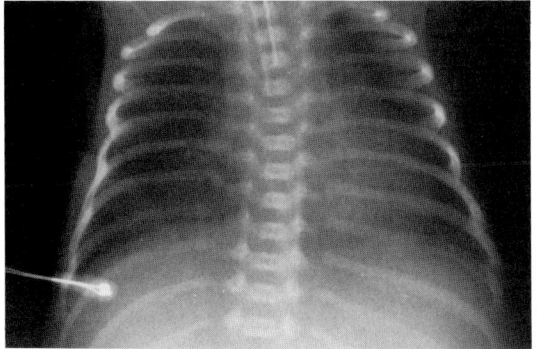

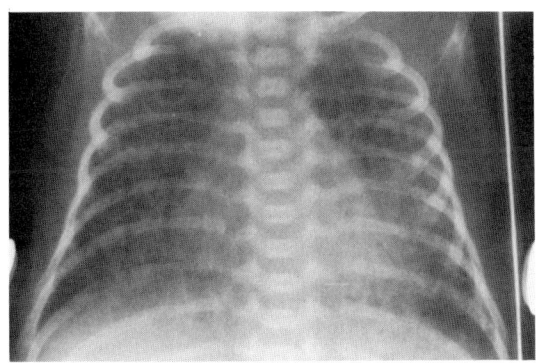

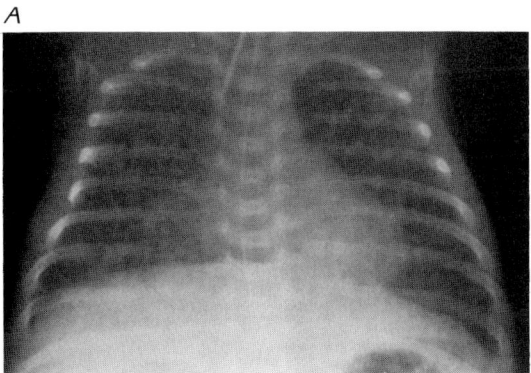

Figure 12.9. Wilson-Mikity syndrome simulated by viral infection. (*A*) Very premature infant with no lung disease ("PALM" infant) at 1 hour of age. (*B*) At 33 hours, a bubbly pattern has appeared. It persists and is still seen at 1 month (*C*). Radiographically and clinically the patient had Wilson-Mikity syndrome, but cytomegalovirus was cultured from the trachea.

peared 3 to 4 days following surfactant administration (92). This phenomenon did not appear related to hydration, and in all cases it disappeared within a week. Like the interstitial pattern sometimes seen with overhydration, the evanescent character of the infiltrate retrospectively excludes BPD, and the early appearance is similarly unlike the relatively delayed appearance of BPD.

Uncommon Radiographic Appearances of Chronic Bronchopulmonary Dysplasia

Asymmetric Bronchopulmonary Dysplasia

Characteristically BPD is a global disease that involves both lungs symmetrically. However, cases of involvement of primarily one lung have been reported (93). The mechanism by which this evidently occurred was "protection" of the relatively spared lung by prolonged collapse secondary to an endobronchial obstruction or pneumothorax. This appearance is unusual, possibly because brisk efforts are usually made to re-expand a collapsed lung as soon as it is identified.

Focal Emphysema in Bronchopulmonary Dysplasia

It is generally recognized that the emphysema associated with BPD is more marked at the lung bases than at the apices (80), although this appears more notable in severe cases than in mild cases. Additionally focal lobar emphysema has been described in BPD, usually involving a lower lobe (94), most commonly the right lower lobe (95). Sometimes this emphysema has been severe enough to warrant lobectomy (95). A variety of mechanisms have been proposed to account for this condition, including preferential gas flow to the lower lobes, the Bernoulli effect drawing gas from upper lobe bronchi, the local stretching effects of diaphragmatic excursions, and relatively early lower lobe maturation increasing lower lung compliance (94).

We have reported similar findings in BPD patients in whom right lower and usually middle lobe emphysema was secondary to endobronchial masses of granulation tissue (96). The mechanism of emphysema appears to be a one-way-valve effect caused by these masses in a manner reminiscent of a foreign body; the masses themselves seemed to result from the mechanical trauma of repeated endotracheal tube suctioning (Fig. 12.10). One recent patient, who exhibited bizarre patterns of lung collapse prior to his demise, proved at autopsy to have masses of these granulomatous polyps at his carina, evidently from the same cause (Fig. 12.10, F). This appearance of BPD is much less prevalent when endotracheal tube suctioning catheters are measured and shortened so that they do not reach the carina.

"Bronchopulmonary Dysplasia Alba"

Preterm infants commonly demonstrate transient periods of pulmonary parenchymal opacity (Table 12.2), most of which presumably have little or nothing to do with BPD, excepting of course Stage II BPD. However, periods of pulmonary opacification or of relative opacification that are poorly understood also occur in preterm infants treated with respiratory support. These episodes of opacification seem to be at least related to BPD, and may indeed be manifestations of BPD; hence "bronchopulmonary dysplasia alba" (white BPD).

In 1975 Rhodes and associates (10) described a "chronic" lung abnormality seen in nine of 150 infants ventilated for RDS; this abnormality was a pattern of diffuse haziness with loss of identifiable lung markings that appeared at 5 to 15 days of life and disappeared in 1 to 5 days. Patients exhibiting this appearance appeared clinically unaffected. While this finding may reflect increased capillary permeability from oxygen toxicity, it is also seen fairly often in the course of healing RDS and may represent nothing more than a manifestation of such healing (97).

In other patients, however, a very similar appearance may be seen that is genuinely chronic, lasting as long as 3 months in my experience (68). The appearance is one of hazy, lint-like opacity that is densest centrally, obscuring the vascular shadows, but not the cardiac silhouette, which remains normal in size. The findings suggest noncardiogenic pulmonary edema so a reasonable speculation is that it represents edema engendered by the edemagenic effects of oxygen toxicity (98). As such, chronic "hazy lung" may be considered a variant of BPD. Clinically such patients generally are essentially healthy but have a mild oxygen requirement that improves with time. To date the relative health of such patients has precluded pathologic verification of the lesion.

Recently several patients have been noted who exhibit an extended period of parenchymal opacification, generally beginning at 2 to 3 weeks of life following the acute phases of RDS and continuing for several weeks, sometimes associated with cardiomegaly. The overall degree of opacity waxes and wanes, and during periods of relatively diminished

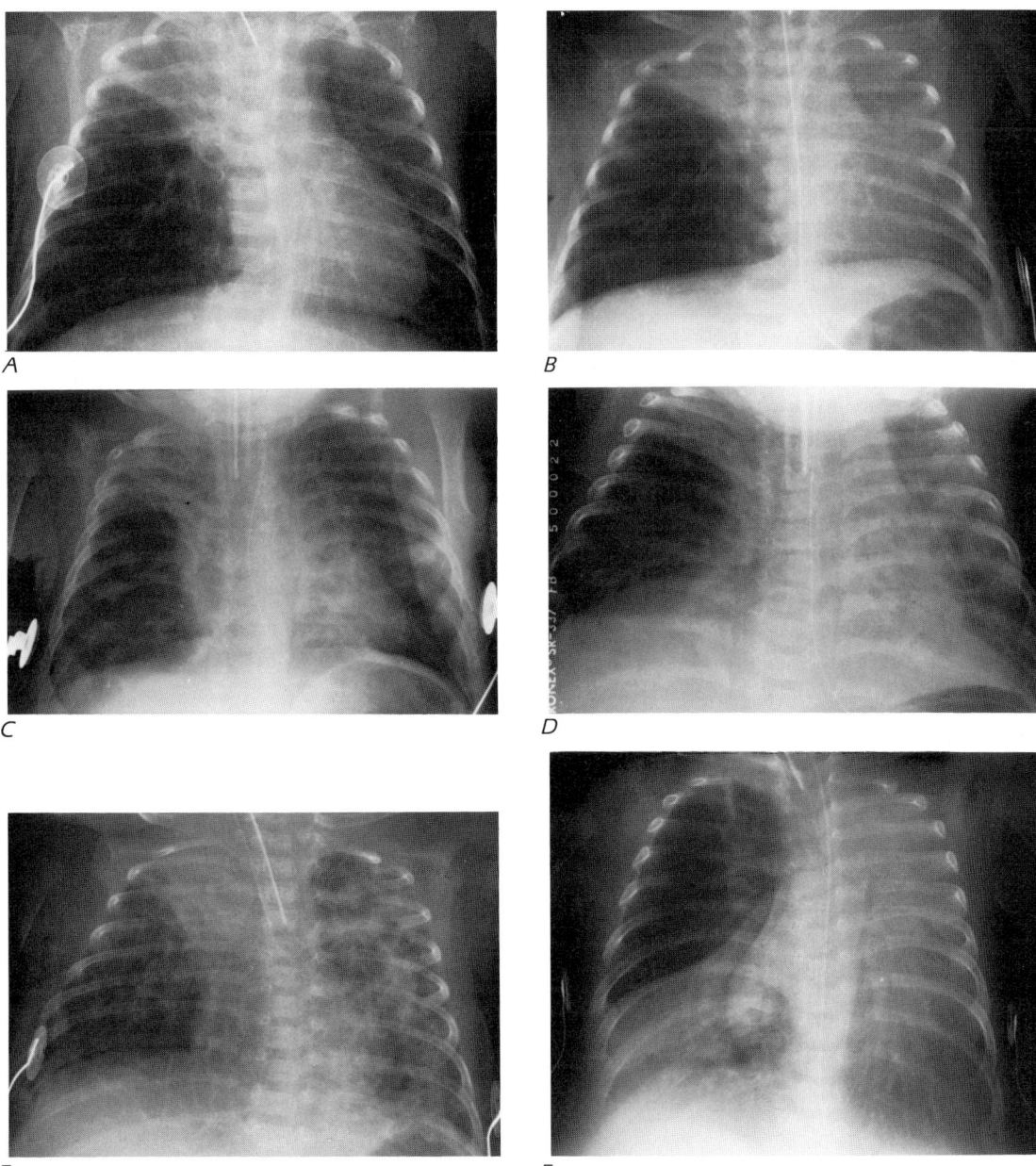

Figure 12.10. Airway polyps in BPD. (*A*) Chest radiograph at 40 days shows right lower and middle lobe emphysema, with associated right upper lobe collapse; assisted expiration view (*B*) confirms focal air trapping. (*C*) Similar case, 4 months of age, with focal air trapping confirmed with assisted expiration view (*D*). (*E*) Similar case at 1 month of age. (*F*) Two month old infant requiring multiple suctionings of the endotracheal tube, with recurrent episodes of extensive, bizarre-appearing collapse leading to demise; at autopsy polyps were heaped over the carina.

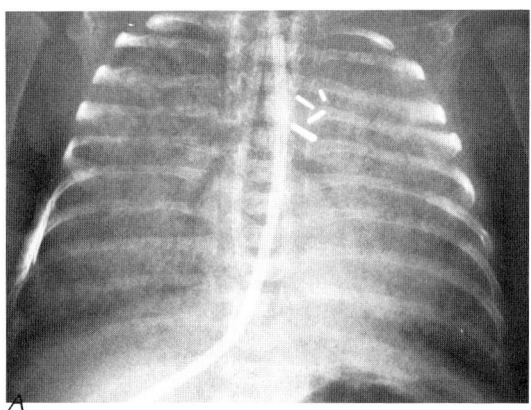 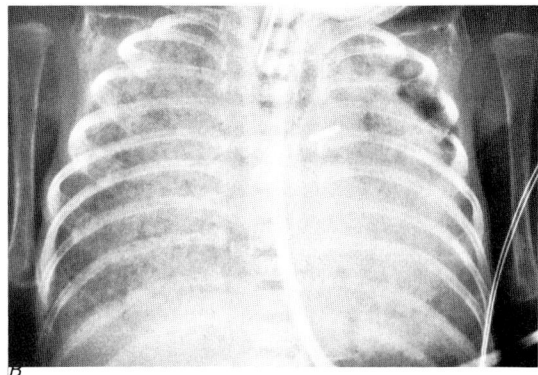

Figure 12.11. "Bronchopulmonary dysplasia alba"; patients whose BPD was characterized by several weeks of parenchymal opacity. Both patients are 2 months old, and both are shown during periods of relative clearing. In *A*, a nasogastric tube is looped in the esophagus.

opacification (Fig. 12.11), a pattern of increasingly irregular aeration is seen. The opacity finally and gradually clears, first at the bases and then the apices, leaving a radiograph suggesting moderate to severe BPD. At the University of California at San Diego Medical Center, we have learned to regard this sort of extended "whiteout" with trepidation.

The Radiographic Evolution of Chronic Bronchopulmonary Dysplasia

Few conditions in medicine remain absolutely static, and this is particularly true in the setting of a growing, developing infant, even an infant with BPD. The chronic radiographic lesions of BPD change with the passage of time, although the changes are noted over periods of weeks to years rather than days.

Once a patient with chronic BPD no longer requires supplemental oxygenation and ventilation, the overwhelming tendency is for the lungs to heal. Radiographic improvement that is often marked is the rule, and patients who stay the same or worsen are relatively uncommon (7, 16, 99–101). This happy outcome is also seen clinically, in that exercise tolerance and pulmonary function tend to approach or reach normal by school age (31, 75, 102, 103).

As might be expected the rate at which the radiograph improves depends on the initial severity of the chronic BPD. With mild BPD the radiograph usually becomes normal at about 1 year of age or sooner, while with severe BPD, normalcy may not be reached until 2 to 3 years (99). The majority of the clearing occurs in the first 2 years (100). In some severe cases the radiograph may never become normal, but the existence of persisting abnormalities does not necessarily (or even commonly) imply impaired function (75).

Despite the generally favorable prognosis, a child with healing BPD is by no means free of danger. Such children are at increased risk for a variety of complications such as pneumonia and even sudden infant death syndrome (104), although it is reasonable to expect that such risks diminish with increasing age. Furthermore the prognosis of BPD survivors in adulthood is unknown, particularly whether or not their risk for chronic obstructive pulmonary disease (31) or other, unsuspected, diseases is increased.

Radiographic Scoring of the Severity of Chronic Bronchopulmonary Dysplasia

When you can measure what you are speaking about, and express it in numbers, you know something about it; but when you cannot measure it, when you cannot express it in numbers, your knowledge is of a meager and unsatisfactory kind. . . . Lord Kelvin, 105

Many authors have succumbed to the temptation to assign numerical values to the pictorial information presented on the radiograph. Often such numbers represent direct measurements, such as the cardiac width or the CT number, and such values appear to be accurate reflections of genuine physical characteristics of the body. Occasionally, however, unitless and essentially subjective values are assigned to radiographic features that are thought to reflect the patient's medical condition. Examples are the severity of RDS (92, 106, 107) and of cystic fibrosis (108, 109) on chest films. Conventionally these values represent a scale of varying severity, so that 5 (for example) may represent very severe RDS, and 1 very mild RDS (92); zero, presumably, is no RDS at all. Usually such numbers are generated either by a "match-the-picture" technique or by summing other numbers that each reflect one of several radiographic features.

The temptation to assign such numbers is understandable. The complexities of a full radiographic report are not amenable to statistical analysis, whereas assigning each radiograph a number would seem to permit statistical comparison of radiographic findings between groups of patients. Thus one could compare treatment modalities, for example, in terms of severity of BPD observed on subsequent chest radiographs. Assigning a number permits a seemingly quantitative measure by which an individual patient's progress might be followed over time.

The prototype of such numbers in pediatrics is the Apgar score. This score is derived by summing individual numbers that are generated by noting five aspects of the infant's physical examination. These aspects form a complex of findings that individually reflect cardiorespiratory and neurologic variables. A perfect score is 10, while zero essentially represents death. Statistical manipulation of Apgar scores, and comparison of groups by Apgar scores, is often reported in the literature.

However, the validity of statistical manipulation of such numbers has been questioned (110). The difficulty is that Apgar scores, and similar scores engendered from radiographs, are not interval measures. Thus the "distance," so to speak, between an Apgar score of 2 and 3 may be quite different from the "distance" between 7 and 8, which is not the case with true interval measures such as those made using a yardstick. In this setting the usual statistical analyses applied to interval measures, such as mean, standard deviation, and t-test, may not be appropriate and should perhaps be replaced entirely by nonparametric techniques.

This objection has in turn been vigorously criticized (111). Although purists may object, it appears that the parametric manipulation of noninterval measures such as Apgar score,

Table 12.5. Radiographic Scoring of Chronic Bronchopulmonary Dysplasia

Variable	Score 0	Score 1	Score 2
Cardiovascular abnormalities	None	Cardiomegaly	Gross cardiomegaly *or* right ventricular hypertrophy *or* enlarged main pulmonary artery
Hyperexpansion	Anterior plus posterior rib count* of 14 or less	Anterior plus posterior rib count of 14½ to 16	Anterior plus posterior rib count of 16½ or more *or* hemidiaphragms flat or concave
Emphysema	No focal areas seen	Scattered small abnormal lucencies	One or more large blebs or bullae
Fibrosis and/or interstitial abnormalities	None seen	Few streaks of abnormal density; interstitial prominence†	Many abnormal strands; dense fibrotic or atelectatic bands
Subjective‡	Appears mildly diseased	Appears moderately diseased	Appears severely diseased

* Rib counts of anterior plus posterior ribs intersecting the dome of the right hemidiaphragm. If the level of the right hemidiaphragm were at the sixth anterior rib and the eighth posterior intercostal space, the total rib count would be 14½.

† Enlarged lymphatics and areas of atelectasis cannot usually be distinguished from fibrosis.

‡ "Subjective" factor is based on overall radiographic judgment of the severity of disease.

(Reproduced, with permission, from Edwards DK. Radiology of hyaline membrane disease, transient tachypnea of the newborn, and bronchopulmonary dysplasia. In: Farrell PM, ed. Lund development: biological and clinical perspectives, vol 2. New York: Academic Press, 1982, p 80.)

clinical scoring systems, staging of malignancies, staging of BPD, etc., introduces relatively little distortion of the data. Furthermore parametric manipulations ". . . are usually more powerful than nonparametric techniques, are generally better understood, and are robust to violations of their assumptions . . ." (111). Still caution might be advocated in making too much of differences in such data that just marginally clear the $p < .05$ level.

In attempting to summarize numerically the radiographic findings in BPD, the four stages of disease initially described (1) may be considered as Arabic numbers and manipulated statistically (42). This is limiting, first, because only four levels of disease may be considered. Second, investigations of outcome involve primarily chronic BPD, of which all cases by definition have Stage IV disease; a better system would permit comparison of severity between different Stage IV patients.

One approach to this problem was adapting a scoring system devised for cystic fibrosis patients for use in BPD (112); an objection to this is that cystic fibrosis, at least in its later phases, is radiographically quite different from chronic BPD. Another approach is grading cases of chronic BPD as mild, moderate, and severe (113). This system has the disadvantage of providing only three grades of disease; furthermore it may err by being overly subjective (114).

Encouraged by the successful reproducibility and the close correlation with pulmonary function tests of the scoring system for cystic fibrosis (109), I devised a somewhat similar system tailored to the common chest radiographic abnormalities in chronic BPD (115). This system is outlined in Table 12.5. In a manner reminiscent of the Apgar score, five features are scored with 0, 1, or 2, and the result summed; unlike the Apgar score, 10 is very bad instead of very good. The scoring system has been used with fair success and apparent utility (116–118), but studies of its reproducibility have not been done.

Using this system (Table 12.5) cardiomegaly can be assessed by standard tables, but these may be inappropriate when the patient is hyperinflated; the trained eye is probably better. Signs of pulmonary hypertension are given a higher score than mild to moderate cardiomegaly. Lung inflation is judged by rib-counting, noting which anterior and which posterior ribs lie at the level of the dome of the right hemidiaphragm and summing these. Fractional values are used when the hemidiaphragm lies at an interspace. Flat or concave hemidiaphragms (Fig. 12.6) are given a score of 2, whatever the rib count. The remaining features of the system are self-explanatory.

The potential advantage of this system is that it offers a numerical value of radiographic severity of chronic BPD (*not* developing BPD) for any given film. Thus a descriptive value is provided for clinical evaluation and statistical comparisons. The range of values available (0 to 10) would seem to permit greater discrimination than other techniques. It is easy to use, not overly time-consuming, and encourages a systemic evaluation of the radiograph. However, its overall value has yet to be demonstrated.

Complications and Associations of Chronic Bronchopulmonary Dysplasia

General

Radiologists who frequently encounter infants with BPD have learned to examine the films for a variety of additional conditions. Some of these conditions are complications of the patient's chronic lung disease; some are only indirectly related to BPD itself, and may be thought of as associations of BPD. This section discusses the most important of these complications and associations that may be observed radiographically.

Cardiopulmonary Problems

Pneumonias

For reasons that are uncertain but may relate to impaired drainage of secretions and other factors, infants with BPD are subject to recurring pneumonias during the early chronic phases of their disease (112, 119–122). Patients with BPD have more severe and more frequent pneumonias that RDS survivors who do not have BPD (117). Bronchopneumonia is a common cause of death in patients with BPD (123). The frequency of infections is greatest during the first 2 years of life, and is increased in patients with the most severe lung disease; the incidence drops dramatically during the next 2 years (100). By school age BPD survivors seem to have no more infections than unaffected children (102, 124).

Wheezing is a frequent component of lower respiratory tract infections in these infants (103, 119, 125, 126); indeed BPD patients are similar to asthmatics not only in their responses to methacholine (127) and to bronchodilators (128, 129) but even in family history (130). A pathologic finding that may be related to this propensity for bronchospasm is smooth muscle hypertrophy around the small airways (66).

The radiographic findings in bronchitis and bronchiolitis in normal children are somewhat reminiscent of BPD itself; increased interstitial markings, frequent appearance of focal areas of atelectasis, and variable hyperinflation. Thus in a child with underlying BPD, the changes of a superimposed bronchitis may be difficult or impossible to appreciate.

Bacterial pneumonias in patients with BPD are usually radiographically nondescript, consisting of focal or sometimes widespread regions of abnormal opacity superimposed on the background changes of BPD. The bacteriology of these infections is varied, with no particular organism predilection reported; in hospitalized infants with BPD, unusual pathogens are sometimes encountered, such as *Candida* and *Pseudomonas*. The abnormal densities of pneumonia may be difficult to distinguish from simple atelectasis (see below); the presence of air bronchograms suggests a consolidative, infectious etiology (Fig. 12.12). It should be borne in mind that patients with severe BPD may survive with a cardiopulmonary status so precarious that even pneumonias that appear small and unimpressive can cause significant clinical decompensation.

The distinction between viral and bacterial pneumonia can be difficult (131), and

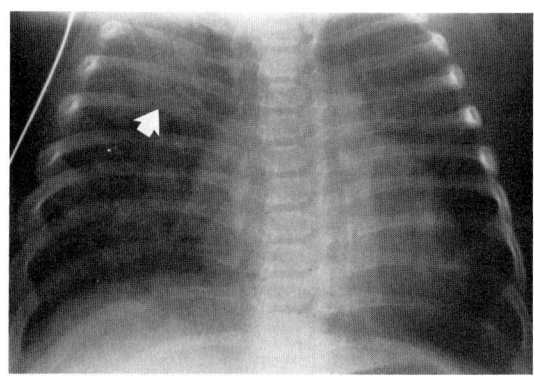

Figure 12.12. Right upper lobe pneumonia in BPD (patient 6 months old). The focal process (above arrow) is hazy and reveals ill-defined air bronchograms. Clinically, aspiration was suspected; no organism was identified, and the process cleared with antibiotic therapy. The patient's left lower lobe is chronically and profoundly collapsed, probably because of cardiomegaly.

probably is more difficult in the setting of BPD. Features that may be helpful include the following: 1) bacterial pneumonias are more often focal, whereas viral pneumonias tend to exhibit global abnormalities; 2) an alveolar process favors bacterial pneumonia, as does an air bronchogram sign; 3) adenopathy and pleural effusion can accompany either, but are more suggestive of bacterial pneumonia; 4) shifting areas of atelectasis favor viral pneumonia; 5) disproportionate hyperinflation favors a viral process; and 6) cavity formation with an air-fluid level suggests a bacterial process.

An acute pneumonia involving the right upper lobe (Fig. 12.12), the superior segment of the right lower lobe, or the left perihilar region should suggest aspiration pneumonia in a supine infant. Indeed it has been suggested that gastroesophageal reflux and aspiration contributes to the prolongation of BPD (132). It is my clinical impression that infants with BPD, when they are studied radiograph-

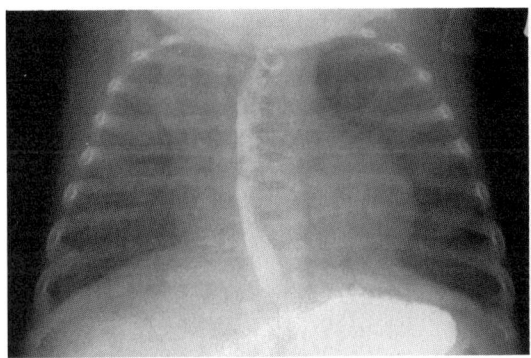

Figure 12.13. Gastroesophageal reflux demonstrated radiographically in a 2 month old patient whose BPD was complicated by frequent episodes of pneumonia.

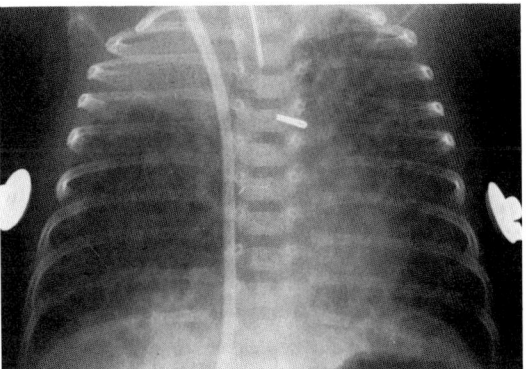

Figure 12.14. Transient right upper lobe atelectasis in a 1 month old patient with BPD. The process elevates the minor fissure, with some associated compensatory emphysema of the lower and middle lobes. No air bronchogram is seen in the density, and the process cleared by the next day after chest physiotherapy.

ically for reflux, commonly exhibit significant gastroesophageal reflux (Fig. 12.13). However, this has not been the case when such infants are studied with a pH probe (133). Although reflux does not seem to be readily documented in many such infants, clinical improvement seems to follow fundoplication (132, 134). The possible contribution of gastroesophageal reflux to the pulmonary lesion of BPD is presently uncertain, but the finding of severe reflux in a BPD patient should prompt strong consideration of corrective surgery.

The normal thymus is sometimes confused with atelectasis or pneumonia. Patients with BPD, at least in their relatively acute phases, generally exhibit little or no thymic shadow, possibly because of stress related thymic involution.

Atelectasis, Transient and Chronic

Areas of segmental or subsegmental lung collapse (Fig. 12.14) are quite common in BPD, particularly in early phases of the disease when an endotracheal tube is in place. Atelectasis can simulate pneumonia, but can often be distinguished from the consolidation of pneumonia by the following characteristics of atelectasis: 1) shifts of fissures toward the abnormal density, 2) shift of mediastinal structures toward the density, 3) compensatory emphysema in the unaffected lung, 4) usually, but not invariably, absence of an air bronchogram in the density, and 5) the fact that atelectasis is generally transient, and may occur in a temporal setting of shifting foci of abnormal density.

The atelectasis seen in BPD most commonly results from a mucus plug. Generally these are readily dislodged, or at least moved from place to place, by pulmonary physiotherapy, but sometimes the mucus plug is recalcitrant, so that the atelectasis threatens to become fixed. In this setting catheter suction and saline lavage under fluoroscopic guidance is often helpful (135). If this fails, bronchoscopy is necessary, because unresolved atelectasis can become permanent (16).

Occasionally atelectasis is secondary to

something other than a mucus plug. A fairly common example is left lower lobe collapse secondary to an enlarged heart compressing the lobar bronchus (79). The only successful way of correcting the ensuing atelectasis is treating the cause of cardiomegaly, if this is possible. Often it is not, and atelectasis in this setting may become permanent (Fig. 12.15).

Another cause of chronic atelectasis in BPD is compression of part of the lung, usually an upper lobe, by marked emphysema in the remainder of the lung (94, 95). If the emphysema is truly intrinsic, perhaps surgery is indicated, as has been suggested (95). However, similar findings are seen when there is lower lobe emphysema secondary to endobronchial polyps, which may be treated in a less drastic fashion (96).

Congestive Heart Failure

Episodes of congestive heart failure are common in patients with BPD (1), and these are often precipitated by iatrogenic fluid overload or by attempting to wean the patient from supplemental oxygen (136). The radiographic picture in BPD complicated by congestive heart failure includes increased cardiac size, which may not reach true cardiomegaly by measurement, but which is generally revealed by comparison with previous films. The lungs tend to become diffusely more opaque. Because of the underlying lung disease, changes in the pulmonary veins, such as engorgement and loss of crisp outlines, can seldom be appreciated (Fig. 12.16).

The radiographic distinction between congestive heart failure and the onset of a global pneumonia can be difficult. Generally, diffuse pneumonia does not enlarge the heart as much as congestive failure. Of course radiographic clearing following fluid restriction or diuretic or inotropic therapy is retrospectively diagnostic.

In acute episodes of congestive heart failure, identification of specific chamber enlargement would be diagnostically helpful. Right ventricular enlargement commonly

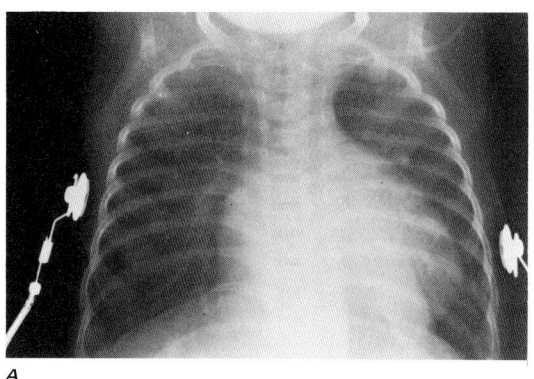
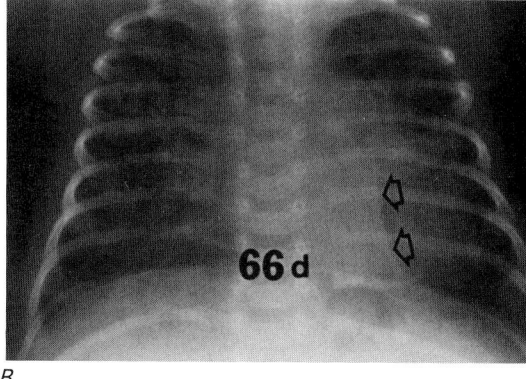

A *B*

Figure 12.15. Chronic left lower lobe atelectasis in BPD, probably secondary to an enlarged heart (see also Fig. 12.12). (*A*) A dense region of increased density is seen in the retrocardiac region in this 3 month old patient. (*B*) Similar but slightly more subtle finding (arrows) in a younger infant with BPD; also of note is an enlarged main pulmonary artery segment, reflecting pulmonary hypertension.

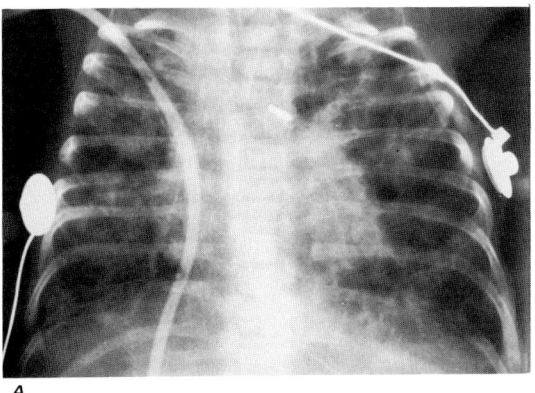 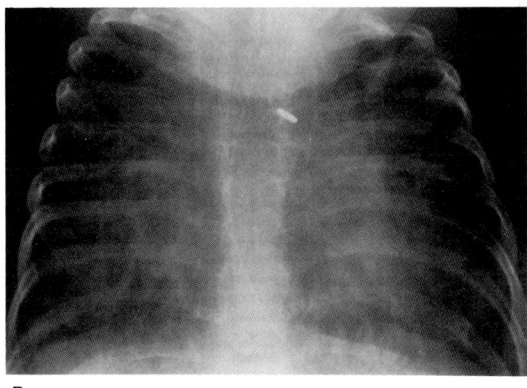

Figure 12.16. Congestive heart failure in BPD. (*A*) Six month old patient with chronic BPD in her baseline state. (*B*) Same patient during an episode of congestive heart failure; the cardiac silhouette is larger, and the lungs diffusely more opaque.

obliterates the lower portions of the retrosternal clear space on the lateral view and straightens the left cardiac margin on the frontal view. These changes are helpful if they can be identified, but in fact focal chamber enlargement is difficult to appreciate in infants; usually their hearts enlarge globally.

Chronic Cardiovascular Changes

Considering the extensive pulmonary abnormalities seen in moderate to severe chronic BPD (66), it is not surprising that the heart and pulmonary vasculature are secondarily affected. Pulmonary arterial hypertension occurs in such infants commonly, and may be diagnosed directly by cardiac catheterization (137) or inferred by echocardiographic (136, 138) or radiographic (68) findings. In a large autopsy series of such patients, nearly half had arterial wall thickening suggesting at least some degree of pulmonary hypertension (73).

Pulmonary hypertension in BPD patients is difficult to diagnose radiographically unless it is severe. The expected finding of an abnormally abrupt tapering of the pulmonary arteries is generally masked by the parenchymal abnormalities; indeed it is usually difficult to see the distal pulmonary arteries at all. The best sign seems to be an enlarged main pulmonary artery segment, which bulges notably from the left mediastinum just below the aortic arch (Fig. 12.15). It has been speculated that this enlarged artery, by stretching the recurrent laryngeal nerve, may be responsible for the sudden infant death syndrome occurring in BPD survivors (104).

Hypertrophy of the right ventricle, presumably secondary to pulmonary hypertension, is also common in patients with chronic BPD (75, 76, 136, 139, 140). Right ventricular hypertrophy may be discerned radiographically by an uptilted cardiac apex that at times can be marked enough to suggest tetralogy of Fallot (68). Ventricular wall thickness can more reliably be assessed by echocardiography (136) or gated magnetic resonance imaging (141).

Left ventricular hypertrophy, diagnosed

echocardiographically and at autopsy, has also been reported in chronic BPD patients (76, 142). None of the patients reported had an anatomic cardiac abnormality, so the association is difficult to understand. However, another report describes a high incidence of systemic hypertension in BPD patients, and three of these hypertensive patients had left ventricular hypertrophy diagnosed electrocardiographically (143). The reason for the systemic hypertension is unclear, but would certainly explain left ventricular hypertrophy in some of these infants. Another possible mechanism is left-to-right shunting through systemic-to-pulmonary collateral vessels, which have been observed in some infants with BPD (144).

Left ventricular hypertrophy is difficult to diagnose from plain films of infants; the major finding on the frontal view is fullness and prominence of the left cardiac border. The lateral view may reveal a backward displacement of the cardiac silhouette. I have seldom seen these findings in BPD patients, and as noted above, imaging modalities other than plain chest films more reliably demonstrate concentric hypertrophy.

Lesions of the Central Airways

Generally BPD is considered to be a disease of the pulmonary parenchyma, specifically the interstitium and the small, distal airways (66). Experience has shown, however, that lesions of the larger, central airways also accompany BPD, although they should probably not be considered aspects of the BPD disease process.

A relatively common lesion of the central airways presents as masses of polypoid granulation tissue that obstruct a main bronchus in a manner suggesting a foreign body, producing a one-way-valve effect by which air enters with inspiration but is trapped during expiration (96). This results in focal emphysema, usually involving the right lower and middle lobes, often with compressive atelectasis of the associated upper lobe. I have also encountered a case in which the polypoid masses were situated at the carina, producing intermittent obstructions to both lungs and ultimately causing the patient's demise (Fig. 12.10).

The location and pathologic character of these masses suggest that they result from the repeated trauma of endotracheal tube suction catheters. The treatment is either with endoscopic extirpation or by simply ensuring that suction catheters do not pass the carina and then waiting for the lesion to resolve.

When the combination of focal lower lobe emphysema and compressive upper lobe atelectasis is noted, the lesion may be pursued radiographically in the same manner as an endobronchial foreign body. The simplest method is the assisted expiration view, by which compression of the infant's abdomen during expiration forces the normal lung to near residual volume, vividly documenting regions of focal air trapping (145). In the setting of BPD the unaffected regions of lung do not collapse as fully as they do in normal infants; nonetheless a diagnostic examination is usually attainable (Fig. 12.10). Of course the assisted expiration view is not helpful if the polyps are situated at the carina, or if they have grown large enough to cause inspiratory as well as expiratory obstruction and hence distal atelectasis.

Subglottic stenosis is a well-known complication of extended endotracheal intubation; the tube causes mucosal necrosis acutely, whose severity seems related primarily to the duration of intubation (146, 147) and to the coexistence of infection (147). This inflammatory change appears more common and more marked in infants treated with high-frequency jet ventilation (148). In some cases the acute lesion progresses to scarring and fixed narrowing of the upper airway. Fortunately this complication is unusual at present.

Radiographically the chronic lesion is best evaluated using ordinary upper airway views, consisting of a soft-tissue-technique lateral view and a high-kilovoltage, filtered-beam frontal view, filmed near the end of quiet inspiration (149). The radiographic findings are somewhat suggestive of croup or focal edema, with tapering subglottic narrowing that is most marked on the frontal view (150); unlike croup, however, there is often some mild, wavy irregularity to the abnormal "steeple" or "pinch" formed by the air column (Fig. 12.17).

Another airway lesion that has been described in the setting of chronic BPD is expiratory collapse of the trachea and upper bronchi (151). This process was first noted on lung scintigraphy and confirmed fluoroscopically. It must be borne in mind that conventional radiography is only indirectly indicative of the motion of structures; perhaps this expiratory collapse is common, but it is seldom suspected on routine radiographs. Certainly such a process would contribute to the expiratory difficulties and air trapping of many BPD patients.

Seemingly BPD is also associated with enlargement of the trachea; tracheal measurements of plain radiographs of extremely small infants who had been ventilated in the newborn period showed significant tracheal enlargement all along the course of the intrathoracic trachea (152). This finding suggests a chronic deformation of the central airway,

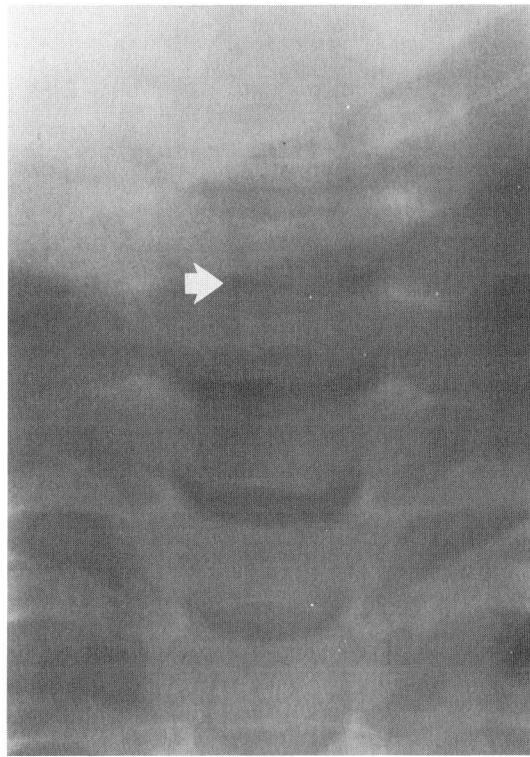

Figure 12.17. Subglottic stenosis a 4 month old infant with BPD. The high-kilovoltage, filtered view shows a focal, smooth, "pinch" narrowing of the airway (arrow) in the subglottic region.

presumably secondary to positive pressure ventilation. The resulting enlarged respiratory dead space would be expected to increase the infant's hypercapnia and work of breathing.

If the airways of some ventilated newborn infants collapse markedly with expiration and are also enlarged in the resting or inspiration state, the resulting situation is reminiscent of tracheomalacia. Indeed tracheobronchomalacia has been noted in survivors of RDS (153). Fluoroscopic diagnosis of tracheomalacia is difficult, and other imaging modalities may prove preferable. One encouraging technique is cine-computerized tomography (cine-CT), which permits real-time cross-sectional viewing of the upper airways during respiration, and direct measurement of airway cross-sectional area at multiple levels (154). The use of this modality has not been described in patients with BPD, but results with other patients suggest considerable promise.

Skeletal Problems

Osteopenia and Rickets

Bone disease is increasingly recognized as an important problem in infants with BPD. The overwhelming majority of infants with chronic BPD are survivors of premature birth, many with birth weights in the extremely low range (below 1000 g). Prematurity and (especially) very low birth weight are associated with subsequent osteopenia that is often severe (155), as well as with frank rickets (156–158). A variety of causative factors have been implicated, including malabsorption of calcium and phosphorus and dietary deficiencies of calcium, phosphorus, and vitamin D.

For a variety of reasons infants with chronic BPD commonly require extended parenteral nutrition. Total parenteral nutrition in adults is associated with a diffuse skeletal disease manifested by considerable bone pain and demineralization (159); it also appears that parenteral nutrition in infants is associated with demineralization and rickets (160, 161). The mechanism seems to involve inadequate phosphate, together with cholestasis secondary to the parenteral protein hydrolysate causing decreased bile acids in the enterohepatic circulation and a resultant diminished absorption of gut calcium and vitamin D.

A further risk factor for the development of osteopenia and rickets in BPD is chronic furosemide administration. In growing rats chronic furosemide administration maintains a negative calcium balance for as long as the drug is continued (162). A similar situation seems to occur in infants with BPD who require long-term furosemide for cor pulmonale; such infants may develop not only marked osteopenia, but also secondary hyperparathyroidism (163).

Finally, sodium bicarbonate, which is usually administered to combat acidosis, also may play a role by causing calciuresis (164).

With all of these risk factors, it is scarcely surprising that many infants with BPD suffer marked osteopenia, and often rickets. The radiograhpic progression of these conditions has been described in detail in the setting of infants weighing less than 1000 g at birth (158), and this progression is summarized as follows. The earliest finding seems to be focal demineralization at the growing ends of long bones, with similar rims of lucency appearing in the scapulae and iliac bones, and a "bone within a bone" appearance of vertebrae; these findings begin at 14 to 30 days and reach a maximum at 40 days. Between about 50 and 80 days, the demineralization progresses along the diaphyses of the bones and becomes generalized. After this some patients undergo a gradual return to normal bone density, while others at 60 to 100 days develop rickets, which subsequently heals (158).

My impression is that this progression is approximately the same as that in similar infants with BPD, but that the progression is more rapid in its onset. Parenthetically it may be noted that nutritional rickets itself is sometimes associated with diffuse lung disease (165). Furthermore preterm infants have been described in whom lung disease appears secondary to the skeletal process (166). The relationship, if any, of these observations to BPD is uncertain.

The chest is the most frequently radiographed portion of BPD patients, so it is reasonable to glean as much information as possible regarding skeletal abnormalities from the chest film. The early demineralization of the growing ends of long bones is readily perceived in the proximal humerus. Poznanski and associates devised a method of evaluating bone loss in premature infants using the middle portion of the humerus as seen on chest radiographs (167). This method relies on standards of normal cortical thickness as a function of gestational age, and seems to be helpful in assessing the extent of osteopenia in these patients (158).

Unfortunately the proximal humeral metaphysis often does not display obvious changes of rickets until the condition is moderately advanced; indeed rib fractures may be the first suggestion of rickets noted on the chest film (161, 168). Flaring of the anterior rib ends, when this occurs, is an even more reliable sign of rickets. Early changes of rickets, such as cupping and then fraying, irregularity, and splaying of the metaphyses, are much better appreciated on a single frontal view of a wrist or knee (Fig. 12.18). These areas are also best for monitoring responses to therapy and healing.

The skull, if it is radiographed, also shows osteopenia vividly (158). The bones of the calvarium may become essentially invisible, and the multiple line shadows of the inner facial bones become fuzzy and effaced. Occasionally the skull base is included on a poorly coned chest film, and marked osteoporosis

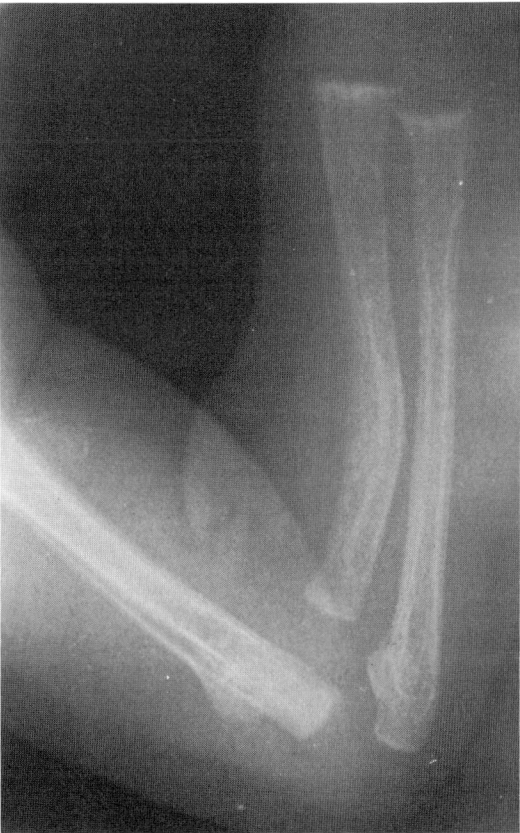

Figure 12.18. Rickets in a 5 month old child with BPD. The wrist demonstrates cupping and frayed irregularity of the distal radius and ulna, findings of rickets. In addition there is a pathologic bowing fracture of the radius, periostitis of the humerus, and gross overall demineralization.

may be noted by seeing the curving, calcific rims of the semicircular canals seeming to float above the petrous bone.

More elaborate techniques for determining bone mineral content are available, such as direct photon absorptiometry (169) and measurement of CT number of vertebral bodies or other regions. The primary utility of these at present seems to be in research endeavors rather than day-to-day patient management.

Fractures

The only time I have seen X-rays of more fractured bones was in an Air Force crash victim. (Physician's note in a case of BPD, 170)

Infants with BPD and severe osteopenia, with or without rickets, sometimes demonstrate skeletal radiographs that suggest nearly eggshell fragility. It is not surprising that fractures are common in such patients. These fractures must be considered pathologic, in that they occur in the setting of abnormal bone whose mineral content is minimal and whose structural integrity is precarious. Furthermore the fractures occur in the course of normal handling. This does not mean that such fractures are not painful as well as potentially deforming, and there are few more pathetic sights in radiology than a bone survey of such an infant.

The most commonly fractured bones are the ribs. The reason for this is probably twofold: first, because the ribs are thin and relatively easily fractured in any case; and second, because the brunt of the chest physiotherapy necessary in BPD is physically directed against the rib cage (168). Rib fractures in BPD may be difficult to discern when acute, unless diligently sought; more often they are seen when bony callus begins to form.

Long bones are somewhat less frequently fractured, or at least fractures of long bones are less commonly noted; sometimes these are occult and may be noted only during the healing phase. Routine skeletal surveys are not generally done, so it is possible for fractures, particularly those causing no marked deformity, to go unsuspected.

Often long bone fractures in these patients are buckling or "torus" fractures near the ends of the bones, usually with some angulation and often a degree of impaction (Fig. 12.19). Less usual are complete fractures of the diaphysis, with or without angulation or over-riding of the fracture fragments, although these certainly occur. Metaphyseal "corner" fractures and bowing deformities (Fig. 12.18) are also seen.

In the general setting of pediatric radiology, of course, multiple fractures in an infant

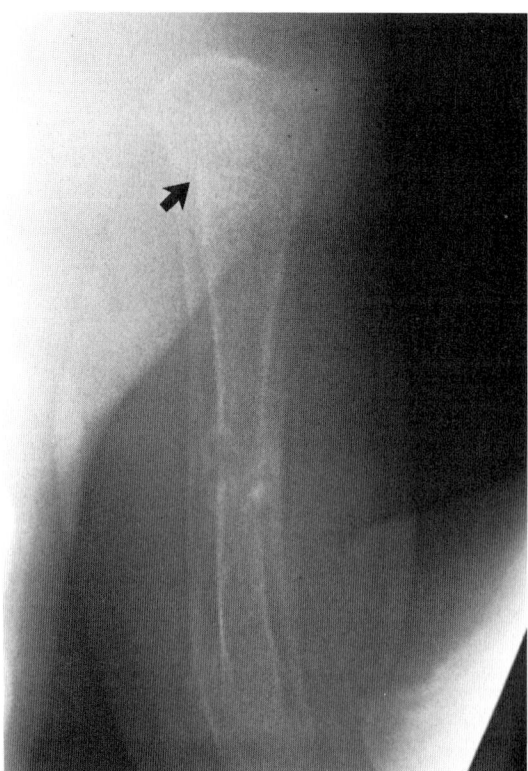

Figure 12.19. Pathologic fractures in a 5 month old child with BPD. The proximal humerus shows an incomplete buckling fracture (arrow) with some impaction medially; there is also a nondisplaced midshaft fracture, exuberant periostitis, and marked demineralization.

strongly suggest child abuse. I and others (158) have had this awkward question raised when seeing films of an unknown "expremie" with unexplained fractures of different ages. The pattern of fractures in child abuse appears subtly different from that encountered in BPD, although this question has not been systematically studied. For example, the rib fractures in child abuse are most commonly posterior, and are usually multiple at about the same spot in three to five adjacent ribs, reflecting the single impact of an adult fist (171). The rib fractures in BPD are more often lateral and tend to present singly or in pairs.

Metaphyseal "corner" fractures occur both in BPD and abuse cases, but are more commonly encountered in the latter. Fractures of the skull are noted considerably more often in abused children. Long bone diaphysial fractures are more frequently spiral or oblique in abused children. Fractures in abused children are more common on the patient's left than the right (171).

Of course none of these diagnostic clues is as important as noting the underlying abnormal bone of BPD patients. A substrate of normally mineralized bone is essential for the radiographic diagnosis of child abuse. Noting marked demineralization, either by eye or by measurement (167), precludes the radiographic diagnosis of abuse; in fact the child may have been abused, but the radiographic evidence is inapplicable. Similarly the radiographic diagnosis is precluded when changes of active or healing rickets are encountered. It should also go without saying that the clinical history is crucial, as is examination of the patient for dermal and other lesions suggesting abuse.

Other differential diagnostic considerations include osteogenesis imperfecta (which should demonstrate wormian bones in the skull), Menkes' kinky-hair syndrome (which should demonstrate wormian bones and distinctive metaphyseal spurs), congenital syphilis and other intrauterine infections (primarily metaphyseal involvement, but may be a close mimic), "physiologic" periostitis (normal underlying bone, bilateral symmetry), metastatic neuroblastoma (lesions focal and often both lytic and blastic), and other, less common lesions. Fortunately, in the clinical setting of BPD, the diagnosis is usually apparent.

Chest Shape Deformity

To spare unnecessary radiation and patient handling, the great majority of chest films of BPD patients are frontal views only. Obviously these views do not provide a full assessment of chest wall configuration. Commonly in cases of severe BPD, the chest on the frontal view assumes a somewhat rounded shape which usually reflects hyperinflation (100). In some cases of BPD associated with severe bone disease, however, this rounded shape becomes unusually pronounced, or there is marked lateral splaying of the inferior ribs. Usually this is first noted at 3 to 5 months of age. If a lateral view is exposed, the chest is seen to be quite flattened along its anteroposterior axis (Fig. 12.20; see also reference 160, Fig. 1). Physical examination of the patient is confirmatory: the chest appears abnormally flattened and splayed in its left-to-right dimension.

The etiology of this appearance is uncertain. It might result from abnormally soft, demineralized bones, with an uncertain contribution from chronic substernal retractions and rib fractures, responding to months of supine or prone position in which the gravi-

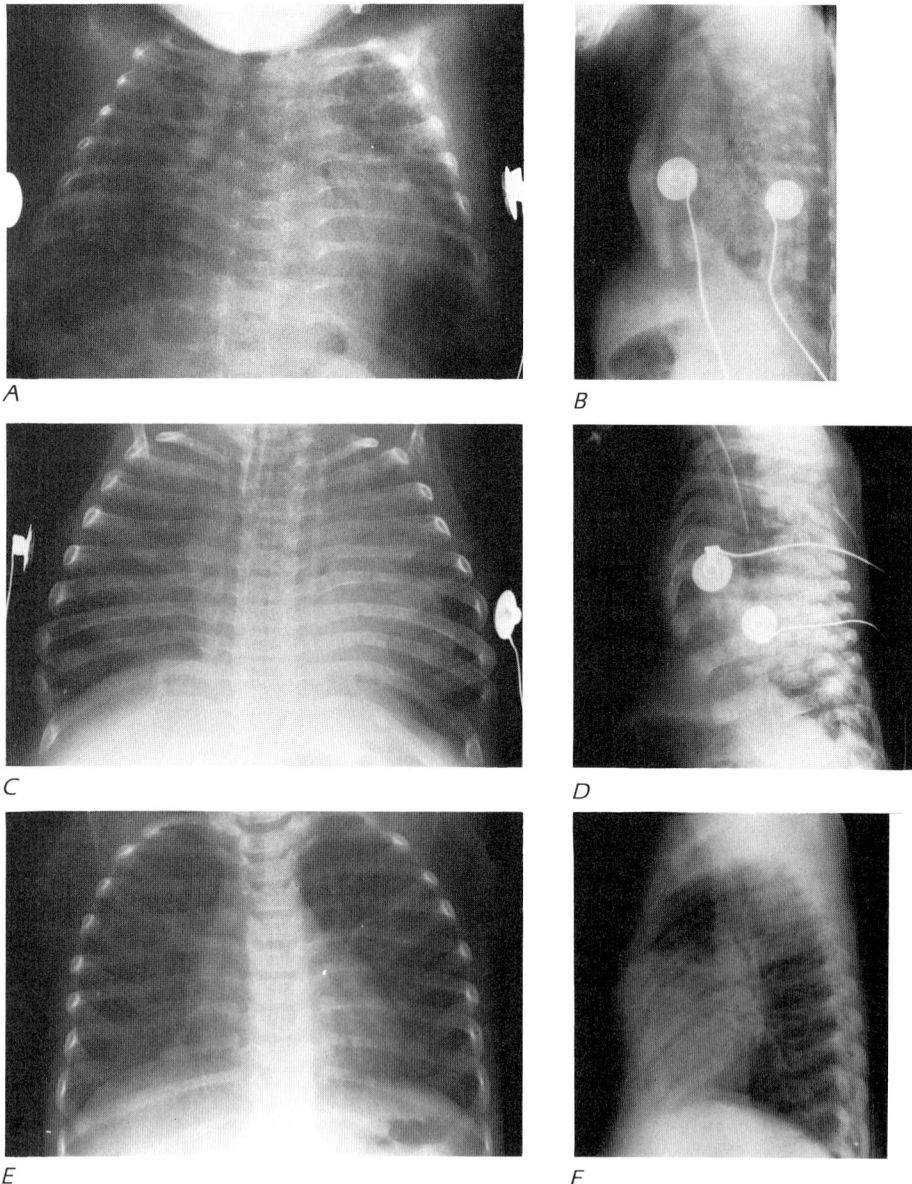

Figure 12.20. Chest shape deformity in BPD. (*A*) Frontal view of this 4 month old patient with severe BPD shows gross demineralization and widely flared lower ribs; (*B*) lateral view shows chest flattening (diminished anteroposterior thickness). (C) Frontal view of a 9 month old infant shows widely spread lower ribs and a rounded chest configuration; (*D*) lateral view reveals flattening of the chest. (*E*) In this 1 year old child with healing BPD, the frontal projection shows a rounded chest configuration; (*F*) lateral view shows slight chest flattening.

THE RADIOLOGY OF BPD

tational vector is anteroposterior. Perhaps the mechanism is analogous to the occipital flattening encountered in severely retarded children. It is uncertain whether or not this chest deformity is associated with additional impairment of pulmonary function. The condition seems to improve with age; as the patient grows the chest acquires a more normal configuration, often suggesting no more than a pectus excavatum deformity.

Abdominal Abnormalities

Cholelithiasis

The etiology of gallstones in the setting of BPD is uncertain. The usual causes of cholelithiasis in infants and children—hemolytic disease, ileal disease, infection, and anatomic deformity of the biliary system (172)—are seldom applicable. The most plausible etiology involves parenteral feeding (173); the hyperalimentation formula generally contains both protein hydrolysate that seems to promote bile stasis by a hepatotoxic effect (174) and fat emulsion that promotes crystalization of bile (175). Even mechanical obstruction of the biliary tree has been reported in the setting of parenteral nutrition (176). A contribution of furosemide has also been suggested in BPD patients (177–180). The composition of these stones, when reported, seems variable from patient to patient and of mixed chemical character (177, 178, 181).

The majority of the stones are radiopaque, although this may merely reflect the fact that radiotransparent stones are less often discovered. The stones are generally multiple. Discovery of the stones is usually a radiographic accident, with the densities noted on a widely coned chest radiograph (Fig. 12.21) in the usual right upper quadrant position

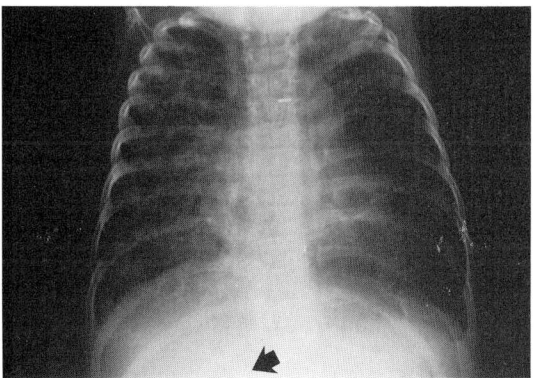

Figure 12.21. Gallstone (arrow) first noted on the edge of this widely coned chest radiograph of a 7 month old child with severe BPD. This is a common presentation of cholelithiasis in such infants.

(177–181). Stones may also be discovered during abdominal sonograms done for other reasons (182), or may be deliberately sought in screening sonograms done on infants treated with parenteral nutrition (183). The reported time at which these are noticed varies between 11 days and 7 months, with an average of about 3 months (177–181).

Radiographically the only important lesion with which gallstones might be confused are right renal calculi (179). Their nonrenal origin can be established by a lateral radiograph of the abdomen, which shows the stones lying far anterior to the renal fossa. Definitive diagnosis is ultrasonographic; the stones are revealed as foci of bright echoes lying in the dependent portion of the gallbladder and casting sharp acoustic shadows (Fig. 12.22).

Once cholelithiasis is diagnosed the question arises of what to do next. In my experience with gallstones in the setting of BPD, no clinical problems referable to the hepatobiliary system have been noted; and in one BPD survivor who received occasional chest films

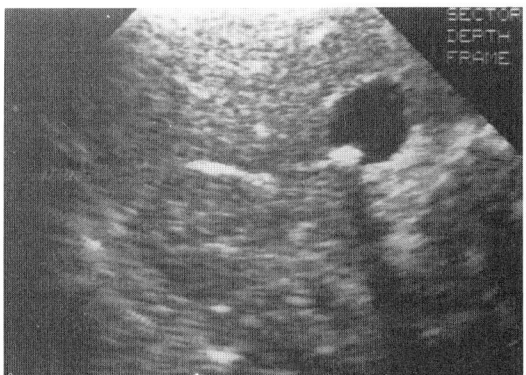

Figure 12.22. Single gallstone in a 4 month old child with BPD. Abdominal sonogram reveals a brightly echoic filling defect in the gallbladder with acoustic shadowing.

to 2 years of age, the gallstones were seen to become smaller and then vanish. Spontaneous resolution of gallstones in infants has also been reported by others (182). It would seem to be prudent to adopt a watch-and-wait attitude, and reserve surgery for patients who develop hepatobiliary abnormalities. The long-term prognosis of such patients in unknown.

Renal Calcifications

Renal calcifications and frank calculi also occur in premature infants, almost invariably in infants who have been treated with furosemide (184–186). Furosemide promotes prolonged calcium excretion and hypercalciuria (162), which, as discussed above, contributes to osteoporosis, and which also exposes the renal collecting system to high concentrations of calcium. Other agents that may be involved are sodium bicarbonate and calcium gluconate (182). Renal calcifications, and indeed abnormal calcification of many soft tissues, are common with hyperparathyroidism, and one infant with primary hyperparathyroidism, and renal calcifications has been reported (185). Secondary hyperparathyroidism also may occur in the setting of long-term furosemide therapy, with similar results (163).

Calcifications in the setting of furosemide therapy may be recognized at an average of 1 month following institution of therapy (185). The calcifications are more common in small premature infants than in larger infants (185). The radiographic character of the renal calcification is variable, including isolated stones, staghorn calculi, and nephrocalcinosis (184). The most common finding is a faint array of curvilinear densities that form the vague outline of a collecting system. These can be difficult to appreciate on plain films, and ultrasonography appears to be superior for diagnosis (Fig. 12.23), revealing abnormally increased echogenicity of the pyramids and distinctive "shadowing" (163).

As with gallstones the question arises as to what should be done about renal calcifications once they are identified. Spontaneous resolution of the calcifications has been noted

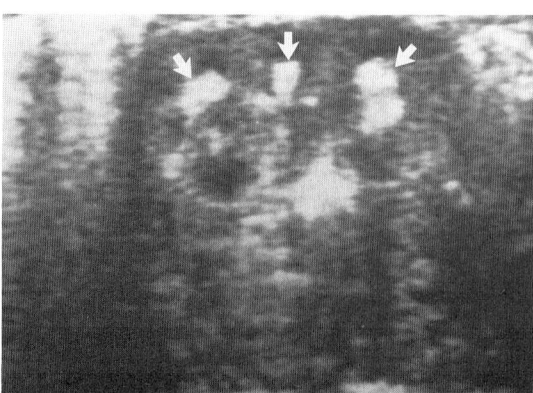

Figure 12.23. Renal calcifications in a 3 month old patient with BPD. Sonogram reveals bright echoes (arrows) in the distribution of the renal pyramids, with acoustic shadowing from the bright echoes.

following discontinuation of furosemide and following changing the diuretic to chlorothiazide (185). The long-term natural history of the calcifications is unknown. One anecdotal report described an obstructing stone that caused hydronephrosis and required surgical removal (187). This does not seem to be a common experience, and it may be hoped that resolution following discontinuation of furosemide is the more usual rule.

Inguinal Hernia

Empirically inguinal hernias are common in infants with chronic BPD, which probably merely reflects the marked increased incidence of these in small premature infants generally (188). While inguinal hernia is not primarily a radiographic diagnosis, in BPD patients shadows of gas over one or both groins permit incidental diagnosis of this association on films of the abdomen or pelvis (Fig. 12.24).

Summary

BPD is a chronic disease of infancy and early childhood that most commonly appears in a preterm infant with the radiographic and clinical findings of respiratory distress syndrome. Less commonly BPD appears in infants with other underlying diseases who require substantial respiratory support with oxygenation and mechanically assisted ventilation. The acute phases during which the chronic disease appears and then develops are radiographically variable, and are poorly monitored by radiographs. The severity of the disease that ultimately appears is also variable, ranging from a few abnormal interstitial markings to a florid picture of gross hyperinflation, with regions of emphysema alternating with streaks of abnormal density, and often cardiomegaly and evidence of pulmonary arterial hypertension. In recent years the appearance of chronic BPD is usually less severe than in the past, with films demonstrating less overall emphysema and less pulmonary inhomogeneity.

Chronic BPD can radiographically be simulated by several other entities, including diffuse pulmonary interstitial emphysema, chronic viral pneumonitis, Wilson-Mikity syndrome, and excessive lung fluid. Superimposed chronic viral infection may worsen the pulmonary abnormalities of BPD. Occa-

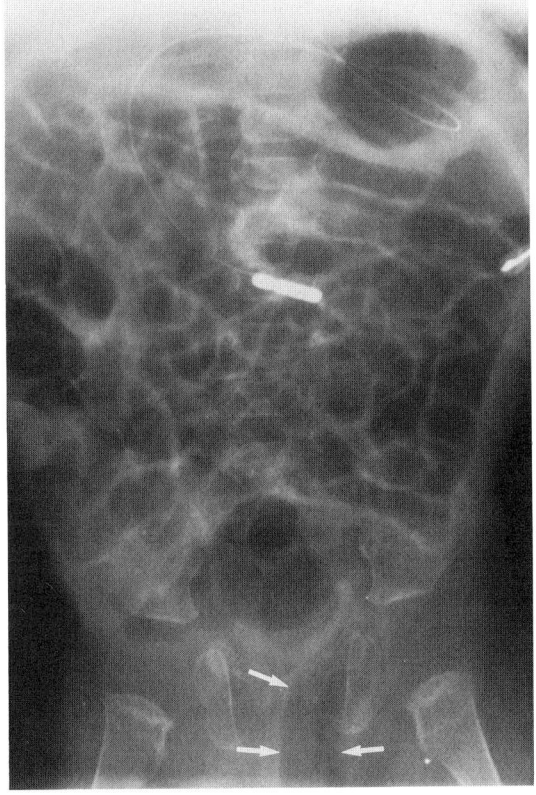

Figure 12.24. Left inguinal hernia in a 3 month old child with BPD. Gas shadows are seen extending into the left scrotum (arrows).

sionally the radiographic appearance of chronic BPD is atypical. BPD that is asymmetric from left lung to right lung has been described following extended collapse of the relatively uninvolved lung. Focal and usually lower lobar emphysema in BPD may be intrinsic or secondary to partially obstructing polypoid, granulomatous airway lesions that seem to result from mechanical trauma. Occasionally BPD is manifested radiographically by extended pulmonary parenchymal opacity whose pathologic character is unclear.

Radiographically, chronic BPD tends to improve slowly once the patient's respiratory assistance (oxygenation and assisted ventilation) is discontinued. A radiographic scoring system is suggested that permits semiquantitative assessment of chronic BPD and its changes over time.

Chronic BPD has several complications and associations that can be diagnosed and monitored radiographically. In the chest these include pneumonias, transient and long-lived atelectasis, congestive heart failure, signs of cor pulmonale, and abnormalities of the central airways. In some affected patients severe bone disease accompanies BPD, with osteopenia, rickets, secondary hyperparathyroidism, and pathologic fractures. In the abdomen some BPD patients have gallstones and renal calcifications; the long-term significance of these is uncertain. Inguinal hernias are relatively common in BPD patients, which probably reflects the increased incidence of these in premature infants.

While plain film radiography remains the cornerstone of radiographic imaging in BPD patients, several other modalities offer potential benefit in particular settings. Of these diagnostic ultrasound is probably the most important, certainly in the abdomen, and also in the brain of infants with open fontanelles. In imaging the brain of children with closed or small fontanelles, magnetic resonance imaging, because of the lack of associated marrow radiation and the excellence of the images produced, appears superior to computerized tomography.

References

1. Northway WH Jr, Rosan RC, Porter DY. Pulmonary disease following respiratory therapy of hyaline-membrane disease: bronchopulmonary dysplasia. N Engl J Med 1967;276:357–368.
2. National Heart, Lung, and Blood Institutes. Report of Workshop on Bronchopulmonary Dysplasia. NIH Publication No. 80-1660. Bethesda, Md: U. S. Department of Health, Education, and Welfare, 1979.
3. Northway WH Jr, Rosan RC. Radiographic features of pulmonary oxygen toxicity in the newborn: bronchopulmonary dysplasia. Radiology 1968;91:49–58.
4. Cashore WJ, Stern L. Neonatal problems of the preterm baby. Clin Obstet Gynecol 1984; 11:391–414.
5. Edwards DK, Jacob J, Gluck L. The immature lung: radiographic appearance, course, and complications. AJR 1980;135:659–666.
6. Loeber NV, Morray JP, Kettrick RG, Downes JJ. Pulmonary function in chronic respiratory failure of infancy. Crit Care Med 1980;8:596–601.
7. Mayes L, Perkett E, Stahlman MT. Severe bronchopulmonary dysplasia: a retrospective review. Acta Paediatr Scand 1983;72:225–229.
8. Philip AGS. Oxygen plus pressure plus time: the etiology of bronchopulmonary dysplasia. Pediatrics 1975;55:44–50.
9. Truog WE, Jackson JC, Badura RJ, Sorensen GK, Murphy JH, Woodrum DE. Bronchopulmonary dysplasia and pulmonary insufficiency of prematurity. Lack of correlation of outcome with gas exchange abnormalities at 1 month of life. Am J Dis Child 1985;139:351–354.

10. Rhodes PG, Hall RT, Leonidas JC. Chronic pulmonary disease in neonates with assisted ventilation. Pediatrics 1975;55:788–796.
11. Bomsel F, Couchard M, Polje J, Larroche JC. Pulmonary sequelae of the hyaline membrane disease: iatrogenic factors? Radiological and anatomical study. Ann Radiol 1973;16:70–74.
12. Pusey VA, MacPherson RI, Chernick V. Pulmonary fibroplasia following prolonged artificial ventilation of newborn infants. Can Med Assoc J 1969;100:451–457.
13. Barnes ND, Glover WJ, Hull D, Milner AD. Effects of prolonged positive-pressure ventilation in infancy. Lancet 1969;2:1096–1099.
14. Campognone P, Singer DB. Neonatal sepsis due to nontypable *Haemophilus influenzae*. Am J Dis Child 1986;140:117–121.
15. Jentzen J, Rockswold G, Anderson WR. Pulmonary oxygen toxic effect. Occurrence in a newborn infant despite low PaO_2 due to an intracranial arteriovenous malformation. Arch Pathol Lab Med 1984;108:334–337.
16. Edwards DK. Radiographic aspects of bronchopulmonary dysplasia. J Pediatr 1979;823–829.
17. Chew DTA, Yin ALS. Oxygen therapy and pulmonary fibroplasia: a review and case reports. Med J Malaya 1971;26:122–128.
18. Oppermann HC, Wille L, Bleyl U, Obladen M. Bronchopulmonary dysplasia in premature infants. A radiological and pathological correlation. Pediatr Radiol 1977;5:137–141.
19. Churg A, Golden J, Fligiel S, Hogg JC. Bronchopulmonary dysplasia in the adult. Am Rev Repair Dis 1983;127:117–120.
20. Dyck DR, Zylak CJ. Acute respiratory distress in adults. Radiology 1973;106:497–501.
21. Ablow RC, Gross I, Effmann EL, Uauy R, Driscoll S. The radiographic features of early onset group B streptococcal neonatal sepsis. Radiology 1977;124:771–777.
22. Leonidas JC, Hall RT, Beatty EC, Fellows RA. Radiographic findings in early onset neonatal group B streptococcal septicemia. Pediatrics 1977; 59:1006–1011.
23. Vollman JH, Smith WL, Ballard ET, Light IJ. Early onset group B streptococcal disease: clinical, roentgenographic, and pathologic features. J Pediatr 1976;89:199–203.
24. Lilien LD, Harris VJ, Pildes RS. Significance of radiographic findings in early-onset group B streptococcal infection. Pediatrics 1977;60:360–363.
25. Weller MH, Katzenstein AA. Radiological findings in group B streptococcal sepsis. Radiology 1976;118:385–387.
26. Foote GA, Stewart JH. The coexistence of pneumonia and the idiopathic respiratory distress syndrome in neonates. Br J Radiol 1973;46:504–511.
27. Jacob J, Edwards D, Gluck L. Early-onset sepsis and pneumonia observed as respiratory distress syndrome: assessment of lung maturity. Am J Dis Child 1980;134:766–768.
28. Wesenberg RL, Graven SN, McCabe EB. Radiological findings in wet-lung disease. Radiology 1971;98:69–74.
29. Finnegan LP, McBrine CS, Steg NL, Williams ML. Respiratory distress in the newborn. Value of roentgenography in diagnosis and prognosis. Am J Dis Child 1970;119:212–217.
30. Rowe RD, Mehrizi A. The neonate with congenital heart disease. Philadelphia: WB Saunders, 1968, p 113.
31. Nickerson BG. Bronchopulmonary dysplasia. Chronic pulmonary disease following neonatal respiratory failure. Chest 1985;87:528–535.
32. Miyatake K, Okamoto M, Kinoshita N, et al. Clinical applications of a new type of real-time two-dimensional Doppler flow imaging system. Am J Cardiol 1984;54:857–868.
33. Higgins CB, Rausch J, Friedman WF, et al. Patent ductus arteriosus in preterm infants with idiopathic respiratory distress syndrome. Radiographic and echocardiographic evaluation. Radiology 1977;124:189–195.
34. Higgins CB, DiSessa T, Kirkpatrick SE, et al. Assessment of patent ductus arteriosus in preterm infants by single lateral film aortography. Radiology 1980;135:641–647.
35. Cleveland RH, Todres ID. Patterns of evolution of x-ray changes in respiratory distress syndrome. Helv Paediatr Acta 1981;36:43–53.
36. Bancalari E, Abdenour GE, Feller R, Gannon J. Bronchopulmonary dysplasia: clinical presentation. J Pediatr 1979;95:819–823.

37. Ponhold VW, Coradello H. Die bronchopulmonale Dysplasie: Rontgensymptomatik und Stadieneinteilung. Fortschr Rontgenstr 1980;133:586–590.
38. Singleton EB. Radiologic considerations of intensive care in the premature infant. Radiology 1981;140:291–300.
39. Tooley WH. Epidemiology of bronchopulmonary dysplasia. J Pediatr 1979;95:851–855.
40. Wung JT, Koons AH, Driscoll JM Jr, James LS. Changing incidence of bronchopulmonary dysplasia. J Pediatr 1979;95:845–847.
41. Heneghan MA, Sosulski R, Baquero JM. Persistent pulmonary abnormalities in newborns: the changing picture of bronchopulmonary dysplasia. Pediatr Radiol 1986;16:180–184.
42. Edwards DK, Dyer WM, Northway WH Jr. Twelve years' experience with bronchopulmonary dysplasia. Pediatrics 1977;59:839–846.
43. Berg TJ, Pagtakhan RD, Reed MH, Langston C, Chernick V. Bronchopulmonary dysplasia and lung rupture in hyaline membrane disease: influence of continuous distending pressure. Pediatrics 1975;55:51–54.
44. Moylan FMB, Walker AM, Kramer SS, Todres ID, Shannon DC. The relationship of bronchopulmonary dysplasia to the occurrence of alveolar rupture during positive pressure ventilation. Crit Care Med 1978;6:140–142.
45. Moylan FMB, Walker AM, Kramer SS, Todres ID, Shannon DC. Alveolar rupture as an independent predictor of bronchopulmonary dysplasia. Crit Care Med 1978;6:10–13.
46. Stahlman MT, Cheatham W, Gray ME. The role of air dissection in bronchopulmonary dysplasia. J Pediatr 1979;95:878–882.
47. Bauer CR, Brennan MJ, Doyle C, Poole CA. Surgical resection for pulmonary interstitial emphysema in the newborn infant. J Pediatr 1978;93:656–661.
48. Drew JH, Landau LI, Acton CM, Kent M, Campbell PE. Pulmonary interstitial emphysema requiring lobectomy: complication of assisted ventilation. Arch Dis Child 1978;53:424–426.
49. Magilner AD, Capitanio MA, Wertheimer I, Burko H. Persistent localized intrapulmonary interstitial emphysema. An observation in three infants. Radiology 1974;111:379–384.
50. Lopez JB, Campbell RE, Bishop HC, Boggs TR Jr. Nonoperative resolution of prolonged localized intrapulmonary interstitial emphysema associated with hyaline membrane disease. J Pediatr 1977;91:653–654.
51. Lindroth M, Jonson B, Svenningsen NW, Mortensson W. Pulmonary mechanics, chest x-ray and lung disease after mechanical ventilation in low birth weight infants. Acta Pediatr Scand 1980;69:761–770.
52. Mortensson W, Lindroth M, Jonsson B, Svenningsen N. Chest radiography and pulmonary mechanics in ventilator treated low birth weight infants. Acta Radiol Diag 1983;24:71–79.
53. Krauss AN, Klain DB, Auld PAM. Chronic pulmonary insufficiency of prematurity (CPIP). Pediatrics 1975;55:55–58.
54. Parker BR, Pinckney LE, Johnson JD, Northway WH. Immature lung syndrome (abstr). Clin Res 1976;24:194A.
55. Fletcher BD, Fanaroff AA. The "immature" lung and RDS (letter). AJR 1981;136:840.
56. Hallman M, Feldman BH, Kirkpatrick E, Gluck L. Absence of phosphatidylglycerol (PG) in respiratory distress syndrome in the newborn. Study of the minor surfactant phospholipids in newborns. Pediatr Res 1977;11:714–720.
57. Bernbaum JC, Russell P, Sheridan PH, Gewitz MH, Fox WW, Peckham GJ. Long-term follow-up of newborns with persistent pulmonary hypertension. Crit Care Med 1984;12:579–583.
58. Hageman JR, Adams A, Gardner TH. Persistent pulmonary hypertension of the newborn. Trends in incidence, diagnosis, and management. Am J Dis Child 1984;138:592–595.
59. Swischuk LE, Richardson CJ, Nichols MM, Ingman MJ. Primary pulmonary hypoplasia in the neonate. J Pediatr 1979;95:573–577.
60. Fox WW, Duara S. Persistent pulmonary hypertension in the neonate: diagnosis and management. J Pediatr 1983;103:505–514.
61. Hallman M, Kankaanpaa K. Evidence of sur-

62. Nussbaum E. Adult-type respiratory distress syndrome in children. Experience with seven cases. Clin Pediatr 1983;22:401–406.
63. Droge MA, Jewett CV, Schmalstieg FC. Adult respiratory distress syndrome in an infant (letter). Pediatrics 1982;70:329–330.
64. Avery GB, Fletcher AB, Kaplan M, Brudno DS. Controlled trial of dexamethasone in respirator-dependent infants with bronchopulmonary dysplasia. Pediatrics 1985;75:106–111.
65. Mammel MC, Green TP, Johnson DE, Thompson TR. Controlled trial of dexamethasone therapy in infants with bronchopulmonary dysplasia. Lancet 1983;1:1356–1358.
66. Bonikos DS, Bensch KG, Northway WH Jr, Edwards DK. Bronchopulmonary dysplasia: the pulmonary pathologic sequel of necrotizing bronchiolitis and pulmonary fibrosis. Hum Pathol 1976;7:643–666.
67. Goetzman BW. Understanding bronchopulmonary dysplasia (editorial). Am J Dis Child 1986;140:332–334.
68. Edwards DK. Bronchopulmonary dysplasia today. In: Milunksky A, Friedman EA, Gluck L, eds. Advances in perinatal medicine, vol 3. New York: Plenum, pp 117–163.
69. D'Ablang G III, Bernard B, Zaharov I, Barton L, Kaplan B, Schwinn CP. Neonatal pulmonary cytology and bronchopulmonary dysplasia. Acta Cytol 1975;19:21–27.
70. Merritt TA, Stuard ID, Puccia J, et al. Newborn tracheal aspirate cytology: classification during respiratory distress syndrome and bronchopulmonary dysplasia. J Pediatr 1981;98:949–956.
71. Merritt TA. Oxygen exposure in the newborn guinea pig lung lavage cell populations, chemotactic and elastase response: a possible relationship to neonatal bronchopulmonary dysplasia. Pediatr Res 1982;16:798–805.
72. Wesenberg RL, Wax RE, Zachman RD. Varying roentgenographic patterns of patient ductus arteriosus in the newborn. AJR 1972;114:340–349.
73. Edwards DK, Colby TV, Northway WH Jr. Radiographic-pathologic correlation in bronchopulmonary dysplasia. J Pediatr 1979;95:834–836.
74. Kwok-Liu JP, Zylak CJ, deSa DJ. Bronchopulmonary dysplasia. A radiologic-pathologic correlation. J Can Assoc Radiol 1980;31:238–241.
75. Harrod JR, L'Heureux P, Wangensteen OD, Hunt CE. Long-term follow-up of severe respiratory distress syndrome treated with IPPB. J Pediatr 1974;84:277–286.
76. Stocker JT. Pathologic features of longstanding "healed" bronchopulmonary dysplasia: a study of 28 3- to 40-month old infants. Hum Pathol 1986;17:943–961.
77. Rubin A, Krepela K, Janouskova A, Biganovska V. Diffuse interstitial lung fibrosis from childhood and adolescence to adult life. Pediatr Radiol 1981;11:125–128.
78. Hodgman JE, Mikity VG, Tatter D, Cleland RS. Chronic respiratory distress in the premature infant. Wilson-Mikity syndrome. Pediatrics 1969;44:179–195.
79. Cochran ST, Gyepes MT, Smith LE. Obstruction of the airways by the heart and pulmonary vessels in infants. Pediatr Radiol 1977;6:81–87.
80. Swischuk LE. Bubbles in hyaline membrane disease. Differentiation of three types. Radiology 1977;122:417–426.
81. Clarke TA, Edwards DK. Pulmonary pseudocysts in newborn infants with respiratory distress syndrome. AJR 1979;133:417–421.
82. Whitley RJ, Brasfield D, Reynolds DW, Stagno S, Tiller RE, Alford CA. Protracted pneumonitis in young infants associated with perinatally acquired cytomegaloviral infection. J Pediatr 1976;89:16–22.
83. Panjvani ZFK, Hanshaw JB. Cytomegalovirus in the perinatal period. Am J Dis Child 1981;135:56–60.
84. Sawyer MH, Edwards DK, Spector SA. Cytomegalovirus infection and bronchopulmonary dysplasia in premature infants. Am J Dis Child, 1987;141:303–305.
85. Paryani SG, Yeager AS, Hosford-Dunn H, et al. Sequelae of acquired cytomegalovirus infection in premature and sick term infants. J Pediatr 1985;107:451–456.
86. Adler SP, Baggett J, Wilson M, Lawrence L,

McVoy M. Molecular epidemiology of cytomegalovirus in a nursery: lack of evidence for nosocomial transmission. J Pediatr 1986;108: 117–123.
87. Nakamura Y, Hosokawa Y, Nakashima T, et al. Pulmonary complications of long-term respirator care in infants: relationship to bronchopulmonary dysplasia. Acta Pathol Jpn 1981;31:75–84.
88. Wilson MG, Mikity VG. A new form of respiratory disease in premature infants. Am J Dis Child 1960;99:489–499.
89. Mikity VG, Taber P. Complications in the treatment of the respiratory distress syndrome. Bronchopulmonary dysplasia, oxygen toxicity, and the Wilson-Mikity syndrome. Pediatr Clin N Am 1973;20:419–431.
90. Thibeault DW, Grossman H, Hagstrom JWC, Auld PA. Radiologic findings in the lungs of premature infants. J Pediatr 1969;74:1–10.
91. Oetgen WJ. Chlamydial pneumonia of infancy vs Wilson-Mikity syndrome (letter). Pediatrics 1979;64:119–120.
92. Edwards DK, Hilton SvW, Merritt TA, Hallman M, Mannino F, Boynton BR. Respiratory distress syndrome treated with human surfactant: radiographic findings. Radiology 1985;157:329–334.
93. Sickles EA, Gooding CA. Asymmetric lung involvement in bronchopulmonary dysplasia. Radiology 1976;118:379–383.
94. Moylan FMB, Shannon DC. Preferential distribution of lobar emphysema and atelectasis in bronchopulmonary dysplasia. Pediatrics 1979;63:130–134.
95. Cooney DR, Menke JA, Allen JE. "Acquired" lobar emphysema: a complication of respiratory distress in premature infants. J Pediatr Surg 1977;12:897–903.
96. Miller KE, Edwards DK, Hilton S, Collins D, Lynch F, Williams R. Acquired lobar emphysema in premature infants with bronchopulmonary dysplasia: an iatrogenic disease? Radiology 1981;138:589–592.
97. Swischuk LE. Radiology of the newborn and young infant. 2nd ed. Baltimore: Williams and Wilkins, 1980, pp 51–52.
98. Charbonneau P, Azoulay E, Brun M, Bernaudin JF, Blayo MC, Pocidalo JJ. Normobaric oxygen toxicity in the adult rat lung: evidence for a non hypoxaemic pulmonary oedema. Bull Eur Physiopathol Respir 1981;17: 117–127.
99. Monset-Couchard M, Henry E, Larroche JC, Moriette G, Bomsel F. Dysplasie bronchopulmonaire. Analyse de 565 cas de ventilation artificielle chez le nouveau-né. Ann Radiol 1981;24:55–65.
100. Mortensson W, Lindroth M. The course of bronchopulmonary dysplasia. A radiographic follow-up. Acta Radiol Diag 1986;27: 19–22.
101. Westgate HD, Fisch RO, Langer LO Jr, Staub HP. Pulmonary and respiratory function changes in survivors of hyaline-membrane disease. Dis Chest 1969;55:465–470.
102. Heldt GP, McIlroy MB, Hansen TN, Tooley WH. Exercise performance of the survivors of hyaline membrane disease. J Pediatr 1980;96: 995–999.
103. Johnson JD, Malachowski NC, Grobstein R, Welsh D, Daily WJR, Sunshine P. Prognosis of children surviving with the aid of mechanical ventilation in the newborn period. J Pediatr 1974;84:272–276.
104. Werthammer J, Brown ER, Neff RK, Taeusch HW Jr. Sudden infant death syndrome in infants with bronchopulmonary dysplasia. Pediatrics 1982;69:301–304.
105. Thomson W (Baron Kelvin). Quoted in Beck EM. Familiar quotations. Boston: Little, Brown, 1980, p 594.
106. Martin-Bouyer F, Monset-Couchard M, Bomsel F, Larroche JC, Amiel-Tison C, Minkowski A. Artificial ventilation in hyaline membrane disease. Analysis of a series (130 cases). Biol Neonate 1970;16:164–183.
107. Tudor J, Young L, Wigglesworth JS, Steiner RE. The value of radiology in the idiopathic respiratory distress syndrome. A radiological and pathological correlation study. Clin Radiol 1976;27:65–75.
108. Chrispin AR, Norman AP. The systematic evaluation of the chest radiograph in cystic fibrosis. Pediatr Radiol 1974;2:101–105.
109. Matthew DJ, Warner JO, Chrispin AR, Norman AP. The relationship between chest radiographic scores and respiratory function

tests in children with cystic fibrosis. Pediatr Radiol 1977;5:198–200.
110. Student (anon). Illegal number crunching. Pediatrics 1983;71:864–865.
111. Davis HC, Robertson A. Number crunching. Pediatrics 1983;72:580.
112. Kamper J. Long term prognosis of infants with severe idiopathic respiratory distress syndrome. II. Cardio-pulmonary outcome. Acta Paediatr Scand 1978;67:71–76.
113. Ehrenkranz RA, Bonta BW, Albow RC, Warshaw JB. Amelioration of bronchopulmonary dysplasia after vitamin E administration. A preliminary report. N Engl J Med 1978;299:564–569.
114. Northway WH Jr. Bronchopulmonary dysplasia and vitamin E. N Engl J Med 1978;299:599–601.
115. Edwards DK. Radiology of hyaline membrane disease, transient tachypnea of the newborn, and bronchopulmonary dysplasia. In: Farrell PM, ed. Lung development: biological and clinical perspectives, vol 2. New York: Academic Press, 1982, pp 47–89.
116. Toce SS, Farrell PM, Leavitt LA, Samuels DP, Edwards DK. Clinical and roentgenographic scoring systems for assessing bronchopulmonary dysplasia. Am J Dis Child 1984;138:581–585.
117. Myers MG, McGuinness GA, Lachenbruch PA, Koontz FP, Hollingshead R, Olson DB. Respiratory illnesses in survivors of infant respiratory distress syndrome. Am Rev Respir Dis 1986;133:1010–1011.
118. Perlman JM, Moore V, Siegel MJ, Dawson J. Is chloride depletion an important contributing cause of death in infants with bronchopulmonary dysplasia? Pediatrics 1986;77:212–216.
119. Bryan MH, Hardie MJ, Reilly BJ, Swyer PR. Pulmonary function studies during the first year of life in infants recovering from the respiratory distress syndrome. Pediatrics 1973;52:169–178.
120. Fitzhardinge PM. Follow-up studies in infants treated by mechanical ventilation. Clin Perinatol 1978;5:451–461.
121. Meisels SJ, Plunkett JW, Roloff DW, Pasick PL, Stiefel GS. Growth and development of preterm infants with respiratory distress syndrome and bronchopulmonary dysplasia. Pediatrics 1986;77:345–352.
122. Sauve RS, Singhal N. Long-term morbidity of infants with bronchopulmonary dysplasia. Pediatrics 1985;76:725–733.
123. Turkel SB, Sims ME, Guttenberg ME. Postponed neonatal death in the premature infant. Am J Dis Child 1986;140:576–579.
124. Lamarre A, Linsao L, Reilly BJ, Swyer PR, Levison H. Residual pulmonary abnormalities in survivors of idiopathic respiratory distress syndrome. Am Rev Respir Dis 1973;108:56–61.
125. Stahlman M. Long time results of respiratory therapy. Biol Neonate 1970;16:133–137.
126. Outerbridge EW, Nogrady MB, Beaudry PH, Stern L. Idiopathic respiratory distress syndrome. Recurrent respiratory illness in survivors. Am J Dis Child 1972;123:99–104.
127. Smyth JA, Tabachnik E, Duncan WJ, Reilly BJ, Levison H. Pulmonary function and bronchial hyperreactivity in long-term survivors of bronchopulmonary dysplasia. Pediatrics 1981;68:336–340.
128. Rooklin AR, Moomjian AS, Shutack JG, Schwartz JG, Fox WW. Theophylline therapy in bronchopulmonary dysplasia. J Pediatr 1979;95:882–885.
129. Kao LC, Warburton D, Platzker ACG, Keens TG. Effect of isoproterenol inhalation on airway resistance in chronic bronchopulmonary dysplasia. Pediatrics 1984;73:509–514.
130. Nickerson BG, Taussig LM. Family history of asthma in infants with bronchopulmonary dysplasia. Pediatrics 1980;65:1140–1144.
131. Swischuk LE, Hayden CK Jr. Viral vs. bacterial pulmonary infections in children (is roentgenographic differentiation possible?). Pediatr Radiol 1986;16:278–284.
132. Lew C, Keens T, O'Neal, et al. Gastroesophageal reflux prevents recovery from bronchopulmonary dysplasia (abstr). Clin Res 1981;29:149A.
133. Sindel BD, Maisels MJ, Ballantine TVN. Gastroesophageal reflux (GER) to the proximal esophagus in neonates with bronchopulmonary dysplasia (abstr). Pediatr Res 1985;19:365A.

134. Sindel BD, Maisels MJ, Ballantine TVN. The effect of a Nissen fundoplication on infants with chronic lung disease (CLD) (abstr). Pediatr Res 1985;19:365A.
135. Wesenberg RL, Struble RA. Selective bronchial catheterization and lavage in the newborn. A new therapeutic procedure for diagnostic radiology. Radiology 1972;105:397–400.
136. Fouron J-C, Le Guennec J-C, Villemant D, Bard H, Perreault G, Davignon A. Value of echocardiography in assessing the outcome of bronchopulmonary dysplasia of the newborn. Pediatrics 1980;65:529–535.
137. Berman W Jr, Yabek SM, Dillon T, Burstein R, Corlew S. Evaluation of infants with bronchopulmonary dysplasia using cardiac catheterization. Pediatrics 1982;70:708–712.
138. Halliday HL, Dumpit BS, Brady JP. Effects of inspired oxygen on echocardiographic assessment of pulmonary vascular resistance and myocardial contractility in bronchopulmonary dysplasia. Pediatrics 1980;65:536–540.
139. Szego E, Shankaran S, Eisert D, Siegel P, Schultz G. Severe bronchopulmonary dysplasia (BPD): morbidity, mortality and follow-up of survivors (abstr). Pediatr Res 1980;14:652.
140. Walsh EP, Lang P, Ellison RC, Zierler S, Harned HS, Miettinen OS. Electrocardiogram of the premature infant at 1 year of age. Pediatrics 1986;77:353–356.
141. Higgins CB, Byrd BF II, McNamara MT, *et al.* Magnetic resonance imaging of the heart: a review of the experience in 172 subjects. Radiology 1985;155:671–679.
142. Melnick G, Pickoff AS, Ferrer PL, Peyser J, Bancalari E, Gelband H. Normal pulmonary vascular resistance and left ventricular hypertrophy in young infants with bronchopulmonary dysplasia: an echocardiographic and pathologic study. Pediatrics 1980;66:589–596.
143. Abman SH, Warady BA, Lum GM, Koops BL. Systemic hypertension in infants with bronchopulmonary dysplasia. J Pediatr 1984;104:928–931.
144. Ascher DP, Rosen P, Null DM, de Lemos RA, Wheller JJ. Systemic to pulmonary collaterals mimicking patent ductus arteriosus in neonates with prolonged ventilatory courses. J Pediatr 1985;107:282–284.
145. Wesenberg RL, Blumhagen JD. Assisted expiratory chest radiography: an effective technique for the diagnosis of foreign-body aspiration. Radiology 1979;130:538–539.
146. Rasche RFH, Kuhns LR: Histopathologic changes in airway mucosa in infants after endotracheal intubation. Pediatrics 1972;50:632–637.
147. Joshi VV, Mandavia SG, Stern L, Wiglesworth FW. Acute lesions induced by endotracheal intubation. Occurrence in the upper respiratory tract of newborn infants with respiratory distress syndrome. Am J Dis Child 1972;124:646–649.
148. Boros SJ, Mammel MC, Coleman JM, *et al.* Neonatal high-frequency jet ventilation: four years' experience. Pediatrics 1985;75:657–663.
149. Joseph PM, Berdon WE, Baker DH, Slovis TL, Haller JO. Upper airway obstruction in infants and small children. Improved radiographic diagnosis by combining filtration, high kilovoltage, and magnification. Radiology 1976;121:143–148.
150. Edwards DK. The child with stridor. In: Hilton SvW, Edwards DK, Hilton J, eds. Practical pediatric radiology. Philadelphia: WB Saunders, 1984, p 13.
151. Gates GF, Dore EK, Markarian M, Takanaka J. Radionuclide imaging of airway obstruction following assisted ventilation. Am J Dis Child 1976;130:1222–1227.
152. Bhutani VK, Ritchie WG, Shaffer TH. Acquired tracheomegaly in very preterm neonates. Am J Dis Child 1986;140:449–452.
153. Sotomayor JL, Godinez RI, Borden S, Wilmott RW. Large-airway collapse due to acquired tracheobronchomalacia in infancy. Am J Dis Child 1986;140:367–371.
154. Frey E, Smith W, Wagener J, Grandgeorge S, Franken E, McCrae P. Evaluation of chronic pediatric airway obstruction with cine-CT. Presented at the 29th annual meeting of The Society for Pediatric Radiology, Washington, DC, April 11, 1986.
155. Steichen JJ, Gratton TL, Tsang RC. Osteope-

nia of prematurity: the cause and possible treatment. J Pediatr 1980;96:528–534.
156. Kulkarni PB, Hall RT, Rhodes PG, et al. Rickets in very low-birth-weight infants. J Pediatr 1980;96:249–252.
157. Chesney RW, Hamstra AJ, DeLuca HF. Rickets of prematurity. Am J Dis Child 1981;135:34–37.
158. Masel JP, Tudehope D, Cartwright D, Cleghorn G. Osteopenia and rickets in the extremely low birth weight infant. A survey of the incidence and a radiological classification. Australas Radiol 1982;26:83–96.
159. Klein GL, Targoff GM, Ament ME, et al. Bone disease associated with total parenteral nutrition. Lancet 1980;2:1041–1044.
160. Toomey F, Hoag R, Batton D, Vain N. Rickets associated with cholestasis and parenteral nutrition in premature infants. Radiology 1982;142:85–88.
161. Gefter WB, Epstein DM, Anday EK, Dalinka MK. Rickets presenting as multiple fractures in premature infants on hyperalimentation. Radiology 1982;142:371–374.
162. Warshaw BL, Anand SK, Kerian A, Lieberman E. The effect of chronic furosemide administration on urinary calcium excretion and calcium balance in growing rats. Pediatr Res 1980;14:1118–1121.
163. Venkataraman PS, Han BK, Tsang RC, Daugherty CC. Secondary hyperparathyroidism and bone disease in infants receiving long-term furosemide therapy. Am J Dis Child 1983;137:1157–1161.
164. Chudley AE, Brown DR, Holzman IR, Oh KS. Nutritional rickets in 2 very low birth-weight infants with chronic lung disease. Arch Dis Child 1980;55:687–690.
165. Khajavi A, Amirhakimi GH. The rachitic lung. Pulmonary findings in 30 infants and children with malnutritional rickets. Clin Pediatr 1977;16:36–38.
166. Glasgow JFT, Thomas PS. Rachitic respiratory distress in small preterm infants. Arch Dis Child 1977;52:268–273.
167. Poznanski AK, Kuhns LR, Guire KE. New standards of cortical mass in the humerus of neonates: a means of evaluating bone loss in the premature infant. Radiology 1980;134:639–644.
168. Geggel RL, Pereira GR, Spackman TJ. Fractured ribs: unusual presentation of rickets in premature infants. J Pediatr 1978;93:680–682.
169. Steichen JJ, Edwards NK, Tsang RC. Adaptation of direct photon absorptiometry for measurement of bone mineral content in small infants. AJR 1976;126:1284–1285.
170. Stinson R, Stinson P. On the death of a baby. Atlantic Monthly 1979;244:64–72.
171. Hilton S. The accidentally injured and abused child. In: Hilton SvW, Edwards DK, Hilton J, eds. Practical pediatric radiology. Philadelphia: WB Saunders, 1984, pp 443–485.
172. Pokorny WJ, Saleem M, O'Gorman RB, McGill CW, Harberg FJ. Cholelithiasis and cholecystitis in childhood. Am J Surg 1984;148:742–744.
173. Roslyn JJ, Berquist WE, Pitt HA, et al. Increased risk of gallstones in children receiving total parenteral nutrition. Pediatrics 1983;71:784–789.
174. Bernstein J, Chang C-H, Brough AF, Heidelberger KP. Conjugated hyperbilirubinemia in infancy associated with parenteral alimentation. J Pediatr 1977;90:361–367.
175. Linden W, Nakayama F. Effect of intravenous fat emulsion on hepatic bile. Increased lithogenicity and crystal formation. Acta Chir Scand 1976;142:401–406.
176. Enzenauer RW, Montrey JS, Barcia PJ, Woods J. Total parenteral nutrition cholestasis: a cause of mechanical biliary obstruction. Pediatrics 1985;76:905–908.
177. Whitington PF, Black DD. Cholelithiasis in premature infants treated with parenteral nutrition and furosemide. J Pediatr 1980;97:647–649.
178. Brill PW, Winchester P, Rosen MS. Neonatal cholelithiasis. Pediatr Radiol 1982;12:285–288.
179. Callahan J, Haller JO, Cacciarelli AA, Slovis TL, Friedman AP. Cholelithiasis in infants: association with total parenteral nutrition and furosemide. Radiology 1982;143:437–439.
180. Boyle RJ, Sumner TE, Volberg FM. Cholelithiasis in a 3-week-old small premature infant. Pediatrics 1983;71:967–969.
181. Wolf P, Hofmann A, Nickoloff B, Mannino F, Edwards D. Neonatal calcium oxalate-phos-

phate gallstones—a new chemical composition of gallstones. Clin Chem 1982;28:1804–1805.
182. Keller MS, Markle BM, Laffey PA, Chawla HS, Jacir N, Frank JL. Spontaneous resolution of cholelithiasis in infants. Radiology 1985;157:345–348.
183. Takiff H, Fonkalsrud EW. Gallbladder disease in childhood. Am J Dis Child 1984;138: 565–568.
184. Hufnagle KG, Khan SN, Penn D, Cacciarelli A, Williams P. Renal calcifications: a complication of long-term furosemide therapy in preterm infants. Pediatrics 1982;70:360–363.
185. Gilsanz V, Fernal W, Reid BS, Stanley P, Ramos A. Nephrolithiasis in premature infants. Radiology 1985;154:107–110.
186. Robinson CM, Cox MA. The incidence of renal calcifications in low birthweight (LBW) infants on Lasix for bronchopulmonary dysplasia (BPD) (abstr). Pediatr Res 1986;20: 359A.
187. Goldsmith MA. Renal calcification in premature infants (letter). Pediatrics 1983;71:992.
188. Peevy KJ, Speed FA, Hoff CJ. Epidemiology of inguinal hernia in preterm neonates. Pediatrics 1986;77:246–247.

Comments

William H. Northway, Jr.

Chronic lung disease is a term that has been used by others to describe infants with mild to moderate BPD as judged by the scoring system developed by Edwards. Infants with this mild to moderate BPD are very small infants who survive. As treatment for respiratory failure continues to improve, the radiographic and pathologic changes of BPD will become even more subtle. There is no evidence that the underlying pathology in such infants differs from the known spectrum of BPD.

13

Contribution of the Patent Ductus Arteriosus to Lung Injury

ROBERT B. COTTON

Introduction

Bronchopulmonary dysplasia (BPD) has become by far the greatest contributor to morbidity in newborn intensive care units. While the proportion of patients with BPD is less than 9% of all infants admitted to the Neonatal Intensive Care Unit at Vanderbilt University Hospital, almost half of the time and effort of medical and nursing personnel is to the care of premature infants who have BPD. In addition to chronic pulmonary insufficiency, other kinds of morbidity, such as intraventricular hemorrhage, retinopathy of prematurity, necrotizing enterocolitis, rickets, bacterial sepsis, acquired cytomegaloviral infection—to name a few—are highly concentrated among patients with BPD.

Likewise symptomatic patent ductus arteriosus (PDA) is highly associated with BPD, occurring as an antecedent event in over half of infants who develop BPD and occasionally as a condition complicating the ongoing management of BPD. Symptomatic PDA is closely linked to the pathogenesis of BPD, both as a contributor to the initial phase of lung injury and, if allowed to persist, as a factor disrupting the orderly healing process necessary for intact recovery of the injured lung. In addition to its role in the pathogenesis of BPD, symptomatic PDA is itself an important cause of pulmonary insufficiency which may require prolonged ventilatory support and oxygen therapy. For these reasons optimal management of symptomatic PDA (or its prevention) will be a requisite of any successful approach toward decreasing the incidence and severity of BPD.

The purpose of this chapter is to consider the role of symptomatic PDA in the pathogenesis of BPD. The beneficial effects of ductus closure on ventilatory failure are reviewed, the recent phenomenal increase in the number of infants with BPD is discussed as to implications regarding management of symptomatic PDA, and the case for preemptive closure of the ductus is addressed. Finally, recommendations for management of symptomatic PDA based on experience in the NICU at Vanderbilt University Hospital are given.

In this chapter the diagnosis of BPD is derived from the criteria of Bancalari (1), and includes four components. First, the infant must have experienced lung injury in the first week after birth. This injury may be either primary, in the form of hyaline membrane disease (HMD), or secondary, due to barotrauma or oxygen injury occurring consequent to the management of ventilatory failure regardless of its etiology. Second, the patient with BPD has sufficiently impaired pulmonary gas exchange at 28 days postnatal age to require added inspired oxygen. Third, the chest radiograph must be persistently abnormal at 28 days postnatal age, showing poor aeration, overdistention (lobar or bilateral), atelectasis, or a combination of these findings. Fourth, examination of the chest will reveal tachypnea and intercostal retractions, usually accompanied by rales (which may be limited to dependent lung fields and heard only on deep inspiration).

Virtually every preterm infant and most full-term infants will experience left-to-right shunting through the ductus arteriosus some time during the first 96 hours after birth. When left-to-right shunting is accompanied by cardiopulmonary compromise, the condition is referred to as symptomatic PDA (2). Infants with symptomatic PDA usually have the characteristic ductus murmur, an active precordium, bounding pulses, rales and radiographic evidence of cardiomegaly and of pulmonary vascular engorgement or pulmonary edema. The presence of left-to-right shunting may be detected by Doppler cardiography, but this procedure cannot substitute for the clinical assessment required to diagnose symptomatic PDA. The most common "symptoms" of symptomatic PDA is pulmonary edema and ventilatory failure. The cardiopulmonary compromise of symptomatic PDA may also include inadequate forward flow of left ventricular output into the systemic circulation. Common clinical manifestations of compromised perfusion include poor cutaneous capillary refill, impaired renal function, and episodic intestinal distention occasionally progressing to frank necrotizing enterocolitis.

Role of Symptomatic Patent Ductus Arteriosus in the Pathogenesis of Bronchopulmonary Dysplasia

The histopathologic hallmarks of developing BPD are necrotizing bronchiolitis of the distal conducting airways followed by the appearance of squamous metaphasia (3–5). There is extensive proliferation of surrounding connective tissue with excessive collagen production (scar tissue formation). Many bronchioles associated with overdistended terminal airways will exhibit peribronchiolar smooth muscle hypertrophy. When pulmonary interstitial air dissection has occurred as an antecedent to BPD, false air spaces created by air dissection into lymphatics may be seen, sometimes becoming newly lined by epithelium, and often compressing neighboring lung tissue (6). One unifying interpretation of these histopathologic features is that BPD results when an injured lung heals in such a way that its structural integrity is preserved at the expense of gas exchange function. The infant whose initial lung injury (*e.g.*, HMD) heals by "first intention" has rapid restoration of gas exchange function, often within 5 to 7 days after birth, and is spared BPD. The infant whose injured lung is repaired by "second intention" develops BPD with prolonged ventilatory failure. Normal gas exchange is achieved only by the orderly growth and development of new lung. This process may require only a few weeks if the initial injury is not extensive and if subsequent repair and new lung growth is not disrupted by repeated injuries. On the other hand, when the initial injury is severe and extensive, when there is ongoing damage to the lung due to barotrauma, free radical excess, and repeated infections, or when repair and new growth are thwarted by nutritional deficiencies, normal gas exchange may never be achieved, and only after months of NICU stay may the pulmonary status be sufficiently stabilized for the patient to be discharged home on oxygen therapy.

Left-to-right shunting through the ductus arteriosus participates in the pathogenesis of BPD in a variety of ways, both at the lung injury stage and during the malappropriate repair by "second intention." Even before shunting becomes clinically apparent as symptomatic PDA, recirculation of left ventricular output back through the pulmonary circulation via the ductus arteriosus is an integral part of the pathophysiology of HMD (7). The contribution of the ductus to the pulmonary congestion of HMD was identified 25 to 30 years ago by Lendrum (8), Burnard (9), Stahlman (10), and Rudolph *et al.* (11). More recently the possibility that early ductus closure will lessen the severity of HMD has been documented by Jacob *et al.* (12) and Johnson *et al.* (13). These investigators showed that intervention to close the ductus within 36 hours of birth by ligation or by the administration of indomethacin resulted in improvements in lung compliance, acidosis, and oxygen and ventilator pressure requirements. In view of the well-established role of the ductus arteriosus in the pathophysiology of HMD and given that early ductus closure will lessen the severity of HMD, one would expect that pre-emptive closure of the ductus would also be a correct step toward preventing or modifying BPD. Experience with such an approach is discussed below.

Continuing with the injury-repair model of the pathogenesis of BPD, symptomatic PDA influences the development of BPD by increasing the lung's susceptibility to interstitial air dissection. Fluid overload and pulmonary edema are closely associated with pulmonary air leak. In our patient population infants who develop symptomatic PDA are more than three times as likely to experience air leak than those in the same weight range without symptomatic PDA.

The biggest contribution of symptomatic PDA to the development of BPD is the accompanying ventilatory failure requiring the use of positive pressure ventilation and oxygen. The prominence and duration of dependence on mechanical ventilation as a characteristic of infants with symptomatic PDA is illustrated by Figure 13.1, which reflects our experience prior to the routine use of ligation or indomethacin to close the ductus. Ongoing barotrauma (14) and the toxic effects of oxygen free radicals (15) experienced by infants with symptomatic PDA are capable of producing both the initial injury to the lung and a continuing disruption of the repair process. In addition to air leak, which is a gross manifestation of pressure damage, barotrauma to small distal conducting airways may occur in two ways. Kotas (16) refers to the direct, static effect of force per unit of surface area as stress, and defines as strain the dimensional changes resulting from applied pressure. A better understanding of the relative effects of stress and strain as forms of barotrauma might allow the development of strategies of mechanical ventilation which minimize the kind of lung injury that leads to BPD. For example high-frequency ventilation would be expected to impart less strain onto conducting airways than conventional ventilation, because intra-airway pressure swings are considerably less during high-frequency ventilation.

Closely coupled to their dependence on mechanical ventilation, infants with symptomatic PDA may also have a prolonged need of oxygen therapy. The potential for high concentrations of inspired oxygen to injure the lung of a variety of experimental animals, adult and newborn, is well established. It is not known whether oxygen free radicals operate directly to produce the lesions of BPD, or indirectly by causing ventilatory failure, which in turn is managed by positive pres-

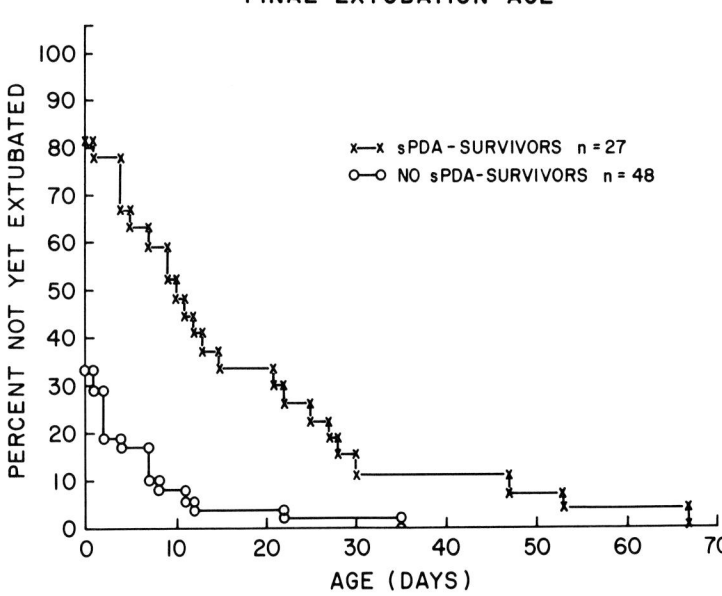

Figure 13.1. Proportion of surviving infants (birth weight ≤ 1500 g) with and without symptomatic PDA requiring endotracheal intubation and mechanical ventilation related to the age at which they were no longer ventilator dependent. (Reprinted, with permission, from Cotton RB, Stahlman MT, Kovar I, Catterton WZ. Medical management of small preterm infants with symptomatic patent ductus arteriosus. J Pediatr 1978; 92:470.)

sure ventilation and the attendant barotrauma.

The endotracheal tube through which the patient with symptomatic PDA and ventilatory failure receives mechanical ventilation may also contribute to the development of BPD. Mechanical trauma from movement of the endotracheal tube up and down against tracheal mucosa will damage the epithelium and grossly interfere with the function of ciliated and goblet cells to maintain proper pulmonary toilet (5). As a result the airways become chronically colonized with opportunistic bacteria, particularly *Staphylococcus epidermidis*. Chronic colonization or recurrent infection of the airway is unavoidable in the symptomatic PDA patient with an endotracheal tube, and may interfere with normal pulmonary and clearance mechanisms.

The patient with symptomatic PDA is at risk for a number of nutritional deficiencies linked to the pathogenesis of BPD. Those with symptomatic PDA whose ductus is allowed to remain open are delayed in achieving any substantial nutritional intake by the enteral route (17). Premature infants who can be fed human milk or commercial formulas are unlikely to become deficient in such antioxidants as vitamin E, selenium, and the sulfur-containing amino acids cysteine and methionine, or in trace elements such as copper, zinc, and manganese, which are required as components of superoxide dismutase, a protective enzyme system against oxygen free radicals (18). The infant with symptomatic PDA who cannot be fed because of recurrent episodes of abdominal distention and is dependent on parenteral nutrition solutions, which are not routinely supplemented, is not ensured an adequate intake of these important antioxidant constituents.

The symptomatic PDA patient who is dependent on parenteral nutrition is also at risk for vitamin A deficiency. Even if the solution is supplemented with vitamin A, it may not reach the patient before being photodegraded or before adsorbing to the plastic intravenous tubing (19). Several lines of evidence incriminate vitamin A deficiency in the pathogenesis of BPD (20, 21). There are striking similarities of epithelial histopathology between vitamin A deficiency and BPD. Premature infants who develop BPD have lower serum vitamin A levels at birth than gestational age matched control infants without BPD.

This section has described how the patent ductus arteriosus contributes to the pathogenesis of BPD, both to the lung injury phase and to the repair phase. Today much of the ductus' role in this form of chronic lung disease has been eliminated by early ductus closure, either pharmacologically with indomethacin or by surgical ligation. The successes in this regard are the subject of the next section. Effort has also been directed toward eliminating any contribution of BPD of the ductus arteriosus by its pre-emptive closure shortly after birth. The mixed success of this tactic is discussed in a subsequent section.

Beneficial Effects of Ductus Closure on Ventilatory Failure

When symptomatic PDA first became recognized as a common complication of premature infants, especially those with HMD, there was considerable ambivalence about recommending ductus closure except for those patients whose lives were immediately threatened by congestive heart failure. The decision whether to transport to the operating room a tiny, ventilator dependent infant for open chest surgery to ligate a ductus that would eventually close spontaneously was a dilemma for many neonatologists. However, the prospect that early ductus closure might curtail the prolonged course of ventilator dependence characteristic of infants with symptomatic PDA (see Fig. 12.1) provided a sufficiently compelling rationale for many to adopt ductus ligation as a standard approach to the management of these patients, a procedure occasionally carried out at the bedside within the NICU. The relative benefits of surgical closure at 1 week postnatal age compared with continued medical management with anticongestive measures alone were evaluated in a randomized, clinical trial conducted at Vanderbilt University Hospital (17). This study demonstrated that infants managed according to the surgical closure protocol could be weaned from the ventilator sooner, suffered fewer complications, could be fed sooner, and had lower hospital bills than those managed according to the medical management protocol. The marked effect of ductus closure on reducing duration of ventilator dependence is illustrated in Figure 13.2.

The demonstration by Friedman *et al.* (22) and by Heymann *et al.* (23) that pharmacologic induction of ductus constriction could be accomplished by the administration of indomethacin opened the door to early ductus closure without the risks and acute pulmonary morbidity of surgical intervention. Although no difference in duration of ventilatory failure or incidence of BPD was demonstrated by a national collaborative randomized trial comparing surgical and pharmacologic intervention, this large study did demonstrate that indomethacin was as safe and effective as ligation in this population of premature infants (24).

Since ventilator dependence among in-

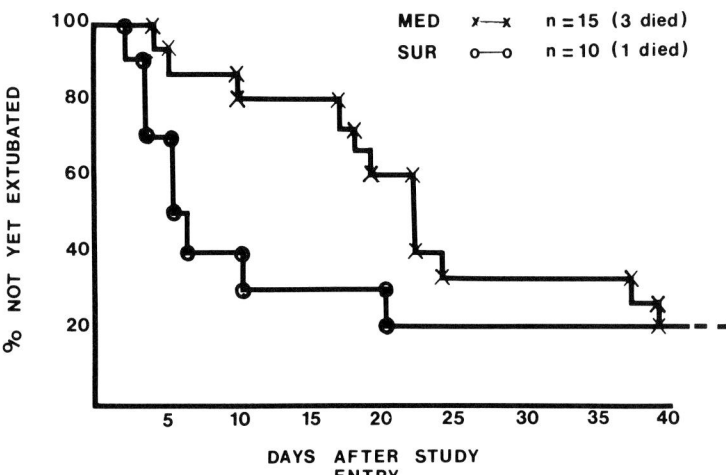

Figure 13.2. Effect of ductus closure on duration of dependence on mechanical ventilation. The patients who died were considered never to have been successfully intubated. (Reprinted, with permission, from Cotton RB, Stahlman MT, Bender HW, Graham TP, Catterton WZ, Kovar I. Randomized trial of early closure of symptomatic patent ductus arteriosus in small preterm infants. J Pediatr 1978;93:649.)

fants with symptomatic PDA was clearly reduced by "early" surgical closure at 7 days postnatal age, it made sense, especially given the availability of noninvasive ductus closure with indomethacin, that even earlier intervention might achieve an additional reduction in pulmonary morbidity. The advantage of earlier intervention to close the ductus was demonstrated by a randomized clinical trial (25) in which one treatment group received indomethacin immediately after the diagnosis of symptomatic PDA was established. The other group received standard anticongestive measures initially, followed by indomethacin, but only in those infants who still had a symptomatic PDA at 1 week postnatal age. Patients in the early indomethacin group experienced ductus constriction at a median postnatal age of 4 days; those receiving only anticongestive measures initially followed later by indomethacin, if necessary, underwent constriction at a median postnatal age of 10½ days. Infants in the early indomethacin group required a significantly shorter duration of ventilator support than those whose indomethacin was delayed pending the outcome of initial anticongestive measures. In this study the shortened requirement of ventilator support resulting from early treatment with indomethacin amounted to almost a 50% reduction in exposure to the hazards of positive pressure ventilation through an indwelling endotracheal tube.

While there is little doubt that early, aggressive intervention to close the ductus will reduce the duration of ventilatory failure experienced by infants with symptomatic PDA, the explosive increase in the number of infants developing BPD makes one question whether we have learned anything in the past 10 years about reducing long-term pulmonary morbidity in premature infants (see Fig. 13.3). Figure 13.4 helps explain where these ever-increasing numbers of infants with BPD are coming from: the steady decline in the mortality rate of very low birth weight

PATENT DUCTUS ARTERIOSUS AND LUNG INJURY 241

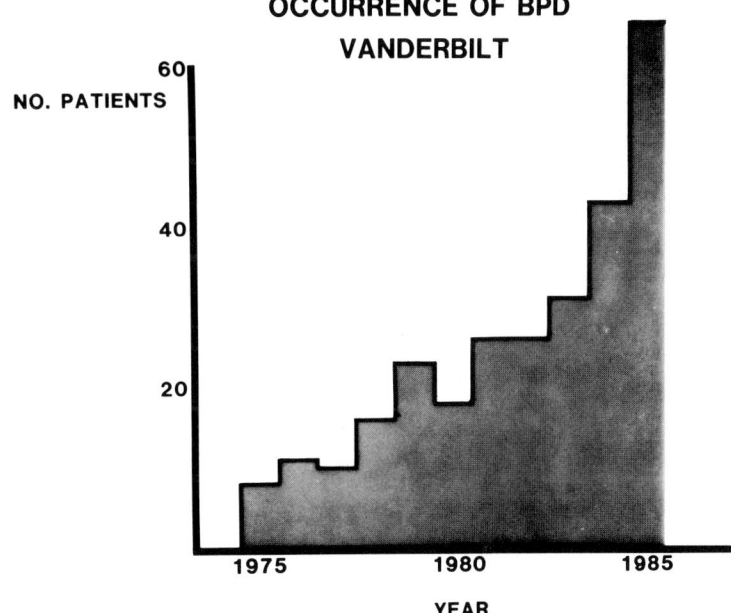

Figure 13.3. Yearly occurrence of bronchopulmonary dysplasia in the NICU at Vanderbilt University Hospital.

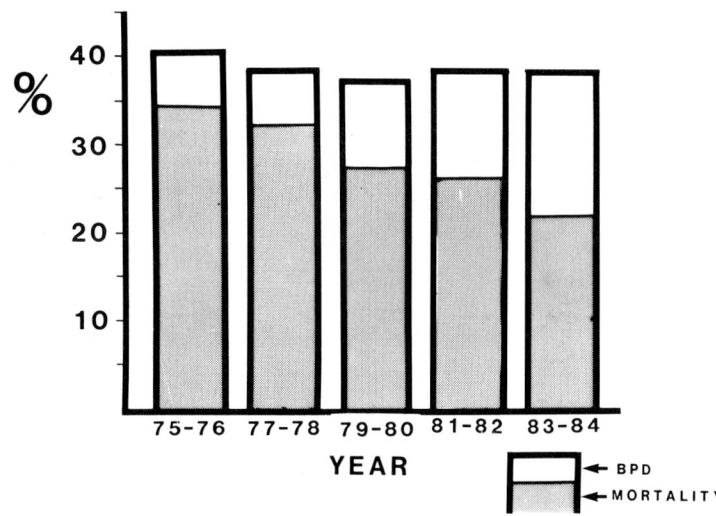

Figure 13.4. Each biennial decrement in mortality among infants with a birth weight less than 1500 g admitted to the Vanderbilt NICU has been replaced by an equivalent increment in incidence of bronchopulmonary dysplasia.

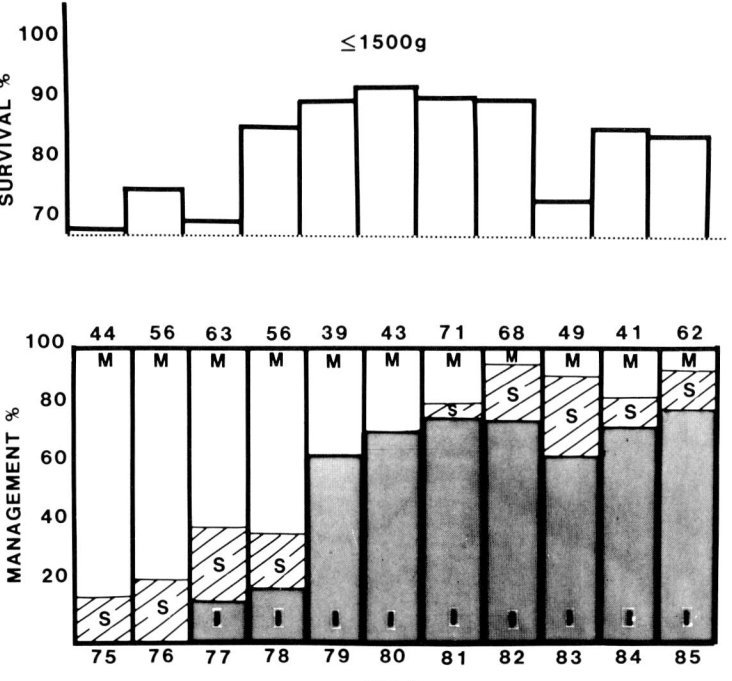

Figure 13.5. Evolution of management of symptomatic PDA for premature infants with birth weights of 1500 g or less admitted to the NICU of Vanderbilt University Hospital between 1975 and 1985. (*Top*) Overall survival by year. (*Bottom*) Proportion of symptomatic PDA patients managed by each of these approaches to therapy: M = medical management (anticongestive measures without intervention to close the ductus); S = surgical closure (includes all patients who underwent ligation regardless of prior management; between 1981 and 1985 almost all patients undergoing ligation had been treated with indomethacin in an unsuccessful attempt to achieve sustained ductus constriction); I = indomethacin treatment. The number of patients treated each year is indicated between the panels.

(VLBW) infants is made up entirely by infants who go on to develop BPD. That our very success in managing VLBW infants, most of whom have symptomatic PDA, is responsible for the burgeoning population of patients with BPD is further illustrated in Figure 13.5. Between 1975 and 1980 reliance on anticongestive measures alone in the management of symptomatic PDA was largely replaced by early intervention to close the ductus, initially by ligation and in later years by indomethacin. Survival of infants with symptomatic PDA improved steadily during this time. Since 1980 survival has declined slightly. At the same time there has been a return to surgical ligation, this time for infants who failed to have a sustained response to indomethacin. The slight decline in survival and the occurrence of indomethacin "failures" requiring ligation share the same common denominator with the concomitant rapid increase in BPD—an increase in both the number and survival rate of extremely immature infants. Among all patients in the Vanderbilt NICU weighing less than 1500 g at birth who develop symptomatic PDA, there has been a steady increase in the proportion under 1000 g, especially in the subgroup under 750 g (see Fig. 13.6).

It would appear that any reduction in the incidence and severity of BPD made by aggressive, early intervention of symptomatic PDA has occurred in infants of more than 1000 g birth weight. However, the ventilatory failure spared these "larger" infants has been far overshadowed by pulmonary morbidity in the extremely immature infants who are admitted in increasing numbers to NICUs because of active high-risk maternal referral programs, and who survive, in part at least,

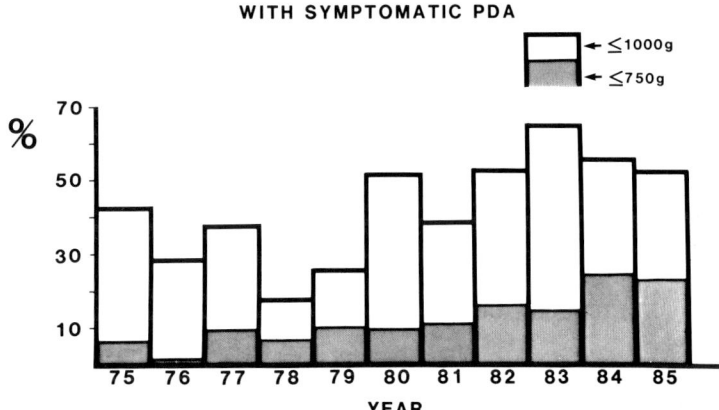

Figure 13.6. Changing birth weight distribution between 1975 and 1985 among patients admitted to the Vanderbilt NICU with birth weights of 1500 g or less who developed symptomatic PDA.

because of aggressive management of symptomatic PDA. Consistent with this description of the impact of successful management of symptomatic PDA vis à vis the epidemiology of BPD is the observation that the median birth weight of infants with BPD in our NICU has dropped from 1219 to 936 g between 1975 and 1985.

Pre-emptive Closure of the Ductus

Guided by the principle "the earlier, the better," several centers have investigated the efficacy of very early intervention to close the ductus arteriosus, either at first evidence of ductus shunting, or prophylactically in premature infants who have a high probability of later developing symptomatic PDA. In addition to the experience at Vanderbilt University Hospital summarized above, there are at least two randomized clinical trials which demonstrate that administration of indomethacin very early in the course of symptomatic PDA will result in an improved pulmonary outcome. Merritt et al. (26) found that BPD occurred less frequently and that the survival rate was higher among infants undergoing early treatment with indomethacin at an average postnatal age of 48.8 hours than among infants who received the drug later (167.4 hours). Among patients with a murmur, but no other evidence of symptomatic PDA, Mahony et al. (27) demonstrated that indomethacin administered at 2.7 days postnatal age was beneficial to infants under 1000 g birth weight in terms of incidence of major left-to-right shunting, number of infants requiring surgical ligation, duration of oxygen therapy, and number of days necessary to regain birth weight.

While the studies just described did reveal a convincing benefit of very early administration of indomethacin, they involved infants who already had evidence of left-to-right shunting. At least six additional studies (28–33) have been reported in which indomethacin was given beginning within the first 24 hours after birth in order to bring about pre-emptive closure of the ductus arteriosus. While all six studies demonstrated the efficacy of indomethacin to prevent symptomatic PDA, none showed any effect on incidence of BPD or on other indicators of pulmonary morbidity such as duration of oxygen therapy or ventilatory support.

There are several explanations why pre-emptive closure of the ductus arteriosus has not been shown to result in a decreased requirement of oxygen therapy and ventilatory support when compared to intervention to close the ductus after development of symptomatic PDA. None of the studies involved a sufficient number of patients to achieve enough statistical "power" to discount the reasonable possibility of a Type II error. Mahony *et al.* (30) calculated that their trial would require more than 400 infants in *each* treatment group to prove any significant difference with a Type II error of 10%. The efficacy of indomethacin to prevent symptomatic PDA is greatest among infants below a birth weight of 1250 to 1500 g, since the incidence of symptomatic PDA rapidly falls off among more mature infants. In extremely low birth weight infants, it is likely that lung immaturity plays such a dominant role in the pathogenesis of BPD that no single contributor, such as symptomatic PDA, can be cleanly implicated when the NICU course of these patients is a minefield of one hazard after another to their vulnerable lungs. It is also possible that a potential beneficial effect of pre-emptive closure on decreasing either the incidence of severity of BPD is offset by other effects of the drug which may aggravate lung injury.

In the initial phase of the randomized clinical trial of prophylactic indomethacin at Vanderbilt University Hospital, we observed that venous admixture during the 24 hours following indomethacin was significantly higher than among control infants (28). We have subsequently attributed this finding to a relative fluid overload due to an indomethacin mediated water retention by the kidneys, in that the difference in venous admixture between patients receiving prophylactic indomethacin and controls disappeared after a practice of more stringent fluid intake following indomethacin administration was instituted. It is interesting in this regard that patients given indomethacin in the study of Mahony *et al.* (30) received the same amount of fluid as the control infants. Since water balance and diuresis are so closely linked to oxygen requirement and lung compliance in HMD (34), administration of indomethacin could readily increase the severity of HMD and be responsible for subjecting vulnerable lungs to additional intensity of oxygen free radical damage and barotrauma, unless the antidiuretic effect of indomethacin is carefully anticipated. Risk of BPD has been shown previously to be related to fluid intake in the first 5 days after birth (35).

Another concern when indomethacin is given in a time frame notorious for the development and extension of intraventricular hemorrhage is that the drug's effect on platelet function will increase the incidence of severity of intracranial bleeding. So far this unacceptable complication of indomethacin has not been detected. To the contrary the experience reported from Miami (36) indicates that prophylactic indomethacin may impart protection against intraventricular hemorrhage. We also observed in our randomized clinical trial that intraventricular hemorrhage of grades III or IV were less frequent in infants receiving prophylactic indomethacin.

In that the efficacy of prophylactic indomethacin to pre-empt the development of symptomatic PDA appears now to be well established, we believe that its routine use is justified among infants who have a 50% or greater risk of developing symptomatic PDA. Unless contraindicated by a serum creatinine greater than 1.5 mg/dL, a platelet count less than 75,000/cu mm, or clinical evidence of coagulopathy (*e.g.*, oozing from puncture sites), we give a single dose of indomethacin, 0.2 mg/kg, intravenously 24 hours after birth, to premature infants weighing 1250 g or less who are ventilator dependent.

Management of Symptomatic Patent Ductus Arteriosus

The definitive treatment of symptomatic PDA is closure of the ductus arteriosus. Unless ductus patency is associated with a primary anatomic defect of the ductus wall that precludes closure (37), ductus constriction and anatomic closure will eventually occur spontaneously. In large, relatively mature infants more than 34 weeks' gestational age who have only minimal ventilatory impairment, or who are rapidly weaning from oxygen therapy and ventilatory support, specific intervention to effect ductus closure is generally unnecessary. In the case of infants with symptomatic PDA of less than 34 weeks' gestational age, and with more mature infants who are not rapidly weaning from oxygen therapy and ventilatory support, we rely on indomethacin as our primary intervention to achieve ductus closure. If indomethacin is contraindicated by impaired renal function (see above), surgical ligation is considered. Regardless of the decision whether or not to intervene to effect ductus closure, management of all infants with symptomatic PDA should include anticongestive measures and steps to maintain adequate systemic perfusion. Details of our recommendations for medical management of symptomatic PDA are published elsewhere (38).

Unless contraindicated by renal or clotting insufficiency, infants for whom indomethacin is indicated receive a single dose of the drug, 0.2 mg/kg, intravenously as soon as the diagnosis of symptomatic PDA is established, usually between 2 and 5 days postnatal age. Fluid intake is decreased by one-third in anticipation of an antidiuretic effect of indomethacin. Fluid balance is re-evaluated 8 to 12 hours later by assessing physical findings, change in body weight, urine output, serum sodium concentration, and hematocrit. Fluid intake is gradually returned to baseline rate as normal water excretion is restored (usually between 24 and 48 hours after indomethacin). Failure to reduce fluid intake in the face of indomethacin induced anti-diuresis will result in fluid overload, which may interfere with achieving sustained ductus closure. This will almost certainly happen if fluid administration is increased in response to diminished urine output.

Almost 90% of infants will experience a major constrictive effect on the ductus following this initial, single dose of indomethacin (39, 40). Those who fail to achieve a major constrictive effect probably have not maintained an adequate plasma level of indomethacin because of rapid clearance of the drug (39). We recommend that these patients receive three additional doses of indomethacin at 12 hour intervals beginning 24 hours after the initial dose (in the absence of contraindication), each dose 0.2 mg/kg. Those patients who fail to undergo a major constrictive effect with the initial single dose of indomethacin will usually experience a major constrictive effect with the series of three follow-up doses.

Some infants who achieve a major constrictive effect will have a recurrence of symptomatic PDA typically 3 to 10 days later. This second kind of indomethacin failure occurs chiefly among extremely immature infants (less than 1000 g birth weight) and is unrelated to rapid clearance of the drug (40). Approximately 30% of infants with birth weight less than 1000 g will have recurrence of symptomatic PDA after an initial major constrictive effect following treatment with indomethacin. Since recurrence of symptomatic PDA does not appear to be related to rapid clearance of indomethacin, we treat recurrence with another single dose. A second recurrence should be managed by immediate surgical closure.

In the National Collaborative Trial (24) of indomethacin, the initial course of treatment involved a series of three intravenous doses of the drug given at 12 hour intervals. A similar regimen is recommended in the package insert provided by the manufacturer. Although this regimen might be more effective for the occasional patient who has an exceptionally rapid clearance of the drug, our experience has indicated that initial treatment with a single dose, followed by additional doses only as necessary, is no less effective in achieving ductus closure. When the initial regimen is designed to provide adequately sustained levels for the small minority of patients who clear the drug rapidly, a large majority of patients will be exposed unnecessarily to excessively high and prolonged drug levels. While indomethacin appears to be safe when used under carefully controlled circumstances, all precautions should be taken to use only the minimal necessary dose in view of reports that gastrointestinal perforation (41), decreased cerebral blood flow (42), and decreased myocardial function (43) may be associated with administration of the drug to premature infants with symptomatic PDA.

Summary

Symptomatic PDA plays an important role in the pathogenesis of BPD, especially if steps are not taken to bring about prompt closure of the ductus. Individual studies have clearly shown the advantages of early closure of the ductus following the appearance of symptomatic PDA. At the same time there has been an explosion in the number of new patients each year who develop BPD. Ironically, successful management of symptomatic PDA, along with many other advances in perinatal and neonatal care, may have done more to contribute to the epidemic of BPD than to alleviate it, by enabling the survival of extremely immature infants who are so vulnerable to the manifold circumstances leading to BPD. While prophylactic indomethacin can be recommended for certain high-risk infants to pre-empt the development of symptomatic PDA, the beneficial effect of this practice on long-term pulmonary morbidity and on the incidence or severity of BPD has not yet been shown.

Success in turning around the tremendous morbidity of BPD will depend on new knowledge and advances directed toward reducing lung injury and promoting orderly repair. Aggressive management (or prevention) of symptomatic PDA will always be a prerequisite for the success of other measures directed toward the prevention of BPD.

Acknowledgments

The author is grateful to Mrs. June Livingstone and Mr. Terry Johnson for their expert help in preparing the manuscript and its illustrations.

This work was supported by National Heart and Lung Institute SCOR Grant HL 14214.

References

1. Bancalari E, Abdenour GE, Feller R, Gannon J. Bronchopulmonary dysplasia: clinical presentation. J Pediatr 1979;95:819–829.
2. Cotton RB, Stahlman MT, Kovar I, Catterton WZ. Medical management of small preterm infants with symptomatic patent ductus arteriosus. J Pediatr 1978;92:467–473.
3. Northway WH Jr, Rosan RC, Porter DY. Pulmonary disease following respirator therapy of hyaline membrane disease. N Engl J Med 1967;276:357–368.
4. Reid L. Bronchopulmonary dysplasia—pathology. J Pediatr 1979;95:836–841.
5. Stahlman MT. Les maladies respiratoires chroniques due nouveau-né. In: Vert P, Stern L, eds. Medecine neonatale. New York: Masson, 1984.
6. Stahlman MT, Cheatham W, Gray ME. The role of air dissection in bronchopulmonary dysplasia. J Pediatr 1979;95:878–882.
7. Stahlman M, Blankenship WJ, Shepard FM, Gray J, Young WC, Malan AF. Circulatory studies in clinical hyaline membrane disease. Biol Neonate 1972;20:300–320.
8. Lendrum FC. The "pulmonary hyaline membrane" as a manifestation of heart failure in the newborn infant. J Pediatr 1955;47:149–156.
9. Burnard ED. A murmur from the ductus arteriosus in the newborn baby. Br Med J 1958;1:806–810.
10. Stahlman MT. Digitalis in hyaline membrane syndrome. In: Oliver TK, ed. Adaptation to extrauterine life. Report of the 31st Ross Conference on Pediatric Research. Columbus, Ohio: Ross Laboratories, 1959.
11. Rudolph AM, Drorbaugh JE, Auld PAM, et al. Studies on the circulation of the newborn period: the circulation in the respiratory distress syndrome. Pediatrics 1961;27:551–566.
12. Jacob J, Gluck L, DiSessa T, et al. The contribution of PDA in the neonate with severe RDS. J Pediatr 1980;96:79–87.
13. Johnson DS, Rogers JH, Null DM, de Lemos RA. The physiologic consequences of the ductus arteriosus in the extremely immature newborn (abstr). Clin Res 1978;26:826A.
14. Taghizadeh A, Reynolds EOR. Pathogenesis of bronchopulmonary dysplasia following hyaline membrane disease. Am J Pathol 1976;82:241–264.
15. Frank L, Massaro D. Oxygen toxicity. Am J Med 1980;69:117–126.
16. Kotas RV. In: Farrell PM, Taussig LM, eds. Bronchopulmonary dysplasia and related chronic respiratory disorders. Report of the 90th Ross Conference of Pediatric Research. Columbus, Ohio: Ross Laboratories, 1986.
17. Cotton RB, Stahlman MT, Bender HW, Graham TP, Catterton WZ, Kovar I. Randomized trial of early closure of symptomatic patent ductus arteriosus in small preterm infants. J Pediatr 1978;93:647–651.
18. Bell EF. Prevention of bronchopulmonary dysplasia: vitamin E and other antioxidants. In: Farrel PM, Taussig LM, eds. Bronchopulmonary dysplasia and related chronic respiratory disorders. Report of the 90th Ross Conference on Pediatric Research. Columbus, Ohio: Ross Laboratories, 1986.
19. Shenai JP, Stahlman MT, Chytil F. Vitamin A delivery from parenteral alimentation solution. J Pediatr 1981;99:661–663.
20. Shenai JP, Chytil F, Jhaveri A, Stahlman MT. Plasma vitamin A and retinol binding protein in premature and term neonates. J Pediatr 1981;99:302–305.
21. Shenai JP, Chytil F, Stahlman MT. Vitamin A status of neonates with bronchopulmonary dysplasia. Pediatr Res 1985;19:185–188.
22. Friedman WF, Hirschklau MJ, Printz MP, Pitlick PT, Kirkpatrick SE. Pharmacologic closure of patent ductus arterious in the premature infant. N Engl J Med 1976;295:526–529.
23. Heymann MA, Rudolph AM, Silverman NH. Closure of the ductus arteriosus in premature infants by inhibition of prostaglandin synthesis. N Engl J Med 1976;295:530–533.
24. Gersony WM, Peckham GJ, Ellison RC, Miettinen OS, Nadas AS. Effects of indomethacin in premature infants with patent ductus arteriosus: results of a national collaborative study. J Pediatr 1983;102:895–906.
25. Cotton RB, Hickey D, Stahlman MT. Management of premature infants with symptomatic patent ductus arteriosus. In: L. Stern, ed.

Intensive care in the newborn, vol 4. New York: Masson, 1983.
26. Merritt TA, Harris JP, Roghmann K, *et al*. Early closure of patent ductus arteriosus in very low-birth-weight infants: a controlled trial. J Pediatr 1981;99:281–286.
27. Mahony L, Carnero V, Brett C, Heymann MA, Clyman RI. Prophylactic indomethacin therapy for patent ductus arteriosus in very-low-birth-weight infants. N Engl J Med 1982;306:506–510.
28. Bratton DL, Mellander M, Krueger ED, Stahlman MT, Cotton RB. Influence of early indomethacin on venous admixture in infants with HMD (abstr). Pediatr Res 1984;18:150A.
29. Setzer ES, Torres-Arraut E, Gomez-del-Rio M, *et al*. Cardiopulmonary effects of prophylactic indomethacin in the very-low-birth-weight infants (abstr). Pediatr Res 1984;18:346A.
30. Mahony L, Caldwell RL, Girod DA, *et al*. Indomethacin therapy on the first day of life in infants with very low birth weight. J Pediatr 1985;106:801–805.
31. Vincer MJ, Allen AC, Stinson DA, *et al*. Early indomethacin (IND) does not prevent bronchopulmonary dysplasia (BPD) in a randomized clinical trial (abstr). Pediatr Res 1985;19:369A.
32. Puckett CG, Cox MA, Haskins KS, Fisher DJ. Prophylactic indomethacin (I) for the prevention of patent ductus arteriosus (PDA) (abstr). Pediatr Res 1985;19:358A.
33. Sola A, Rogido M, Lezama C, Urman JE. Effects of ''prophylactic'' I.V. indomethacin (P INDO) in VLBW infants with HMD (abstr). Pediatr Res 1986;20:361A.
34. Langman CB, Engle WD, Baumgart S, Fox WW, Polin RA. The diuretic phase of respiratory distress syndrome and its relationship to oxygenation. J Pediatr 1981;98:462–466.
35. Brown ER, Stark A, Sosenko I, Lawson EE, Avery ME. Bronchopulmonary dysplasia: possible relationship to pulmonary edema. J Pediatr 1978;92:982–984.
36. Setzer ES, Morse BM, Goldberg RN, Smith M, Bancalari E. Prophylactic indomethacin and intraventricular hemorrhage (IVH) in the premature (abstr). Pediatr Res 1984;18:345A.
37. Gittenberger-de Groot AC. Persistent ductus arteriosus: most probably a primary congenital malformation. Br Heart J 1977;39:610–618.
38. Cotton RB. Patency of the ductus arteriosus—its etiologic and pathogenetic relationship in the respiratory distress syndrome. In: Stern L, ed. Hyaline membrane disease. New York: Grune and Stratton, 1984.
39. Brash AR, Hickey DE, Graham TP, Stahlman, MT, Oates JA, Cotton, RB. Pharmacokinetics of indomethacin in the neonate: the relationship of indomethacin plasma levels to response of the ductus arteriosus. N Engl J Med 1981;305:67–72.
40. Mellander M, Leheup B, Lindstrom DP, *et al*. Recurrence of symptomatic patent ductus arteriosus in extremely premature infants treated with indomethacin. J Pediatr 1984;105:138–143.
41. Alpan G, Eyal F, Vinograd I, *et al*. Localized intestinal perforations after enteral administration of indomethacin in premature infants. J Pediatr 1985;106:277–281.
42. Lundell BPW, Sonesson SE, Cotton RB. Ductus closure in preterm infants: effects on cerebral hemodynamics. Acta Paediatr Scand 1986;Suppl 329:140–147.
43. Appleton RS, Graham TP, Cotton RB, Moreau GA, Boucek RJ. Abnormal diastolic cardiac function following indomethacin therapy of patent ductus arteriosus. Pediatr Res 1986;20:167A.

Comments

T. Allen Merritt

A major issue confronting the neonatologist and cardiologist is determining when the ductus arteriosus has responded to pharmacologic closure, and thus whether left-to-right shunting through it can be removed from the complex equation producing lung injury. While increasing numbers of very low birth weight infants with lung immaturity are surviving through the first week of assisted ventilation, due in part to ductal closure attempts, it remains conceivable that early surfactant deficiency and pulmonary edema are only partially responsible for the lung injury responsible for BPD. Even after ductal closure these infants require supplemental oxygen and remain sensitive to fluid and nutritional advances.

Dr. Cotton's evaluation of studies demonstrating the efficacy of indomethacin (and pharmacologic failures) should stimulate a rethinking of whether ductal constriction after indomethacin is sufficient to eliminate the effects ascribed to left-to-right shunting in the presence of an agent that alters renal function, promotes an antidiuretic response, and may reduce myocardial and brain blood flow. Perhaps evolving color Doppler echocardiographic techniques will enable more precise differentiation of accelerated ductal closure from reduced ductal shunting in these tiny infants.

Certainly other anti-prostanoids may be as efficacious than indomethacin. Indeed agents with similar effects on ductal closure might be more potent anti-inflammatory agents and serve to promote endothelial integrity, reduce inflammatory mediators such as the leukotrinenes, and promote lung healing.

Although transvascular ductal obliteration is being used in selected cases of PDA in older infants, microrefinements in this technology might enable the neonatologist to plug the ductus at the time of umblical artery catheterization. Much remains to be learned about the inter-relation between ductal shunting, intrapulmonary shunting, and lung injury resulting in BPD.

14

Cor Pulmonale

FREDERICK S. SHERMAN

Introduction

The World Health Organization defines the chronic form of cor pulmonale as a combination of right ventricular hypertrophy and dilatation secondary to pulmonary hypertension. The pulmonary hypertension is caused by a disease of the pulmonary parenchyma or pulmonary vascular system (1). This chapter analyzes the pathophysiologic consequences of bronchopulmonary dysplasia (BPD) on the heart, describes ways to evaluate noninvasively the presence and degree of cor pulmonale, and discusses the frustrating aspect of treatment for cor pulmonale.

Pathophysiology

The lung of the normal newborn is quite different from that of the adult. There is extensive remodeling and growth of the pulmonary vascular bed during the newborn period. With increasing age muscle is observed in arteries located more peripherally within the acinus. At birth these muscularized arteries in the acinus are very thick-walled. Within days the smallest muscular arteries will dilate, and they are like thin-walled adult pulmonary arteries by 4 months of age. Arteries in the newborn also grow in number and size. The ratio of alveoli to arteries decreases from the newborn value of 20:1 to the adult value of 8:1, indicating a tremendous growth in vasculature (2).

BPD thoroughly disrupts the normal pulmonary vascular maturation. The primary insult is most likely hypoxia, which causes the muscular arteries to become much thicker, and there is also extension of the musculature to arteries that are nonmuscular (3, 4). There is a failure of the smallest muscular arteries to dilate. Furthermore hypoxia leads to pulmonary vasoconstriction and increased pressure. Both hypoxia and pressure tend to abbreviate the growth and development of alveoli and vessels in the newborn with BPD. In fact there is a tremendous decrease in the concentration of small peripheral arteries, leading to abrupt tapering of the axial arteries. This decreases the size of the vascular bed, leading to increased vascular resistance in the lungs (5, 6).

In summary, there are two basic physiologic events that lead to right ventricular hypertension in these infants. The first, which is present immediately from birth, is profound hypoxia, which leads to pulmonary vasoconstriction, which in turn will lead to poor development of distal pulmonary arteries. The second process involves the anatomic changes described in Chapter 3, which further leads to loss of development of alveoli and vessels that would have occurred normally. The final results are increased pulmonary vascular resistance and pulmonary hypertension, which lead to right ventricular hypertension and dilatation (2).

The heart of the newborn, however, is well suited to compensating for the pulmonary changes. The right ventricle is the predominant ventricle *in utero* and pumps two-thirds of the combined cardiac output in the fetus (7). At birth it is the stronger and more highly developed ventricle. In the normal infant a rapid physiologic change occurs as the pulmonary vascular resistance diminishes and the systemic resistance increases. Since the newborn's right ventricle is prepared for pressure and volume overload, the immediate stresses of increased pulmonary resistance from respiratory distress syndrome and, later, BPD do not lead to acute right ventricular failure. In fact the newborn has the capability of developing new cardiac muscle since pulmonary hypertension induces a myosin isoenzyme pattern suited to adapting to a pressure overload (8). Signs of right ventricular failure, therefore, do not develop until extremely severe lung disease has developed. Even then signs of right ventricular failure are very variable. Some infants with severe BPD by blood gas and radiographic evaluation have no signs of right ventricular failure, whereas others with what appears to be disease not as severe will have respiratory distress, hepatomegaly, and peripheral edema. The ability of the newborn to develop new cardiac myocytes in response to a stimulus differentiates the infant substantially from the older child or adult who develops chronic lung disease and cor pulmonale. The latter situation will lead to the signs and symptoms of right ventricular failure much sooner than in the newborn. The increase in preload and afterload on the right ventricle does not lead to the dysfunction that is seen in older children and adults, or in an animal model (9).

The manifestations of cor pulmonale in infants with BPD are the signs of right ventricular failure which are described below. There is also evidence that there is a right ventricular–to–left ventricular interdepen-

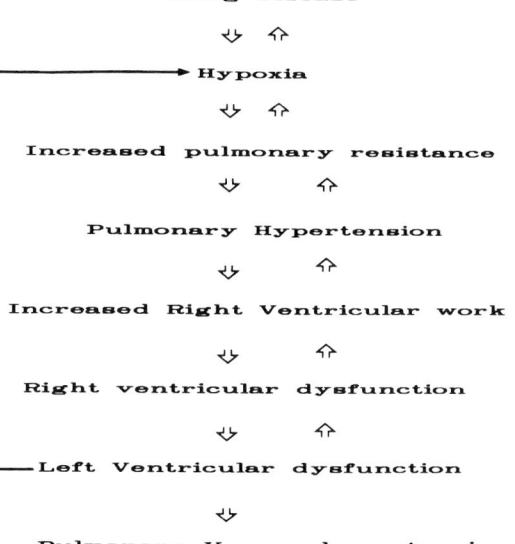

Figure 14.1. Schematic representation of the physiology and lung disease causing left ventricular dysfunction.

dence such that a pressure or a volume overload on the right ventricle can significantly interfere with normal left ventricular function. Hence infants with cor pulmonale may also have left ventricular dysfunction and failure (9, 10). When left ventricular dysfunction occurs, with or without overt failure, the following changes occur. Left atrial pressure increases and leads to increased pulmonary venous pressure, which causes increased transudation of fluid into alveoli, which further causes an increase in hypoxia and pulmonary vasoconstriction. This cycle further advances right ventricular failure, which will make the left ventricular dysfunction worse, and the vicious circle continues (Fig. 14.1) Ultimately cor pulmonale makes management of these infants more difficult and often signals the terminal phase of the disease.

COR PULMONALE

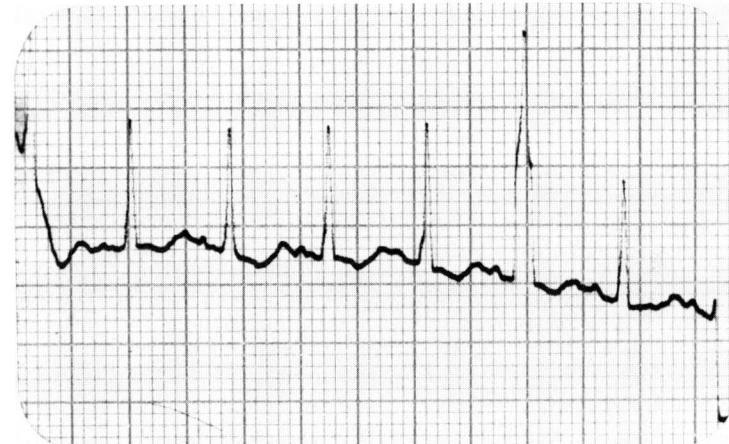

Figure 14.2. Lead V, from an electrocardiogram of a patient with pulmonary hypertension. There is a qR pattern with an R-wave of 44 millivolts. This correlates with systemic right ventricular pressure.

Evaluation

Physical Exam

Even in the technologically sophisticated 1980s, physical examination still has a role in the evaluation of pulmonary hypertension. A normally split second heart sound is a strong argument against pulmonary hypertension. Likewise, in a patient with known chronic lung disease, a single second heart sound raises the spectre of pulmonary hypertension. Sometimes these patients will have a murmur of tricuspid regurgitation. Rarely a murmur of pulmonary regurgitation can be appreciated. The liver is felt below the right costal margin in nearly all these patients because their lungs are hyperexpanded. The pulsatile liver, often described with tricuspid insufficiency, is rarely, if ever, appreciated in these patients since the onset of tricuspid regurgitation is insidious, and the right atrium dilates gradually and becomes very compliant, thereby not transmitting pulsatile V-waves to the systemic veins and liver.

Electrocardiogram

The electrocardiogram may be helpful in estimating right ventricular pressure. From the natural history study of congenital heart defects (11), the ECG gives good correlation with the severity of pulmonary stenosis, which is a pressure overload on the right ventricle. From this study, a Q in lead V_1 invariably means that the pressure was systemic in the right ventricle. In addition the greater the R in V_1, the greater the right ventricular pressure. A 20 mm or greater deflection of the R-wave in V_1 correlates strongly with a systemic right ventricular pressure. An R-wave of less than 10 in lead V_1 is essentially normal. These data were gleaned largely from patients with pulmonary stenosis. It is reasonable to apply these findings to the pressure overload situation that develops on the right ventricle from bronchopulmonary dysplasia (Fig. 14.2). The ECG, therefore, gives a good indirect assessment of the severity of right ventricular hypertension secondary to pulmonary artery hypertension in this disease.

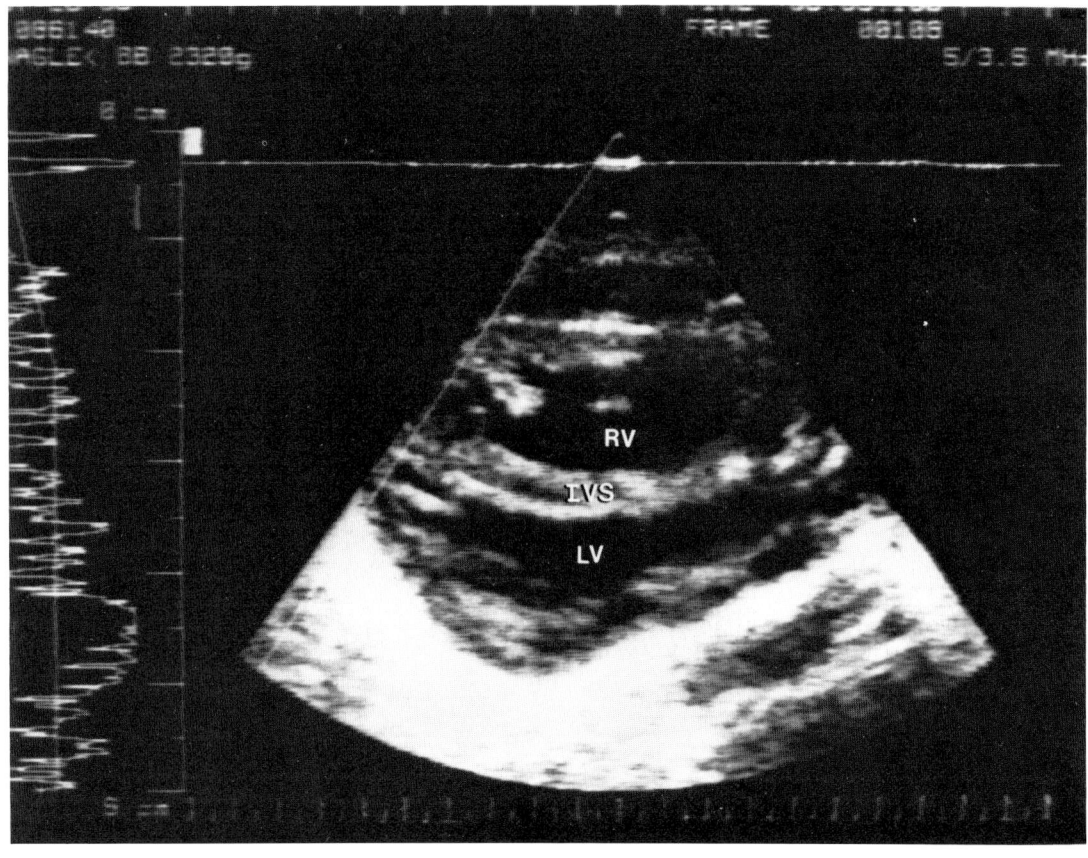

A

Figure 14.3. (A) Parasternal long-axis, two-dimensional echocardiographic view from a baby with bronchopulmonary dysplasia. The interventricular septum (IVS) bows posteriorly to compress the left ventricle (LV). The right ventricle (RV) is dilated.

Echocardiography

There have been many attempts to correlate pulmonary artery pressure with echocardiographic findings. This is understandable since a noninvasive assessment of pulmonary artery pressure is much preferred to an invasive method. Unfortunately the only sure method of knowing the pulmonary artery pressure is to measure it. The correlation between pulmonary artery pressure measured at catheterization and conclusions drawn from echocardiographic measurements has not been good (12). There is no parameter that is entirely reliable for predicting the degree of pulmonary artery hypertension. Nevertheless, important information can be obtained from the echocardiogram. Systolic time intervals can be a valuable adjunct to the physical examination and EKG for evaluation of pulmonary hypertension

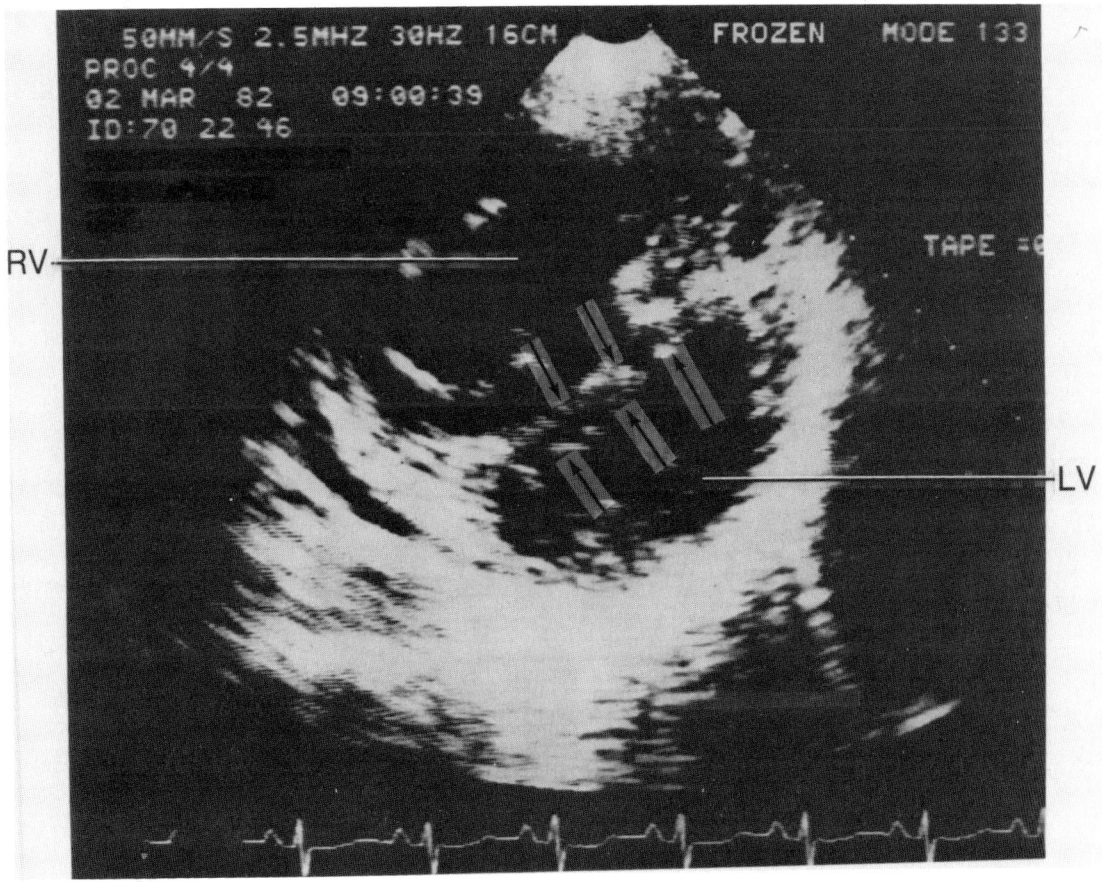

B

Figure 14.3. (B) Parasternal short-axis, two-dimensional echocardiographic view of the patient in A. The arrows indicate the interventricular septum that is straight and compressing the left ventricle (LV). The right ventricle (RV) is quite large.

(13, 14). Hirschfeld found a good correlation between the pulmonary artery diastolic pressure and the ratio of the right-sided pre-ejection period (RPEP) to the right ventricular ejection time (RVET). Systolic time intervals in and of themselves do not give an absolute prediction of the degree of pulmonary artery hypertension or the degree of pulmonary vascular resistance (12). However, if followed over time in a particular infant, they are quite valuable for assessing changes in severity. Hirschfeld found that when the ratio of RPEP to RVET was prolonged, the chances of getting BPD were increased. Furthermore the clinician can follow changes in this ratio as a means of measuring efficacy of his therapy in a particular infant. Another echocardiographic sign of increased right ventricular pressure is the contour of the interventricular septum.

There is a normal contour of the interventricular septum. Since the pulmonary resistance is normally lower than the systemic resistance, the left ventricle is circular on the two-dimensional echocardiogram and the right ventricle takes on a crescentic shape (Fig. 14.3). As the right ventricular pressure increases, the right ventricle loses this shape and the interventricular septum becomes straight. The interventricular septum becomes virtually straight when the right ventricular pressure reaches systemic levels. When the right ventricular pressure is greater than systemic levels, then the interventricular septum bows into the left ventricle and causes "pancaking" of the left ventricle. It is easy to appreciate left ventricular dysfunction in the face of right ventricular hypertension when viewing these striking echocardiograms in these infants.

Azancot and coworkers have developed a quantitative method for assessing the left ventricular shape and various right ventricular volume and pressure overload conditions (15). With a fast Fourier transform technique, shape factors from 1 to 7 are assigned to left ventricular shapes ranging from a circle to an indented banana elipse. This is a mathematical way of assessing what has been mentioned previously. This technique, however, is cumbersome and complicated. Its value most likely is with serial measurements in the same patient.

Another way to assess pulmonary artery pressure is the motion-mode (M-mode) echocardiogram. The so-called flying "W" indicating early systolic closure of the pulmonary valve correlates well with increased pulmonary artery pressure (Fig. 14.4). This method, however, is not reliable in assessing the severity of pulmonary hypertension. It merely indicates whether it is present. There are patients in everyone's experience in whom the flying W was not present on M-mode and who indeed had severe pulmonary hypertension. This method, therefore, is not useful in serial measurements. It is essentially a finding that is present or absent.

Lastly, Doppler echocardiography can be valuable. Continuous wave Doppler measures a velocity that can be incorporated into the modified Bernoulli, equation, which states that the pressure gradient can be predicted by squaring the peak velocity and multiplying that value by 4 (16). This methodology has been validated in aortic stenosis and pulmonary stenosis (17, 18). Patients with BPD, however, may have tricuspid regurgitation secondary to right ventricular dilatation. The peak velocity of the regurgitant jet allows an estimate of right ventricular systolic pressure. Many with severe right ventricular hypertension, however, may not have tricuspid insufficiency if their tricuspid valve annulus is not dilated. Those patients that do have tricuspid insufficiency can be assessed by Doppler, and the Bernoulli equation can be applied. A peak velocity across the tricuspid valve can be measured, and hence an estimate of the transvalvular pressure gradient made. If the right atrial pressure is estimated and then added to this gradient, an indirect assessment of right ventricular pressure and therefore pulmonary artery pressure can be made (19). It is easy to obtain the patient's blood pressure, and therefore the pulmonary artery pressure can be related to the systemic pressure. In the example shown (Fig. 14.5) there is tricuspid insufficiency with a 3.2 m/sec peak velocity across the tricuspid valve. Using the Bernoulli equation a transvalve pressure drop of 41 mmHg ($3.2 \times 3.2 \times 4$) is calculated. If the

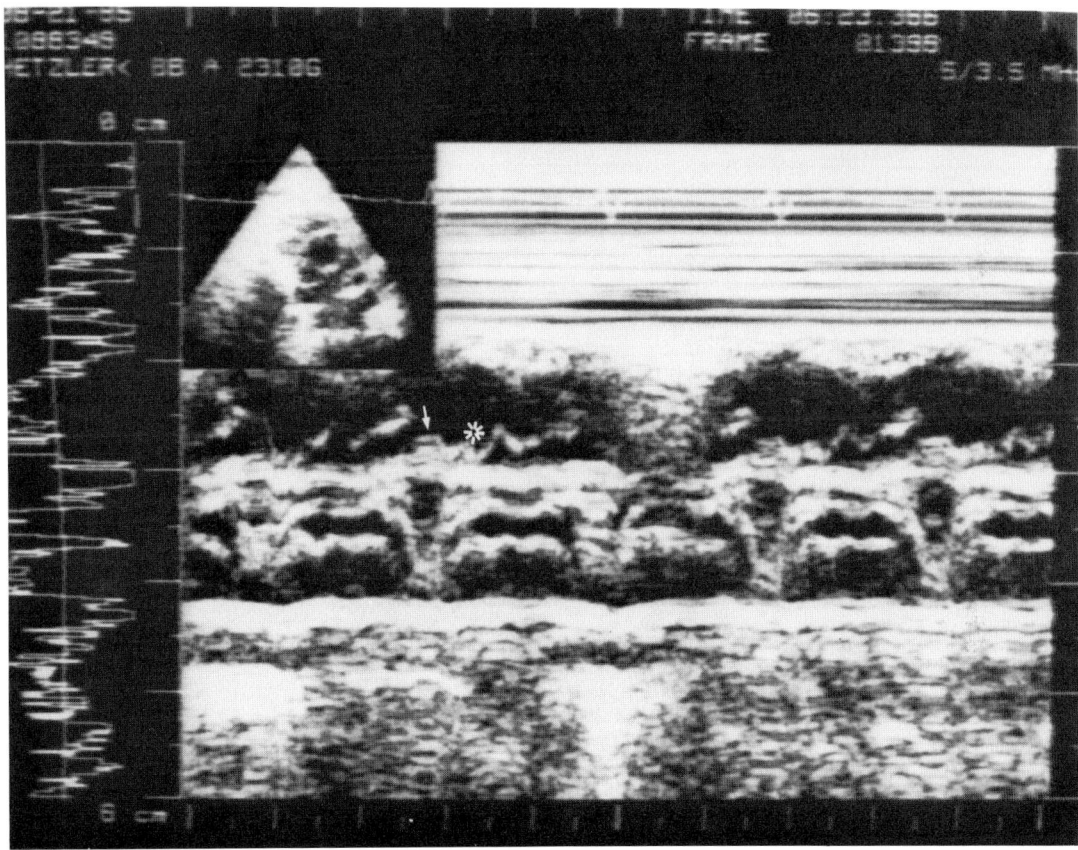

Figure 14.4. Motion-mode echocardiogram of the pulmonary valve (arrow) in a patient with bronchopulmonary dysplasia and pulmonary hypertension. There is early systolic closure of the valve (*). This pattern makes the systolic period of pulmonary valve motion appear like a flying W and is associated with increased pulmonary artery pressure.

mean right atrial pressure is 4, then the right ventricular pressure is 45 mmHg (41 + 4).

In summary, there are many echocardiographic techniques for making an indirect assessment of pulmonary artery hypertension. None of these techniques is useful in giving an absolute prediction of the severity of pulmonary hypertension. They are quite useful in suggesting and strongly implying the presence of pulmonary artery hypertension. In addition these techniques are extremely useful in serial evaluations of a particular patient.

Using the physical examination, electrocardiogram, and echocardiogram with Doppler, a clinician can get a very accurate idea of whether a patient has pulmonary artery hypertension. Furthermore, by utilizing all these techniques. the physician can make a reasonable estimate of the severity of the pulmonary hypertension. From that initial evaluation of the assessment of cor pulmo-

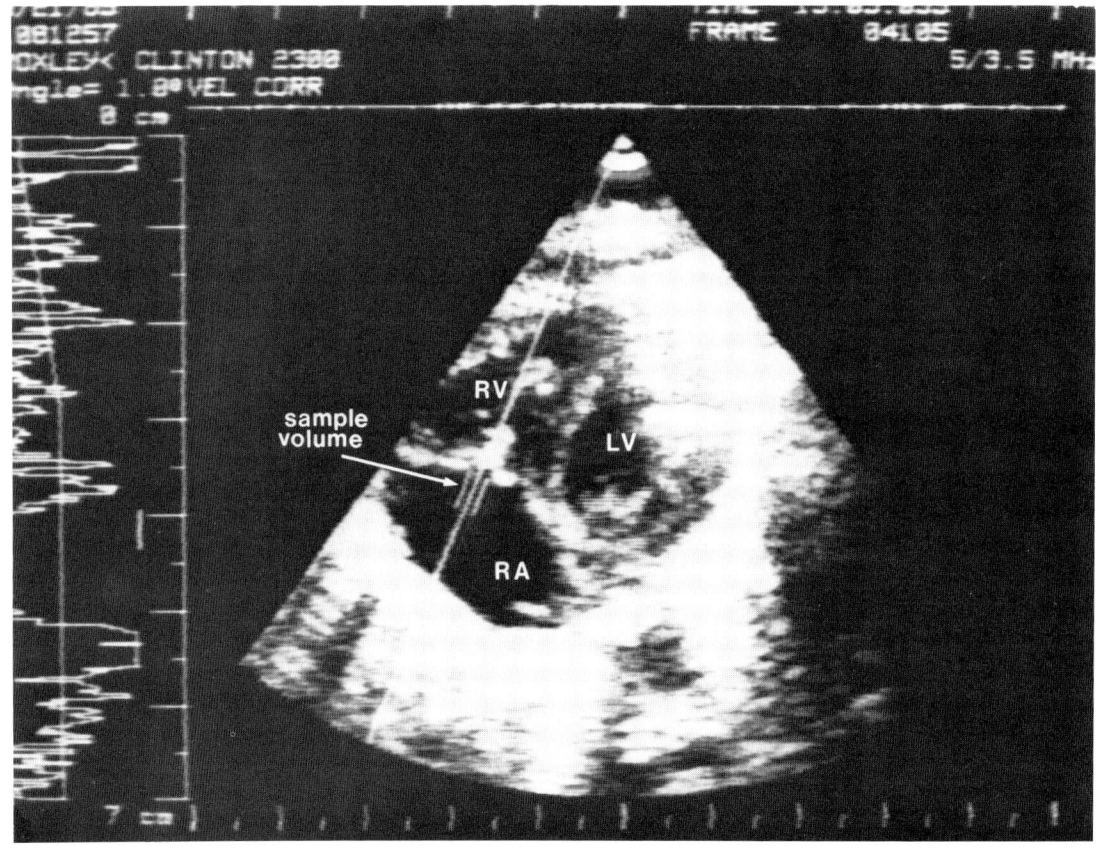

Figure 14.5. (A) Four-chamber apical, two-dimensional echocardiographic view with Doppler sample volume located in right atrium (RA).

nale, the follow-up serial evaluations by physical exam, electrocardiography, and echocardiography can indicate whether the disease process is progressive, static, or improving. The emphasis must be on the entire clinical picture and not on one or two modalities alone.

Cardiac Catherization

Cardiac catheterization is not routinely indicated in these babies. The diagnosis is clear, and treatment is standard, albeit inadequate. If there is a question about the diagnosis, if therapy has been woefully and surprisingly inadequate, and if an experimental drug trial is needed, then cardiac catheterization is indicated.

A hemodynamic evaluation of these babies should measure a cardiac output. Usually the Fick method is inadequate since the patients require oxygen. Thermodilution, therefore, is the preferred method to determine cardiac output. The pulmonary artery

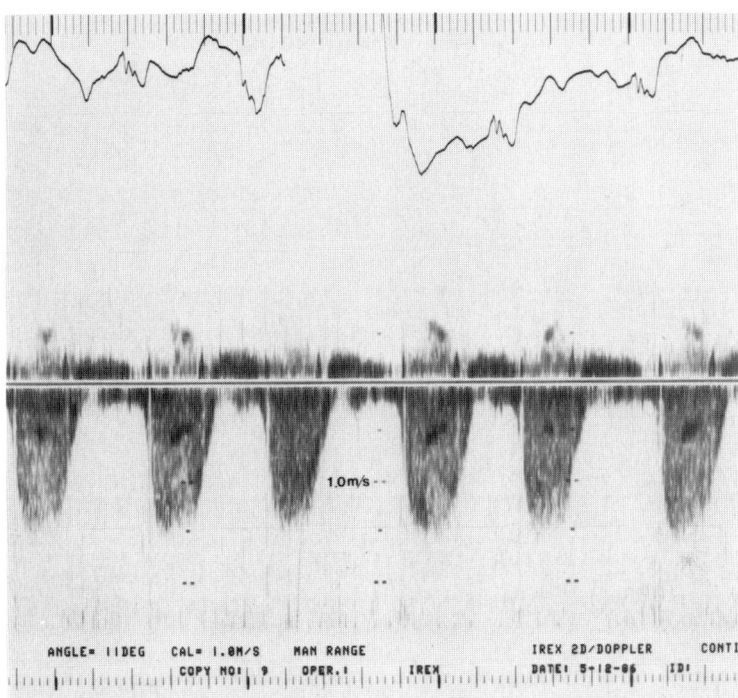

Figure 14.5. (*B*) Continuous wave spectral flow analysis from patient in *A*. Systolic flow recorded going away from transducer at peak velocity of 3.2 m/sec. Using the modified Bernoulli equation this velocity corresponds to a pressure gradient of 41 mmHG (3.2 × 3.2 × 4 = 41). RV = right ventricle. LV = left ventricle.

pressure must be measured in room air or low ambient oxygen and compared with the pulmonary artery pressure in 100% oxygen to ascertain lability of pulmonary vasculature and usefulness of oxygen therapy. Pulmonary artery wedge pressure should be low. If it is not, then left ventricular dysfunction is present or there is pulmonary vein stenosis or mitral stenosis. An arterial catheterization is then indicated to evaluate the possibility of those lesions by comparing simultaneous pulmonary artery wedge and left ventricular end-diastolic pressures.

Finally, if a drug trial is warranted, then hemodynamic parameters should be measured before and after the agent is given to determine hemodynamic efficacy.

Catheterization of these babies is hazardous, and the mortality risk is probably the same as for a sick newborn with congenital heart disease, about 3% to 5%. If an arterial study is done, there is a significant risk of losing the pulse in that leg since the vessel is diminutive.

Treatment

The treatment of cor pulmonale is the most frustrating aspect in the management of these unfortunate infants. It is also the aspect that may strain the relationship between the neonatologist and the cardiologist since the neonatologists are growing weary of hearing the cardiologists repeatedly say, "treat the lung disease." The cardiologists are tired of being called to consult on these infants and not have anything to offer in terms of their management. The problem that caused the cor pulmonale should be the basis of the treatment plan. What is good for the lungs will be good for the heart. The best proven therapy for pulmonary hypertension is oxygen. Abman found that infants with BPD and pulmonary hypertension had labile pulmonary artery pressure that decreased significantly with high inspired oxygen. Continuous supplemental oxygen therapy by nasal cannula is probably useful, therefore, in the treatment of pulmonary hypertension in these children (20).

The question is raised often whether digitalis should be used. There is no definite answer. The issue becomes more pressing when the infant has developed signs of left ventricular dysfunction and left-sided heart failure. Nevertheless there is probably no role for digitalis in cor pulmonale, since there is some evidence that digitalis increases pulmonary vascular resistance (21). If this is indeed the case, then digoxin would be contraindicated. As a desperate measure in a child who is doing very badly, a carefully monitored trial of digoxin may be warranted. New inotropic agents, such as amrinone and milrinone, are being released for human trials, and some of these may offer some benefit to the left ventricle, but they first must undergo strict clinical trials in this specific patient population before therapeutic benefit can be expected (22).

Summary

- Cor pulmonale is an expected and dreaded complication of severe bronchopulmonary dysplasia. Its presence greatly alters a patient's prognosis.
- Right ventricular hypertension interferes with left ventricular function which can make the lung disease worse.
- Noninvasive evaluation is very useful for documenting the presence of pulmonary hypertension, but it is not accurate in determining the severity of the pulmonary hypertension. Serial evaluations are helpful in following the progress of the hypertension in individual infants.
- Occasionally, cardiac catheterization is helpful in evaluating the severity of disease and determining whether left ventricular dysfunction exists.
- There is no effective therapy for cor pulmonale other than the obvious treatment of the underlying lung disease. New inotropic agents may offer some benefit to left ventricular dysfunction, but these have not been used in clinical trials in children to this date.

References

1. Chronic cor pulmonale: report of an expert committee. World Health Organization Technical Report Series. 1961;213:1–12
2. Rabinovitch M. Pulmonary hypertension. In: Adams F, Emmanoulides G, eds. Heart disease in infants, children, and adolescents. 3rd ed. Baltimore: Williams & Wilkins, 1983.
3. Davies G, Reed L. The growth of alveoli and pulmonary arteries in childhood. Thorax 1970;25:669–681.
4. Tauweryns JM. Pulmonary arterial vasculature in neonatal hyaline membrane disease. Science 1966;153:1275–1277.
5. Hislop A, Reid L. Formation of the pulmonary vasculature. In: Hodson WA, ed. Develop-

ment of the lung, vol 6. New York: Marcel Dekker, 1977.
6. Tomashefski JF Jr, Oppermann HC, Vawter GF, Reid LM. Bronchopulmonary dysplasia: a morphometric study with emphasis on the pulmonary vasculature. Pediatr Pathol 1984;2:469–487.
7. Rudolph AM. Congenital diseases of the heart. Chicago: Yearbook Medical Publishers, 1974.
8. Morkin E. Contractile proteins of the heart. Hospital Practice 1983;97–112.
9. McFadden ER, Braunwald E. Cor pulmonale and pulmonary thromboembolism. In: Braunwald E, ed. Heart disease: a textbook of cardiovascular medicine. Philadelphia: WB Saunders, 1984.
10. Robtham JL. Cardiovascular disturbances in chronic respiratory insufficiency. Am J Cardiol 1981;47:941–949.
11. Ellison RC, Freedom RM, Keane JF, Nugent EW, Rowe RD, Miettinen OS. Indirect assessment of severity in pulmonary stenosis. Circulation 1977;56(suppl):I14–I20.
12. Newth CJ, Gow RM, Towe RD. The assessment of pulmonary arterial pressures in bronchopulmonary displasia by cardiac catheterization and M-mode echocardiography. Pediatr Pulmonol 1985;1:58–62.
13. Hirschfeld SS, Meyer RT, Schwarty DC, et al. The echocardiographic assessment of pulmonary artery pressure and pulmonary vascular resistance. Circulation 1975;52:642–648.
14. Riggs T, Hirschfeld SS, Borkat G, et al. Assessment of the pulmonary vascular bed by echocardiagraphic right ventricular systolic time intervals. Circulation 1977;57:939–944.
15. Azancot A, Candell T, Allen HD, et al. Echocardiographic ventricular shape analysis in congenital heart disease with right ventricular volume and pressure overload. Am J Cardiol 1985;56:520–527.
16. Hatle L, Angelsen B. Doppler ultrasound in cardiology. Philadelphia: Lea and Febiger, 1985.
17. Oliveira-Lima C, Sahn DJ, Valdez-Cruz LM, et al. Noninvasive prediction of transvalvular pressure gradient in patients with pulmonary stenosis by quantitative two-dimensional echo Doppler studies. Circulation 1982;67:4;866–871.
18. Smith MD, Kwan OL, DeMaria AN. Value and limitations of continuous-wave Doppler echocardiography in estimating severity of valvular stenosis. J Am Med Assoc 1986;255:3145–3157.
19. Yock PG, Popp RL. Noninvasive estimation of right ventricular systolic pressure by Doppler ultrasound in patients with tricuspid regurgitation. Circulation 1984;70:657–662.
20. Abman SH, Wolfe RR, Accurso FJ, et al. Pulmonary vascular response to oxygen in infants with severe bronchopulmonary dysplasia. Pediatrics 1985;75:80–84.
21. Hoffman BF, Bigger JF Jr. Digitalis and allied cardiac glycosides. In: Gilman AG, Goodman LS, Rall TW, Murad F, eds. The pharmacological basis of therapeutics. New York: MacMillan, 1985.
22. Colucci WS, Wright RF, Braunwald E. New positive inotropic agents in the treatment of congestive heart failure: mechanisms of action and recent clinical developments. N Engl J Med 1986;314:349–358.

Comments

T. Allen Merritt

Maintenance of adequate tissue oxygen delivery is the aim of therapy in infants with bronchopulmonary dysplasia. Determination of the adequacy of myocardial and pulmonary artery oxygenation is a clinical challenge that is at best only periodically assessed. Reports by Halliday and coworkers suggest that the adequacy of cardiac and pulmonary vessel oxygenation can be serially reflected by echocardiographic assessment of pulmonary pressures and systolic time intervals. These observations have not been supported in other studies. Precisely how hypoxemia stimulates pulmonary vasculature myogenesis is not well understood, and the role of prostanoids (or their inhibitors) in facilitating a postnatal decline in pulmonary vascular pressure is incompletely understood. However, as carefully described by Sherman, once these changes occur and are reflected by cardiac muscle hypertrophy and hyperplasia with impaired biventricular output, treatment is difficult and frequently only palliative. The obvious strategy is to prevent hypoxemia from developing. Data are as yet unavailable to suggest that continuous skin surface oxygen tension measurement or oxygen saturation monitoring have prevented intermittent or even chronic mild hypoxemia in infants with BPD.

Thus a major challenge to neonatologists and cardiologists must be to gain insights into factors that regulate vascular and myocardial cellular response to changes in the ambient oxygen. Sensitive markers for intracellular oxygenation must be identified, and clinical skills enhanced toward providing that fine margin of optimal oxygen delivery in the neonate—neither too much nor too little!

15

Assessment of Pulmonary Function in the Postneonatal Period

ROBERT S. TEPPER

Introduction

In 1967 Northway and colleagues (1) first described a constellation of chest radiographic and pathologic findings associated with the persistence of respiratory symptoms in premature infants following the acute phase of the respiratory distress syndrome (RDS). These investigators employed the term bronchopulmonary dysplasia (BPD) to describe the chronic respiratory disease present in these infants. The most frequently employed clinical definition of BPD was proposed by Bancalari *et al.* (2) in 1975 and includes the presence of an abnormal chest radiograph, chronic respiratory symptoms, and an oxygen requirement at 30 days of life. This description of BPD allows us to identify infants with overt clinical symptoms and severe chronic lung disease but may neglect those infants with either mild or moderate pulmonary dysfunction.

Our assessment of the respiratory status of infants with BPD has frequently been limited to physical and radiographic examinations, and to blood gas analysis. After the first month of life, chest radiographic abnormalities in infants with BPD remain relatively constant and do not accurately reflect either the acute or the chronic changes in their respiratory status. In addition the oxygen requirement at 1 month of life has been found not to correlate with respiratory symptoms and illness during the first year of life (3).

Pulmonary function testing in infants with BPD offers the potential 1) to define the pulmonary pathophysiology and the spectrum of pulmonary dysfunction, 2) to describe the natural history of this chronic lung disease and the effects upon the subsequent growth and development of the lung, and 3) to evaluate the efficacy of therapeutic interventions. In this chapter several different methodologies for assessing the lung function of infants with BPD are reviewed along with the results of several studies.

Lung Volume

The lung volume most frequently measured in infants is the air in the lungs at end-expiration or functional residual capacity (FRC). In 1973 Bryan *et al.* (4) first reported the measurement of FRC in infants with BPD. These investigators employed the helium dilution method and found that in the first month of life infants with BPD had lower values for FRC than healthy controls, but that between 6 and 12 months of age the BPD infants had elevated FRC values. Eight of the 11 infants died by 5 months of age, suggesting that the subjects enrolled in that study represented infants most severely affected by BPD. Therefore their conclusion that BPD infants have an elevated FRC should be viewed in light of the limited population of three subjects between 6 and 12 months of age and the severity of disease. More recently

Tepper et al. (5) measured FRC by helium dilution in 20 BPD infants only one of whom died in the first year of life. A low FRC was demonstrated in the perinatal period, a finding similar to that of Bryan et al. (4); however, between 6 and 12 months of age, there was no significant difference in FRC when the BPD infants were compared with controls. Employing nitrogen washout, another equilibration technique, to measure FRC, Gerhardt et al. (6) also reported no significant difference in FRC between BPD and control infants. In contrast to the helium dilution method, which determines the volume of air in the lungs at end-expiration that equilibrates with the inspired gas mixture, the thoracic gas volume (TGV) can be measured plethysmographically by the application of Boyle's pressure-volume law (7). Ideally the difference in the lung volumes measured by these two different methods represents the volume of noncommunicating or "trapped" gas. Although these two measurements should yield the same volume in normal subjects, in the presence of obstructive airways disease, the plethysmographic assessment of lung volume (TGV) should exceed that obtained by dilutional techniques (FRC-He).

Radiographically, infants with BPD demonstrate both noncommunicating cystic regions and regions of volume loss, and the plethysmographic measurement of lung volume in these infants has been reported to be elevated. There has been increasing concern that plethysmography, which has previously been the "gold standard" for measuring lung volume, may overestimate true lung volume in both adults and infants, particularly in the presence of obstructive airways disease (8, 9, 10, 11). No studies have yet measured both TGV and FRC-He in the same infant with BPD or attempted to correlate these measured lung volumes with a more detailed analysis of the pulmonary mechanics.

Distribution of Ventilation

The presence of diffuse airways disease in infants with BPD results in a maldistribution of ventilation within the lung, the mismatching of ventilation ($\dot{V}$) to perfusion ($\dot{Q}$), and hypoxemia. Watts et al. (12) were the first to quantitate the maldistribution of ventilation in infants with BPD. From the nitrogen washout curve obtained while the subject is breathing 100% oxygen, these investigators described the very slowly ventilated compartments within the lungs of infants with BPD. Another method of assessing the nonhomogeneity of the distribution of ventilation is by measuring the mixing index (MI). This measurement was first described by Bates and Christie for assessing intrapulmonary gas mixing in adults (13). The mixing index is the ratio $\times$ 100, of the predicted number of breaths to the actual number of breaths to reach 90% of the final helium concentration, as a subject breathes into a closed circuit employed for the measurement of FRC. The predicted number of breaths to reach 90% equilibration is calculated from a single-compartment model of the lung using the infant's measured FRC and tidal volume. The greater the actual number of breaths required to equilibrate with the helium, the lower is the mixing index, and the less uniform is the distribution of ventilation. Infants with BPD demonstrated lower mixing indices than controls, as illustrated in Figure 15.1. For the BPD infants MI increased with increasing age and higher MIs were associated with higher oxygen saturations (5). This association probably reflects an improved distribution of ven-

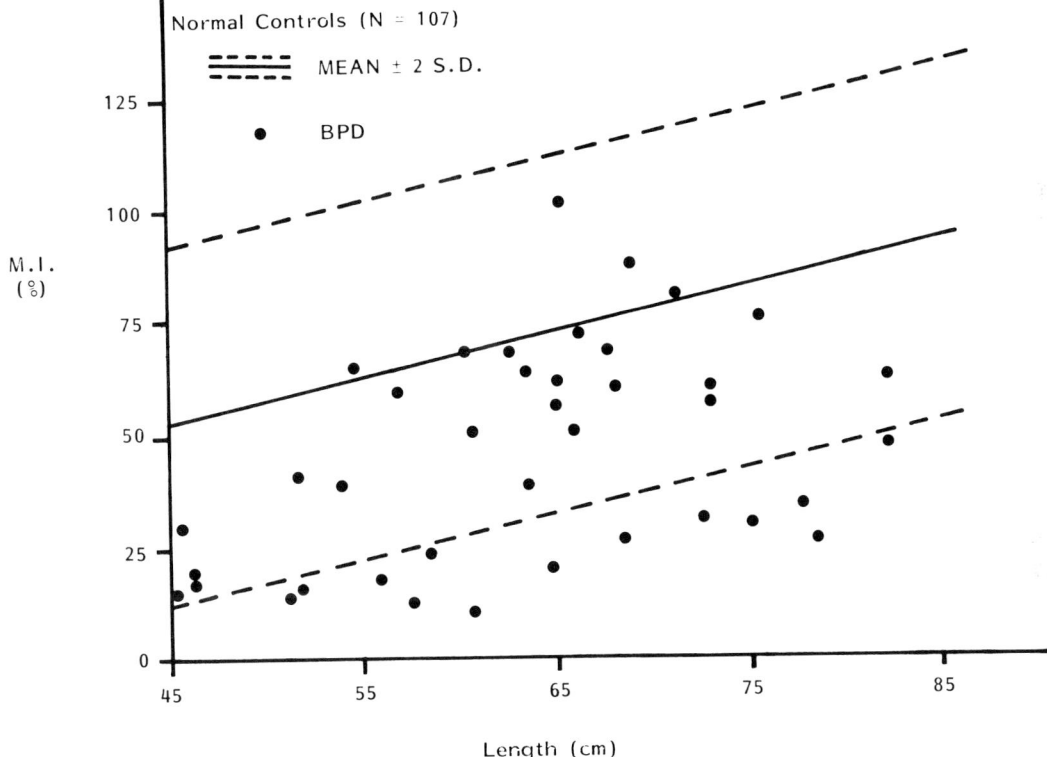

Figure 15.1. Mixing index (M.I.) vs. body length (cm) for infants with BPD vs. the linear regression equation for normal infants.

tilation in the older infants and a better matching of ventilation to perfusion within the lungs.

Compliance

The elastic properties of the lungs have been difficult to evaluate in infants because of the lack of subject cooperation. Although compliance should be measured under static conditions (C_{st}) in order to reflect the elastic properties of the lung, dynamic lung compliance (C_{dyn}) has frequently been measured during tidal breathing with an esophageal catheter used to estimate the changes in pleural pressure. Although several studies have reported a low C_{dyn} in infants with BPD (4), the presence of obstructive airways disease, a maldistribution of ventilation and tachypnea may result in C_{dyn} underestimating C_{st} because of its frequency dependence. It has therefore been unclear whether the low C_{dyn} in infants with BPD reflects an abnormality of the elastic properties of their lungs or primarily the presence of airways disease. In addition to the frequency dependence of C_{dyn}, the use of esophageal catheters in this age group represents an invasive procedure, and there has been increasing concern about the accuracy of this methodology in infants, particularly in the presence of obstructive airways disease (14, 15). These concerns have led investigators to search for other methods to evaluate compliance in infants.

The weighted spirometer method represents a noninvasive technique for measuring total respiratory system compliance (C_{rs}) in infants (16). Because of the infant's highly compliant chest wall, the compliance of the total respiratory system and the compliance of the lung are similar. The measurement of C_{rs} is performed while the infant breathes into the water-sealed spirometer circuit that is used for the measurement of FRC. After establishing a constant end-expiratory level by adjusting the oxygen supply, a weight is placed on the spirometer bell, producing a continuous positive pressure within the respiratory-spirometer circuit and increasing the end-expiratory level as indicated in Figure 15.2. After the new end-expiratory level has remained constant for at least seven breaths, the weight is removed and the subject's end-expiratory level returns to baseline. The infant's total respiratory system compliance (C_{rs}) is obtained by dividing the change in the end-expiratory volume (mL) by the pressure change in the circuit (cm H_2O) and then subtracting the compliance of the spirometer circuit. This measurement of C_{rs} represents a quasi-static compliance. Although the infants are still breathing spontaneously during the measurement, the new end-expiratory level is maintained by a constant distending pressure for at least seven breaths and should provide sufficient time for pressure equilibration within the respiratory system. When total respiratory system compliance was assessed by the weighted spirometer method in groups of BPD and normal full-term infants matched for age and size, infants with BPD had significantly lower values of C_{rs} (.047 ± .008 vs. .073 ± .011 mL/cm H_2O/cm body length). The low values for C_{rs} obtained in the BPD infants suggests that there are changes in the intrinsic elastic properties of their lungs, a finding which is consistent with the fibroproliferative changes observed at necropsy and the strands of increased density observed radiographically.

Airway Function

Most studies evaluating airway function in infants have employed plethysmography to measure airways resistance or esophageal manometry to measure pulmonary resistance. These methods assess the combined upper and lower airways. In infants it has been estimated that the large central airways and the extrathoracic airways may account for approximately 80% of the total airways resistance, thus making it difficult to assess changes in the smaller, more peripheral airways. In addition there has been increasing concern as to the accuracy of these techniques in assessing airway function in infants, particularly in the presence of airways disease.

Forced expiratory flow is routinely employed in older children and adults to assess lower airway function. Recently Adler and Wohl (17) and Taussig and coworkers (18) described methods for obtaining maximal forced expiratory flows in healthy newborn infants by rapidly applying an external pressure around the infant. Tepper and coworkers modified the methodology and extended

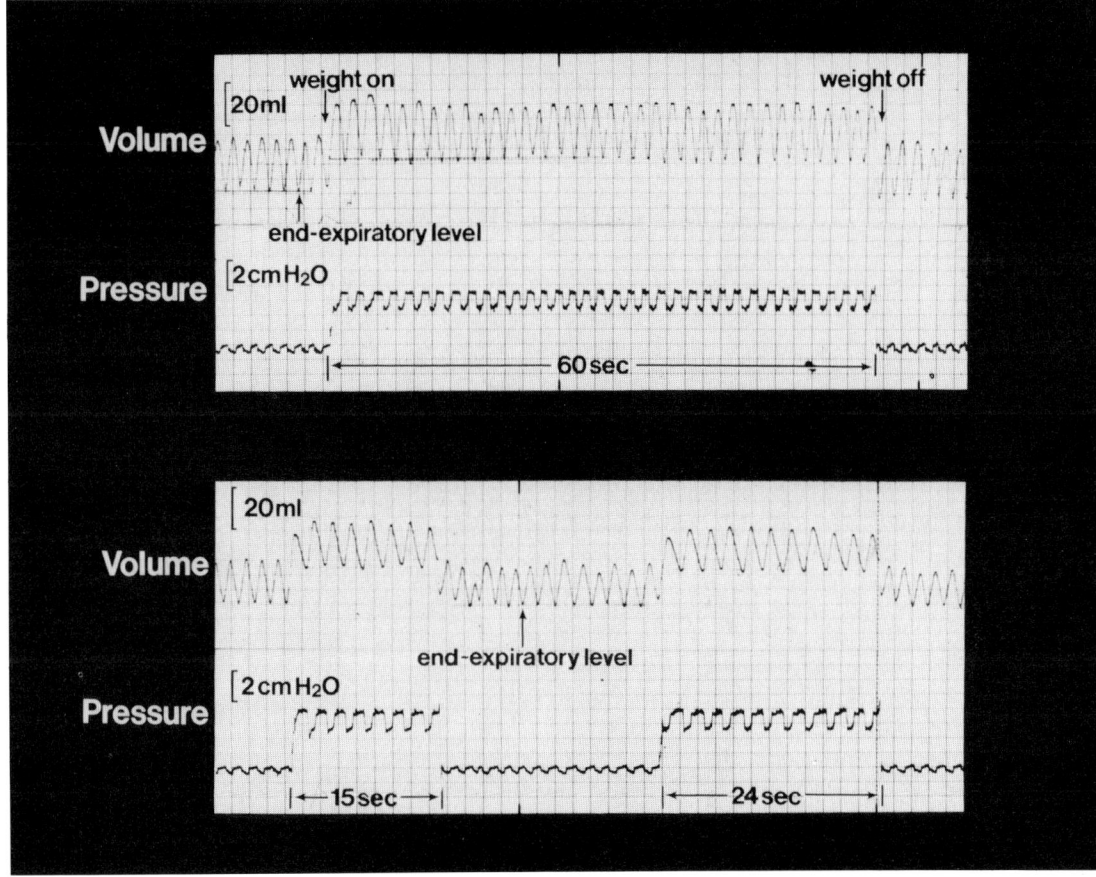

Figure 15.2. Measurement of total respiratory system compliance by the weighted spirometer method. Volume-pressure tracings showing a constant end-expiratory level during a prolonged application of the weight to the spirometer bell (*top*) and reproducible changes in the end-expiratory level during repetitive application and removal of the weight (*bottom*).

the assessment of lung function with partial expiratory flow-volume (PEFV) curves to healthy and ill infants in the first year of life (5, 19, 20, 21, 22). The maximal expiratory flow rates are generated by rapidly (<100 msec) inflating at end-inspiration a plastic bag that is wrapped around the infant's chest and abdomen. The infant breathes through a face mask attached to a #0 Fleisch pneumotachometer, and care is taken to prevent upper airway obstruction either from compression of the nose and mandible with the face mask or by improper positioning of the head and neck. The volume signal is obtained by integration of the flow signal and the flow-volume curves are displayed on a storage oscilliscope. A PEFV curve is schematically illustrated in Figure 15.3. The smaller, inner curve represents tidal breathing, and the larger, outer curve is the maximal expira-

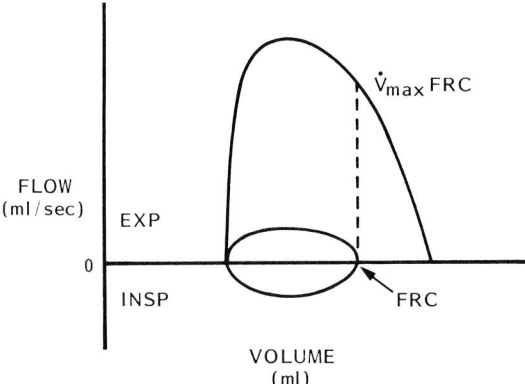

Figure 15.3. Partial expiratory flow-volume curves. The smaller inner curve is the infant's tidal breathing; the larger outer curve is the infant's maximal expiratory flow generated by the rapid compression technique. The separation between these two curves represents the infant's expiratory flow reserve. $\dot{V}_{max}FRC$ = maximal flow at functional residual capacity.

tory flow (flow limitation) generated by the rapid compression technique. The separation between these two curves represents the expiratory flow reserve. The PEFV curve is quantitated by the expiratory flow at functional residual capacity (end-expiration). The PEFV curves are repeated at increasing applied bag pressures until a maximal flow at functional residual capacity ($\dot{V}_{max}FRC$) is obtained.

The PEFV curves from a normal control infant and two infants with BPD are illustrated in Figure 15.4. The normal control infant's PEFV curve (Fig. 15.4, A) demonstrates a convex shape (bowing out) of the expiratory flow relative to the volume, and there is a large expiratory flow reserve between tidal breathing and the maximal expiratory flows. The BPD infant whose PEFV curve is depicted in Figure 15.4, B, had clinically obvious respiratory symptoms consisting of tachypnea, soft tissue retractions, abnormal auscultatory findings, and an oxygen

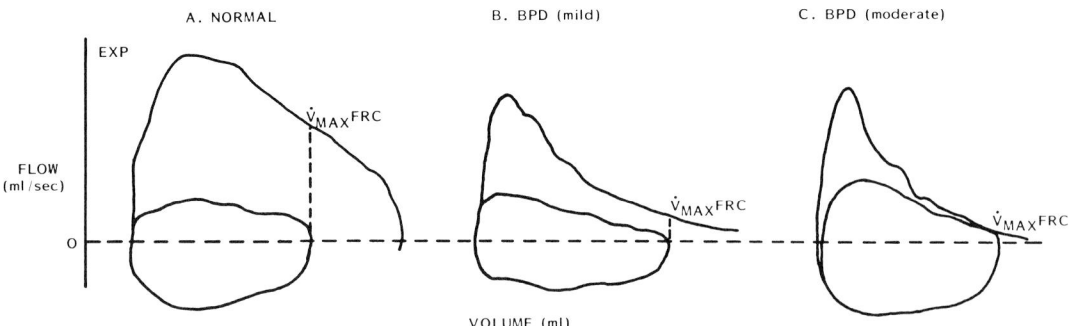

Figure 15.4. Partial expiratory flow-volume curves. (A) Normal infant with a convex (bowing out) flow-volume curve with large expiratory flow reserve between tidal breathing and maximal flows. (B) Infant with mild chronic lung disease (BPD) and no clinical systems at the time of evaluation. Concave shape (bowing inward) of flow-volume curve with decreased expiratory flow reserve as compared to normal, A. (C) Infant with moderate chronic lung disease (BPD) and overt respiratory symptoms. Greater concavity of flow-volume curve, as compared to B, with the tidal breathing curve at maximal expiratory flow limitation and the absence of any expiratory flow reserve.

requirement, in addition to a chronically abnormal chest radiograph. This infant's tidal breathing curve is at his maximal expiratory flow limitation, and the absence of any expiratory flow reserve is consistent with his overt clinical symptoms. Also shown is the PEFV curve of an infant with BPD who also has a chronically abnormal chest radiograph but had a normal physical examination and no oxygen requirement at the time of testing. Although the PEFV curve demonstrates a concave shape (a bowing in toward the volume axis) and a decreased $\dot{V}_{max}FRC$, this infant is not flow limited during tidal breathing, and there is an expiratory flow reserve present.

The limited activity and the limited demands placed upon the ventilatory system of infants during normal daily activity frequently make the clinical assessment of either respiratory function or reserve in infants very difficult. Lower respiratory illness is probably the most significant clinical challenge to the respiratory system of infants. The BPD infant who appeared to be clinically well (Fig. 15.4, C) was subsequently rehospitalized in acute respiratory distress associated with a lower respiratory illness. The abnormal PEFV curve in this infant and the decreased expiratory flow reserve, even when he was clinically well, help to explain his acute deterioration, and the high incidence of rehospitalization of infants with BPD during the first year of life (5, 23–25). In addition this example illustrates the potential dichotomy between the clinical and physiologic assessments of pulmonary function in infants.

The concave shape of the PEFV curve and the decreased flow rates at relatively low lung volumes (FRC) are consistent with the presence of more peripheral than central airways disease in the infants with BPD. The change in maximal expiratory flow rates when the subject is breathing a less dense gas such as Heliox (80% helium and 20% oxygen) has been employed in older children and adults to localize the site of airways obstruction (26, 27). Turbulent flow in the central airways and convective acceleration associated with the movement of flow from the peripheral to the central airways are both density dependent. Therefore, when the subject is breathing Heliox as compared with air, maximal expiratory flows should increase when flow is limited primarily by one of these two flow regimes. The low flow rates in the more peripheral airways are associated with a laminar flow profile which is density independent but is a function of the viscosity of the gas mixture. Figure 15.5 illustrates the PEFV curves obtained from a normal, healthy infant and an infant with BPD when breathing air and Heliox. The normal infant (A) demonstrates a convex flow volume curve, a large expiratory flow reserve, and a significant increase in the PEFV curve when breathing Heliox as compared with air. In contrast the BPD infant demonstrates a markedly concave flow volume curve, no expiratory flow reserve, and no increase in flow while breathing Heliox. The BPD infant actually exhibits a small decrease in $\dot{V}_{max}FRC$ which is consistent with the greater viscosity of the Heliox mixture as compared with that of air. The very low flow rates at FRC and the absence of an increase in flow rate when breathing a less dense gas mixture demonstrates in this infant the presence of a laminar flow profile at this lung volume and the presence of severe peripheral airways disease. This finding is consistent with the pathologic reports of obstructive airways disease in infants with BPD.

Wheezing is a common respiratory symptom in infants with BPD and represents the

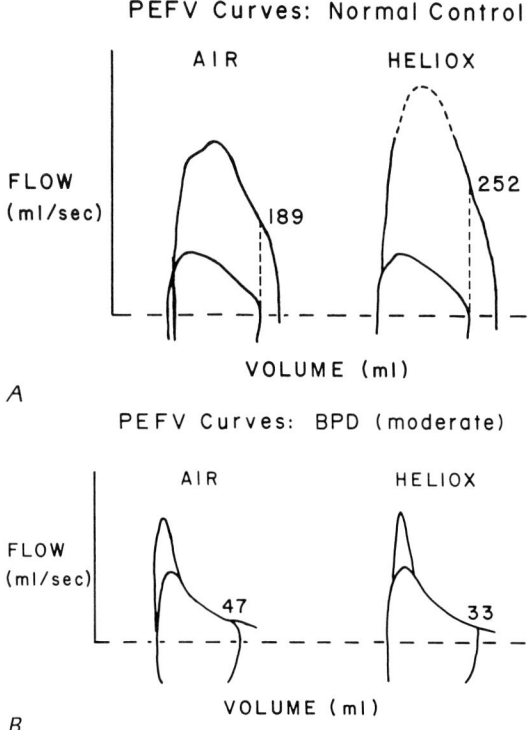

Figure 15.5. Partial expiratory flow-volume curves obtained while subject is breathing room air and Heliox (20% oxygen and 80% helium). (A) Normal infant demonstrates a 33% increase in maximal expiratory flow at functional residual capacity, $\dot{V}_{max}FRC$ (ml/sec). (B) Infant with BPD had a 30% decrease in $\dot{V}_{max}FRC$.

presence of airways obstruction that may be secondary to bronchospasm, mucosal edema of the airways, mucus secretions, or dynamic compression of the airways. The relative contributions of these factors to the airways obstruction and wheezing that occur in infants with BPD has been difficult to assess. Autopsies of infants with BPD have demonstrated the presence of airway smooth muscle hypertrophy, and older children with a history of BPD as infants have hyper-reactive airways as demonstrated by the presence of a positive methacholine bronchial provocation test. Both of these findings suggest that bronchospasm contributes to the presence of airways obstruction in infants with BPD. Several recent studies have demonstrated an improvement in the pulmonary function of infants with BPD following the administration of a bronchodilator (28, 29). Figure 15.6 illustrates the positive response of the inhaled bronchodilator, metaproterenol, as demonstrated by the improvement in the PEFV curves obtained from an infant with BPD. As the PEFV curve still demonstrated a concave shape and a decreased expiratory flow reserve following administration of the bronchodilator, bronchospasm represents only one component of the airways obstruction in this infant.

Nickerson and Taussig (30) have reported an increased incidence of asthma and allergies in first degree relatives of infants with BPD as compared with a control population of healthy full-term infants. This observation raises the possibility that a genetic predisposition along with injury to the airways may contribute to the presence of airway hyperreactivity in infants with BPD. In fact the predisposition to airway reactivity may be one of the factors that contributes to the development of BPD in certain infants.

Early Prediction of BPD

Although the complex pathogenesis of BPD is not fully understood, there is a transition of the pulmonary pathophysiology from the acute illness of respiratory distress syndrome which represents a parenchymal disease with low lung compliance and low lung volumes to the development of chronic lung disease with airways obstruction, hyperinflation, parenchymal fibrosis, and cyst formation. Pul-

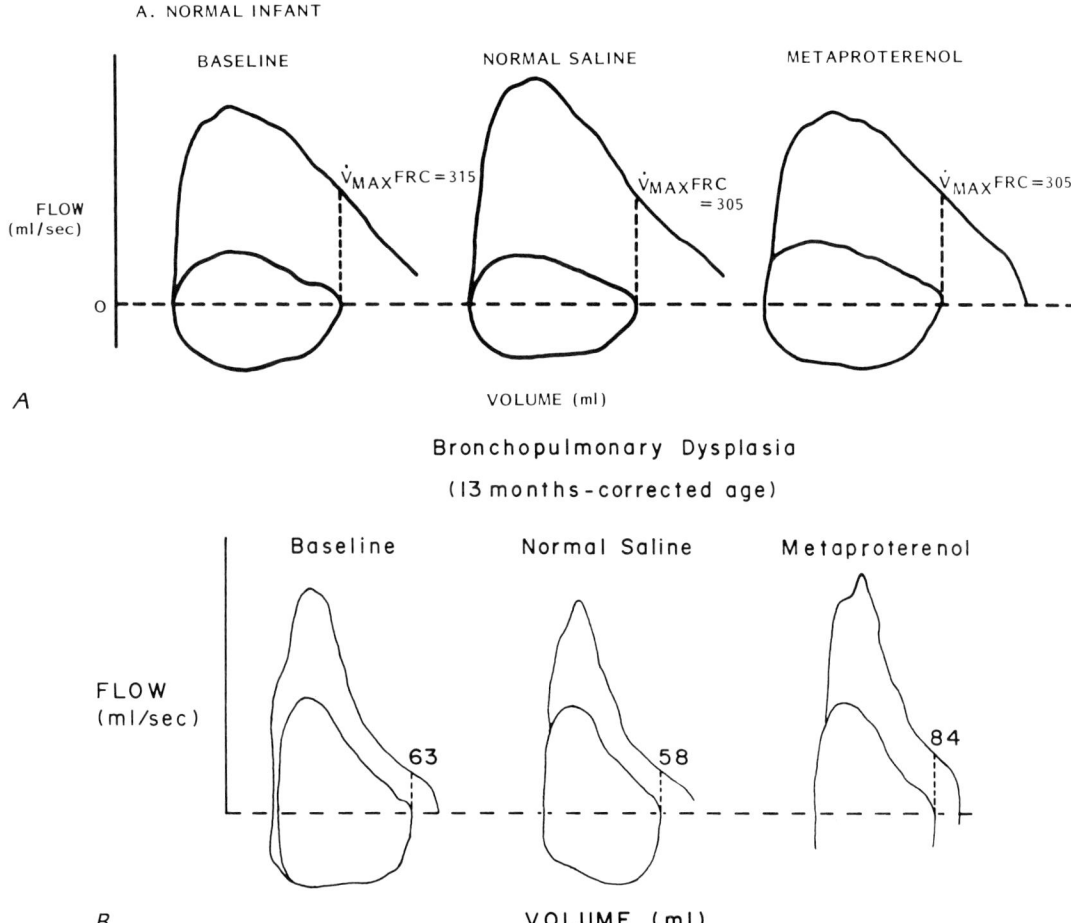

Figure 15.6. Partial expiratory flow-volume curves obtained at baseline, after inhaling normal saline, and 10 minutes following inhalation of the bronchodilator metaproterenol. (*A*) Normal control infant demonstrates no significant change in the maximal expiratory flow at functional residual capacity $\dot{V}_{max}FRC$. (*B*) Infant with BPD demonstrates no significant change in $\dot{V}_{max}FRC$ following normal saline, but a 33% increase in $\dot{V}_{max}FRC$ following the bronchodilator.

monary function testing early in the neonatal period has not yet been successful in the prospective identification of those premature infants who will develop BPD. Goldman *et al.* (31) have reported that when premature infants were assessed in the first week of life, there was no difference in dynamic compliance, but a higher pulmonary resistance in the group who subsequently developed BPD as compared with those infants without evidence of chronic lung disease at 28 days of life. However, the former group was significantly younger and smaller at the time of testing, and the difference in body size between the two groups probably account for the differences in pulmonary resistance, a measurement which is significantly affected by the size of the more central airways (nasal, pharyngeal, and tracheal) and influenced by the presence and size of an endotracheal tube. In contrast to pulmonary resistance, maximal expiratory flows at low lung volumes are independent of the central and upper airways, reflecting the function of the more peripheral airways (32). Maximal expiratory flow rates can be obtained in intubated premature infants by transiently applying a negative pressure to the endotracheal tube to evacuate the air in the lungs (33). This measurement may prove to be more sensitive than pulmonary resistance in the early detection of obstructive airways disease as premature infants progress from RDS to BPD. The large intersubject variability of most pulmonary function tests will make it difficult for a single measurement to identify an individual as abnormal, and therefore longitudinal evaluation will be more sensitive in detecting the development of obstructive airways disease.

During the first year of life many infants with BPD improve with respect to their respiratory symptoms even though their chest radiographs demonstrate no significant changes. The clinical improvement is most likely related to their somatic growth and the absolute increase in the size of their larger, more central airways, an observation consistent with the decline in total airways resistance during the first year of life (34). As indicated above these infants have significant peripheral airways disease, which as the infants grow contributes an ever smaller fraction to the total airways resistance. Figure 15.7 illustrates the longitudinal evaluation of $\dot{V}_{max}FRC$ in a group of BPD infants. With increasing body length most of the infants demonstrate an increase in $\dot{V}_{max}FRC$ but remain below the regression equation for the normal controls (5). In addition the slope of the regression equation for the infants with BPD is significantly ($p < .05$) smaller than that for the normal controls (2.25 vs. 4.52). Although the infants with BPD are growing and their clinical symptoms are improving, the persistently low flow rates at FRC illustrate the abnormal functional development of their airways, with no evidence of "catch-up" growth during the first year of life.

Summary

The finding of abnormal airway function in infants with BPD is consistent with several follow-up studies that have evaluated the lung function of children with a history of BPD as infants. Those studies have reported the persistence of airways obstruction into childhood as evidenced by decreased flow rates at relatively low lung volumes (35, 36, 37, 38). In addition follow-up studies of children with a history of prematurity requiring respiratory support for the respiratory distress syndrome, but without evidence of BPD, have also been demonstrated to have lower values of lung function when compared with children who were full-term at the time of birth (39). As the number of conducting airways is fixed by the 24th week of fetal development, it is not surprising that injury to the airways early in life might result in a spectrum of chronic abnormalities of the airways, which could vary from infants who are clinically asymptomatic to those with overt chronic respiratory disease. The persistent abnormalities in lung function may reflect the fixed residua from injury to the lung during the neonatal period as well as an alteration of the subsequent growth and development pattern of the infant's lung secondary to the initial injury. As the survivors from newborn

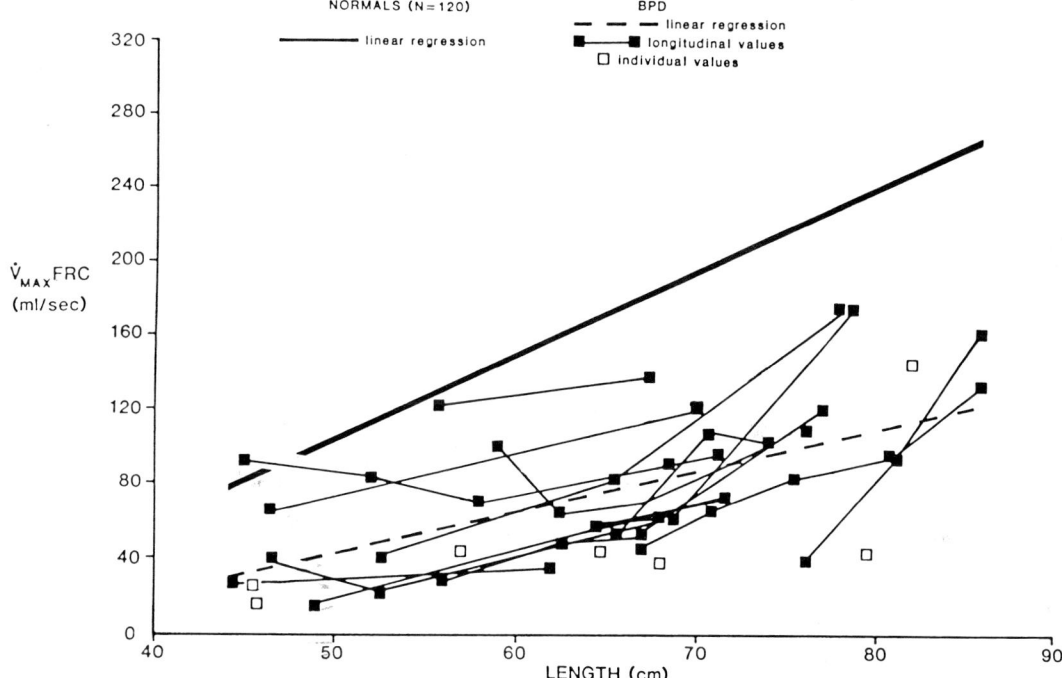

Figure 15.7. $\dot{V}_{max}FRC$ (ml/sec) vs. body length (cm). Individual values for infants with BPD followed longitudinally, along with the linear regression equation for these values and those obtained in normal controls (19).

intensive care units of 20 years ago are just entering adulthood, it is not known whether insults to the respiratory system in the neonatal period will accelerate the normal age related decline in pulmonary function that occurs during adulthood (35, 40). It will be very important to monitor the long-term outcome of these infants.

During the past few years there has been a significant increase in the number of studies that have employed pulmonary function testing in the evaluation of infants with BPD. These studies have helped to define the pulmonary pathophysiology associated with BPD and to evaluate our medical management of these infants. The ability to detect the earliest abnormalities of lung function, prior to the presence of chronic lung disease, might allow for early therapeutic interventions and would offer the potential to minimize the progression and severity of pulmonary disease.

References

1. Northway W, Rosan R, Porter D. Pulmonary disease following respiratory therapy of hyaline membrane disease. N Engl J Med 1967; 276:357–368.
2. Bancalari E, Abdenour G, Feller R, Giannon J. Bronchopulmonary dysplasia: clinical presentation. J Pediatr 1979;95:819–823.
3. Truog W, Jackson C, Badura R, et al. Bronchopulmonary dysplasia and pulmonary insufficiency of prematurity—lack of correlation of

outcome with gas exchange abnormalities at 1 month of age. Am J Dis Child 1985; 139:351–354.
4. Bryan M, Hardie M, Reilly B, et al. Pulmonary function studies during the first year of life in infants recovering from the respiratory distress syndrome. Pediatrics 1973;52:169–178.
5. Tepper RS, Morgan WJ, Cota K, Taussig LM. Expiratory flow limitation in infants with bronchopulmonary dysplasia. J Pediatr 1986; 109(6)1040–1046.
6. Gerhardt T, Hehre D, Feller R, et al. Long-term study of pulmonary function in infants surviving with chronic lung disease (CLD). Pediatr Res 1984;392A:1776.
7. DuBois A, Botelko S, Bedell G, Marshall R, Comroe J. A rapid plethysmograph method for measuring TGV. J Clin Invest 1956;35:322–326.
8. Rodenstein DO, Stanescu DC, Francis C. Demonstration of failure of body plethysmography in airway obstruction. J Appl Physiol 1982;52:949–954.
9. Beardsmore C, Stocks J, Silverman M. Problems in measurement of thoracic gas volume in infancy. J Appl Physiol 1982;52:995–999.
10. Helms P. Problems with plethysmographic estimation of lung volume in infants and young children. J Appl Physiol 1982;53:698–702.
11. Godfrey S, Beardsmore C, Moayan C, Baryishay E. Can thoracic gas volume be measured in infants with airways obstruction? Am Rev Respir Dis 1986;133:245–251.
12. Watts J, Ariagno R, Brady J. Chronic pulmonary disease in neonates after artificial ventilation: distribution of ventilation and pulmonary interstitial emphysema. Pediatrics 1977; 60:273–281.
13. Bates D, Christie R. Intrapulmonary mixing of helium in health and in emphysema. Clin Sci 1950;9:17–27.
14. LeSouef P, Lopes J, England S, et al. Influence of chest wall distortion on esophageal pressure. J Appl Physiol 1983;55:353–358.
15. Thomson A, Elliott J, Silverman M. Pulmonary compliance in sick low birthweight infants. How reliable is the measurement of esophageal pressure? Arch Dis Child 1983; 58:891–896.
16. Tepper RS, Pagtakham RD, Taussig LM. Noninvasive determination of total respiratory system compliance in infants by the weighted-spirometer method. Am Rev Respir Dis 1984; 130:461–466.
17. Adler S, Wohl ME. Flow-volume relationship at low lung volumes in healthy term newborn infants. Pediatrics 1978;61:636–640.
18. Taussig L, Landau L, Godfrey S, et al. Determinants of forced expiratory flows in newborn infants. J Appl Physiol 1982;53:1220–1227.
19. Tepper RS, Morgan W, Cota K, Taussig LM. Physiologic growth and development of the lungs during the first year of life. Am Rev Respir Dis 1986;134:513–519.
20. Tepper RS, Morgan WJ, Wright A, Cota K, Taussig LM. Persistent airways obstruction and bronchodilator responsiveness in infants following a lower respiratory infection (abstr). Am Rev Respir Dis 1984;129(4, part 2):217A.
21. Hiatt P, Tepper RS, Eigen H. Bronchodilator response in infants with cystic fibrosis (abstr). Am Rev Respir Dis 1985;131(4, part 2):240A.
22. Tepper R, Hiatt P, Eigen H, Wyszomierski D, Meyers J. Flow limitation in infants with cystic fibrosis. Am Rev Respir Dis 1985;131(4, part 2):240A.
23. Lewis S. A follow-up study on the respiratory distress syndrome. Proc Roy Soc Med 1968; 61:771–773.
24. Outerbridge E, Nogrady B, Beaudry P, et al. Idiopathic respiratory distress syndrome. Recurrent respiratory illness in survivors. Am J Dis Child 1972;123:99–104.
25. McCormick M, Shapiro S, Starfield B. Rehospitalization in the first year of life for high-risk survivors. Pediatrics 1980;66:991–999.
26. Despas P, Leroux M, Macklem P. Site of airways obstruction in asthma as determined by measuring maximal expiratory flow breathing air and a helium-oxygen mixture. J Clin Invest 1972;51:3235–3243.
27. Dosman J, Bode F, Urbonetti J, Martin R, Macklem P. The use of a helium oxygen mixture during maximum expiratory flow to demonstrate obstruction in small airways in smokers. J Clin Invest 1975;55:1090–1099.

28. Kao LC, Warburton D, Platzker ACG, Keens TG. Effect of isoproterenol inhalation on airway resistance in chronic bronchopulmonary dysplasia. Pediatrics 1984;73:509–514.
29. Kao L, Durand D, Birch M, Phillips B, Nickerson B. Oral theophylline and diuretics improve pulmonary mechanics in infants with bronchopulmonary dysplasia. Am Rev Respir Dis 1986;133(4, part 2):A207.
30. Nickerson B, Taussig L. Family history of asthma in infants with bronchopulmonary dysplasia. Pediatrics 1980;65:1140–1144.
31. Goldman S, Gerhardt T, Sonni R, Feller R, et al. Early prediction of chronic lung disease by pulmonary function testing. J Pediatr 1983; 102:613–617.
32. Hyatt RE. Expiratory flow limitation. J Appl Physiol: Respirat Environ Exercise Physiol 1983;55:1–8.
33. Motoyama E, Fort M. Evidence of bronchial reactivity in premature infants with bronchopulmonary dysplasia. In: Farrell PM, Taussig LM, eds. Bronchopulmonary dysplasia and related chronic respiratory disorders. Report of the 90th Ross Conference on Pediatric Research. Columbus, Ohio: Ross Laboratories, 1986, pp 53–57.
34. Stocks J. The functional growth and development of the lung during the first year of life. Early Hum Dev 1977;285–309.
35. Borkenstein J, Borkenstein M, Rosegger M. Pulmonary function studies in long-term survivors with artificial ventilation in the neonatal period. Acta Paediatr Scand 1982;69:159–163.
36. Lamarre A, Linsao L, Reilly B, Swyer P, Levison H. Residual pulmonary abnormalities in survivors of idiopathic respiratory distress syndrome. Am Rev Respir Dis 1973;108:56–61.
37. Coates A, Bergsteinsson H, Desmond K, et al. Respiratory distress syndrome. J Pediatr 1977; 90:611–616.
38. Smyth J, Tabachnik E, Duncan E, et al. Pulmonary function and bronchial hyperreactivity in long-term survivors of bronchopulmonary dysplasia. Pediatrics 1981;69:336–340.
39. Bertrand JM, Riley SP, Popkin J, et al. The long term pulmonary sequelae of prematurity: the role of familiar airway hyperreactivity and the respiratory distress syndrome. N Engl J Med 1985;312:742–745.
40. Knudson R, Clark D, Kennedy T, Knudson D. Effect of aging alone on mechanical properties of the normal adult human lung. J Appl Physiol: Respirat Environ Exercise Physiol 1977; 43(6):1054–1062.

Comments

Bruce R. Boynton

What will be the future role of pulmonary function tests in clinical neonatology? Ideally such tests will distinguish infants destined to develop BPD from those who will recover normally from their primary lung injury. Detection of high-risk infants would allow clinicians to use new techniques such as antioxidants or high-frequency ventilation to prevent or modify further lung damage. It is doubtful whether currently available pulmonary function tests will live up to this expectation. The process of tissue destruction and abnormal repair leading to clinically overt BPD may be well established before abnormalities can be detected with tests of pulmonary mechanics. A more realistic expectation is that pulmonary function testing will be useful in patients with established BPD for the purpose of selecting and monitoring the efficacy of treatments such as steroids, bronchodilators, and diuretics.

16

Diuretic Therapy in Bronchopulmonary Dysplasia

T. F. YEH

Introduction

Bronchopulmonary dysplasia (BPD) is a spectrum of chronic lung disease commonly seen in premature infants as sequelae of respiratory distress syndrome (RDS), oxygen therapy, and mechanical ventilation. The incidence of BPD reported in infants with RDS was about 20% but could vary from 5% to 68% (1–4). BPD is characterized by abnormal gas exchange, increased airway resistance, and decreased lung compliance (5–7). These functional changes are caused by interstitial pulmonary edema, bronchial smooth muscle hypertrophy, and bronchoconstriction. Once the diagnosis of BPD has been established, management is essentially supportive.

Excessive lung water and interstitial edema have been verified pathologically in premature infants recovering from RDS (8). Diuretics may decrease pulmonary arterial pressure by volume depletion and could minimize pulmonary edema and thus may be beneficial to infants recovered from RDS. This chapter presents an overview of diuretic therapy of BPD. Several diuretic agents are available commercially; however, only a few have been tried in infants with BPD.

Furosemide

Furosemide is the most common diuretic used in neonates and small infants. It has been used in infants with BPD, pulmonary edema, congestive heart failure, and fluid overload, and occasionally in infants with hypertension.

Pharmacology

Furosemide is an anthranillic acid derivative (Fig. 16.1). The bioavailability of oral absorption of furosemide has not been well studied in neonates and small infants. It is generally believed that despite incomplete oral absorption, the diuretic effect of furosemide following an oral dose is probably not different from that given intravenously except in the first 2 hours, when a larger response is produced by the intravenous route. Thus the principal advantage of the intravenous route is a rapid early response (9, 10).

About 91% to 99% of plasma furosemide binds with albumin (11–13). The apparent volume of distribution in neonates and small infants is larger than that of adults and ranges from 0.17 to 0.24 L/kg. In small infants with fluid overload, the apparent volume of distribution may increase to as high as 0.82 L/kg (14).

Elimination of plasma furosemide is essentially through the kidney as intact furosemide. It is generally believed that the liver in the newborn infant is immature in microsomal enzymes and is unable to metabolize furosemide. Tuck *et al.* demonstrated in the neonate 90% intact furosemide in the urine at 24 hours following one intravenous dose of

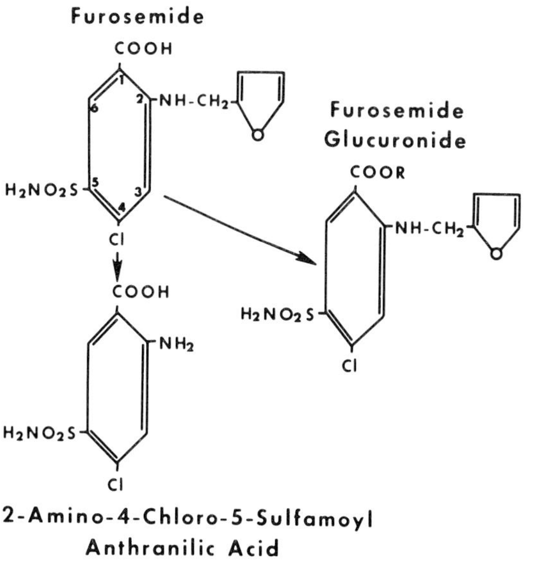

Figure 16.1. Furosemide and Its Metabolites

Table 16.1. Drug Therapy in Bronchopulmonary Dysplasia (BPD)

Agents Possibly Protective Against BPD

   Surfactant therapy
   Vitamin E
   Vitamin A
   Selenium
   Sulfur-containing amino acids
   Superoxide dismutase
   Catalase

Drugs for Cardiopulmonary Distress

   Oxygen therapy
   Bronchodilators
   Dexamethasone
   Diuretics
   Digoxin (?)

Drugs for Infection

   Drugs for upper respiratory tract infection
   Appropriate antibiotics for bacterial pneumonia

furosemide (12). On the other hand Aranda *et al.* were able to detect furosemide gluconide and acid metabolites in urine of infants who had previous exposure to furosemide (15) (Fig. 16.1). The elimination half-life of plasma furosemide ranged from 7.7 to 19.9 hours (13, 14) in infants of 1–40 days. A good correlation between the urinary elimination and plasma clearance of furosemide was observed by Prandota and Houin (16). Renal excretion of furosemide is essentially through the proximal convoluted tubules, similar to that of excretion of para-aminohippuric acid. Because of the extensive protein binding, furosemide is usually not eliminated from the glomerulus. Poor renal and liver function may affect elimination of furosemide.

Mechanism of Action

Ross *et al.* (17) and Woo *et al.* (18) noted a peak diuretic effect within 1 to 3 hours after intravenous injection of furosemide, and this effect persisted above the baseline for approximately 6 hours. The diuretic action of furosemide is directly related to the concentration of intact furosemide in the renal tubule, particularly in the ascending limb of loop of Henle, where it inhibits active reabsorption of chloride and results in a decrease in passive sodium reabsorption and diuresis. At high concentrations furosemide may have an effect on the proximal tubule through inhibition of carbonic anhydrase (10). Furosemide has also been shown to act against antidiuretic hormone (19). This action may be important in infants with BPD in whom vasopressin has been shown elevated (20). Furosemide may stimulate renal prostaglandin synthesis (21), and the renal hemodynamic action of furosemide may be mediated by the prostaglandins. The role of furosemide glucuronide and acid metabolites is not known.

Table 16.2 Diuretic Agents

Drug (Trade Name)	Mechanism of Action	Route of Administration	Onset of Action	Dose
Furosemide (Lasix)	Loop diuretics; inhibits sodium and chloride reabsorption in proximal tubule	IV or IM PO	15–30 min 30–60 min	1 mg/kg/dose 1–3 mg/kg/dose
Chlorothiazide (Diuril)	Inhibits sodium and chloride reabsorption along the distal tubules	PO	1–2 hrs	20–40 mg/kg/24 hrs
Hydrochlorothiazide (Hydrodiuril)	Similar to chlorothiazide	PO	1–2 hrs	2–4 mg/kg/24 hrs
Spironolactone (Aldactone)	Competitive antagonist of aldosterone	PO	3–5 days	1.5–3.0 mg/kg/day
Ethacrynic acid (Edecrin)	Similar to furosemide	IV PO	10–20 min 1 hr	1 mg/kg/dose 1–3 mg/kg/day

(From Oh. W. Diuretic therapy. In T. F. Yeh (ed). *Drug Therapy in Neonate and Small Infant.* Chicago: Year Book Medical Publishers, 1985, with permission.)

Furosemide has been shown to have systemic vascular effects that are independent of its diuretic action. In adult patients with myocardial infarction and congestive heart failure, furosemide increases venous capacitance, resulting in reduced left ventricular filling pressure (22). Furosemide may also diminish the permeability of the microvasculature to protein (23). Thus the mechanisms by which furosemide improves cardiopulmonary status in BPD could be due to the diuretic effect and/or the vascular effect of the drug.

Effects in Infants with BPD

Table 16.3 shows the effects of furosemide therapy on infants with BPD in studies by various investigators (24–30). Although the mechanism is not known, in most of the studies an acute improvement in lung compliance and decrease in airway resistance has been demonstrated following furosemide therapy. Some clinical improvement and decreases in venous admixture were also noted. However, most of these improvements were transient and did not last for more than 6 hours. Kao et al. (28) demonstrated that within 1 hour after intravenous administration of furosemide, 1 mg/kg, to infants with BPD, airway resistance fell 38% (Fig. 16.2) and dynamic compliance increased 54% (Fig. 16.3), associated with an increase of urine output of 226%. The airway resistance and lung compliance returned to baseline values in 2 hours. In a study from our nursery (30), we found that although the use of furosemide (1 mg/kg IV) is associated with an increase in urine output at 0–24 hours following the drug administration, a decrease in PCO_2 and in respiratory distress score were not seen until 2 hours after starting the drug

Table 16.3 Summary of Effects of Furosemide Therapy on Infants with Bronchopulmonary Dysplasia.

Study	Postnatal Age (days)	Dosage and Route of Administration	Clinical Respiratory Distress	pH	PO$_2$	PCO$_2$	A-aDO$_2$	C$_L$	R$_L$	Time (hrs) Evaluated after Initiation of Therapy
Sniderman et al. (24)										
Najak et al. (25)	7–13	1 mg/kg IV single dose				↓	↓	↑		2 hrs
Tapia et al. (26)		2 mg/kg q 12 h IM or IV 2 doses		±	±	±		↑	↓	18 hrs and 36 hrs
Singhal et al. (27)	23–101	1 mg/kg q 12 h IM 3 doses	Improved	↑	±	±		↑		2 hrs and 38 hrs
Kao et al. (28)	77 (mean)	1 mg/kg IV single dose						↑	↓	1 hr
McCann et al. (29)	36–72	1 mg/kg IV q 12 h or 2 mg/kg PO q 12 h for 7 days	Improved	±	±	±	↓	↑	±	48 hrs and 7 days
Patel et al. (30)	217 (mean)	1 mg/kg and 2 mg/kg IV, in 24 hrs for 2 doses	Improved	±	±	↓	±			2 hrs and 26 hrs

↑ Increase.
↓ Decrease.
± No change.

(Fig. 16.4). Similar improvements were seen 2 hours after the second dose of furosemide (2 mg/kg IV), given 24 hours later (Fig. 16.4). If the pulmonary effect of furosemide was related to the diuretic action of the drug, a sustained improvement in respiratory distress would have been seen, since the fluid intake had been kept constant throughout the study. The results of our study and those of Kao *et al.* (28) and Najak *et al.* (25) suggest that furosemide may have direct vascular effects independent of diuretic action in infants with BPD. McCann *et al.* (29) studied the effects of furosemide on BPD following a week of therapy. These investigators reported an improvement in clinical status, an increase in dynamic lung compliance and aveolar ventilation, and a decrease in venous admixture. Infants treated with furosemide could be weaned from mechanical ventilation earlier than the control group.

Indication and Recommended Dosage

Current dosing schedule and indication are somewhat variable. Furosemide may be indicated under three conditions:

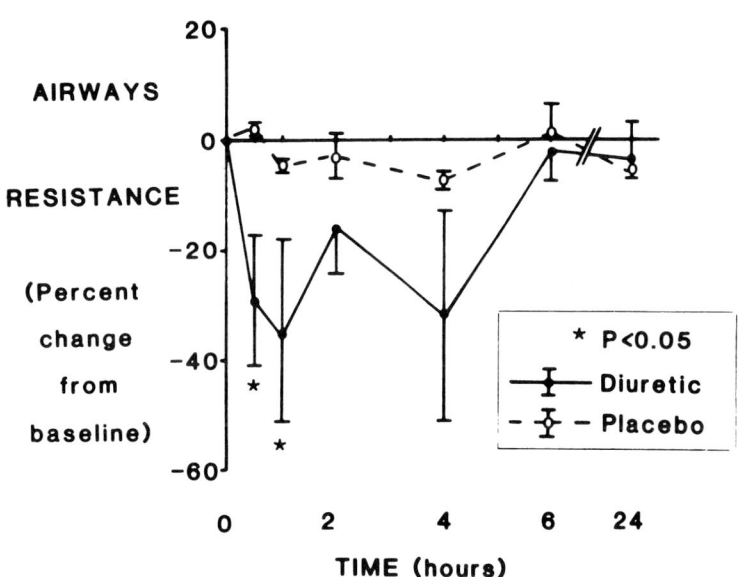

Figure 16.2. Changes of airway resistance following furosemide or placebo administration. Infants in furosemide group had significantly lower airway resistance than the placebo group at a half hour and 1 hour. (Reprinted, with permission, from Kao LC, Warburton D, Sargent CW, Platzker ACG, Keen TG. J Pediatr 1983;103:624–629.)

1. In the early stage of BPD (*e.g.*, Stage II BPD) when pulmonary edema is the main feature.
2. In the late stage of BPD (Stage III-IV) when there is an acute exacerbation of respiratory distress (*e.g.*, following fluid overloading).
3. In the late stage of BPD when there is evidence of pulmonary hypertension, cor pulmonale, or congestive heart failure.

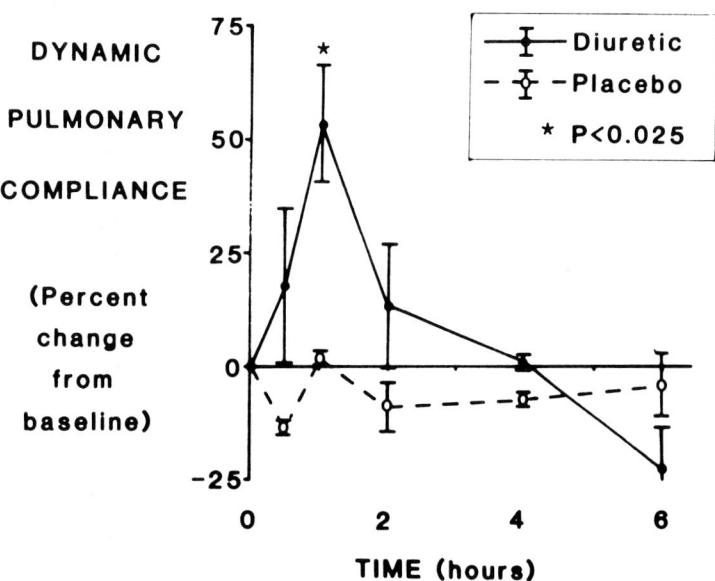

Figure 16.3. Changes of dynamic lung compliance following furosemide or placebo administration. Infants in the furosemide group had significantly higher lung compliance than placebo group at 1 hour after drug administration. (Reprinted, with permission, from Kao LC, Warburton D, Sargent CW, Platzker ACG, Keen TG. J Pediatr 1983;103:624–629.)

Figure 16.4. Changes of RDS score, PCO_2, alveolar-arterial DO_2, pH, and base deficit following 1 mg/kg and 2 mg/kg of furosemide in 24 hour intervals. Significant ($p < 0.05$) decrease in RDS score and PCO_2 was seen at 2 hours. (Reprinted, with permission, from Patel H, Yeh TF, Jain R, Pildes RS. Am J Dis Child 1985;139: 917–920. Copyright 1985, American Medical Association.)

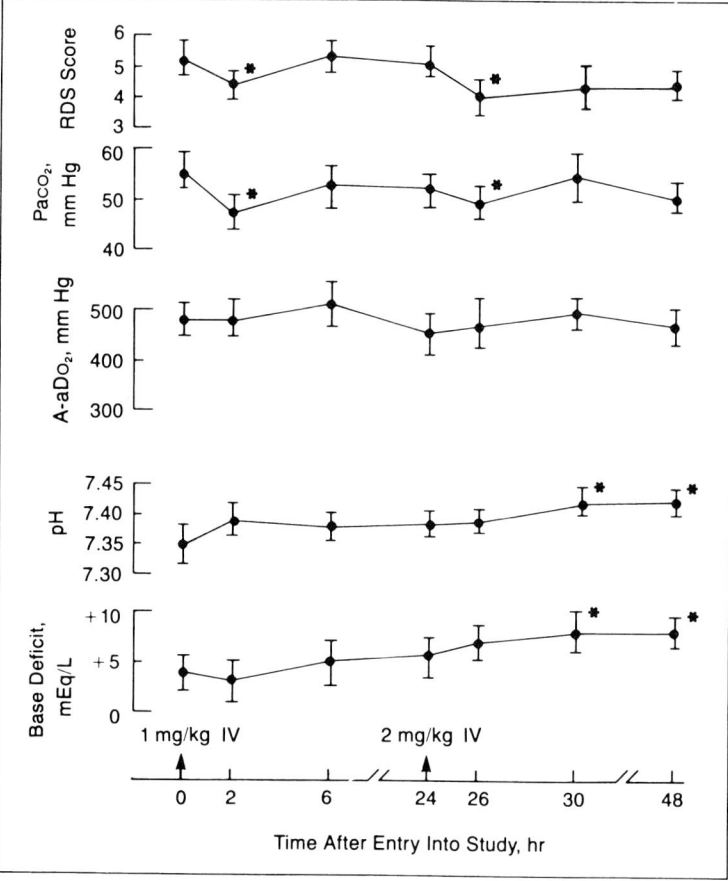

In the first two conditions furosemide 1 mg/kg intravenously every 12 hours can be given for a short period of time if needed. In infants with cor pulmonale or congestive heart failure, furosemide 1 mg/kg can be given intravenously for acute relief of distress, then 1–2 mg/kg orally every 12 hours can be given for 1 week. This can be followed by intermittent weekly courses of therapy if necessary. It was recently suggested that a combination of diuretic and theophylline is very effective for acute decrease of airway resistance and may be recommended in an urgent situation for acute relief of respiratory distress (31).

Side Effects

The side effects following a short period (*e.g.*, 2–3 days) of furosemide therapy are probably not clinically important. However, following prolonged furosemide therapy, the complications could be serious. These include the following:

1. hypercalciuria, renal calcification, urolithiasis and nephrolithiasis

2. electrolytes and fluid imbalance
3. metabolic alkalosis and compensatory hypoventilation
4. secondary hyperparathyroidism
5. cholelithiasis
6. osteopenia and rickets
7. ototoxicity
8. displacement of bilirubin from albumin binding sites

Among these side effects renal calcification and renal stone formation appear to be the most clinically significant.

Hypercalciuria, Renal Calcification, Urolithiasis, and Nephrolithiasis

Furosemide is known to cause increases in urinary excretion of calcium in adults, small infants, and neonates. Although the mechanism is not completely understood, hypercalciuria may play an important role for renal stone formation. Chemical analysis of the stones associated with prolonged furosemide therapy indicated that they are essentially composed of calcium oxalate and calcium phosphate (32). Microscopic examination of the kidney frequently showed calcium deposits in the interstitial area of renal papillae (32).

Table 16.4 lists various reports of renal calcification and/or stone formation (32–38). The highest daily dose of furosemide administered ranged from 1.0 to 16 mg/kg. Duration of furosemide therapy ranged from 11 to 81 days. Age at the time of diagnosis varied from 23 days to 5½ months. Most of the infants did not have symptoms or signs of renal stone formation, but in two infants hematuria and urinary tract infection were presented as initial signs. Renal calcification was usually suspected in plain abdominal roentogenograms, and the diagnosis was confirmed by ultrasound. In some cases the diagnosis was made by postmortem examination at autopsy. In a retrospective study by Robinson *et al.* (38), the incidence of renal calcification in BPD infants who received furosemide therapy was 48%. In this study the average age at the time of diagnosis was 56 days, and the average duration of furosemide therapy was 38 days. Infants who developed renal calcification were smaller, less mature, and received furosemide longer, especially by intravenous route, than the group without calcification. Renal calcification can be resolved spontaneously following discontinuance of furosemide; however, the addition of chlorothiazide therapy (20 mg/kg/d) appeared to be beneficial in the dissolution of the calculus (32).

From these reports some suggestions and recommendations can be made.

1. The incidence of renal calcification is probably high, and the diagnosis is based largely on suspicion or awareness of this complication. Therefore a routine ultrasonogram should be performed on infants who receive furosemide for 2 weeks or longer.
2. An intermittent weekly use of furosemide, followed by complete evaluation of complications, appears to be safer than continuous prolonged use of furosemide.
3. Once renal calcification occurs, furosemide should be discontinued, or a combination of furosemide and chlorothiazide (20 mg/kg/d) should be initiated.
4. Since the etiology of stone formation appears to be related to furosemide induced hypercalciuria, the appropriate medical therapy is to reduce urinary calcium excretion. This can usually be achieved by giving chlorothiazide and withdrawing furosemide. Once the massive calcium excretion has been reversed with chloro-

Table 16.4. Summary of Reports of Furosemide Therapy Administered to Infants with Renal Calcification and/or Stone Formation.

Study	No. of Infants Reported	Highest Daily Dose	Duration of Therapy	Age at Diagnosis of Calcification	Supplemental Ca	Complication(s)	Symptoms and Signs	Diagnosis	Lab findings	Treatment
Hufnagle et al. (32)	10	2–16 mg/kg	12–44 days	23–105 days	—	Nephrolithiasis Urinary tract infection	Urinary tract infection	Radiograph ultrasound	Alkaline phosphatase ↑ Urine Ca ↑	Thiazide
Glasier et al. (33)	2	—	2 months	$2\frac{1}{2}$–$5\frac{1}{2}$ months	Vitamin D Oral Ca	Nephrolithiasis Rickets	Rickets	Radiograph ultrasound	Hematuria Urine Ca ↑	Surgery D/C furosemide
Venkataraman et al. (34)	4	1–6 mg/kg	6–12 weeks	12–15 weeks	Through special care formula	Renal calcification osteopenia	—	Radiograph ultrasound postmortem	Serum parathyroid hormone ↑ Urine Ca ↑ 25-DH Vitamin D ↑ Bone mineral content ↓	—
Noe et al. (35)	1	2–5 mg/kg	5 weeks	5 weeks	—	Urolithiasis hydronephrosis	Hematuria	Ultrasound IVP	Hematuria pyuria	Thiazide and D/C furosemide
Pearse et al. (36)	2	2 mg/kg	13–81 days	3 weeks and 3 months	—	Nephrocalcinosis	—	Ultrasound postmortem	—	—
Gilsanz et al. (37)	9	1–6 mg/kg	11–50 days	—	Through TPN	Nephrolithiasis	—	Radiograph postmortem	—	Thiazide and D/C furosemide
Robinson and Cox (38)	14	5.8 mg/kg (mean)	36 days (average)	56 days (average)	—	Renal calcification	—	Ultrasound	—	Thiazide

↑ Increase.
↓ Decrease.
TPN = total parenteral nutrition.
D/C = discontinue

thiazide, dissolution of even multiple discrete stones can occur. This is a situation not commonly seen in other instances of calcium-containing stone disease. Furthermore renal stones that accompany nephrocalcinosis are usually small and may pass spontaneously or remain without causing serious trouble. Indications for surgical intervention in stone disease have been determined in adults. The infant with BPD presents a special problem in that he has pathologic lungs, posing great risk of complications under general anesthesia. However, if a patient is severely obstructed and infected, then one must relieve the obstruction. Fortunately this is usually not the case with nephrocalcinosis, in which the stones are punctate. Thus medical therapy is the key to correcting the underlying problems, and surgery is reserved for when renal function is jeopardized or the patient is septic from an infected stone and obstruction. In children the technique of extracorporeal shock wave lithotripsy (ESWL) has not been perfected, so that children affected by obstructive stone disease will require open or percutaneous intervention.

Electrolytes and Fluid Imbalance

Furosemide increases the urinary excretion of sodium, chloride, and potassium and may cause hyponatremia and hypokalemia. However, the effects of prolonged use of furosemide on electrolyte balance has not been well studied in infants with BPD. Studies from Najak *et al.* (25) and McCann *et al.* (29) indicated that except for hypochloremia severe electrolyte imbalance did not occur, even though furosemide had been given for 1 week. My clinical impression is consistent with these findings. It is not clear why prolonged use of furosemide in BPD does not produce severe hyponatremia and/or severe dehydration. An alteration in sodium and potassium homeostasis or an alteration in adrenal or renal hormones may occur following prolonged use of furosemide (39). At present I recommend monitoring serum electrolytes closely to ensure that hypokalemia and hyponatremia do not occur.

Metabolic Alkalosis and Compensatory Hypoventilation

Furosemide may cause metabolic alkalosis (40). In adult patients with chronic obstructive lung disease who receive furosemide, compensatory hypoventilation to metabolic alkalosis has been observed, and its potential for hypercarbia has been described (41). Hazinski tested this hypothesis in young rabbits by giving furosemide, 4 mg/kg per day, for 8 to 10 days, and concluded that furosemide induced metabolic alkalosis could indeed cause hypoventilation and hypercarbia (42). If this is also true in infants with BPD, the hypercarbia could obscure the beneficial effects of furosemide and could lead to longer intubation than necessary. Provision of extra chloride would theoretically prevent the hypercarbia. It is therefore advisable to provide extra potassium chloride to the infant if furosemide is to be given for a long duration.

Secondary Hyperparathyroidism

Furosemide therapy is associated with hypercalciuria and hyperparathyroidism in adults (43). Venkataraman *et al.* (34) reported four premature infants who received long-term furosemide therapy because of BPD; three of them showed high serum concentrations of parathyroid hormone and low mineral content of the bone. It was thought that hypocalcemia, resulting from urinary calcium losses, might occur but be transitory and not detected by the usual laboratory methods; secondary parathyroidism might be a reflection of the reaction of the parathyroid glands to small changes in serum calcium concentration, in an attempt to maintain calcium homeostasis. However, the same group of investigators in the results of a later animal experiment, reported no change in serum calcium and bone mineralization (44). They speculated that there might be an increase in calcium absorption from the gastrointestinal tract to compensate for the renal loss of calcium.

Cholelithiasis

Cholelithiasis has been reported in six infants who have received long-term furosemide therapy and total parenteral nutrition (45, 46). Cholestasis is a known complication of prolonged total parenteral nutrition. Furosemide could further alter bile stability or enhance excretion of calcium into the bile, leading to the stone formation. Cholelithiasis in these infants is usually asymptomatic, and is diagnosed by ultrasonogram. Every effort should be made to increase oral feeding and decrease parenteral nutrition. Surgery may be indicated if persistent obstruction of the bile flow or infection occur.

Rickets

Rickets or "osteopenia of prematurity" has been described in premature infants with chronic lung disease. The basic factors resulting in the occurrence of rickets in infants with BPD are not known, but it could be related to the low initial stores of calcium and phosphorus of the bone, the relatively low intakes of calcium and phosphorus, and the increased urinary losses of calcium. Prolonged use of furosemide with excessive losses of urinary calcium has been considered one of the possible causes of rickets in infants with BPD.

Ototoxicity

The ototoxicity of furosemide appears to be related to plasma concentration (47). In adults the plasma level associated with reversible ototoxicity is about 25 μg/mL or greater (48, 49). Since ototoxicity from furosemide is more frequently observed in patients with impaired renal function, and therefore presumably longer half-lives, the prolonged half-life observed in the premature infants should caution against large or repeated doses. Furthermore an apparently synergistic interaction of furosemide with aminoglycosides to produce ototoxicity has been demonstrated in children (50). There are no data available regarding the use of furosemide in premature infants with RDS or BPD and the long-term morbidity of hearing impairment. Peterson *et al.* (13) suggested that furosemide, 1 mg/kg, given parenterally with a frequency of more than twice daily to premature infants in the immediate neonatal period, or in parenteral doses of more than 2 mg/kg, may lead to plasma levels associated with toxicity. I suggest that all infants who receive prolonged furosemide therapy should have audiologic assessment periodically.

Displacement of Bilirubin from Albumin Binding

Furosemide has been shown *in vitro* to displace bilirubin from the albumin-binding site, causing a potential hazard in neonates with hyperbilirubinemia. However, studies from Wennberg et al. (51) and Aranda et al. (14) indicated that a single dose of furosemide (1–1.5 mg/kg) did not displace bilirubin from the albumin-binding site. Since the majority of the infants with BPD are beyond the age of hyperbilirubinemia, this risk is probably not clinically significant.

Chlorothiazides

Thiazides exert their major diuretic effect by inhibiting sodium reabsorption in the distal nephron (10). The resultant sodium retention in the lumen of the distal segment enhances the exchange of sodium for potassium, consequently increasing the excretion of potassium. Chloride is also lost in association with the inhibition of sodium reabsorption. The thiazides also inhibit carbonic analydrase activity in the proximal tubule, but this mechanism is not considered a major contribution to diuresis. Unlike furosemide, the thiazides do not enhance, but decrease, the renal excretion of calcium (10). The excretion of magnesium is also increased by the thiazides; this may lead to hypomagnesemia. The thiazides may also have direct action on renal vasculature, particularly when administered intravenously. Glomerular filtration may be reduced by the thiazides (10). Chlorothiazide (Diuril) and hydrochlorothiazide (Hydrodiuril) are the most common thiazides used in neonates and small infants. The precise mechanism and pharmacokinetics have not been well studied in these age groups. Walker and Cumming (52) administered chlorothiazide to normal infants (75 mg orally); the peak diuresis occurred between 2 and 6 hours, and diuresis lasted about 8 hours after administration. Green et al. (53) demonstrated a diuretic response equivalent to that of furosemide in infants with patent ductus arteriosus who received hydrochlorothiazide (20 mg/kg). Both chlorothiazide and hydrochlorothiazide are given orally; duration of action is about 6–12 hours, so that the dose must be repeated every 12 hours.

Table 16.2 gives indications and dosages for thiazide therapy in BPD. Thiazides have been suggested to replace or to combine with furosemide in the treatment of BPD infants with hypercalciuria and nephrolithiasis (32). Thiazides have also been used in BPD infants with systemic hypertension (54). Chlorothiazide can be given in dosage of 10 to 20 mg/kg orally every 12 hours and hydrochlorothiazide 1 to 2 mg/kg orally every 12 hours.

Side effects of thiazides have rarely been reported in small infants. Hypokalemia is probably the most common electrolyte disturbance associated with chronic therapy. Other side effects include renal and hepatic insufficiency, glucose intolerance and hyperglycemia, increased serum uric acid, hypercalcemia, and magnesium deficiency (10).

Spironolactone

Spironolactone (Aldactone) is a competitive antagonist of aldosterone. As a consequence of interfering with aldosterone binding in the distal segment of the nephron, it increases sodium excretion and decreases potassium excretion (10). The diuretic effect of spironolactone is not as great as that of furosemide and thiazide because the aldosterone dependent distal mechanism for sodium excretion involves only a small fraction of excreted sodium. The diuretic effect of spironolactone is usually not evident until 3–5 days after initiation of therapy. Spironolactone has been suggested to be particularly effective in situations of increased aldosterone secretion. Spironolactone can be given in a daily dose of 1.5–3.0 mg/kg orally.

Summary

The pathogenesis of BPD is probably initiated very early in the neonatal period. Once the underlying pathology has been established, any subsequent treatment is only supportive. Therefore every effort should be directed at the prevention of BPD. Use of furosemide shortly after birth does not appear to be beneficial in reducing BPD morbidity (54, 55). However, furosemide, particularly when given in association with theophylline, is very effective in acute relief of respiratory distress. Whether prolonged use of furosemide would affect the mortality or morbidity of infants with BPD remains to be determined.

References

1. Northway WH Jr. Observations on bronchopulmonary dysplasia. J Pediatr 1979;95:815–818.
2. Edwards DK, Dyer WM, Northway WH. Twelve years' experience with bronchopulmonary dysplasia. Pediatrics 1977;59:839–846.
3. Farrell PM, Palta M. Clinical presentation and pathogenesis: bronchopulmonary dysplasia. Presented at the 90th Ross Conference on Pediatric Research: Bronchopulmonary dysplasia and related chronic respiratory disorders, March 17–20, 1985, Arizona.
4. Avery ME, Hurd SS, Tooley WH. Is chronic lung disease in prematurely-born infants preventable? Pediatr Res 1986;20:341A(abstr).
5. Stocks J, Godfrey S, Reynolds EOR. Airway resistance in infants after various treatments for hyaline membrane disease: special emphasis on prolonged high levels of inspired oxygen. Pediatrics 1978;61:178–183.
6. Morray JP, Fox WW, Kettrick RG, Downes JJ. Improvement in lung mechanics as a function of age in infant with severe bronchopulmonary dysplasia. Pediatr Res 1982;16:290–294.
7. Moylan FMB, Shannon DC. Preferential distribution of lobar emphysema and atelectasis in bronchopulmonary dysplasia. Pediatrics 1979;63:130–134.
8. Rosan RC. Hyaline membrane disease and a related spectrum of neonatal pneumopathies. In: Rosenberg HS, Bolande RP, eds. Perspectives in pediatric pathology, vol 2. Chicago: Year Book Medical Publishers, 1975, pp 15–60.
9. Roberts RJ. Diuretics. In: Roberts RJ, ed. Drug therapy in infants. 1st ed. Philadelphia: WB Saunders, 1984, pp 226–249.
10. Weiner IM, Mudge GH. Diuretics and other agents employed in the mobilization of edema fluid. In: Gilman AG, Goodman LS, Rall TW, Murad F, eds. The pharmacological basis of therapeutics. 7th ed. New York: Macmillan, 1985, pp 887–907.
11. Turmen T, Thorn P, Louridas AT, LeMorvan P, Aranda J. Protein binding and bilirubin displacing properties of Bumetanide and furosemide. J Clin Pharmacol 1982;22:551–556.
12. Tuck S, Morsell P, Broquaire M, Vert P. Plasma and urinary kinetics of furosemide in newborn infants. J Pediatr 1983;103:481–485.
13. Peterson RG, Simmons MA, Rumack BH, Levine RL, Brooks JG. Pharmacology of furosemide in the premature newborn infant. J Pediatr 1980;97:139–143.
14. Aranda JV, Perez J, Sitar DS, et al. Pharmacokinetic disposition and protein binding of furosemide in newborn infants. J Pediatr 1978;93:507–511.
15. Aranda JV, Lambert C, Perez J, Turmen T, Sitar D. Metabolism and renal elimination of furosemide in the newborn infant. J Pediatr 1982;101:777–781.
16. Prandota J, Houin G. Kinetics of urinary furosemide elimination in infants. Dev Pharmacol Ther 1984;7:273–284.
17. Ross BS, Pollak A, Oh W. The pharmacologic effects of furosemide therapy in the low birth weight infant. J Pediatr 1978;92:149–152.
18. Woo WCR, Dupont C, Collinge J, Aranda JV.

Effect of furosemide in the newborn. Clin Pharmacol Ther 1978;23:266–271.
19. Chrysant SG, Baxter PR, Miller RF, Amonette RL. Acute renal function changes induced by furosemide and meclofenamate in the rat. Curr Ther Res 1980;28:741–749.
20. Rao M, Eid N, Mitchell M, Herod L, Parekh A, Steiner P. Antidiuretic hormone (ADH) secretion during respiratory distress in children with bronchopulmonary dysplasia (BPD) (abstr). Pediatr Res 1985;19:413A.
21. Ahallah AA. Interaction of prostaglandin with diuretics. Prostaglandins 1979;18:369–375.
22. Dikshit K, Vyden JK, Forrester JS, Chatterjee K, Prakash R, Swan HJC. Renal and extrarenal hemodynamic effects of furosemide in congestive heart failure after acute myocardial infarction. N Engl J Med 1973;288:1087–1090.
23. Bland RD, McMillan DD, Bressack MA. Decreased pulmonary transvascular fluid filtration in awake newborn lambs after intravenous furosemide. J Clin Invest 1978;62:601–609.
24. Sniderman S, Clyman RI, Chung M, Roth R, Ballard R. Treatment of neonatal chronic lung disease with furosemide (abstr). Pediatr Res 1981;15:682A.
25. Najak ZD, Harris EM, Lazzara A, Pruitt AW. Pulmonary effects of furosemide in premature infants with lung disease. J Pediatr 1983;102:758–763.
26. Tapia JL, Gerhardt T, Goldbert RN, Gomez-del-Rio M, Hehre D, Bancalari E. Furosemide and lung function in neonates with chronic lung disease (CLD) (abstr). Pediatr Res 1983;17:338A.
27. Singhal N, McMillan DD, Rademaker AW. Furosemide improves lung compliance in infants with bronchopulmonary dysplasia (abstr). Pediatr Res 1983;17:336A.
28. Kao LC, Warburton D, Sargent CW, Platzker ACG, Keen TG. Furosemide acutely decreases airway resistance in chronic bronchopulmonary dysplasia. J Pediatr 1983;103:624–629.
29. McCann EM, Lewis K, Deming DD, Donovan MJ, Brady JP. Controlled trial of furosemide therapy in infants with chronic lung disease. J Pediatr 1985;106:957–962.
30. Patel H, Yeh TF, Jain R, Pildes RS. Pulmonary and renal responses to furosemide in infants with Stage III-IV bronchopulmonary dysplasia. Am J Dis Child 1985;139:917–920.
31. Kao LC, Durand DJ, Phillips BL, Lyon MN, Nickerson BG. Comparison of drug therapy in infants with bronchopulmonary dysplasia (abstr). Pediatr Res 1986;20:351A.
32. Hufnagle KG, Khan SN, Penn D, Cacciarelli A, Williams P. Renal calcification: a complication of long-term furosemide therapy in premature infants. Pediatrics 1982;70:360–363.
33. Glasier CM, Stoddard RA, Ackerman NB, McCurdy FA, Null DM, deLemos RA. Nephrolithiasis in infants: association with chronic furosemide therapy. Am J Radiol 1983;140:107–108.
34. Venkataraman PS, Han BK, Tsang RC, Daugherty CC. Secondary hyperparathyroidism and bone disease in infants receiving long-term furosemide therapy. Am J Dis Child 1983;137:1157–1161.
35. Noe HN, Bryant JF, Roy S III, Stapleton FB. Urolithiasis in pre-term neonates associated with furosemide therapy. J Urol 1984;132:93–94.
36. Pearse DM, Kaude JV, Williams JL, Bush D, Wright PG. Sonographic diagnosis of furosemide-induced nephrocalcinosis in newborn infants. J Ultrasound Med 1984;3:553–556.
37. Gilsanz V, Fernal W, Reid BS, Stanley P, Ramas A. Nephrolithiasis in premature infants. Radiology 1985;154:107–110.
38. Robinson CM, Cox MA. The incidence of renal calcifications in low birthweight (LBW) infants on Lasix for bronchopulmonary dysplasia (BPD) (abstr). Pediatr Res 1986;20:359A.
39. Sulyok E, Varga F, Nemeth M, Tenyi I, Csaba IF, Ertl T, Gyory E. Furosemide-induced alterations in the electrolyte status, the function of renin-angiotensin-aldosterone system, and the urinary excretion of prostaglandins in newborn infants. Pediatr Res 1980;14:765–768.
40. DeRubertis FR, Michelis MF, Beck N, Davis BB. Complications of diuretic therapy: severe alkalosis and syndrome resembling inappropriate secretion of anti-diuretic hormone. Metabolism 1970;19:709–719.
41. Tuller MA, Mehdi F. Compensatory hypoven-

tilation and hypercapnia in primary metabolic alkalosis. Am J Med 1971;50:281–290.
42. Hazinski TA. Furosemide decreases ventilation in young rabbits. J Pediatr 1985;106:81–85.
43. Coe FL, Canterbury JM, Firpo JJ, Reiss E. Evidence for secondary hyperparathyroidism in idiopathic hypercalciuria. J Clin Invest 1973;52:134–142.
44. Koo WWK, Guan ZP, Tsang RC, Laskarzewski P, Neumann V. Growth failure and decreased bone mineral of newborn rats with chronic furosemide therapy. Pediatr Res 1986;20:74–78.
45. Whitington PF, Black DD. Cholelithiasis in premature infants treated with parenteral nutrition and furosemide. J Pediatr 1980;97:647–649.
46. Callahan J, Haller JO, Caccianelli AA, Slovis TL, Friedman AP. Cholelithiasis in infants. Association with total parenteral nutrition and furosemide. Radiology 1982;143:437–439.
47. Rybak LP. Pathophysiology of furosemide ototoxicity. J Otolaryngol 1982;11:127–135.
48. Cutler RE, Forrey AW, Christopher TG, Kimpel BM. Pharmacokinetics of furosemide in normal subjects and functionally anephric patients. Clin Pharm Ther 1974;15:588–596.
49. Wigand ME, Heidland A. Ototoxicity side-effects of high dose of furosemide in patient with uraemia. Postgrad Med J 1970;47:54–59.
50. Lynn AM, Redding GJ, Morray JP, Tyler DC. Isolated deafness following recovery from neurologic injury and adult respiratory distress syndrome—a sequela of intercurrent aminoglycoside and diuretic use. Am J Dis Child 1985;139:464–466.
51. Wennberg RP, Rasmussen LF, Ahlfors CE. Displacement of bilirubin from human albumin by three diuretics. J Pediatr 1977;90:647–658.
52. Walker RD, Cumming GR. Response of the infant kidney to diuretic drug. Can Med Assoc J 1964;91:1149–1153.
53. Green TP, Johnson DE, Bass JL, Landrum BG, Ferrara TB, Thompson TR. Prophylactic furosemide in severe respiratory distress syndrome: a blinded prospective study (abstr). Pediatr Res 1986;20:430A.
54. Abman SH, Warady BA, Luni GM, Koops BL. Systemic hypertension in infants with bronchopulmonary dysplasia. J Pediatr 1984;104:928–931.
55. Yeh TF, Shibli A, Leu ST, Admani M, Pildes RS. Early furosemide therapy in premature infants (≤2000 g) with respiratory distress syndrome: a randomized controlled study. J Pediatr 1984;105:603–609.

Comments

T. Allen Merritt

The major challenge in selecting diuretic therapy for infants developing or with diagnosed BPD is achieving a lessening in pulmonary interstitial fluid and transvascular filtration with minimum side effects. Whether furosemide is necessary for protracted periods (often 2 to 3 months) or adequate diuretic effect can be achieved with thiazides, spironolactone, methylxanthines, or combinations of these has not been adequately studied. The addition of steroids only further complicates the pharmacokinetics of these diuretics. Furosemide in doses similar to those used in infants with BPD also exerts nondiuretic functions including a preferential perfusion of nonedematous alveolar units, decreased pulmonary venous resistance and decreased fluid filtration, and effects on gas exchange in the presence of pulmonary edema. Clearly the multiple effects of this potent agent and its interaction with other agents offer a complexity to the determination of mechanism(s) of action in the premature infant. Yet furosemide will continue to be the major drug used in the acute and convalescent phases of BPD.

The adverse side effects of furosemide have been well documented by Dr. Yeh. Anticipatory determination of calcium, potassium, and phosphate balance, periodic abdominal ultrasound for nephrolithiasis, and careful assessment of bony calcification density permit intervention prior to the emergence of major metabolic derangements. Unfortunately the ototoxicity is more problematic, and the interaction of multiple factors influencing sensoryneural hearing loss is less well understood.

Recent evidence supports the enhanced production of atrial naturetic peptide when fluid volumes distend the atria or evidence of congestive heart failure exists, such as in patency of ductus arteriosus. It may be possible to determine optimal diuretic effect by assessing the response of this peptide level to various dosages of diuretics and effectively determine the pharmacologic effect using atrial naturetic peptide measurements. Yet scrutiny of fluid intake, daily weights, presence of edema, and awareness of the adverse effects of these agents on mineral metabolism, remain the current criteria for effective diuretic therapy.

17

Bronchodilators and Anti-inflammatory Agents

ROBERT KATZ AND SHIRLEY MURPHY

Introduction

Bronchodilators are frequently used in the management of infants with bronchopulmonary dysplasia (BPD). Initially this was based on the clinical observation that many of these infants had recurrent episodes of bronchospasm. In the last several years data have been gathered that support this empiric approach. Bonikos et al. showed pathologically that infants who died of BPD had hypertrophied peribronchial smooth muscle even at a young age (1). Nickerson and Taussig showed that infants who developed BPD had first degree or second degree relatives with asthma severe enough to require hospitalization more commonly than controls did (2). Finally, physiologic measurements have confirmed that airway reactivity develops as early as 26 weeks postconception (3). Other studies have demonstrated the presence of airway hyper-reactivity in BPD children from a few months of age until 10 years (4,5). Thus the combination of clinical impressions and physiologic data makes bronchodilator therapy a rational approach in the management of selected infants with BPD.

Theophylline

There have been few objective measurements of the effect of theophylline in infants with BPD. Rooklin et al. performed serial pulmonary function measurements in 11 neonates with BPD after intravenous aminophylline therapy (6). In those infants less than 30 days of age there was a trend (although not statistically significant) toward increases in compliance and decreases in both inspiratory and expiratory resistance. Infants more than 30 days of age had no change in their pulmonary functions. The authors speculated that the lack of response in the older infants may have been due to extensive pulmonary fibrosis which caused irreversible airway obstruction. Kao et al. studied 18 infants with BPD treated with theophylline (7). At the end of the 4 day study period, oral theophylline produced significant improvements in airway resistance, specific conductance, V_{max}, functional residual capacity and maximal expiratory flow. When a diuretic was added to the theophylline an additive effect was noted in most pulmonary functions and compliance compared with placebo.

Theophylline may have other beneficial effects in patients with chronic lung disease. In infants theophylline decreases the frequency and duration of respiratory pauses that occur in association with BPD and may be related to the increased risk of sudden infant death syndrome reported in BPD patients (8). In adults with chronic obstructive pulmonary disease, theophylline improves diaphragmatic function and decreases pulmonary artery pressure (9,10). Infants have been shown to have less fatigue resistant (type 1) fibers in their diaphragm and fatigue

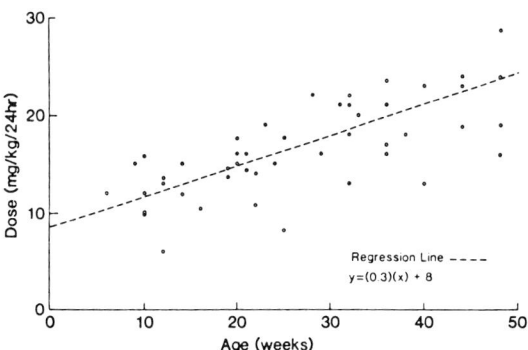

Figure 17.1. Relationship of age and dose required to achieve a steady state peak serum theophylline concentration within the 10–20 μg/mL range among 50 infants 6–48 weeks old ($r = 0.78$, $p < .001$). The linear relationship between age and dose requirements is a function of progressively increasing clearance over the first year of life as the mixed function oxidative enzyme system slowly matures. The formula for the regression of dose on age (dashed line), dosage in mg/kg/24 hr = (0.3)(age in weeks) + 8.0, allows prediction of age specific mean dosage.

Table 17.1 Loading Doses of Aminophylline

Patient Group	IV Dose*	Oral Dose†
Neonates	5–6 mg/kg	4–5 mg/kg
Children		
No previous theo	9 mg/kg	7.5 mg/kg
Previous theo‡		
>6 hr	6 mg/kg	5.0 mg/kg
<6 hr	3 mg/kg	2.5 mg/kg
Previous sustained release theo		
>12 hr	6 mg/kg	5.0 mg/kg
<12 hr	3 mg/kg	2.5 mg/kg

*Based on aminophylline that contains 80% anhydrous theophylline. (From Oglivie RI. Clinical pharmacokinetics of theophylline. Clin Pharmacokinet 1978; 3:267–293.)

†Based on 100% anhydrous theophylline. (From Hendeles L, Massanari M, Weinberger M. Theophylline. In: Evans WE, Schenta JJ, Jusko WJ, eds. Applied pharmocokinetics: principles of therapeutic drug monitoring. 2nd ed. Spokane: Spokane Applied Therapeutics, 1986; pp 1105–1188.)

‡It is recommended that any patient with a history of previous theophylline administration have blood drawn for a serum theophylline determination.

may play a large role in the respiratory manifestations of BPD. The reduction of pulmonary artery pressure may decrease transvascular filtration, and has the potential of minimizing pulmonary edema in BPD infants.

Pharmacokinetics

Studies of theophylline pharmacokinetics in young infants indicate that under the age of 6 months the elimination half-life of theophylline is considerably longer than that found in infants and older children (11). Elimination increases in a linear fashion during the first year of life (Fig. 17.1). However, there have been no specific studies on the pharmacokinetics of theophylline in infants with BPD. This lack of knowledge, combined with the potential for hepatic or cardiac failure in BPD patients, requires careful monitoring of plasma theophylline concentrations.

In an acute attack of wheezing, a loading dose of theophylline is used to obtain a desired plasma concentration quickly. A loading dose may be administered intravenously or orally. General loading dose recommendations when the current theophylline concentration is unknown are given in Table 17.1. The loading doses are based on a mean volume of distribution (V_d) for theophylline of 0.5 L/kg (range 0.3–0.7 L/kg). This relationship would give a 2 mg/L increase in serum theophylline concentration for every 1 mg/kg increment in dose.

$$\text{Plasma concentration (2 mg/L)} = \frac{\text{Dose (1 mg/kg)}}{V_d \text{ (0.5 L/kg)}}$$

After the loading dose is given maintenance theophylline dosages can be given orally or as aminophylline infusions. Recommended infusion rates are listed in Table 17.2 based on the amount of intravenous aminophylline (80% theophylline) required to achieve a steady state theophylline concentration of 15 μg/mL. Regardless of the route of administration, the wide interpatient variability in theophylline clearance mandates that theophylline plasma concentrations be routinely monitored and the dosages adjusted accordingly. This is particularly true in light of the paucity of pharmacokinetic data in infants with BPD.

There are numerous methods for monitoring plasma theophylline concentrations. Most children will be within 95% of their steady state concentration within 12–16 hours on continuous dosing. On continuous intravenous infusions dosages can be adjusted based on one steady state level. Alternatively one can obtain a level 30 minutes after the loading dose and then a second level at 4–8 hours. This will give the clinician what the loading dose achieved and an estimate of whether the infusion rate should be increased or decreased based on whether the second level is increased or decreased from the first.

In regards to chronic therapy with oral theophylline, the doses listed in Table 17.3 conform to the maximum dosage recommended before it is necessary to monitor theophylline blood levels. While theophylline levels maintained between 10 and 20 μg/mL will provide optimal results for the majority of patients, each patient's treatment should be individualized, and whatever plasma theophylline concentration provides optimal effects with minimum side effects is the therapeutic range for a given individual.

A large number of theophylline preparations are available for chronic oral dosing. For neonates and small infants liquid preparations must be used. However, they are the most expensive and least palatable method of administering theophylline and require dosing every 6 hours. Even with this short dosing interval, it may be difficult to achieve consistent therapeutic levels. A liquid preparation without alcohol, sugar, or dyes will be best tolerated. Sustained release formulations improve patient compliance through their ease of administration. Sustained release capsules can be opened and the beads sprinkled on food for the young child; for the older patients there are numerous sustained release tablets available.

Patients may be monitored by beginning them on an average dose based on the patient's age. After at least 3 days on that dose, a theophylline level is determined. If the patient is taking a rapid release product, a trough (lowest) theophylline level is obtained, and should be maintained between 5 and 10 μg/mL. With sustained release theophylline the slow absorption provides a lower peak–trough difference, so that the

Table 17.2. Infusion Rates of Aminophylline

Patient Age	Infusion Rate
1 mo–6 mo*	0.5 mg/kg/hr
6 mo–1 yr	1.0 mg/kg/hr
1 yr–9 yr	1.5 mg/kg/hr

*This age range has the widest interpatient variability and is based on the fewest number of patients.

Table 17.3. Chronic Oral Dosing of Theophylline

Patient Age	Dosage
Neonates	3–9 mg/kg/d
1 mo–6 mo	10 mg/kg/d
6 mo–1 yr	15 mg/kg/d
1 yr–9 yr	24 mg/kg/d

peak level is a better estimate of the steady state plasma level. Therefore peak concentrations should be monitored when using these preparations. If patients are having symptoms at the end of a dosing interval, a serum theophylline determination at that time will help guide the decision whether to administer the drug every 8 hours.

Multiple factors may affect the metabolism and elimination of theophylline. The changes in theophylline clearance that occur with age have been mentioned previously. Of particular relevance to infants with BPD is the fact that clearance of theophylline can be reduced in the presence of cor pulmonale and also during febrile viral respiratory tract infections.

Several drugs affect theophylline clearance, but the clinical relevance of these interactions is variable. For example the concurrent administration of erythromycin decreases theophylline clearance. In contrast chronic administration of phenobarbital or phenytoin increases theophylline clearance, and in patients receiving these drugs theophylline doses may have to be adjusted. The reader is referred to an extensive review for more detail on drug interactions involving theophylline (11).

Toxicity

Theophylline has the potential for a wide range of adverse effects. Caffeine-like side effects, including minor degrees of central nervous system stimulation and gastrointestinal upset, occur frequently after a loading dose and appear to have little direct relationship to serum concentrations (12). More severe and persistent adverse effects generally are associated with serum concentrations above 20 μg/mL and include nausea, vomiting, headache, diarrhea, irritability, and at higher serum levels hyperglycemia, hypokalemia, hypotension, cardiac arrythmias, seizures, brain damage, and death. Among infants and children severe toxicity including death most commonly has resulted from therapeutic mistakes whereby inappropriate dosages have been administered. Irritability, vomiting of coffee-ground-appearing material, and seizures from which the patient never regained consciousness characterize the clinical course in many such patients.

Another major concern with theophylline therapy is in regards to chronic and subtle central nervous system effects. In a study comparing theophylline and cromolyn therapy in asthmatic children, many of the children receiving theophylline were reported to have behavioral problems in school and other subtle CNS effects (13). Although this has not been studied in BPD infants, one could speculate that in this group of infants with a high incidence of development delays and pre-existing brain damage theophylline may have more serious CNS side effects.

β_2-Agonists

Selective β_2-adrenergic agonist aerosols are playing an increasingly greater role in the management of bronchospasm in children. Several studies on the effects of these drugs in infants and children with BPD have been published recently. Kao *et al.* (4) studied the

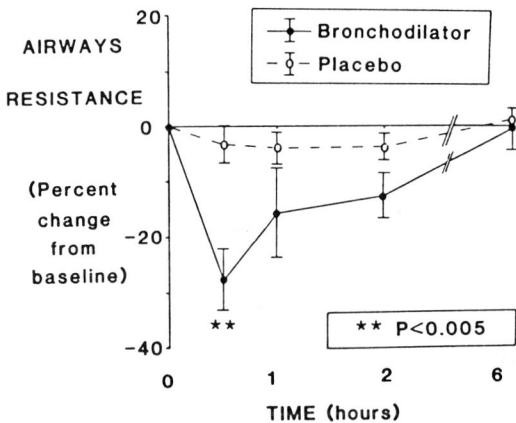

Figure 17.2. Effect of bronchodilator aerosol and placebo on airway resistance. Airway resistance is plotted in percent change from baseline, on the ordinate. Time after administration of bronchodilator aerosol or placebo is plotted on the abscissa in hours. Means ± SEM are shown. There was significant decrease in airway resistance 30 minutes after administration of bronchodilator aerosol.

effect of inhaled isoproterenol, a nonselective β-agonist, on lung mechanics in 10 BPD infants with a mean age of 41 weeks. Thirty minutes after inhalation of the drug, airway resistance dropped by 28% and specific conductance increased by an average of 53% (Fig. 17.2). The fact that the decrease in airway resistance was only significant at 30 minutes may be related to the short duration of action of isoproterenol. Motomoya studied 35 ventilator dependent premature infants who had a mean postnatal age of 45 days (3). After inhalation of isoetharine 42% of the infants had a significant increase in forced vital capacity (FVC), and almost all infants older than 28 weeks postconceptional age had marked increases in $V_{max}25$. Logvinoff studied six infants 5–43 months of age who had moderate to severe BPD and found that inhaled isoproterenol produced a decrease in pulmonary resistance and work of breathing, although the responses were not statistically significant (14). Similar improvements in pulmonary functions have also been seen after the administration of subcutaneous terbutaline and inhaled salbutanol (68,69). Smyth studied an older group of children with BPD (mean age 8.4 years) and found that five of eight improved their flow rates after salbutamol inhalation (5).

The route by which β_2-agonists are delivered is of great importance since it affects onset, duration of action, and selectivity. Inhalation is usually the preferred route of administration for β_2-agonists since the onset of action is rapid, and it provides greater bronchoselectivity than systemic administration (15,16). Studies in asthmatics of direct comparisons of aerosolized β-agonists versus the oral form demonstrated that the aerosolized form was significantly more effective in increasing FEV_1 than the oral administration (16,17). For young infants and children β_2-agonists can be delivered with a jet nebulizer driven by air or oxygen. Older children who can be taught the proper technique can use a metered dose inhaler. Tables 17.4 and 17.5 list the most commonly used β_2-agonists by nebulizer and metered dose inhalers.

The nebulized solution of albuterol has recently become available for use in the United States and is probably the β_2 agonist of choice in most circumstances. Because of β_2 selectivity, more bronchodilation is achieved with less tachycardia than with higher doses of the nonselective metaproterenol (18). For older children a wide variety of metered dose inhalers are available including metaproterenol, terbutaline, albuterol, and bitolterol. It is crucial that these inhalers be used properly to achieve optimal results. Due to the high incidence of developmental de-

Table 17.4. β_2-Adrenergic Aerosols

Drug	Preparation	Dosage
Metaproterenol		
Alupent	5% (50/mg/mL) Sol'n for nebulization	0.25–0.5 mg/kg every 2–4 hr
Metaprel	0.6% Unit dose vial of 2.5 mL (15 mg)	
Terbutaline		
Brethaire	0.1% (1 mg/mL) Sol'n in 0.9% NaCl for injection (not approved for this use)	0.1–0.3 mg/kg every 2–6 hr
Isoethranine		
Isoetharine hydrochloride	0.1%, 0.125%, 0.2%	0.1–0.2 mg/kg every 2–4 hr
Bronkosol	0.25%	
Albuterol		
Proventil	0.5% (5 mg/mL) Sol'n for nebulization	0.05–0.15 mg/kg every 2–4 hr
Ventolin		

(Adapted from Kelly WH. New β_2-adrenergic agonist aerosols. Clin Pharm 1985; 4:393–413.)

Table 17.5. β_2-Adrenergic Metered Dose Inhalers

Drug	Preparation	Dosage
Metaproterenol		
Alupent	0.65 mg/puff (300 puffs)	2–3 puffs every 4–6 hr
Albuterol		
Ventolin Proventil	90 µg/puff (200 puffs)	1–2 puffs every 4–6 hr
Terbutaline		
Brethaire	0.2 mg/puff (300 puffs)	1–2 puffs every 4–6 hr
Fenoterol		
Berotec	0.16 mg/puff (300 puffs)	1–2 puffs every 4–6 hr
Bitolterol mesylate		
Tornalate	0.37 mg/spray (300 sprays)	1–3 sprays every 4–6 hr

(Adapted from Kelly WH. New β_2-adrenergic agonist aerosols. Clin Pharm 1985; 4:393–413.)

lays in children with BPD, many of the patients may have difficulty mastering the use of an inhaler and must add a spacer or continue to use a nebulizer.

Side effects from β_2-agonists are largely due to β-adrenoceptor stimulation and depend on dose, selectivity, and route of administration. The most commonly seen adverse effects include tachycardia, tremor, CNS stimulation, palpitation infrequently, and occasional gastrointestinal side effects. Systemic administration produces an increase in serum glucose and a drop in serum potassium. Overall, side effects are minimal and rarely result in discontinuation of therapy. However, there have been no detailed studies on the side effects of these drugs in infants and children with BPD.

Oral preparations of metaproterenol and albuterol are also available in elixir form for infants and children. However, because of the increased frequency of side effects such as tremor, tachycardia, and hyperexcitability, administration by the inhaled route is preferred for treating acute and chronic bronchospasm in these patients.

Steroids

Since 1983 multiple studies have looked at the effect of steroids on the ventilator dependent infant with BPD. Most of the study

Table 17.6. Use of Steroids in Bronchopulmonary Dysplasia

Study	No. Patients	Design	Results	Comments
Pomerance & Puri (70)	10	Retrospective, uncontrolled	2/10 – Weaned 8/10 – ↓ PIP	Multiple complications, sepsis, NEC, ↑ BP, osteo, pneumothorax
Grylack et al. (71)	14	Retrospective, uncontrolled	8/14 – ↓ A-aO_2 9/14 – ↓ Vent Tx	Hypertension, glucosuria
Kramer & Hultzan (72)	11	Uncontrolled	11/11 – ↑ C_L ↓ A-aO_2 ↓ Vent Tx	Multiple complications
Shick et al. (73)	23	Retrospective, uncontrolled	13/23 – ↓ A-aO_2 ↓ PCO_2	Prednisone, no mention of complications
Mammel et al. (19)	6	Double-blind, crossover, randomized	6/6 – ↓ A-aO_2 ↓ PIP ↓ Vent Tx	Sequential analysis—study terminated after only 6 patients; multiple septic complications
Avery et al. (20)	14	Randomized	7/7 – ↑ C_L 7/7 – Weaned	Sequential analysis; minimal complications
Mammel et al. (21)	8	Controlled, prospective	8/8 – Weaned 8/8 – ↓ FiO_2	"Control" group had less significant lung disease

↓ = decrease; ↑ = increase; PIP = peak inspiratory pressure; A-aO_2 = alveolar-arterial oxygen gradient; Vent Tx = ventilatory therapy; C_L = pulmonary compliance; PCO_2 = arterial carbon dioxide tension; FiO_2 = fraction of inspired oxygen; NEC = necrotizing entolocolitis; BP = blood pressure.

designs were retrospective and uncontrolled. To date only two randomized prospective studies have been published, and they involved small numbers of patients (Table 17.6). Mammel et al. administered dexamethasone (0.5 mg/kg/d) to six infants with long-established BPD and noted a marked improvement in clinical status and pulmonary function (19). Significant improvement in ventilator determined respiratory rate, peak-inspiratory pressure, supplemental oxygen, and alveolar-arterial oxygen tension gradient occurred in all infants receiving dexamethasone (Table 17.7). Although the study was double-blind and randomized, the use of sequential analysis and marked short-term improvement resulted in a very small study group. In addition, three of the six infants died from septic complications after the acute part of the study was completed while they were on "weaning" doses of dexamethasone.

Avery and coworkers used a shorter course of steroids in a group of premature infants who remained ventilator dependent at 2 weeks of life (20). The patient population consisted of seven pairs of matched infants of 1500 g birth weight and less than 6 weeks postnatal age who were refractory to weaning from ventilatory support despite diuretic

Table 17.7. Dexamethasone Treatment Versus Placebo in Six Infants with BPD

Variable	Baseline	Dexamethasone	Placebo
Rate	19 ± 10	5 ± 7*	17 ± 15
PIP (cm H_2O)	26 ± 7	14 ± 15	23 ± 13
PEEP (cm H_2O)	3.5 ± 1.0	2.7 ± 1.5	3.3 ± 0.8
FiO_2	0.49 ± 0.13	0.31 ± 0.06*	0.45 ± 0.25
$A-aO_2$ (torr)	236 ± 82	159 ± 55*	271 ± 183

*$p < 0.05$
PIP = peak inspiratory pressure; PEEP = positive end-expiratory pressure; FiO_2 = fraction of inspired oxygen; $A-aO_2$ = alveolar-arterial oxygen tension difference.

therapy and fluid restriction. All seven pairs favored dexamethasone therapy in weaning from ventilatory support within 72 hours. Dynamic pulmonary compliance improved significantly in infants receiving dexamethasone, as compared with the control infants. There were few complications in this short-term study, which demonstrated that dexamethasone was relatively safe and resulted in extubation within 3 days. However, the number of infants studied was small, the steroid group tended to require less ventilatory support, criteria for extubation were not defined, and the study was not blinded.

Mammel and his colleagues have recently treated another eight infants with BPD with a 2 week course of dexamethasone (21). Significant improvements were noted in ventilatory status and in supplemental oxygen needs for all treated infants within 7 days. The incidence of septicemia, rickets, and retinopathy of prematurity were similar in patients with BPD or uncomplicated respiratory distress syndrome. Most dexamethasone-treated patients developed arterial hypertension which returned to normal after therapy was discontinued. Two patients had decreased responses to infusion of 0.25 mg cosyntropin 1–2 months after dexamethasone was discontinued; however, their responses returned to normal 6 months later.

The mechanism whereby steroid improves lung function is unknown. Multiple hypotheses have been suggested including decreased polymorphonuclear cell recruitment to the lungs, decreased leukotriene production, increased surfactant synthesis, and perhaps enhanced β_2-adrenergic receptor responsiveness.

It appears from these two controlled studies and other uncontrolled trials that dexamethasone treatment leads to significant acute, short-term improvement in pulmonary functions with BPD and facilitates weaning from ventilatory support and supplemental oxygen. However, significant morbidity may occur, including septic complications, systemic hypertension, and possibly adrenal suppression. Many questions remain about steroid therapy in BPD: 1) which subgroup of patients will benefit the most; 2) what is the optimal dosing schedule; and 3) what are the long-term effects on the developing infant? It is clear that further studies are required before widespread use of steroids can be recommended.

Cromolyn Sodium

Cromolyn sodium (disodium cromoglycate) was discovered in 1965 and has been used for the treatment of asthma in the United Kingdom since 1968 and in the United States since 1973 (22).

Cromolyn sodium is synthesized by link-

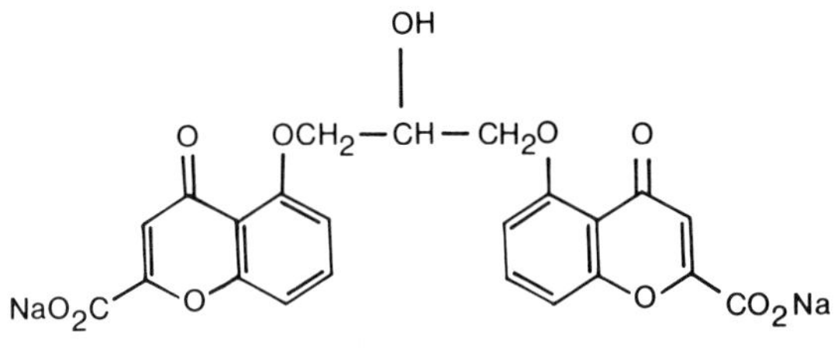

Figure 17.3. Cromolyn sodium is synthesized by linking two monochrome nuclei with a shared alkyl residue.

ing two monochromone nuclei with a shared alkyl residue (23). It is a white hydrated powder that is a lipophobic, highly polar, acidic molecule with a pka of 2 and a molecular weight of just over 500 daltons (Fig. 17.3).

Mechanisms of Action

Despite intensive research, a precise mechanism that explains cromolyn sodium's clinical activity has not been completely delineated. The primary mode of action of cromolyn sodium is considered to be that of stablizing mast cells, which prevents the subsequent release of mediators. Early laboratory studies of antigen challenge of tissues presensitized with reaginic (IgE) antibodies demonstrated that cromolyn sodium inhibited the release of biologically active chemical mediators (23).

Further experiments established that cromolyn sodium exerted an inhibitory effect on rat mast cells degranulated by other nonimmunologic substances including phospholipase A compound 48/80, and the calcium ionophore A 23,187 (23).

Cromolyn sodium appears to exhibit tissue specificity, preventing release of mediators from lung mast cells, but not circulating basophils or skin mast cells (23).

Recent studies have confirmed that cromolyn can block both the release of β-hexosaminidase and leukotrienes from mast cells (24). However, in some *in vitro* models coculturing mast cells with cromolyn for 5 to 7 days may be required to obtain the maximum inhibitory effect (24).

The effect of cromolyn sodium has been examined in cells obtained by bronchoalveolar lavage, which may be more representative of mast cells which come into contact with allergens (25). Cromolyn sodium is more effective in blocking mast cell mediator release in these lavage cells than in chopped lung mast cells (25).

Administration of cromolyn sodium prior to antigen challenge blocks both the antigen induced bronchospasm and the serum rise of neutrophil chemotactic activity (26). Neutrophil chemotactic factor (NCF-A) has a molecular weight of 500,000 daltons and is considered to be of mast cell origin (26). This *in vivo* inhibition of NCF-A adds to the confirmation of *in vitro* inhibition of mast cell mediator release by cromolyn sodium.

In a clinical study, 3 months of cromolyn sodium therapy resulted in a significant decrease in the number of eosinophils recovered in bronchoalveolar lavage fluid (27) (Fig. 17.4). Thus cromolyn sodium, by blocking the release of mast cell mediators such as eosinophil chemotactic factor (ECF-A), and leukotriene E_4 (LTB_4), may prevent recruitment of eosinophils into the lungs.

Several theories have been proposed and investigated as to the exact cellular mechanisms by which cromolyn sodium inhibits mast cell mediator release, but none has been definitely established. Like many other secretory systems the antigen induced release of

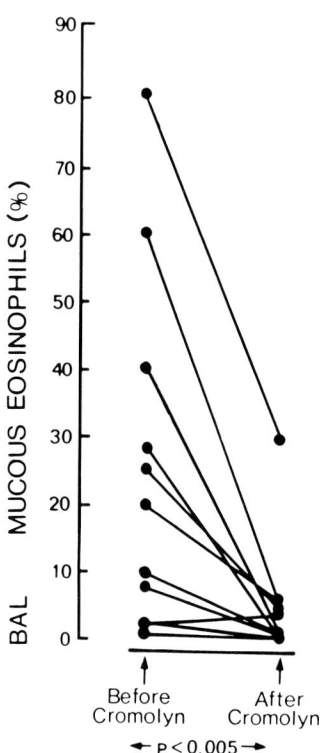

Figure 17.4. Three months of cromolyn sodium therapy resulted in a significant decrease in the number of eosinophils recovered in bronchoalveolar lavage fluid. (Reprinted, with permission, from Diaz P, Galleguillo FR, Gonzalez MC, Poutin CFA, Kay AB. Broncheolar lavage in asthma. J Allergy Clin Immunol 1984;74:41–48.)

histamine and other mediators from mast cells requires extracellular calcium. The secretory process is initiated by aggregation of Fc receptors bound to mast cell membranes. After this trigger a series of biochemical events occur resulting in the transient increase in permeability of the mast cell's plasma membrane to calcium ions. Although no direct evidence is available, this calcium influx may occur via membrane channels (28). Cross-linking of membrane bound IgE by antigen results in opening the ion channels. Incubation of mast cells with cromolyn sodium abolishes or inhibits the channel conductance (28).

A biochemical basis by which cromolyn prevents mast cell mediator release may be through its ability to induce phosphorylation of a protein with a molecular weight of 78,000 daltons (29). Phosphorylation of this specific protein occurs 30 to 60 seconds after stimulation of rat peritoneal mast cells, and coincides with the termination of the entire secretory process. These experiments suggest that cromolyn sodium activates a naturally occurring cell mechanism which is thought to represent an off switch to mast cell mediator release (29).

Although the key cell type affected by cromolyn has usually been considered to be the mast cell, cromolyn has been shown to inhibit the activation of other cell types (30). Cromolyn sodium at a concentration of 10^{-7} mol/L inhibits peripheral blood leukocyte activation as measured by formyl-methionyl-leucyl-phenylalanine (FMLP) induced enhancement of complement and IgG rosettes (30). Inhalation of cromolyn sodium prior to exercise challenge will also inhibit the enhanced neutrophil and monocyte activation that occurs in asthmatic patients (31).

Cromolyn sodium has been shown to reduce significantly platelet-activating factor (PAF-acether) induced immediate and delayed inflammatory responses in the skin of nonatopic volunteers (32).

Besides acting on mast cells these new observations suggest that cromolyn sodium may have a direct suppressive effect on other inflammatory cells, which could result in modulating inflammatory mechanisms in asthma.

In animal pharmacologic experiments cromolyn sodium has not demonstrated smooth muscle relaxant properties (either *in vitro* or *in vivo*). However, cromolyn sodium administered by nebulization in stable asthmatic children was shown to be an effective bronchodilator comparable in degree and duration of effect to salbutamol (33). However, other investigators have not shown this (34,35).

In isolated guinea pig tracheal strips, cromolyn attenuates the acetycholine, histamine, serotonin, bradykinin, and $PGF_{2\alpha}$ induced contractile responses in a dose dependent response (36). On the other hand cromolyn potentiates isoproterenol, epinephrine, PGE_2, and salbutamol induced relaxation responses and shifts these dose-response curves downward (36). These experiments suggest that cromolyn may have a direct action on smooth muscle or may potentiate the relaxation induced by other pharmacologic agents.

Cromolyn has been shown to inhibit bronchoconstriction induced in man by a number of nonimmunologic triggers, including exercise, inhalation of cold air, sulfur dioxide, and ultrasonically nebulized distilled water or fog, suggesting that it could have a neuropharmacologic effect (23).

Cromolyn sodium inhibits excitatory responses of "C" fiber sensory nerve endings in the dog lung, which initiate reflex bronchoconstrictor responses in the dog (37). Cromolyn sodium also inhibits a component of the bronchoconstriction induced by leukotriene D_4 which is mediated by vagal reflex. These data indicate that cromolyn may exert an effect through a neuropharmacologic mechanism.

Pharmacokinetics

Intravenous administration of cromolyn shows that it is rapidly cleared from plasma and excreted unchanged, with 50% in the urine and 50% in the bile. The disposition of cromolyn sodium following intravenous administration fits a two-compartment open pharmacokinetic model (22) (Table 17.8).

Oral dosing shows that oral absorption is less than 1%. Therefore the amount of drug in plasma after inhalation is a good estimate of total dose to the lung. Because of the relatively short terminal half-life of cromolyn sodium (11–20 minutes) and its low bioavailability, there is no significant accumulation during therapy (22). The amount of cromolyn absorbed after inhalation varies according to the delivery system and the dose.

Adverse Reactions and Toxicity

Long-term, worldwide clinical experience with the use of cromolyn sodium in various forms has shown that adverse reactions are rare. The most common side effects are transient cough and mild wheezing with use of the powder formulation which rarely require treatment or discontinuation of the drug.

According to experience accumulated since the availability of cromolyn sodium in the United States in 1973, the following incidence of adverse reactions to cromolyn sodium has been reported in less than 1 in

Table 17.8. Pharmacokinetics of Intravenous Cromolyn Sodium

Alpha:	22.5 ± 10 hr^{-1}
Beta:	1.85 ± 0.13 hr^{-1}
T ½:	0.32 hr
Clp	0.35 ± 0.1 L/kg hr^{-1}
Vd$_{Beta}$	0.2 ± 0.04 L/kg

Clp = plasma clearance
Vd$_{Beta}$ = Volume of distribution beta phase

10,000 patients: laryngeal edema, swollen parotid gland, angioedema, bronchospasm, joint swelling and pain, dizziness, dysuria and urinary frequency, nausea, cough, wheezing, headache, nasal congestion, rash, urticaria, and lacrimation.

Other adverse reactions have been reported in less than 1 in 100,000 patients, and it is unclear whether these were attributable to the drug: anaphylaxis, nephrosis, periarteritic vasculitis, pericarditis, peripheral neuritis, pulmonary infiltrates with eosinophilia, polymyositis, exfoliative dermatitis, hemoptysis, anemia, myalgia, hoarseness, photodermatitis, and vertigo.

Although most side effects are mild, there are a few case reports of more serious adverse experiences with cromolyn (38,39,40). Anaphylaxis with inhaled cromolyn sodium was reported in a 7 year old timothy sensitive asthmatic girl after 1 week of inhalation (41). In a prospective study of adverse reactions to cromolyn in 375 patients, the frequency of side effects of the drug was 2% (8/375), and these were all not serious and completely reversible.

Acute toxicity studies have demonstrated an extremely low order of toxicity. Parenteral administration in mice, rats, guinea pigs, hamsters, and rabbits demonstrated an LD_{50} of 4000 mg/kg. With oral administration no deaths have occurred at the highest doses given to rats and mice (8000 mg/kg). By inhalation, even in long-term studies, it has proved impossible to achieve toxic dose levels of cromolyn sodium in a range of mammalian species.

Animal studies have demonstrated no effect on urinary, endocrine, or central nervous systems of doses up to 10 mg/kg intravenously. In most species the drug has no effect on the cardiovascular and respiratory systems. However, in marmosets and dogs there was an effect with intravenous administration. In marmosets, intravenous doses of 1 μg/kg produced an increase in blood pressure and heart rate, while with higher doses there was also transient apnea. In contrast intravenous doses of 10 μg/kg and above in dogs produced bradycardia and hypotension, with apnea occurring in some cases.

Cromolyn sodium is listed as Pregnancy Category B, and no chromosomal damage, mutagenesis, or impaired fertility has been shown. Also six to 18 month studies in animals have shown no neoplastic effect (package insert 1985). Cromolyn sodium was used to treat 296 asthmatic women throughout pregnancy. Malformations occurred in four newborns (1.35%), which represented a frequency less than that reported for the population as a whole (2%–3%) (42).

Clinical Effectiveness

Cromolyn sodium protects against challenge with a variety of antigens in man and animals (23). It also blocks the effect of antigen challenge on mucociliary clearance and returns impaired mucociliary function found in asymptomatic asthmatics to normal (43). The effect of sulfur dioxide challenge is also blocked by cromolyn and shows dose dependency (44). Inhalation of cromolyn sodium blocks a variety of occupational substances including toluene diisocyanate, western red cedar, laboratory animal sensitivity, and metabisulfites. Exercise and cold air challenge have also been shown to be blocked by cromolyn (23).

The occurrence of late asthmatic response has been shown to correlate with more severe asthma and has been associated with a pulmonary inflammatory response (45). Cromolyn sodium inhaled before challenge will block both the early and the late asthmatic response in man and in animal models (46,47). Long-term therapy with cromolyn also will decrease nonspecific bronchial hyper-reactivity as measured by both histamine and methacholine (48).

Nebulizer Solution

Cromolyn sodium has been available in the United States as a 1% nebulizer solution since 1982. It contains 20 mg cromolyn sodium in 2 mL of purified water with no preservatives and is packaged in 2 mL unit dose glass ampules. The clear, colorless solution has a pH of 4.0–7.0 and is administered from a power operated nebulizer having an adequate flow rate via face mask or mouthpiece. The face mask has the potential of delivering the medication to the entire upper airway, which may be an advantage in patients who also have allergic rhinitis.

Cromolyn sodium nebulizer solution has been shown to be physically and chemically compatible for up to 60 minutes when mixed *in vitro* with metaproterenol sulfate solution, isoproterenol hydrochloride solution, isoetharine hydrochloride 0.25% inhalation solution, epinephrine hydrochloride solution, terbutaline sulfate sterile aqueous solution, and 20% acetyl-cysteine solution (49). Therefore it is possible to make a mixture of medications which can be simultaneously nebulized to the patient.

Cromolyn sodium as a 1% solution has been studied in several clinical trials in very young asthmatic patients. Hiller and coworkers (50) studied 17 asthmatic children under 5 years of age in a double-blind placebo controlled randomized 2 month crossover trial. Daily symptom scores kept by the parents showed improvement in 11 children during active treatment.

Mellon and colleagues (51) studied 1% cromolyn sodium nebulizer solution in 19 young asthmatic children (1–7 years of age) who required daily oral bronchodilators but not corticosteroid therapy. During the 8 week active treatment phase, significant reductions in asthmatic symptoms, physician assessment of asthma severity, and concomitant bronchodilator usage were observed in 16 of 19 children. These 16 patients continued to receive nebulizer cromolyn sodium treatment for at least 1 year after completion of the study. During the 6 months of cromolyn maintenance, there was a marked reduction in emergency visits ($p < .01$), corticosteroid courses, and hospitalizations (51).

In an open study 50 children under 4 years of age with severe chronic asthma were treated with nebulized cromolyn sodium (20 mg inhaled for 10 minutes four times a day) for 6 months (52). Thirty-three children showed marked improvement with no attacks occurring during the treatment period while 13 showed partial improvement. There was also a marked decrease in the use of other medications and in hospital admissions.

Newth and coworkers (53) compared 1% nebulized cromolyn sodium given four times a day with liquid theophylline given every 6 hours to maintain serum concentrations of approximately 10–20 mg/L in controlling symptoms of chronic asthma in pre-school-children in a double-blind crossover study with each treatment period lasting 8 weeks. Patients had an average of 61% symptom-free days while on cromolyn sodium compared with only 46.5% for days free of symptoms when on theophylline alone ($p < .05$) (Fig. 17.5). Numerous adverse side effects from

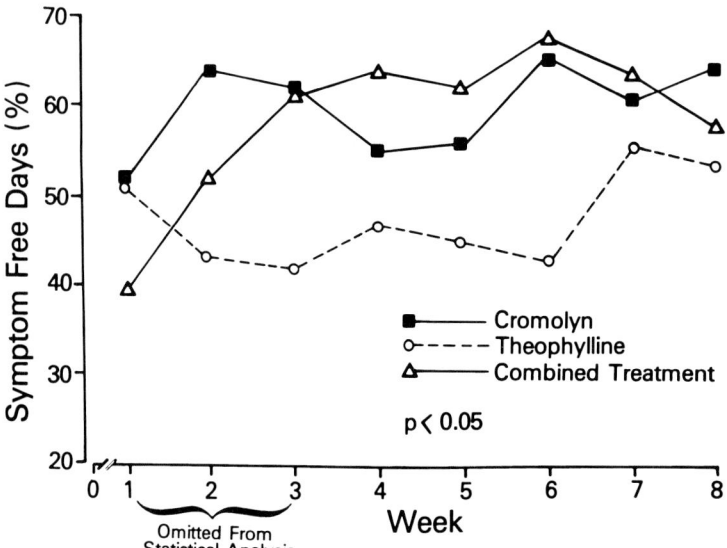

Figure 17.5. Preschool children treated with either nebulized cromolyn or theophylline in a double-blind crossover study with each treatment period lasting 8 weeks. Patients had an average of 61% symptom free days while on cromolyn sodium compared with only 46.5% when on theophylline alone. ($p < .05$) (Reprinted, with permission, from Newth CJL, Newth CV, Turner JAP. Comparison of nebulized sodium cromglucate and oral theophylline in controlling symptoms of chronic asthma in pre-school children. Aust NZ J Med 1982;12:232.

theophylline were reported, but none was recorded while patients were receiving cromolyn sodium.

Cromolyn in Bronchopulmonary Dysplasia

Lavage studies have shown a prolonged increase in numbers of neutrophils and neutrophil derived elastase in the lavage fluids of infants who develop BPD (54,55). Lavage studies in older infants (1 to 9 months of age) still requiring mechanical ventilation also demonstrated a marked leukocytosis with a predominance of polymorphonuclear cells (56). These lavage fluids contained leukotriene-like bioactivity in five of eight infants and platelet activating factor in nine of nine (56).

Cromolyn sodium (20 mg nebulized every 6 hours) was administered to 10 infants who required prolonged mechanical ventilation. Eight of the 10 demonstrated clinical improvement with decreased FiO_2, decreased wheezing, decreased respiratory rate, and decreased ventilatory pressures (56). Lavage in four of four infants after treatment showed decreases in total white cell counts, neutrophil counts, and alveolar macrophage counts (56).

Airway reactivity develops early in BPD patients and is still present years later at follow-up (5). Also, infants with advanced pulmonary changes due to BPD have a significant family history of reactive airway disease (2). Thus cromolyn sodium may play an important role in the long-term management of BPD either by its anti-inflammatory effect or through its ability to reduce nonspecific bronchial hyperreactivity. The exact role of cromolyn sodium in the management of BPD awaits further controlled clinical trials.

Atropine

Mechanism of Action

Current concepts of the control of airways caliber in humans demonstrate the apparent dominance of the parasympathetic system. In normal subjects there is a level of bronchomotor tone caused by tonic parasympathetic activity (57). In animals stimulation of the distal end of cut vagal branches to the lung results in bronchoconstriction (58). This parasympathetic bronchoconstriction can be prevented by blocking vagal conduction or by atropine (3) and can be potentiated by cholinesterase inhibitors. The site of airways narrowing is almost entirely ipsilateral to the vagal stimulation and principally in airways of intermediate size (59).

The parasympathetic efferent pathway functions as the motor limb of a reflex arc whose afferents originate as sensory receptors that have been found immediately beneath the tight junctions between epithelial cells, the "irritant receptors" (57).

Pharmacology

Atropine is well absorbed from the gastrointestinal tract and mucosa. It is distributed throughout the body and crosses the blood-brain barrier. It is largely excreted in the urine, and its serum half-life is 3 hours in young adults and two to three times as long in children (60).

The systemic side effects of antimuscarinic agents are dose related (57). Dryness of the mouth and skin occur at an absorbed dose of 0.5 mg in adults. At about 2.0 mg tachycardia and blurred vision occur, and at 5.0 mg problems with speech, swallowing, micturition, and flushing of the skin occur. At higher doses mental changes occur. The smallest dose of inhaled atropine sulfate that produces significant bronchodilation in adults is about 0.4 mg, which is the level at which side effects may occur.

Inhaled nebulized atropine produces optimal bronchodilation at a dose of 0.05 mg/kg in children (61). After inhalation absorption from the respiratory and gastrointestinal tract is erratic and blood levels are highly variable (62). After optimal doses a significant proportion of subjects experience side effects (62).

Clinical Trials

Most of the clinical trials conducted in the last 10 years with anticholingeric agents have utilized ipratropium bromide, a synthetic quaternary ammonium, which is poorly absorbed and does not cross the blood-brain barrier. This gives it a wider therapeutic margin than atropine. Ipratropium bromide has recently been approved for use with a metered dose inhaler in the United States and is available in Canada, the United Kingdom, and Europe in both a metered dose inhaler and nebulizer form (Fig. 17.6).

In the majority of clinical trials in adult asthmatics, ipratropium bromide has been found to be as effective as β_2-agonists in the treatment of acute and chronic asthma (57). In adults the combination of ipratropium bromide with β_2-agonists has produced an additive and often a more prolonged effect (57). In chronic bronchitis patients it may be more effective than β_2-agonists (57,63).

Studies in children have shown ipratropium to be an effective and safe drug. Lin et al. (64) demonstrated that the combination of orally administered metaproterenol and inhaled ipratropium bromide in children with stable asthma produced significantly better bronchodilation than either drug alone. Mann and Miller (65) showed that ipratropium bromide significantly improved symptoms in children with asthma maintained with inhaled cromoglycate or beclomethasone. A dose-response curve for ipratro-

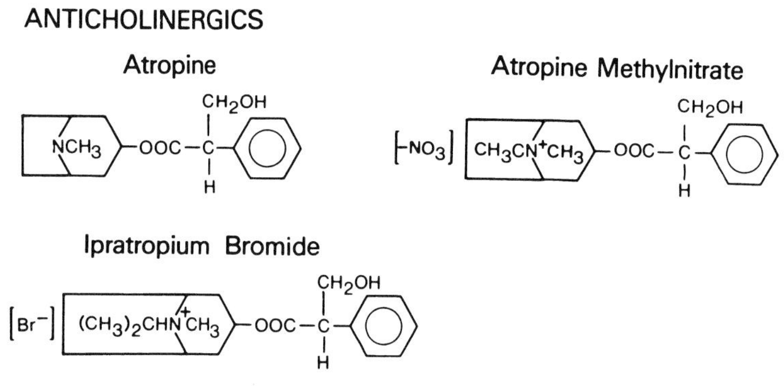

ANTICHOLINERGICS

Figure 17.6. Comparison of structures of atropine, atropine methylnitrate, and ipratropium bromide.

pium bromide for children showed that the optimal nebulized dose was 75 to 250 mg (66).

Beck and coworkers studied the addition of 250 mg of nebulized ipratropium bromide after maximum β_2 bronchodilation was obtained from salbutamol in acute asthma (67). They found that the inhaled ipratropium produced a significant additional increase in FEV_1 after maximum effect from salbutamol had been reached. These results imply that in children there is a significant cholinergic component to their bronchospasm.

Studies in Bronchopulmonary Dysplasia

Logvinoff and coworkers (14) obtained pulmonary function tests during the course of a self-controlled study of six children, 5 to 43 months of age, who had moderate to severe BPD. Inhaled atropine (0.05 mg/kg) significantly ($p < .05$) increased dynamic compliance (C_L). Total work of breathing decreased after atropine, but the change was not significant. The significant improvement of small airway function seen in this study following atropine inhalation suggests increased baseline small airway tone secondary to increased vagal activity (14).

Using a noninvasive passive flow volume technique to measure respiratory system resistance and compliance, the effects of 25 micrograms/kg delivered over 10 to 15 minutes using a hand ventilation circuit was studied in 5 premature infants ranging in age from 19 to 103 days. In all five infants there was a significant decrease in respiratory system resistance ($p < .001$) and an increase in compliance ($p < .001$) at one hour compared to baseline values. There was no significant change in heart rate and transcutaneous oxygen tension which were measured continuously during the study (68).

Further studies are needed in both the acute and chronic phases of BPD to determine the exact role of anticholinergics.

References

1. Bonikos DS, Bensch KC, Northway WH. Bronchopulmonary dysplasia: the pulmonary pathologic sequel of necrotizing bronchilitis and pulmonary fibrosis. Hum Pathol 1976; 7:643.
2. Nickerson BG, Taussig LM. Family history of asthma in infants and children with bronchopulmonary dysplasia. Pediatrics 1980;65:1140.
3. Motoyama EK, Fort MD, Klesh WK, et al. Early onset of airway reactivity in premature infants with bronchopulmonary dysplasia. Am Rev Resp Dis 1987;136:50–57.
4. Kao LC, Warburton D, Platzker ACG, Keens TG. Effect of isoproterenol inhalation on air-

way resistance in chronic bronchopulmonary dysplasia. Pediatrics 1984;73:509.
5. Smyth JA, Tabachnik E, Duncan WJ. Pulmonary function and bronchial hyperreactivity in long term survivors of bronchopulmonary dysplasia. Pediatrics 1981;68:336.
6. Rooklin AR, Moomjiian AS, Fox WW. Theophylline therapy in bronchopulmonary dysplasia. J Pediatr 1979;95:882.
7. Kao LC, Durand DJ, Dhillias BL, Nickerson BG. Oral theophylline and diuretics improve pulmonary mechanics in infants with bronchopulmonary dysplasia (abstr). J Pediatrics 1987;111:439–444.
8. Werthhammer J, Brown BR, Neff RK. Sudden infant death syndrome in infants with bronchopulmonary dysplasia. Pediatrics 1982;69:301.
9. Merciano D, Aubier M, Pariente R. Effects of theophylline on diaphragmatic strength and fatigue in patients with COPD. N Engl J Med 1984;311:349.
10. Foy T, Marion J, Harris TR. Isoproterenol and aminophylline reduced lung capillary filtration during high permeability. J Appl Physiol 1979;46:146.
11. Hendeles L, Weinberger M. Theophylline: a state of the art review. Pharmacotherapy 1983;3:2.
12. Hendeles L, Weinberger M. Disposition of theophylline after a single intravenous infusion of aminophylline. Am Rev Respir Dis 1978;118:97.
13. Furukawa CT, Shapiro GG, Bierman W. A double blind study comparing the effectiveness of cromolyn sodium, and sustained release theophylline in childhood asthma. Pediatrics 1984;74:453.
14. Logvinoff MM, Lemen RJ, Taussig LM, Lamont BA. Bronchodilators and diuretics in children with bronchopulmonary dysplasia. Pediatr Pulmonol 1985;1:198.
15. Walker SR, Evans ME, Richards AJ. The clinical pharmacology of oral and inhaled salbutamol. Clin Pharmacol Ther 1971;13:861–867.
16. Larsson RS, Svedmyr N. Bronchodilating effect and side effects of β_2-adrenoceptor stimulants by different modes of administration. Am Rev Respir Dis 1977;116:861.
17. Shim C, Williams MH. Bronchial response to oral versus aerosol metaproterenol in asthma. Ann Intern Med 1980;93:428.
18. Nelson HS. Beta-adrenergic therapy. In: Middleton G, Reed CB, Ellis EF, eds. Allergy: principles and practice. 2nd ed. St. Louis: CV Mosby, 1983, p 511.
19. Mammel MC, Green TP, Johnson DE. Controlled trial of dexamethasone therapy in infants with bronchopulmonary dysplasia. Lancet 1983;1:1356.
20. Avery GB, Fletcher AB, Brudno DS. Controlled trial of dexamethasone in respirator-dependent infants with bronchopulmonary dysplasia. Pediatrics 1985;75:106.
21. Mammel MC, Fiterman C, Coleman JM, Boros SJ. Short term dexamethasone therapy bronchopulmonary dysplasia: acute effects and 1-year follow-up. Dev Pharmacol Ther 1987;10:1–11.
22. Cox JSG. Review of chemistry, pharmacology, toxicity, metabolism, specific side-effects, antiallergic properties in vitro and in vivo of disodium cromoglycate. In: Pepys J, Frankland AW, eds. Disodium cromoglycate in allergic airway disease. London: Butterworths, 1970, p 13.
23. Cox JSG. Disodium cromoglycate: mode of action and its possible relevance to the clinical use of the drug. Br J Dis Chest 1971;65:189–204.
24. Marguardt DL, Walker LL, Wasserman SI. Cromolyn inhibition of mouse bone marrow–derived mast cell mediator release. J Allergy Clin Immunol 1985;75(2):193.
25. Flint KC, Leung KBP, Pearce FL, Hudspith BN, Brostoff J, Johnson NM. Human mast cells recovered by bronchoalveolar lavage: their morphology, histamine release and the effects of sodium cromoglycate. Clin Sci 1985;68:427–432.
26. Atkins PC, Norman ME, Zweiman B. Antigen-induced neutrophil chemotactic activity in man. Correlation with bronchospasm and inhibition by disodium cromoglycate. J Allergy Clin Immunol 1978;62:149–155.
27. Diaz P, Galleguillo FR, Gonzalez MC, Pantin CFA, Kay AB. Bronchoalveolar lavage in asthma: the effect of disodium cromoglycate

(cromolyn) on leukocyte counts, immunoglobulins, and complement. J Allergy Clin Immunol 1984;74:41–48.
28. Mazurek N, Berger G, Pecht I. A binding site on mast cells and basophils for the antiallergic drug cromolyn. Nature 1980;286:722–723.
29. Theoharides TC, Sieghart W, Greengard P, Douglas WW. Anti-allergic drug cromolyn may inhibit histamine secretion by regulating phosphorylation of a mast cell protein. Science 1980;207:80–82.
30. Kay AB, Walsh GM, Mogbel R, et al. Disodium cromoglycate inhibits activation of human inflammatory cells in vitro. 1985, submitted for publication.
31. Mogbel R, Durham SR, Carroll M, et al. Enhanced neutrophil and monocytotoxicity after exercise-induced asthma. Thorax 1985;40:218–219.
32. Basran GS, Page CT, Paul W, Morley J. Cromoglycate inhibits the responses to platelet-activating factor (PAF-acether) in man: an alternative mode of action for DSCG in asthma? Eur J Pharmacol 1983;86(1):143–144.
33. Chung JTN, Jones RS. Bronchodilator effects of sodium cromoglycate and its clinical implications. Br Med J 1979;11:1033.
34. Hasham F, Kennedy JD, Jones RS. Actions of salbutamol, disodium cromoglycate and placebo administered as aerosols in acute asthma. Arch Dis Child 1981;56:722.
35. Thomson NC, Clark CJ, Boyd G, Oran F. Effect of sodium cromoglycate on bronchial smooth muscle. Br J Clin Pharm 1981;12:440.
36. Kitamura S, Ishihara Y, Takaku F. Effect of disodium cromoglycate on the action of bronchoactive agents in guinea pig tracheal strips. Arzneim-Forsch/Drug Res 1974;34(11):1002–1004.
37. Harries MG. Bronchial irritant receptors and a possible new action for cromolyn sodium. Ann Allergy 1981;46:156–158.
38. Sheffer AL, Rocklin RE, Goetzel BJ. Immunologic components of hypersensitivity reactions to cromolyn sodium. N Engl J Med 1975;293:1220–1224.
39. Kus J, Ciszek JA, et al. Immediate allergic reaction to Intal in a patient with bronchial asthma. Pneumonal Pol 1978;46:745–749.
40. Menon MPS, Das AK. Asthma and urticaria during disodium cromoglycate treatment. Scand J Respir Dis 1977;58:145–149.
41. Brown LA, Kaplan RA, Benjamin PA, Hoffman LS, Shearer WT. Immunoglobulin E-mediated anaphylaxis with inhaled cromolyn sodium. J Allergy Clin Immunol 1981;68:416–420.
42. Wilson J. Use of sodium cromoglycate during pregnancy (French). J Pharm Med 1982;8(2, suppl):45–51.
43. Mezey RJ, Cohn MA, Fernandez RJ, Januszkiewicz AJ, Wanner A. Mucociliary transport in allergic patients with antigen-induced bronchospasm. Am Rev Respir Dis 1978;118:677–684.
44. Sheppard D, Nadel JA, Boushey HA. Inhibition of sulfur dioxide–induced bronchoconstriction by disodium cromoglycate in asthmatic subjects. Am Rev Respir Dis 1981;124:257–259.
45. Warner JC. Significance of late reactions after bronchial challenge with house dust mite. Arch Child Dis 1976;51:905–911.
46. Booij-Noord H, Orie NGM, deVries K. Immediate and late bronchial obstructive reactions to inhalation of house dust and protective effects of disodium cromoglycate and prednisolone. J Allergy Clin Immunol 1971;48:344–354.
47. Abraham WM, Delehunt JC, Yerger L, Marchette B. Characterization of a late phase pulmonary response after antigen challenge in allergic sheep. Am Rev Respir Dis 1983;128:839–844.
48. Furukawa CT, Shapiro CG, Kraemer MJ, Pierson WE, Bierman CW. A double-blind study comparing the effectiveness of cromolyn sodium and sustained-release theophylline in childhood asthma. Pediatrics 1984;74:453–459.
49. Lesko LJ, Miller AK. Physical-chemical compatibility of cromolyn sodium nebulizer solution—bronchodilator inhalant solution admixtures. Ann Allergy 1984;53(3):236–238.
50. Hiller EJ, Milner AD, Lenney W. Nebulized sodium cromoglycate in young asthmatic children. Arch Dis Child 1977;52:875–876.
51. Mellon MH, Harden K, Zeiger RS. The effectiveness and safety of nebulized cromolyn

solution in the young childhood asthmatic. Immunol Allergy Practice 1982;4:168–172.
52. Zareceansky S, Nadel G, Yahav J, Katznelson D. Treatment of asthmatic patients under four years of age with sodium cromoglycate. Harefuah 1983;105:257–258.
53. Newth CJL, Newth CV, Turner JAP. Comparison of nebulized sodium cromoglycate and oral theophylline in controlling symptoms of chronic asthma in pre-school children: a double blind study. Aust NZ J Med 1982;12:232.
54. Ogden BB, Murphy SA, Saunders GC, Pathak D, Johnson J. Neonatal lung neutrophils and elastase/proteinase inhibitor imbalance. Am Rev Respir Dis 1984;130:817–821.
55. Merritt TA, Cochrane CC, Holcomb K, et al. Elastase and α_1-proteinase inhibitor activity in tracheal aspirates during respiratory distress syndrome. J Clin Invest 1983;72:656–666.
56. Stenmark KR, Eyzaguirre M, Remigio L, Seccombe J, Henson PM. Recovery of platelet activating factor and leukotrienes from infants with severe bronchopulmonary dysplasia: clinical improvement with cromolyn treatment. Am Rev Respir Dis 1985;13:A236.
57. Cross NJ, Skorodin MS. Anticholinergic, antimuscarinic bronchodilators. Am Rev Respir Dis 1984;129:856–870.
58. Olsen CR, Colebatch HJH, Mebel PE, Nadel JA, Staub NC. Motor control of pulmonary airways studied by nerve stimulation. J Appl Physiol 1965;20:202–208.
59. Nadel JA, Widdicombe JG. Reflex control of airway size. Ann NY Acad Sci 1963;108:712–722.
60. Virtanen R, Kanto J, Tisalo F, Salo M, Sjovall. Pharmacokinetic studies on atropine with special reference to age. Acta Anaesth Scand 1982;26:297–300.
61. Cavanaugh MJ, Cooper DM. Inhaled atropine sulfate: dose response characteristics. Am Rev Respir Dis 1976;114:517–524.
62. Kradjan WA, Lakshminarayan S, Hayden PW, Larson SW, Marini JJ. Serum atropine concentrations after inhalation of atropine sulfate. Am Rev Respir Dis 1981;123:471–472.
63. Pabes CP, Progdin PN, Heel RC, Speight TM, Avery GS. Ipratropium bromide: a review of its pharmacological properties and therapeutic efficacy in asthma and chronic bronchitis. Drugs 1980;20:237.
64. Lin MT, Lee-Hong E, Collins-Williams C. A clinical trial of the bronchodilator effect of SCH 1000 aerosol in asthmatic children. Ann Allergy 1978;40:326.
65. Mann NP, Hiller FJ. Ipratropium bromide in children with asthma. Thorax 1982;37:72.
66. Davis A, Vickerson F, Worsley G, Mindorff C, Kazim F, Levison H. Determination of dose-response relationship for nebulized ipratropium in asthmatic children. J Pediatr 1984;105:1002–1005.
67. Beck R, Robertson C, Galdis-Debaldt M, Levison H. Combined salbutamol and ipratropium bromide by inhalation in the treatment of severe acute asthma. J Pediatr 1985;107:605–608.
68. Sosulski R, Abbasi S, Bhutani VK, et al. Physiologic effects of Terbutaline on pulmonary function of infants with bronchopulmonary dysplasia. Pediatr Pulmonol 1986;2:269–273.
69. Wilkie RA, Bryan MH. Effect of bronchodilators on airway resistance in ventilator dependent neonates with chronic lung disease. J Pediatr 1987;111:278–282.
70. Pomerance J, Puri AP. Treatment of neonatal bronchopulmonary dysplasia with steroids. Pediatr Res 1980;14:649A.
71. Grylack LI, Scanlon KB, Scanlon LW. Corticosteroid treatment of fourteen newborns with bronchopulmonary dysplasia. Clin Res 1979;2:819A.
72. Kramer LI, Hultzen C. The role of steroids in early bronchopulmonary dysplasia. Pediatr Res 1978;12:564A.
73. Schick JB, Goetzman BW. Corticosteroid response in chronic lung disease of prematurity. Am J Perinatol 1983;1:23–27.

Comments

T. Allen Merritt

Pulmonary mechanic measurements in infants with BPD clearly demonstrate increased resistance in the airways. Airway hyper-reactivity in these infants is well recognized by neonatologists, yet in few nurseries are pulmonary mechanics assessments performed prior to and after pharmacologic treatment with agents targeted to improve airway conductance. Indeed clinical response, usually assessed by blood gas changes (primarily a reduction in $PaCO_2$, improved auscultation of airway turbulence, and finally improved oxygenation are the usual clinical parameters. Clinical management could, however, probably be improved by application of cribside pulmonary function assessment in a serial fashion to better ascertain individual response to theophylline, β_2-agonists, cromolyn sodium, and the anticholinergic agents. Studies evaluating the efficacy of various β_2-agonists and other bronchodilatory agents are lacking, and thus the relative benefit of one mixture of polypharmacy over another is lacking in infants with BPD. Various β_2-agonists, including albuterol, have regional preference over other agents by some neonatologists; however, albuterol is not recommended by the manufacturer for children under 12 years of age.

Although well studied as an effective treatment for apnea of prematurity, theophylline has multiple effects at the cellular level (as a phosphodiesterase inhibitor and an adenosine inhibitor). While affecting both intercostal and diaphragmatic muscle activity, presumably from its calcium channel blocking actions, theophylline continues to be a mainstay treatment for infants with BPD. The levels at which specific effects are predicted (*i.e.*, bronchodilatation, enhanced diaphragmatic contraction) are still imprecisely known.

Management of infants with chronic pulmonary insufficiency with inhalation agents will continue to be a major responsibility of neonatologists and will undoubtedly consume the energies of pediatric pulmonologists for the next several years. Better methods of neonatal inhalation of these agents with predictable doses of particle or droplet size to reach the conducting airway require refinement in present technology.

18

Nursing Care of the Infant with Bronchopulmonary Dysplasia

CAROLE A. BOYNTON AND BARBARA JONES

Introduction

Over the past 15 years the increased survival rate of very immature infants with respiratory distress syndrome (RDS) has led to the emergence of a new form of chronic lung disease, bronchopulmonary dysplasia (BPD). BPD was first described in 1967 by Northway and his associates (1) and is characterized by hypoxemia, hypercapnia, respiratory distress, and chronic radiographic changes. It develops in about 20% of all infants who require mechanical ventilation for RDS and is even more common in extremely immature infants. Although our understanding of the pathogenesis is incomplete, most authorities consider that BPD is caused by exposure of the immature respiratory system to high concentrations of inspired oxygen and to barotrauma from intermittent positive pressure ventilation (2, 3). If we accept that BPD is caused by therapy and that the nurse is the person who carries out that therapy, it becomes clear that the nurse is in a position to ensure that the infant receives optimal care. There is evidence that innovative nursing care can reduce the time infants spend on the ventilator (4). The application of innovative nursing care may also reduce the risk of developing BPD.

Once BPD develops the focus and timing of care must change. Nutrition becomes a major focus of care, and the pace of weaning from respiratory support must be slowed. When the infant's medical condition is stable, planning for discharge should be started. The primary nurse team teaches the family the individual characteristics of their infant and helps them assume some of the routine infant care in the hospital. After discharge the primary nurse remains in telephone contact with the family to assist in transition of care to the appropriate home care nurse or public health clinic. Readmission of BPD patients is common in the first year of life, and these nurses will be an important link between the hospital and family.

Primary Nursing and BPD

The role of the neonatal nurse has expanded as our ability to treat infants has improved. In addition to routine care the nurse is expected to manage complex equipment, provide life support measures, deal with families in crisis, and understand and participate in medical management decisions. This level of nursing practice is best suited to the primary nursing model. This allows the family and infant to have two or three nursing staff members with whom they may become comfortable during the long hospitalization.

Primary nursing is not a new staffing pattern or way of assigning patients but a philosophy of nursing practice (5). It provides a framework for nurses to meet the needs of the infant with BPD and his family in a comprehensive and satisfying manner.

Generally neonatal intensive care units are staffed by nurses who function as primary nurses, coprimary nurses, or associates. Nursing tasks are best performed by a knowledgeable person who is able to see directly the consequences of the care provided. This is especially true in the case of infants with BPD, who require long-term, consistent care. Problems related to elements of the health care system experienced by the patient or his family can be handled by the primary nurse acting as a patient advocate. The primary nurse provides direct care, produces a written nursing care plan with measurable goals and outcomes, and facilitates communication between the family and other staff members. In caring for infants with BPD, it is important to evaluate the patient's response to the planned medical interventions and nursing care and to be responsible for discharge planning and parent teaching. The primary nurse arranges and attends all patient care conferences and places a written summary of those meetings in the patient's chart. She collaborates with other team members to organize and direct the care of the infant.

Infants with chronic lung disease especially benefit from having a primary care team. Benefits include stable observers and caregivers who are sensitive to that infant's physical condition and behavior, thereby allowing the detection of early signs of fluid overload or feeding intolerance. Nurses who can read physiologic and behavioral cues can modify the care plan to meet the infant's changing needs. Because physician team members rotate monthly, the members of the primary nursing team serve as constant caregivers who become expert observers of the patient's changing condition. The primary nurses take an active role in discharge planning by preparing an individualized discharge care plan based on their assessment of the family and infant. From this a teaching plan is developed for the parents. The primary nursing team coordinates follow-up visits and remains a resource to answer questions after discharge. The primary nurse also makes referrals to appropriate outpatient and community resources needed for ongoing care.

Parents of infants with BPD especially benefit from the primary nursing approach and will be able to establish trust and rapport more quickly with team members who know them and understand their child's problems.

Nursing Care of the Acutely Ill Ventilated Infant

An important function of the NICU nurse is to assess continuously the infant's need for, and response to, mechanical ventilation. The primary care team establishes guidelines for ventilator management, and the primary nurse uses these guidelines to make decisions about ventilator support. Prevention of BPD by limitation of barotrauma and oxygen toxicity is a major goal during the acute phase of treatment. It requires that respiratory support be tailored to meet the needs of the individual infant. Two reports suggest that some very immature infants can tolerate much lower arterial oxygen tensions and much higher carbon dioxide tensions than previously thought (6, 7). If such changes in respiratory support could be made safely, it would permit a reduction in exposure to elevated concentrations of oxygen and high peak airway pressures. Immature infants can maintain aerobic metabolism at a PaO_2 as low as 35 to 40 torr if perfusion is normal. Development of metabolic acidosis may signal a shift to anaerobic metabolism and indicate a need for increased concentrations of inspired oxygen. If the pH is greater than 7.25, carbon dioxide tensions as high as 65 torr may be safely tolerated. These guidelines are inappropriate for term or near-term infants, who are at much greater risk for pulmonary hypertension and should be maintained at higher levels of arterial oxygen.

It is the responsibility of the nurse to determine how well the ventilator support is meeting the needs of the infant. The first step of this process is an evaluation of the infant's own respiratory efforts. Infants who are not breathing may be overventilated while infants who are "fighting" the ventilator are often inadequately ventilated and have air hunger. It is not unusual for infants who are breathing asynchronously with the ventilator to be inappropriately treated with paralyzing drugs, rather than changes in ventilator settings, from the assumption that ventilation would be adequate if only the baby would cooperate. Often after administration of pancuronium ventilator settings must be increased, suggesting that the infant's own respiratory efforts were contributing to his ventilation. Morphine or fentanyl citrate injection are often used to sedate very ill stress sensitive infants who require high ventilatory pressures. In assessing the need for peak-inspiratory pressure, it is important to watch chest excursions, listen to breath sounds and aeration, and evaluate lung volumes on the chest radiograph. Babies with decreased lung compliance need higher peak-inspiratory pressures to inflate the lungs adequately. If the ribcage does not move, tidal volume is inadequate. Excessive peak-inspiratory pressure places the infant at risk for air leaks (pneumothorax or interstitial emphysema) (8). In babies ventilated with high peak-inspiratory pressures, it is useful to transilluminate the chest at the beginning of the nursing shift in order to establish a baseline examination so that it will be easier to make a determination of air leak. Air leaks can develop as compliance improves if peak pressures are not reduced appropriately.

If there is evidence of inadequate gas exchange (e.g., abnormal arterial blood gas values or a sudden change in transcutaneous oxygen monitors or oximeter), it is important to consider all the possible etiologies rather than automatically increasing ventilatory support. The nurse should check to make sure the ventilator is working properly, listen for breath sounds, and ensure the patency of the tracheal tube. Any recent changes in patient care such as increased fluid intake, blood transfusions, suctioning, ventilator changes, repositioning of the endotracheal tube or of the infant, and administration of medications should be considered.

Weaning from Mechanical Ventilation

Effective weaning requires an active plan on the part of the primary care team, with both physician and nurse constantly thinking about, and making appropriate changes in, ventilator settings. It is not a process that can be relegated to a low priority. From the moment the child is intubated and placed on the ventilator, all energy should be focused on weaning him as quickly as possible. The following are general principles to consider in weaning an infant from ventilatory support:

1. Weaning should be tailored to the needs of the individual patient. Very immature infants with RDS require an approach different from that for more mature infants with RDS, whose course may in-

clude an element of pulmonary hypertension.
2. If several ventilator settings can be decreased, the inspiratory pressure and oxygen concentration should be decreased first.
3. Reduction in peak pressure should be a priority in order to reduce the risk of pneumothorax and pulmonary interstitial emphysema.
4. If the infant's oxygenation or ventilation deteriorate after a ventilator change he should be allowed to rest for a few hours before further attempts to wean him.
5. A balance should be struck; peak-inspiratory pressure should not be reduced to barely tolerable levels before reducing FiO_2. Conversely, FiO_2 should not be reduced to .21 before reducing peak pressures.
6. Inspiratory time should be reduced as lung compliance improves.
7. If the infant is paralyzed, the effects of pancuronium must be reversed before reducing the ventilator rate too far. It may take as long as 24 hours for the effects of pancuronium to disappear.

Detection of the Complications of Mechanical Ventilation

Nurses caring for mechanically ventilated infants must understand the complications of mechanical ventilation and be able to assess immediately and treat those complications when they occur.

Pneumothorax is pulmonary rupture with escape of air into the intrapleural space. Usually with a pneumothorax there is rapid decompensation in clinical status manifested by rapid decline in the transcutaneous oxygen or oxygen saturation by pulse oximeter. Loss of breath sounds or a change in chest wall movement may occur. In cases of severe pneumothorax, severe hypotension with bradycardia requires immediate treatment such as needle aspiration or placement of a chest tube to evacuate the air. In the presence of a pneumothorax, the chest appears hyperlucent when the affected side is transilluminated. The lung is poorly expanded on chest radiograph. Once the chest tube is inserted and sutured and taped in place, a small petrolatum gauze dressing and a small amount of tape can be used to cover the insertion site. A large, heavy dressing or lots of tape could further restrict chest wall movement and increase the work of breathing.

Pulmonary interstitial emphysema (PIE) is not a rupture of the alveolus itself but results from small tears in the terminal bronchioles (9). It is usually detected by chest radiograph and may cause crackling breath sounds. Splinting of the lungs occurs, so that the chest may appear overdistended. The goal in treating PIE is to reduce peak pressures while preserving adequate gas exchange. This may be done by increasing the ventilatory rate and using a short inspiratory time, by selective bronchial intubation, or by using one of the high-frequency ventilation techniques. There is no treatment that works in all children with PIE.

Impaired cardiac function as a result of excessive ventilatory pressures is another complication of mechanical ventilation. High mean airway pressures can decrease the pulmonary venous return to the heart and decrease diastolic filling, resulting in a fall in cardiac output. This complication may be difficult to detect but can prolong the ventilatory course.

Nursing Care of Infants with a Patent Ductus Arteriosus

More than 20 years ago the systemic-to-pulmonary shunt through the patent ductus arteriosus (PDA) was thought to be an important factor in the pathophysiology of RDS (10). Over time this theory fell by the wayside and the biochemical etiology of RDS came to the forefront. As survival rates of very low birth weight infants improved, large numbers of these infants developed congestive heart failure secondary to shunting through the PDA. These were infants recovering from RDS who were no longer surfactant deficient. It is now believed that left-to-right shunting complicates the majority of cases of RDS, especially in the more immature infants (11). Clinicians speak of a symptomatic PDA, and this term implies the presence of clinical signs of the shunt as well as compromise of cardiac or pulmonary function. Some researchers have proposed that in the very immature infant the dominant clinical problem may be one of the shunt rather than surfactant deficiency (12).

Specifically there is an increase in pulmonary blood flow or pulmonary pressure and the development of alveolar edema. As this occurs the infant may require increased peak-inspiratory pressure or concentration of inspired oxygen in order to maintain adequate gas exchange. Recently it has been realized that many cases are clinically significant without the classical signs of the PDA such as a murmur (10–13). What should the nurse look for in this case? First, one must have a high index of suspicion, because the ductus arteriosus is the normal route for blood flow in late fetal life and the immature newborn is not able to close it like the normal full-term newborn. Signs of a hemodynamically significant shunt include apparent worsening of clinical course by increasing the requirement for pressure and FiO_2, a persistent metabolic acidosis, a hyperactive precordium, a widened pulse pressure, visible axillary pulses, or palpable palmar or pedal pulses. Increasing heart size or engorgement of the pulmonary vasculature is often seen on chest radiographs. A murmur develops only late in the course. The diagnosis may be confirmed by the use of echocardiography. Definitive treatment for a clinically significant PDA is closure by indomethacin or ligation. Infants treated with indomethacin must be monitored for thrombocytopenia and azotemia. Oliguria is common during treatment, so intake and output must be carefully monitored (14). Dopamine (2 to 5 $\mu g/kg/min$) is often used to increase renal blood flow in infants who become oliguric after indomethacin administration.

Suctioning the Infant with BPD

The purpose of chest physiotherapy (PT) and suction is to reinflate collapsing small airways and to loosen, mobilize, and remove debris in the lungs that could impair respiration and occlude the tracheal tube. The procedure is the responsibility of the nurse providing clinical care, and the frequency is determined by the infant's clinical condition and the amount of secretions present. To begin the procedure the nurse notes the reading on the pulse oximeter or transcutaneous monitor, counts the respiratory rate, and auscultates the chest to determine the presence of rales, rhonchi, and aeration throughout the lung fields. She then increases the FiO_2, positions the infant, and begins chest PT and/or vibrations, noting the effect the procedure is having on heart rate and oxygenation. If nebulized bronchodilators are prescribed, she gives the treatment at this time. Following chest PT she puts on sterile gloves, assembles the suction catheter, disconnects the ventilator, and instills saline into the endotracheal tube. The infant is then hand ventilated at pressures slightly greater than the peak-inspiratory pressure and generally at a faster rate. The anesthesia bag is disconnected, and a sterile suction catheter is inserted into the endotracheal or tracheostomy tube for a distance predetermined not to exceed the tip of the tube. This ensures that undue pressure and trauma are not applied to the very delicate tracheal epithelium. Improper suctioning technique may contribute to the formation of bronchial granulomas. The catheter is slowly withdrawn while the tip is rotated to collect secretions within the endotracheal tube. The color, viscosity, and volume of the secretions are noted, and the infant is reconnected to the ventilator.

In children who tolerate pulmonary care poorly, efforts must be made to minimize stresses associated with chest PT and suctioning. Some form of noninvasive monitoring, such as pulse oximetry, is useful in determining short-term and long-term consequences for the baby.

Developmental Issues and Their Implications for Nursing Care of Infants with BPD

Although little is known about the psychologic needs of preterm infants, neonatal nurses have long been aware of the adverse effects of the NICU environment on the developing preterm baby. Effects of bright lights, loud noises, and painful procedures are clinically apparent to the nurse at the bedside. These stimuli cause dramatic changes in color, tone, breathing pattern, and heart rate. This view of infant suffering has not always been shared. In the 1970s infants were viewed as purely reflexive beings, functioning basically at the brainstem level, without the capacity to feel pain or communicate with their caregivers. Surgical procedures were routinely performed without analgesia. It was thought that infants felt no pain because their nerve fibers were unmyelinated. Subsequently it was discovered that myelination was not necessary for sensory nerve tract functioning (15). In 1973 T. Berry Brazelton, a developmental pediatrician from Harvard, published the Neonatal Behavioral Assessment Scale (NBAS) (16). This contribution was important because Brazelton viewed the term neonate as having the ability to interact with caregivers, eliciting an organization from them which he still lacks and simultaneously giving them feedback. The NBAS examiner asks the infant to perform a series of reflex and motor responses that are graded in difficulty. These tasks require that the infant regulate his state, motor behavior, and social interaction. The NBAS, although not standardized, allows the user to quantify, document, and give a numerical score to infant behavior, allowing its use as a research tool for comparing infant behavior. Many of the items used in the NBAS were drawn from neurologic findings of previous investigators, but Dr. Brazelton popularized its use and stimulated interest in infant behavior.

In 1975 Parmelee compared the behavior of a preterm infant at 40 weeks postconceptional age with that of newly born term infants (17). In 1979 Martin *et al.* related the positioning of infants to arterial oxygen tension (18). In 1980 Long *et al.* described handling as a cause of hypoxemia (19). These early observations established a direct link between the environmental stimulus and the infant's physiologic response. As technology progressed so did our ability to detect effects of the caregiving environment and the caregiver.

Als, and her coworkers have developed theories about preterm infants and created instruments to use in quantifying infant behavior (20). In 1979 Gorski and others presented a three-stage model of neurologic and behavioral development of the high-risk neonate (21). These authors attempted to present a way to understand infants' behavior as they recover from illness. The first stage in their model is the development of physiologic organization. This means that the baby has developed some control over his digestive, respiratory, cardiovascular, motor, and state systems. Babies with BPD who are immature or very ill have difficulty attaining this control. Their illness leaves them with little energy for cognitive or affective responses. For example they have poor state regulation and experience difficulty staying either awake or asleep in an NICU environment unlike well-organized term infants who exhibit well-defined sleep and awake periods. At the next stage organized behavioral responses begin. This is the level at which the infant begins to respond by blocking out unpleasant stimuli and seeking out positive stimuli. There is a fine line between providing positive stimulation for CNS development and CNS overload. If the action, sound, or light is intense, or if there are abrupt changes, the infant will have difficulty responding in a positive manner. In contrast a gentle touch, quiet voice, or soft light allows the infant to come to an alert state and engage in interaction. As the infant improves and grows, so does his ability to shut out, or not respond to, disturbing stimuli and respond favorably to appropriate stimuli. As the infant recovers he enters the third stage and is able to show active reciprocity with his social environment. In terms of the infant's response (overt or covert) to specific aspects of his environment, this means he is able socially to give and take. Does he have the ability to engage his caregivers and get his needs met? Does he provide positive feedback for his caregiver? Dr. Barnard, in a follow-up study on the long-term effects of stimulation of preterm infants, found improved growth and higher mental and motor scores on the Bayley Infant Assessment Scale in infants who had received increased stimulation (22). She believes the infant has the ability to turn on mothering behavior in the mother. This concept is important because infants who are unable to relate to their caregivers may be at increased risk for neglect or abuse. Infants with BPD have physiologic instability, making it difficult for them to engage in reciprocal behavior with their caregivers. They may have increased extensor muscle tone, making them irritable, difficult to console, and hard to cuddle. Infants with BPD often have problems with gastroesophageal reflux and apnea when they are overstimulated or attempt excessive social interaction. Because of a lack of reciprocity with the caregiver and environment, infants are placed at a developmental risk. In 1977 Hunter *et al.* found a high incidence of maltreatment in a prospective study of 255 infants admitted to an NICU (23). Maltreated infants were less mature at birth and more likely to have congenital defects. Because infants with BPD have inadequate responses and poor social skills, they may be at greater risk for abuse and neglect.

Using the NBAS as a prototype over a period of 8 years, Heidi Als and others adapted it to include the behavior of preterm infants based on her theory of syntactive development. This theory holds that the developing infant has various subsystems which allow him to control his behavior. These subsystems are autonomic, motor, state organization, attentional interactive and self-regulatory ability. The more immature the baby, the more difficulty he has with behavioral organization of the various subsystems. This adaptation of the NBAS is called the Assessment of Preterm Infant Behavior (APIB) (20). The APIB maneuvers begin with mild distal stimulation presented during sleep. The maneuvers progress from mild tactile to medium tactile and vestibular stimulation, and finally to massive tactile and vestibular stimulation. The attentional interactive portion is given priority and may be presented whenever the infant is awake and alert. If the infant is unable to attain an alert state, he is penalized during scoring. Throughout the exam the infant's need for support and ability to self-regulate are measured. The examiner is then able to use this information in a positive manner to adjust the environment and care provided to support the infant optimally (24).

Many researchers have suggested that preterm infants are abnormally stimulated in the NICU (19, 22–27). The goal of some infant intervention programs has been to combat the supposed sensory deprivation of the NICU by applying blanket sensory stimulation while other programs have focused on stress reduction, providing almost no stimulation. Which is best for the developing brain? In 1977 Lawson and others observed the NICU environment at 15 minute intervals (25). They found acoustic stimuli present in 95% of the measurements and consistently high illumination levels. These findings led them to conclude that premature infants received inappropriate patterns of stimulation rather than inadequate levels of stimulation. In 1979 Bess *et al.* measured noise levels in incubators (26). The operation of life support equipment increased noise by 15 to 20 dB above background levels while opening and closing the incubator door caused an increase of 93 to 114 dB. A report on noise pollution published in 1974 by the American Academy of Pediatrics Committee on Environmental Hazards suggested that ill effects from ototoxic drugs may be potentiated by hospital noise (27).

If one adds to the noisy, bright, cold, rough, and confusing NICU environment an infant who is not only preterm but also has a chronic lung disease, one can appreciate the plight of the infant with BPD. Infants with BPD are behaviorally very disorganized, stress intolerant, and irritable. Often they have greatly increased tone and are difficult to hold. Their tendency toward gastroesophageal reflux and vomiting can be a major problem. The nurse must allow adequate time to feed, position, and return the infant to a relaxed sleep state before leaving the bedside. The ability to provide care in a relaxed and careful manner requires excellent organization and planning skills.

Als conducted a pilot study of the use of individualized behavioral and environmental care for very low birth weight infants at risk for BPD (4). The study group consisted of eight experimental and eight control infants with birth weights less than 1250 g who were mechanically ventilated with FiO_2 greater than 0.6 when the study began. The experimental infants had a clinical behavioral description entered in their charts highlighting specific reactions to stress and suggestions made to modify nursing care. Compared with control infants the study infants had less ventilator and oxygen dependence, improved feeding behavior, and higher mental and motor scores on the Baley Scale. This study is currently being repeated with the addition of brain electrical activity mapping.

Until recently nursing has had a limited role in actually altering the environment and care of infants in the NICU. Most published observations have been made by developmentalists, and suggestions for change have been given to the nurse (4, 24). The direct care and support of infants with BPD in the NICU is the primary responsibility of the nurse, and creative nurses find ways to alter care and the environment to meet individual needs by becoming familiar with the current literature on BPD and behavioral intervention and implementing these strategies in their care. Use of an observation period followed by a written care plan that includes some measurement of outcome is the best approach. The primary nurse can serve as a role model for other health care personnel and parents. The nurse can model gentle handling and sensitivity to the infant's needs, taking opportunities to point out signs of stress. She can control an infant's schedule and limit his interactions, thereby allowing for maximum rest and prevention of unnecessary stress. As his stimulation needs change she can alter his care plan to reflect that change.

As the infant improves clinically and matures, his ability to tolerate stress and desire to interact increase. It is important to provide for the infant's need for increased sensory input and social interaction. Intubated infants have more difficulty signaling their distress or discomfort. Being unable to make a sound, they often cry unnoticed until they become bradycardic or tachycardic, vomit, or become apneic, or until their transcutaneous oxygen level drops. Only then does someone appear to comfort them or change their position. It may be that caregivers foster the development of the BPD personality and abnormal physiologic responses by unknowingly reinforcing them.

Infants who are ready for increased sensory input begin by showing evidence of alertness. They exhibit autonomic stability and have improved motor behavior. They are able to inhibit movements and quiet themselves. They often have a relaxed facial posture and engage in "ooh" face or smiling. They respond to stimulation by moving toward the stimulus and seeking out more (4, 20, 24).

Signs of stress or overstimulation include irregular respirations, gagging, hiccoughs, spitting-up or vomiting, finger splay, yawning, coughing, straining, and sneezing. They may have alterations in tone with either extreme flacidity or hypertonicity, extension of extremities, grimacing, tongue extensions, or frantic, diffuse activity. These infants are often fussy and irritable without clear states. They may appear worried, refuse to focus, and avoid social interaction. It is important to recognize these alterations in behavior and respond appropriately to allow the infant to develop control over his environment, thus facilitating future interactions. Parents are excellent observers when taught these signals and will modify their caregiving almost immediately. It is helpful to have taped to each infant's incubator a developmental plan listing his strengths, stress signals, helpful interventions, and environmental stressors (24).

Stimulus Reduction for Stress Intolerant Infants

Environmental

1. Place sign on incubator indicating extreme stress intolerance.
2. Place incubator in quiet area, away from traffic, telephones, and noisy machinery.
3. Make a personalized developmental care plan for the infant.
4. Provide signs that encourage staff and visitors to speak quietly.

Auditory

1. Eliminate radios, loud laughter, and loud conversations.
2. Place felt strips on portholes, wastecans, and drawers.
3. Provide appropriate stimulation such as quiet rattles, soft music, or tapes of parents' voices when the infant is alert.
4. Provide protection for ears (cotton balls) if environmental noise is unavoidable.
5. Present auditory stimulation alone without visual and vestibular stimulation to assess tolerance.
6. Alter voice to observe the effect of changes in tone and frequency on the infant. Watch for symmetrical reactions; hearing impaired infants may have better hearing on one side than the other and require appropriate modification of auditory stimuli.

Visual

1. Place blanket over incubator to shield infant from bright light or make a canopy for an open crib.
2. Limit visual input by presenting a simple face on incubator or some stable visual pattern.
3. Avoid massive visual overload such as colorful sheets and blankets with complicated designs or multiple, brightly colored stuffed animals.
4. Observe infant for signs of sensory overload such as a hyperalert state, hypervigilant stare, or withdrawal.
5. Visual stimulation should be given at an appropriate distance (8 to 12 inches from face) and timed to coincide with the baby's natural rhythms. It is not appropriate to awaken a sleeping baby to provide stimulation.

Tactile

1. Provide maximal postural support with blanket rolls and provide physical boundaries by encasing the limbs in a flexed position on the body. The trunk should be held in flexion without airway compromise.
2. Change the infant's position slowly with gentle unwrapping and undressing. During bathing expose only the area being washed.
3. Use heat lamps to prevent cold stress. Take care to avoid overheating.
4. Use a pacifier and bundle the infant during any painful procedure.
5. Position the infant properly to help prevent gastroesophageal reflux.
6. Remain with the infant after a procedure until his motor activity returns to the baseline level.
7. Allow the infant to grip your finger or a small roll of gauze.
8. Awaken the infant slowly; first speak

quietly to him, then touch him, and finally unwrap him.
9. If infant is able to suck on his fingers, position hand near face to allow him to do so.
10. Use fabrics with different textures (silk, satin, velvet) for stimulation.

Olfactory

1. Use sterile gauze to protect the mouth and eyes from alcohol and tincture of benzoin during reintubation. Uncap bottles of adhesive remover away from the bedside.
2. Place mild, pleasant-smelling substances such as mother's lotion, perfume, or breast milk on gauze pad in the incubator. Scratch-and-smell books and stickers can also be placed in the incubator.
3. Check the incubator and linen for unpleasant smells. Remove soiled diapers immediately after changing.

Nutritional Support of the Infant with BPD

Nutritional support is a major problem in the management of infants with BPD (28). Among the many factors that conspire to cause malnutrition in these children are low birth weight, increased caloric needs because of increased work of breathing, the use of calciuric diuretics such as furosemide, the need for fluid restriction, and gastroesophageal reflux. Feeding these infants may be difficult, and the success of any nutritional plan depends largely on the skill of the primary care team.

Infants with BPD encounter many of the same feeding problems as other low birth weight infants. In addition BPD infants have three problems that further complicate feeding. They need more calories for growth than the average preterm infant, they are intolerant of normal volumes of fluid, and their irritability, decreased tolerance for stress, and tendency to vomit make feeding both difficult and frustrating.

Infants with BPD usually need between 120 and 150 kcal/kg every 24 hours to achieve an acceptable weight gain. The best procedure to use when beginning feeds is to advance the concentration from diluted formula to normal 20 kcal/30 mL formula. If more calories are required, formula with a higher caloric density can be used. It is usually best to start with a proprietary 24 kcal/30 mL formula such as Similac SC-24 or Enfamil LBW 24. If still more calories are needed, MCT oil (7.7 kcal/mL) or Polycose (2 kcal/mL) may be added. Human milk fortifier may be used if the infant is receiving breast milk. Supplements should be added one at a time and given in divided doses over 24 hours. If intolerance develops (*e.g.*, diarrhea) the supplements should be discontinued and then restarted one at a time.

Infants with BPD can be extremely sensitive to increases in feeding volume, and often small increases (*e.g.*, 5 ml per feed) can cause respiratory distress. Although most preterm infants can tolerate 180 mL of fluid/kg/24 hr, infants with BPD seldom tolerate more than 150 mL/kg/24 hr. These infants tend to retain fluid in the pulmonary interstitium, and inappropriate increases in feeding volume may cause pulmonary edema and acute respiratory distress. Occasionally fluids are restricted to less than 120 ml/kg/24 hr in an attempt to alleviate the child's respiratory distress. However, infants will seldom grow on such a regimen, and it may be preferable to increase the amount of diuretics in order to give the child more free water. When calculating the total volume of fluids received, it is important to include the volume of medications and supplements.

Most infants with BPD are difficult to feed. There are multiple reasons for this. The immature or motor damaged infant may be unable to coordinate sucking, swallowing, and breathing. Infants may also have poor autonomic regulation as evidenced by bradycardia, color changes, and the inability to maintain state. Inappropriate sensory input (*e.g.*, bright lights, loud noises, and painful procedures) and the absence of appropriate sensory input (*e.g.*, cuddling, holding, and soothing) coupled with the infant's inability to control the responses of his caregivers leads to frustration, depression, and learned inappropriate behavior (*e.g.*, vomiting, refusal to suck, arching, and inconsolable crying). These infants may become so difficult to care for and be so unrewarding that they are viewed as a burden by the nursing staff. Consequently it may be difficult to find consistent and appropriate caregivers. This, of course, compounds the infant's problems.

However, these infants can thrive if they receive expert and consistent nursing care (4). The ideal caregiver is very familiar with the infant, provides care in a relaxed, unhurried manner, and is aware of the infant's behavioral cues. The feeding should be given in a quiet, darkened room if possible. There must be adequate time for frequent rest periods during the feed. Before the feed begins an assessment should be made of respiratory status, abdominal girth, and bowel sounds. If the child will be gavage fed, the volume of gastric aspirate is recorded. If the aspirate volume is greater than expected, the aspirate is replaced and an appropriate amount is subtracted from the feeding. All other care such as suctioning, chest percussion, and bathing should be completed well before feeding time to allow the infant to rest. If possible, the baby should be wrapped in ventral flexion during the feed and allowed to suck on a pacifier if not nipple feeding. A pulse oximeter is useful in determining the infant's need for increased oxygen during the feeding. The caregiver should avoid making eye contact and talking during the feed. Multiple stimuli may cause sensory overload, fatigue, and behavioral disorganization and result in poor feeding. When the feeding is completed the infant should be placed in an upright prone or right lateral position in ventral flexion. The infant may continue to suck if he wishes, but it is important to avoid excessive handling and stimulation after eating. It is important to involve the parents in the feeding of their baby as early as possible. They will be the most consistent caregivers and must be confident in their ability by the time of discharge.

Some infants with BPD have problems with the mechanics of feeding. Infants that have poor or uncoordinated suck may be helped by massage of their lips and gums before the feeding. Using a nipple for premature infants may also be helpful, but there is danger of aspiration if the flow exceeds the baby's ability to swallow. Infants who are unable to form a tight seal around the nipple may benefit from a larger diameter nipple and chin support from the caregiver's index finger.

The feeding of BPD infants is very frequently (about 18%) complicated by gastroesophageal reflux (29). Symptoms of this disorder include vomiting, apnea, irritability, deteriorating pulmonary function, failure to thrive, and refusal to eat. The diagnosis may be made by barium swallow, pH monitoring of the lower esophagus, or nuclear medicine milk scan. Medical management includes frequent small feedings, upright prone position, thickened feeds, and drug therapy. It is important for the nurse to document the success or failure of medical management. Without good clinical observation ineffective medical management is sometimes continued for months. Failing medical management, the infant may be helped by fundoplication and placement of a gastrostomy tube.

The true measure of success in feeding infants with BPD is appropriate weight gain. A consistent weight gain of 15 g per 24 hours is excellent in these infants. Weight gains of more than 30 g per 24 hours are almost always caused by fluid retention and often herald the onset of increased respiratory distress. It is important to keep a record of weight, length, and head circumference by the bedside, where it can be reviewed daily by the primary care team. Making the infant with BPD grow is an art. Success requires consistent, thoughtful care and cooperative management by both the nursing and the medical staff.

Discharge Planning

Discharge planning for the infant with BPD is especially challenging and includes not only screening tests and parent education but also a comprehensive plan for ongoing care of these infants and their families (30). Because of the complexities of medical care needed by these infants, discharge planning must begin well ahead of the anticipated discharge date.

The discharge planning process should include standardized care for all infants in planning for their eventual discharge. This may be done through a regular weekly discharge planning conference or an individually scheduled meeting of the primary care team.

Most nurseries have similar criteria for discharge of high-risk infants. The infant must be medically stable, and the parents must be able to provide adequate home care by themselves or with the help of visiting nurses. The infant must weigh about 2000 g and must have an appropriate weight gain. Finally, the family must have selected a primary care physician.

At the time of discharge most infants with BPD are being treated with multiple medications such as theophylline and diuretics. The primary nurse reviews the infant's medications with the parents before discharge. This discussion includes side effects, need for refrigeration, what to do if the child vomits the medications, and the need to monitor drug levels, if appropriate. The parents practice administering the medication in the nursery with supervision. Discharge medications are ordered from the pharmacy the day before discharge and together with measuring syringes are given to the parents to take home with the infant. The parents should be provided with a written chart that lists the medication name, route, dose, and time of administration. The parents are encouraged to bring the chart and all medications to medical appointments.

Infants with BPD have increased caloric needs and may fail to gain weight on standard 20 kcal/30 mL formula. Formulas that supply 24 or 27 kcal/oz are available from the manufacturer as ready-to-feed preparations or can be made from 20 kcal/30 mL formula concentrate by adding less water during preparation. If this method is used, it is important for the parents to practice reconstituting the formula before going home. Feeding overly dilute formula may lead to caloric insufficiency and poor weight gain while overly concentrated formula may cause azotemia or osmotic diarrhea.

Formulas and feeding schedules should not be switched on the day of discharge. The infant's weight, length, head circumference, and hematocrit should be measured on the day of discharge and recorded on a summary sheet for reference at follow-up visits. If the child receives chronic diuretics, serum electrolytes should also be measured.

Screening examinations are an integral part of discharge planning for infants with BPD. These include an ophthalmologic examination, brainstem auditory evoked response, and developmental/neurologic assessment in addition to routine newborn screening for hypothyroidism, phenylketonuria, and other inborn errors of metabolism. All infants who weighed less than 1500 g at birth are screened for intracranial hemorrhage with cranial ultrasonography in the first few days of life. Those with documented intraventricular hemorrhage are studied repeatedly to detect progressive ventricular dilatation. If hydrocephalus is present, the infant should be screened a few weeks after discharge whether or not the ventricular dilatation is thought to be arrested.

A thorough parent teaching program is important in successful discharge planning. In addition to instruction about feeding and medications, each parent is taught the rudiments of well-child care and basic cardiopulmonary resuscitation. We suggest using a standard teaching plan. Topics for discharge teaching are outlined in the appendix.

Discharge of infants with BPD who need supplemental oxygen is especially challenging. The infant must be stable on low-flow oxygen (≤ 1 L/min) for at least a week before discharge and must demonstrate an appropriate weight gain. Ideally the primary nurse will make a home visit before discharge. If there is a question about whether oxygen equipment can be used safely, the equipment supplier and gas and electric company will evaluate the home. The parents must have a telephone. The local paramedics are notified of the home location and the plans to use home oxygen. The medical equipment supplier is contacted by the primary nurse and told what equipment the infant needs for home care. The supplier brings the equipment to the hospital and teaches the parents to use it. On the day of discharge the supplier goes to the home and sets up the equipment, and then services it until oxygen therapy is discontinued. The supplier keeps a written record of his services that is included in the infant's medical record. We have found liquid oxygen systems more convenient than those that use compressed gas; portable oxygen packs are also available. The parents are taught to evaluate the infant for cyanosis, tachypnea, retractions, and edema. Infants with BPD often need to be rehospitalized during the first year of life, and the parents should be reassured that readmission does not represent a failure on their part. It may be helpful for the parents to obtain a handicapped parking sticker to use while the infant requires supplemental oxygen.

Home nursing care is necessary for some infants. The prospect of caring for an infant with a tracheostomy or one needing supplemental oxygen is frightening for many families. If home nursing care will be needed, the primary nurse must contact the agency before discharge. This will allow the agency to send appropriate employees to the hospital to be trained with the parents. After discharge the primary nurse should be available for telephone consultation with family members or the home care nurses. In the week following discharge a call or visit by the primary nurse will provide an opportunity to assess the adequacy and safety of home care for the infant.

Summary

Nurses come in contact with infants with BPD and their families in many settings including the intensive care unit, the ward, the clinic, and the home. All nurses must understand the pathophysiology, treatment, and complications of BPD. Nurses provide specific nursing interventions along with emotional support for the family unit. By developing specific assessment guidelines for nursing care and teaching, continuity and consistency of care will be enhanced.

Appendix

Discharge Teaching Goals for Parents of BPD Infants

1. Understanding of BPD pathophysiology.
2. Assessment of respiratory rate and effort. Detection of cyanosis. Ability to suction the airway, perform chest physiotherapy, and use oxygen equipment.
3. Assessment of weight changes and fluid overload.
4. Role of bronchodilators, diuretics, and electrolyte supplements.
5. Recognition of emergency situations. Knowledge of basic cardiopulmonary resuscitation.
6. Ability to prepare formula and feed infant with respiratory compromise.
7. Understanding of infant behavioral responses and ability to provide environmental and behavioral support.
8. Understanding of basic infant care.

Questions Frequently Asked by Parents of BPD Infants

1. Will my baby outgrow BPD? When? How long will he need a monitor and supplemental oxygen?
2. Can the baby travel by plane? Can we travel with oxygen equipment?
3. What should I do if he spits up his medications?
4. Can visitors come to the home?
5. What do I do if a family member catches a cold?
6. What should I do about cigarette smoking in the home?

Teaching Plan for Parents of Infants with BPD

Upon discharge from the hospital the parent(s) will
1. Be able to verbalize their understanding of BPD, its chronic nature, the course of the illness, and the need for follow-up.
2. Demonstrate their ability to evaluate their infant's respiratory status:
    a. Count respirations.
    b. Identify retractions.
    c. Identify color changes.
    d. Identify fluid overload (puffiness, irritability, refusal of feeds).
3. Describe the key aspects of feeding their infant:
    a. Importance of high caloric intake and the need for rest periods during feeding.
    b. Importance of positioning in "head up" posture.
    c. How to obtain formula supplements.
    d. How to fix formula.
    e. Technique of spoon feeding and plan for introduction of solids when instructed by pediatrician.
    f. Understanding the need for fluid restriction.
    g. Awareness of possible need for increased FiO_2 during feeding.
4. Explain the purpose, dose, schedule, and method of administration for each medication as well as precautions and side effects.

a. Demonstrate how to draw up medications in a syringe accurately.
   b. Demonstrate how each type of medication (oral, inhaled, etc.) is to be administered to the infant.
5. Demonstrate and describe care and use of oxygen equipment.
   a. Demonstrate how to change and secure catheter or cannula.
   b. Describe how to adjust oxygen flow rate and know appropriate levels for infant.
   c. Describe precautions for use of home oxygen.
   d. Understand how oxygen flow rate will be decreased for weaning.
   e. Know what to do if oxygen supply runs out.
6. Describe the special care needs of infant.
   a. Obtain handicapped parking sticker for motor vehicle.
   b. Understand the need for rest periods and protection from infection.
   c. Understand the need to avoid smoking in the home.
   d. Understand the need for developmental evaluation.
   e. Have a means of transportation (public or private) to medical appointments.
7. Describe indications for emergency action and the steps that need to be taken.
   a. Know signs and symptoms of respiratory distress and which problems should be referred to the pediatrician and which to the pulmonologist.
   b. Have phone numbers of pediatrician, pulmonologist, paramedics, oxygen supply company, monitor company, fire department, and police department.
   c. Know cardiopulmonary resuscitation.
   d. Understand the operation and use of the home monitor.
   e. Know the location of the nearest emergency room.

References

1. Northway WH Jr, Rosan RC, Porter DY. Pulmonary disease following respirator therapy of hyaline membrane disease: bronchopulmonary dysplasia. N Engl J Med 1967;276: 357–368.
2. Taghizadeh A, Reynolds EOR. Pathogenesis of bronchopulmonary dysplasia following hyaline membrane disease. Am J Pathol 1976;82: 241–264.
3. Philip AGS. Oxygen plus pressure plus time: the etiology of bronchopulmonary dysplasia. Pediatrics 1975;55:44–50.
4. Als H, Lawhon G, Brown E, et al. Individualized behavioral and environmental care of the VLBW preterm infant at high risk for bronchopulmonary dysplasia: NICU and developmental outcome. Pediatrics 1986;78:1123–1132.
5. Zander KS. Primary nursing. Germantown, Md: Aspen Systems, 1976.
6. Rhodes PG, Graves GR, Patel DM, Campbell SB, Blumenthal BI. Minimizing pneumothorax and bronchopulmonary dysplasia in ventilated infants with hyaline membrane disease. J Pediatr 1983;103:634–637.
7. Boynton BR, Mannino FL, Randel RC, et al. Minimizing bronchopulmonary dysplasia in VLBW infants. J Pediatr 1984;104:962.
8. Heicher DA, Kasting DS, Harrod JR. Prospective clinical comparison of two methods for mechanical ventilation of neonates: rapid rate and short inspiratory time versus slow rate and long inspiratory time. J Pediatr 1981;98: 957–961.
9. Ackerman NB, Kuehl TJ, Coalson JJ, et al. Distal airway rupture during high frequency ventilation (HFV) in the premature baboon with hyaline membrane disease (HMD). Crit Care Med 1983;11:223.
10. Cotton RB. Patency of the ductus arteriosus—its etiology and pathogenetic relationship to respiratory distress syndrome. In: Stern L, ed. Hyaline membrane disease. Orlando, Fla: Grune and Stratton, 1984.
11. Stark AR, Frantz ID. Respiratory distress syndrome. Pediatr Clin N Am 1986;33:533–544.
12. Jacob J, Gluck L, DiSessa T, et al. The contribution of the PDA in the neonate with severe RDS. J Pediatr 1980;96:79–87.
13. Gersony WM. Patent ductus arteriosus in the neonate. Pediatr Clin N Am 1986;33:545–557.
14. Gersony WM, Peckham GJ, Ellison RC, Miettinen OS, Nadas AS. Effects of indomethacin

in premature infants with patent ductus arteriosus: results of a national collaborative study. J Pediatr 1983;102:895–906.
15. Schulte FJ. Neurophysiology aspects of brain development. Mead-Johnson Symposium on Perinatal and Developmental Medicine, 1975; 6:38–47.
16. Brazelton TB. Neonatal behavioral assessment scale. Philadelphia: JB Lippincott, 1973.
17. Parmelee AH. Neurophysiological and behavioral organization of premature infants in the first months of life. Bio Psych 1975;10(5):501–512.
18. Martin R, Herrell N, Rubin D, Fanaroff A. Effect of supine and prone positions on arterial oxygen tension in the preterm infant. Pediatrics 1979;63:528–531.
19. Long JG, Lucey JF, Philip AG. Excessive handling as a cause of hypoxemia. Pediatrics 1980;65:203–207.
20. Als H, Lester BM, Tronick EZ, Brazelton TB. Manual for the assessment of preterm infant behavior (APIB) In: Fitzgerald HE, Lester BM, eds. Theory and research in behavioral pediatrics, vol. 1. New York: Plenum, 1982.
21. Gorski PA, Dovison MF, Brazelton TB. Stages of behavioral organization in the high-risk neonate: theoretical and clinical considerations. Sem Perinatol 1979;3:61–72.
22. Barnard KE. The effects of stimulation on the sleep behavior of the premature infant. In: Batey M, ed. Communicating nursing research. Boulder: Western Interstate Commission for Higher Education, 1974.
23. Hunter RS, Kilstrom N, Kraybill EN, Loda F. Antecedents of child abuse and neglect in premature infants: a prospective study in a newborn intensive care unit. Pediatrics 1978; 78:629–635.
24. Cole JG. Infant stimulation reexamined: an environmental and behavioral based approach. Neonatal Network April 1985, pp 24–31.
25. Lawson K, Paum C, Turkewitz G. Environmental characteristics of a neonatal intensive care unit. Child Dev 1977;48:1633–1639.
26. Bess FH, Peck BF, Chapman JJ. Further observations on noise levels in infant incubators. Pediatrics 1979;63:100–106.
27. Committee on Environmental Hazards, American Academy of Pediatrics. Noise pollution: neonatal aspects. Pediatrics 1974;54:476–478.
28. Farrell PM. Nutrition and infant lung functions. Report of a National Heart, Lung, and Blood Institute symposium. Pediatr Pulmonol 1986;2(1):44–59.
29. Hrabovsky EE, Mullett MD. Gastroesophageal reflux and the premature infant. J Pediatr Surg 1986;21(7):583–587.
30. Boynton BR, Boynton CA. Discharge planning for high risk infants. J Perinatol 1985; 5(4):44–48.

19

Home Respiratory Care

HENRY L. DORKIN

Introduction

Advances in neonatal intensive care have allowed us to save smaller and more critically ill infants than in previous decades (1). While some children eventually have only minor respiratory residua, significant numbers are manifesting more severe morbidity, which in turn requires close follow-up and, in many cases, home oxygen with or without ventilator assistance. In this chapter we discuss the care of these latter infants.

The stresses involved in chronic, complicated home care of the pediatric respiratory patient have been presented at length both in this monograph and elsewhere (2, 3). Despite the child's improving enough to be considered for home therapy, the family has undergone the emotional trial of the acute illness followed by the prolonged, gradual improvement phase of bronchopulmonary dysplasia. The cadre of physicians, nurses, allied health and social workers assembled to support the child in the home may inadvertently cause or amplify the parents' feelings of inadequacy and/or loss of control over their environment or child's care. Guilt and anger over the unfortunate chronic illness may be exacerbated by confusion, conflicting information, and resultant setbacks. A well-organized team approach to home care (3) is crucial to both minimizing parental anxiety and maximizing the chance for successful transfer.

Level of Respiratory Impairment

Patients with BPD may manifest prolongation of either Type I (hypoxemic) or Type II (hypoxemic and hypercarbic) respiratory failure and resultant failure to thrive. If these infants are inadequately supported, they have signs of respiratory distress, including tachypnea, mild or moderate retractions, nasal flaring, borderline or overt cyanosis, mild wheezing, tachycardia, and often decreased appetite. Failure to gain weight (other than fluid retention) can be one of the earliest and most important signs of impairment, with inability to maintain the caloric intake needed for growth (approximately 1½ times normal). These patients often will vacillate between a status of stable fluid balance with inadequate calories and one of adequate calories but excessive fluid intake. Because these children have a limited respiratory reserve, a mild viral respiratory illness occurring in a borderline, compensated child may precipitate overt Type II respiratory failure. Certainly a significant proportion of patients with BPD (in one study as many as 50%) will be rehospitalized within the first 2 years of life (4).

From a respiratory medicine standpoint, therefore, home care begins by not discharging an unstable patient (3). Unreliable airway access, fluctuating oxygen and/or ventilator requirements, inadequate pulmonary toilet, fluid–electrolyte imbalance, and poor growth are factors that will cause even the most organized and motivated attempt at home care to fail.

Home Oxygen Therapy

Supplemental oxygen without ventilator support may suffice for the child who exhibits good growth and stable fluid–electrolyte status, without significant carbon dioxide retention, but who has on room air either a hemoglobin saturation less than 90% or a PaO$_2$ less than 60 torr (1). When evaluating oxygen needs, hemoglobin saturation should be measured while the child is awake, asleep, and during feedings. The advent of oximeters has allowed less invasive, more frequent, and continuous assessment of gas exchange. If only a particular activity results in significant desaturation, then oxygen may need to be administered only at the time of that activity. Care must be taken that a child is not given excess oxygen as, at least theoretically, a child on hypoxic respiratory drive could have suppressed respirations from excessive oxygen administration. Even a child not routinely receiving supplemental oxygen may need such help during an intercurrent respiratory illness.

The route of oxygen administration is important, and the amount delivered may derive directly from the chosen method. Delivery by nasal cannula is the simplest method and allows freedom of movement. The cannula must be taped firmly in place and checked periodically for obstruction. There are two methods to determine the correct flow rate. In the first method the child is placed in a headbox or oxygen tent, the desired hemoglobin saturation is obtained by varying the oxygen flow, and then (after removing the tent or headbox) the nasal cannula is reapplied. Oxygen flow is varied until the desired hemoglobin saturation is duplicated. A variation on this empiric approach has been documented (5). In the second method a complex calculation can be made involving respiratory rate, inspiratory time, tidal volume, inspiratory waveform, and administered oxygen flow rate. This requires several respiratory parameter measurements and/or assumptions, all of which can affect the result. Variations in respiratory rate, degree of mouth breathing, tidal volume, and oxygen consumption, all conspire to alter the actual delivered or required oxygen. It is important to realize that a range of saturations, rather than a specific value, will be the best that can be achieved and is usually adequate for the task.

As is always the case with oxygen therapy, the least amount of this "drug" which allows for growth, retards cor pulmonale or pulmonary hypertension (6), and does no further lung injury is the correct amount. While no FiO$_2$ upper limit has been proven as absolute threshold for prevention of these complications, most pulmonologists would be concerned if the FiO$_2$ could not be reduced below 0.5. Failure to keep this in mind can have serious consequences.

For the patient without a tracheostomy, either the external or internal nasal cannula remains the preferred route of administration (7, 8, 9). The advantage of the indwelling-catheter cannula is more secure placement, while the advantage of the external nasal prong cannula is less nasopharyngeal irritation and increased acceptance, especially as the child ages. The nasal prongs on the cannula can be excised to enchance acceptance, but this requires more careful positioning. For the child who will not tolerate the cannula, less desirable methods may be tried.

A full face mask is usually less well tolerated than the nasal cannula. An oxygen tent or hood confines the child to one location and decreases interactive play with the family. A scoop mask makes maintenance of predetermined FiO_2 almost impossible. Success with the chosen method should be achieved in the hospital before discharge, however, as one cannot ask the parents to accomplish that which eludes the nursing staff.

Oxygen administration to the patient with a tracheostomy is performed by either a tracheostomy mask, a coupled fitting such as a T-piece, or an indwelling tracheostomy catheter. Low profile, circular swivel fittings have been constructed and are often used with good success (R. G. Kettrick, personal communication). The tracheostomy mask can occasionally be less confining but is more readily dislodged than a T-piece or swivel fitting. With either device it is important to determine if, when dislodged, the infant can occlude the tracheostomy with his or her chin. Asphyxia could occur in such a case if there were little air movement around the uncuffed tracheostomy tube while the lumen was obstructed.

Patients with BPD who need long-term ventilatory, support can be divided into three groups. The first group is incapable of supporting life without some augementation or assistance in minute ventilation. Disconnection of the ventilator or rapid reduction in ventilator rate leads to respiratory acidosis and eventual arrest. The second group is not breath-to-breath ventilator dependent and could survive such abrupt or rapid weaning by increasing intrinsic respiratory rate and work of breathing, but at the expense of growth cessation. The third group is a combination of the first two. These patients are able to tolerate transiently the cessation of support, but they lapse into overt respiratory failure with minimal further increases in respiratory work load, such as occur with a mucus plug, large bolus feeding, or viral respiratory tract infection.

Before deciding on home ventilation it is assumed that case review suggests little hope of weaning the patient from the ventilator before discharge. This decision takes into account 1) the degree of BPD and ventilator dependence and 2) the estimated time to train the home caregivers and logistically establish the equipment, service, and ancillary personnel in the home. Obviously it is much easier to care for a child who does not require a ventilator, and every reasonable effort to wean a child completely should be made. It is unrealistic to expect logistics and training to take less than 3–4 weeks from the day the decision is made to ventilate at home. Over the short term cost savings from hospital discharge do not justify the more invasive and complex home therapy.

Of necessity a child ventilated at home will have a tracheostomy. Tracheostomy care, chest physical therapy, and suctioning will be routine aspects of care. For the child unable to sustain his or her own ventilation adequately in the face of respirator breakdown, a second reserve respirator should be kept in the home. The choice of ventilator will be based on familiarity with a given device, size of the patient (patients less than ~10 kg/1 year of age are often more easily managed on time cycled, pressure limited ventilation), and degree of airway leak. If this decision necessitates a switch to a unit different from the one used in the hospital, the switch should be made early enough before discharge to ensure that the child is stable on the new ventilator.

In certain cases complete weaning from

oxygen, continuous positive airway pressure, the ventilator, or some combination of these therapies becomes the rate-limiting step in hospital discharge. Overly aggressive removal of such support usually combines short-term success with failure to grow and gain weight. If the family is eager to have the child home and is undismayed by continued oxygen or ventilator requirements, there can be good success in the home (3). The degree of home nursing support is important, and prolonged family training is essential. We have had parents come into a family participation room in the hospital and under observation assume full care of the child and ventilator. This type of experience has helped parents develop a realistic attitude toward their child's needs during those periods when nurses and home health care workers will not be present. Borderline situations can be assessed in detail, providing the extra assistance needed to avoid failure at home and return to the hospital for long-term care.

The process of weaning from the ventilator continues at home as it did in the hospital, although a grace period should occur during the transition. Once the FiO_2 has been lowered below 0.5, one usually weans from the support most cumbersome to institute: the intermittent mechanical ventilator. Weaning rates greater than 1 or 2 breaths per minute per week have a greater chance of inhibiting growth. In the situation of a child doing well, it takes restraint to avoid weaning him from the ventilator too rapidly. During intercurrent respiratory illness it may be necessary to increase ventilator assistance temporarily. After the illness resolves one can return rapidly (over 2–3 days) to the lowest rate of ventilation previously tolerated.

Once intermittent mandatory ventilation is unnecessary, continuous positive airway pressure is maintained. Continuous positive airway pressure is then gradually lowered until a level of 2 or 3 cm H_2O is reached, at which time portable oxygen without a significant end-expiratory pressure can be substituted. Again one may briefly have to increase the level of support during intercurrent illness. By this point, however, the family may begin to lead a more normal life, taking the child for short excursions using portable oxygen.

Still mindful of somatic growth, the oxygen can be weaned slowly as long as the hemoglobin saturation remains approximately 90% or higher at all times. As the child grows tidal volume and respiratory rate will change. The child will entrain more room air on inspiration, both through the oropharynx and through the tracheostomy. Maintenance of a given oxygen flow rate may in reality represent a gradual decrease of inspired oxygen content. On occasion it may be necessary to increase the oxygen administration modestly to account for these parameter changes (5). Large increases in supplemental oxygen are usually not necessary and warrant search for an underlying problem.

Complications

Medical complications of long-term respiratory care can occur even in the most carefully watched infants. The tracheostomy site may become infected topically, or a bacterial tracheitis may develop. Appropriate attention to tracheostomy care will diminish, but not eliminate, these entities. Laryngeal and/or subglottic stenosis, airway granulomata or cysts, and even acquired tracheomalacia (10) can occur; these complications develop more commonly in the child who underwent traumatic, repetitive, and/or prolonged intubation (11) prior to the decision for surgical tracheostomy. Such patients may have difficulty with decannulation; initial failure rate is as high as 60% (12). Coordinated care with the otorhinolaryngologist and cricoid splitting or endoscopic laser techniques may resolve the problem and lead to successful decannulation.

Ventilator related problems such as extraalveolar air leak are less common once the child has gone home. However, disconnection from the ventilator or oxygen supply must be avoided even if the child is not breath-to-breath dependent. When oxygen is administered through long lengths of tubing, so that the child can play on the floor, flow rates of the respiratory mixture must be sufficient to avoid rebreathing of dead space gas with concomitant rise in inspired CO_2. One must balance humidification between that necessary to avoid inspissation of airway secretions and that which will constitute excess fluid administration or condensed water inhalation.

Outpatient Follow-up

Follow-up physician care is a combination of that provided by the tertiary center personnel (pulmonologist or neonatologist) and that provided by the child's personal physician. In addition to the usual aspects of pediatric primary preventive and maintenance care, special emphasis is placed on growth and nutrition, respiration, and development parameters. Weight should be checked every 7–14 days (for excessively rapid loss or gain). Interval history and physical exam should be initially every 14–28 days, depending on degree of home support, stability of patient, and assessment of parental support needs. It may be helpful to have one of the home health workers accompany the family in order to provide an external perspective. As time passes support decreases, and if the child is doing well, longer intervals between visits may be appropriate.

History should include, as a minimum, assessment of caloric and fluid intake, cyanosis, resting respiratory rate/retractions, cough, wheeze, respiratory accessory muscle use, activity, playfulness, developmental milestones or characteristics, and response to medication. The physical exam should at a minimum evaluate for interval decrease or increase in air trapping, wheezing, cyanosis, nasal flaring/retractions, resting respiratory rate, muscle mass, weight, edema, and developmental milestones. Hemoglobin oxygen saturation should be noninvasively determined, preferably both during activity and at rest. This is necessary to confirm acceptability of continued weaning of oxygen or ventilation support. If CO_2 retention is a concern, serum bicarbonate, venous blood gas (with correction for difference between arterial and venous PCO_2), and end tidal CO_2 or transcutaneous CO_2 measurements can be determined. Other electrolytes, blood urea nitrogen, and creatinine may be measured to assess fluid and electrolyte status in response to diuretics.

Other Aspects of Therapy

Previous chapters have dealt with diuretics and bronchodilators in detail. These drugs should certainly be continued at home if proven efficacious in an individual child. So that we can remove the most complex therapy first, we use these drugs to help support the child while weaning him from the oxygen and/or ventilator. Discontinuation of drug support can then be entertained. Reinstitution during respiratory tract illness may be necessary.

Chest physical therapy is taught to families and its use encouraged. We suggest that it be given 2–3 times daily when the child has an intercurrent respiratory illness, and once daily at other times in order to maintain parental proficiency and patient compliance.

Antibiotics are indicated for bacterial infections. However, there are no data to support the use of continuous or prophylactic therapy. Sputum cultures, throat swab, and other indices of bacterial infection (chest x-ray, counter-immunoelectrophoresis, blood counts, etc.) should be used to guide therapy.

Example Case

LR underwent chronic positive pressure ventilation for congenital cardiorespiratory disease and developed bronchopulmonary dysplasia. Surgical procedures by 1 year of age included repaired coarctation of the aorta, ligation of a patent ductus arteriosus, and tracheostomy. Despite chronic oxygen supplementation to maintain $PaO_2 \geq 60$ torr, growth was poor during the second year of life. She was maintained on diuretics with a mild to moderate hypercarbia. Although formula of high caloric content was used, fluid restriction inhibited desired caloric intake. Periodic attempts to increase fluid intake led to tachypnea, wheezing, and increased work of breathing. At 23 months of age she was referred for evaluation of her pulmonary disease and failure to thrive.

Physical exam revealed a small child weighing 7000 g. The respiratory rate was 45–50 per minute, with marked hyperinflation, intermittent bilateral wheezing, and crackles. She had mild nasal flaring. Other findings included a mildly protruberant abdomen with 6 cm liver span (all below the right costal margin) and spleen tip 3 cm below the left costal margin. The extremities were cachectic, and there was mild clubbing. Pertinent laboratory data were as follows: Hgb = 12.8 g/dL; HCO_3 = 39 mEq/L; Cl = 85 mEq/L; arterial blood gas (0.9 FiO_2), pH 7.41, PaO_2 = 80 torr $PaCO_2$ = 64 torr; creatinine = 0.3 mg/dl; and chest x-ray revealing a hyperinflated, cystic pattern consistent with BPD.

Hosptial course was one of furosemide diuresis and bronchodilator therapy, with significant improvement in her respiratory rate, effort, and gas exchange. She was begun on intermittent mandatory ventilation and oxygen, with further diuresis, a decrease in her CO_2 retention, and modest improvement in her hypochloremia. Her FiO_2 was reduced to 0.4 and she was discharged to home.

This was a highly motivated, involved family. Round-the-clock nursing was provided in the home, and a close working relationship was established between the pulmonologist, primary pediatrician, primary nurse, and parents. The family purchased an oximeter for home monitoring of the child's hemoglobin saturation. The child was seen weekly by the primary pediatrician, and initially every 2 weeks by the pulmonologist.

Fluid and calories were liberalized, and the child was maintained on diuretics and bronchodilators. Her weight gain was approximately 30 g per day over the first 3 months, then 15 g per day over the next 6 months. Five kilograms were gained in the year ventilation was begun. Nine months after inception of the program, she was tolerating room air. Ventilation support continued part of the day for 22 months. Occasional exacerbation of respiratory insufficiency by intercurrent viral infections required transient increases in ventilator and/or oxygen support. By age 5 her tracheostomy was surgically closed and she was in the fifth percentile for height, and tenth percentile for weight. She currently is a neurogically normal, healthy child in the top 25% of her school class.

Part of the cause of this patient's poor initial growth was that she was too rapidly weaned from ventilator and oxygen assistance. The fact that she needed ventilator assistance even *after* her supplemental oxygen requirement had resolved is evidence that the usual pattern of weaning (ventilator, oxygen, diuretics) is not always the best. The rapid but controlled catch-up growth was gratifying to this highly motivated family. Their involvement and commitment were crucial to the success of this case.

Summary

- Home respiratory care is a feasible form of care for the patient with bronchopulmonary dysplasia.
- Only a motivated and organized team of physicians, parents, nurses, respiratory therapists, and case managers or social workers will be successful.
- Patients may have symptoms of respiratory insufficiency and failure to thrive may develop *if* respiratory support is truncated or weaned abruptly in order to send a child home without such support.
- For some patients oxygen and diuretics will be sufficient for discharge. For other patients partial or continuous ventilator assistance will also be needed.
- Various methods of oxygen administration have been developed to provide as much normal activity and parental interaction as possible. Care must be taken to avoid both inadequate support and oxygen toxicity.
- Complications from long-term intubation or tracheostomy are common and are best addressed in consultation with the pediatric otorhinolaryngologist.
- When a patient is sent home on respiratory support, careful, unhurried weaning from the support in conjunction with close medical follow-up is crucial to maintain good growth and developmental progress.

References

1. O'Brodovich HM, Mellins RB. Bronchopulmonary dysplasia. Am Rev Respir Dis 1985; 132(3):694–709.
2. Feinberg EA. Family stress in pediatric home care. Caring 1985;4:38–44.
3. Schreiner MS, Donar ME, Kettrick RG. Pediatric home ventilation. Pediatr Clin N Am 1987;34(1):47–60.
4. Markestad T, Fitzhardinge PM. Growth and development in children recovering from bronchopulmonary dysplasia. J Pediatr 1981; 98(4):597–602.
5. Sotomayor JL, Godinez RI, Borden S, Wilmott RW. Large-airway collapse due to acquired tracheobronchomalacia in infancy. Am J Dis Child 1986;140:367–371.
6. Halliday HL, Dumphit FM, Brady JP. Effects of inspired oxygen on echocardiographic assessment of pulmonary vascular resistance and myocardial contractility in bronchopulmonary dysplasia. Pediatrics 1980;65:536–540.
7. Campbell AN, Zarfin Y, Groenveld M, Bryan MH. Low flow oxygen therapy in infants. Arch Dis Child 1983;58:795–798.
8. Pinney MA, Cotton EK. Home management of bronchopulmonary dysaplasia. Pediatrics 1976;58:856–859.
9. Abman SH, Accurso FJ, Koops BL. Experience with home oxygen in the management of infants with bronchopulmonary dysplasia. Clin Pediatr 1984;23(9):471–476.
10. Sasaki CT, Gaudet PT, Peerless A. Tracheos-

tomy decannulation. Am J Dis Child 1978;132: 266–269.
11. Sherman JM, Lowitt S, Stephenson C, Ironson G. Factors influencing acquired subglottic stenosis in infants. J Pediatr 1986;109:322–327.
12. Solimano JA, Smyth JA, Mann TK, Albersheim SG, Lockitch G. Pulse oximetry advantages in infants with bronchopulmonary dysplasia. Pediatrics 1986;78:844–849.

Comments

Bruce R. Boynton

Successful home respiratory care requires extensive planning. The first and most important step is to select a family that is capable of providing home care. The family must be able to master the necessary nursing techniques, be emotionally mature, and have the financial resources to pay for home care with some form of comprehensive insurance. The home must be safe (*e.g.*, no open flames or fireplaces near the infant), have a telephone, and have a reasonable amount of floor space that can be dedicated to the infant and ventilatory equipment. There must be a means of transporting the infant to and from medical appointments. Finally, the family must have financial coverage for outpatient care. Home respiratory care is expensive and may be needed for months to years, although it is cheaper in the long run than continuous hospitalization. An insurance plan that covers only 80% of home care costs may leave the family financially destitute; thus coverage for home care should be negotiated with third party payers and medical providers with this in mind. Certainly the financial advantage of home care over hospital care can be brought to their attention.

Home respiratory care is best managed by a team approach. The home care team should include the family pediatrician, pulmonologist or neonatologist, home care nurses, respiratory therapist, and a social worker.

The pediatrician provides health care maintenance and may manage the day-to-day oxygen and ventilatory care in collaboration with the pulmonologist. Some pediatricians may wish to defer this care solely to the pulmonologist.

The pulmonologist manages in-hospital care when the infant is readmitted, makes the overall plan for weaning from oxygen and the ventilator, and periodically (usually bimonthly) sees the child in clinic to assess his progress. It is of utmost importance for a physician intimately involved in the child's care to be available for consultation 24 hours a day. Failure to provide this resource frequently leads to night or weekend care by physicians unfamiliar with the case (or with the disease) who may misinterpret signs of impending respiratory failure, sometimes with disastrous results. Communication between the physicians and home care nurses is critical for effective implementation of management plans.

We recommend that the parents keep a care diary, a drug dose list, a copy of the child's outpatient records, and a copy of a contemporary chest radiograph to use in the event of emergency rehospitalization.

The primary nurse will help train and supervise the other caregivers, whether these be the parents or nurses from an outside agency. Home care agencies frequently supply nurses who have limited experience in caring for high-risk infants. In-service training and periodic inspections may be necessary to ensure that nursing care is optimum and the management plan is being followed.

The respiratory therapist provides supplies such as nasal cannulas and helps train parents and nursing personnel in the use of ventilators and oxygen equipment. It is useful for the respiratory therapist to measure the infant's hemoglobin saturation by pulse oximeter weekly. This information will be very helpful in weaning the child from respiratory support. Equipment suppliers provide and maintain the ventilator and oxygen equipment, and monitor and train the parents in their use. The nurse and respiratory therapist must ensure that these services are adequate.

The social worker assists the family in finding community resources and dealing with the stress that home care engenders. Resourceful families will often muster the assistance of family, friends, religious groups, or other care groups for babysitting or "time-out" periods.

Home respiratory care offers many advantages over prolonged hospitalization. The infant is with his family, the care may be less expensive, and there is decreased risk of nosocomial infection. There are some disadvantages as well. Home respiratory care is stressful for the family. The large number of caregivers involved may cause communication problems and lead to inconsistencies in care. It may be difficult to find qualified caregivers, and emergencies may be poorly handled. These problems can often be avoided through thoughtful planning.

Home respiratory care is not for everyone. Success requires the right patient, the right family, and a well-organized team that is invested in the continuing care of these fragile infants and their families.

IV

New Approaches to Treatment and Prevention of Bronchopulmonary Dysplasia

20

Impact of Surfactant Therapy for Respiratory Distress in Preventing or Reducing Bronchopulmonary Dysplasia

T. ALLEN MERRITT AND MIKKO HALLMAN

Infants with respiratory distress syndrome (RDS) from a deficiency or inadequate pool size of pulmonary surfactant are at greatest relative risk for developing bronchopulmonary dysplasia (BPD). Immaturity of the airways and acini, the limited quantity and immature composition of surfactant (phospholipids, apoproteins, and low molecular weight proteins), and the requirement for intermittent mandatory ventilation and supplemental oxygen contribute to the pathogenesis of lung injury.

Since the primary characteristic of RDS pathogenesis is the expression of surfactant deficiency with end-expiratory alveolar collapse, it should be possible to prevent, or at least moderate, the development of RDS by replacing the fetal lung fluid in the airways with an instillation of concentrated surfactant at birth or soon after the clinical manifestations of RDS develop. Surfactant administered to the airways must be able to reach the distal airways and to concentrate on the air-liquid interphase once the lung liquid is absorbed. This stabilizing monolayer at the air-liquid interphase, once formed, should decrease the surface tension characteristics of the acini and allow a surfactant reserve in the hypophase to be re-established, while allowing endogenous surfactant synthesis and secretion to develop normally after birth.

Early attempts to restore a low and variable surface tension to the lungs with aerosolized dipalmitoyl phosphatidylcholine were not successful in reducing either mortality or morbidity in preterm infants (1, 2).

Enhorning and Robertson (3) first demonstrated the anticipated improvement in pulmonary function by restoring surfactant in a series of fetal animal studies using pharyngeal and/or tracheal deposition of natural surfactant derived from lung lavage. Tracheal deposition of the natural surfactant (approximately 30 mg/mL) prior to lung aeration resulted in increased compliance, improved histologic as well as radiologic expansion, and an increased survival rate (4). These short-term studies demonstrated dramatic resolution of hypoaerated "whiteout" on chest radiographs characteristic of RDS, but unfortunately were not carried out until the animal survived the newborn period or had the opportunity to develop changes characteristic of chronic lung disease or resolution of lung disease. When the same surfactant preparation was tested on preterm rhesus monkeys (130–132 day gestation), there was improved gas exchange and survival compared with controls (5). Unfortunately the results of sequential chest radiographs were not reported, and these primate studies were of short duration.

Adams and coworkers found that treating preterm lambs (120 day gestation) with tracheal instillation of natural surfactant in a dose of 50–170 mg total lipid per kilogram of body weight prevented the early features of RDS (4). Jobe et al. gave natural sheep surfactant to 120 day fetal lambs either at birth or at about 20 minutes after birth when respiratory failure was established. Used in a preventative approach or to rescue an animal in respiratory failure, surfactant treatment dramatically increased the PaO_2 from approximately 50 to 270 ± 35 torr in 100% O_2 (6). Although the lambs were ventilated using infant ventilators, they deteriorated within 8 hours as demonstrated by increase in PCO_2 and decrease in PaO_2 and in lung-thorax compliance. Nonetheless natural surfactant deposition improved gas exchange sufficiently to enable a substantial lowering of FiO_2. Egan and associates (7) found similar improvements in fetal sheep given a natural lipid extract of cow lung lavage, while animals treated with synthetic phospholipid mixtures actually fared worse than controls. Surfactant deficient fetal animals not only have increased arterial-alveolar oxygen tension ratios, hypercarbia and acidosis, but also have increased solute permeability (primarily plasma proteins) into the endothelial junctions into the pulmonary interstitium and then through epithelial "tight junctions" into the alveolar air space. Overdistention of the lung by mechanical ventilation in surfactant deficiency was also shown not only to increase the protein solute "leak" into the air spaces but also to cause extensive bronchiolar epithelial desquamation with necrosis and protein transudation into the terminal bronchioles. As plasma proteins "leak" into the alveolus, they can aggregate the surfactant and inhibit its biophysical function of lowering surface tension. Exogenous surfactant instillation is reported by Jobe et al. (8) to decrease protein flux into the alveoli in ventilated preterm lambs, and to reduce the epithelial disruption in rabbits as described by Nilsson and coworkers (9).

Thus when anticipating beneficial clinical responses from surfactant instillation to preterm infants, based on animal studies, one should observe: 1) improvement in PaO_2 sufficient to permit a reduction in supplemental oxygen to near room air levels; 2) lowered $PaCO_2$; 3) reduced peak airway pressures (and therefore a probable reduction in extraalveolar air leaks); 4) reduction in transudation of proteins into the alveoli; 5) reduction in both the duration of assisted ventilation and the need for supplemental oxygen; 6) lower mean airway pressures; and 7) sustained improvement in arterial-alveolar oxygen tension ratios as endogenous surfactant synthesis and release becomes sufficient (Fig. 20.1). If present concepts regarding barotrauma and oxygen exposure and oxidant generation are correct, a reduction in the number of infants developing BPD or a lessening of its severity should accompany the use of an effective surfactant. Several controlled trials are underway to illustrate the beneficial outcome in infants treated with exogenous surfactant.

However, for these beneficial effects to result, a surface active, nonantigenic surfactant should function better when administered prior to the occurrence of lung epithelial injury or protein transudation, and must be delivered in such a way as to provide for as uniform a deposition as possible (10). Complicating factors, including left-to-right ductal shunting requiring increased ventilation, interstitial reaction to surfactant, or uneven distribution with hyperaeration/atelec-

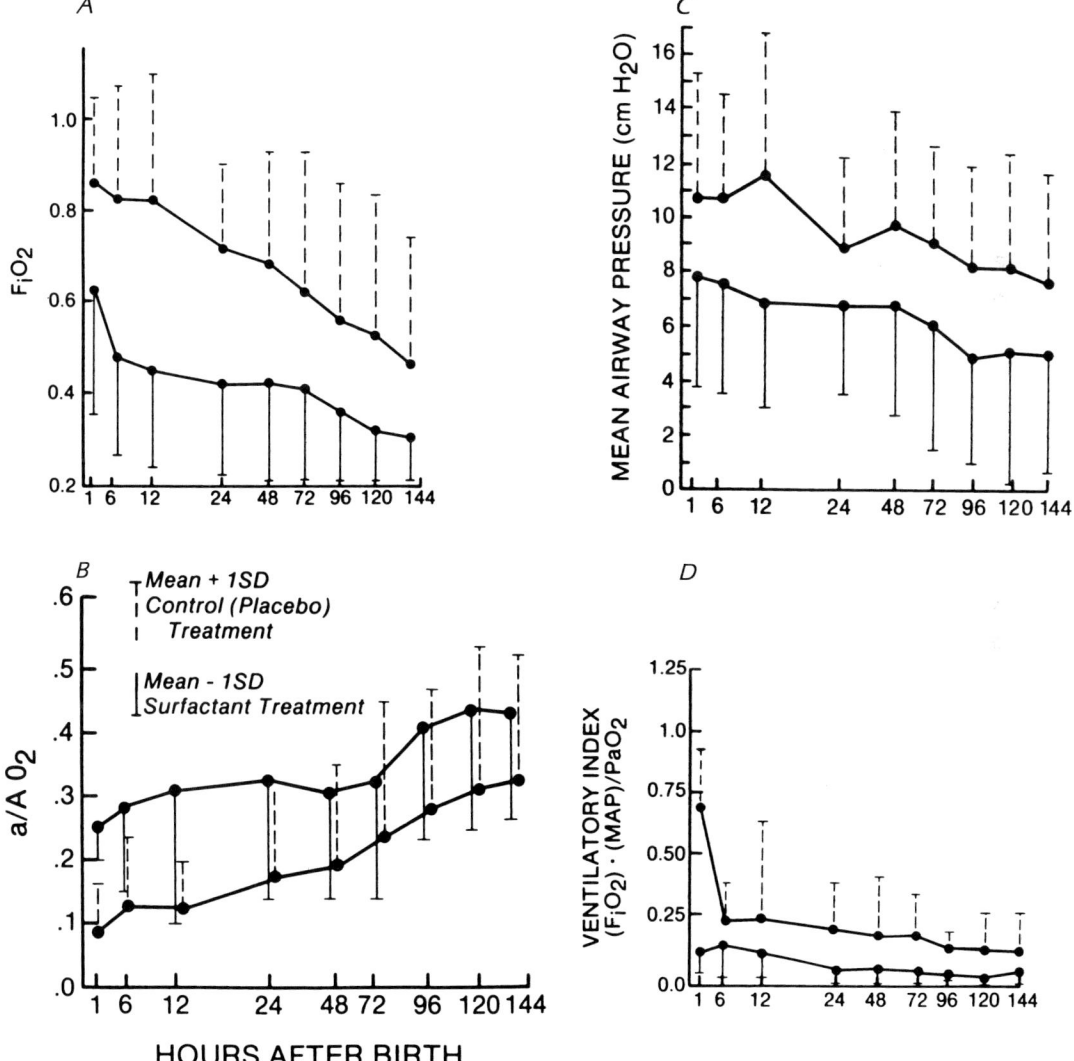

Figure 20.1. Human surfactant-treated infants compared to infants receiving conventional ventilatory treatment compared over the 48 hours after birth. Surfactant-treated = solid lines; conventional ventilation = dashed lines. (Reprinted, with permission, from N Engl J Med 1986;315:785–790.)

tasis, might attenuate the clinical efficacy of surfactant and permit lung injury. Differences in surfactant preparations, immunologic reaction to intratracheally administered heterologous surfactant antigens, or inactivation by protein inhibitors in the airways might also reduce the beneficial effects of surfactant in preventing or moderating RDS. Thus meaningful clinical studies that evaluate the efficacy of surfactants in human infants are obligated to include the occurrence of BPD as a clinical endpoint determining efficacy.

Table 20.1 reviews the reported experiences of controlled studies using surfactant preparations in clinical trials. As stressed by Boynton (Chapter 2) the incidence of BPD following RDS treatment with surfactant treatment must be compared with more conventional ventilation therapies to assess properly the effects of new treatment in terms of reducing the incidence of BPD. Not all of these studies were truly randomized or "blinded" in terms of surfactant therapy versus placebo therapy.

Wilkinson et al. (11) have pointed out that when assessing the efficacy of surfactant therapy, it is essential that only infants demonstrating surfactant deficiency (as assessed by lung effluent phospholipid profiles, or amniotic fluid maturity studies, lecithin/sphingomyelin ratio < 2.0, and absence of phosphatidylglycerol, or similar tests documenting lung surfactant immaturity) have their positive outcomes attributed to administration of "surfactant" under study. Thus reporting disorder specific (RDS vs. ventilation for other disorders) occurrence of BPD in "surfactant" treatment groups versus infants receiving conventional ventilation permits an assessment of the clinical value of its use in reducing lung injury. Indeed infants receiving surfactant for established lung immaturity with recovery from RDS may have other complications of prematurity including apnea or pneumonia. These confounding outcome variables must be controlled when comparing outcomes of groups requiring "surfactant" therapy.

Clinical trials using surfactant derived from human amniotic fluid as an intervention to rescue infants with established RDS demonstrated a significant reduction in BPD and/or death among infants of 24–29 weeks' gestation (12). In a randomized prospective clinical trial using up to three doses of human surfactant given at birth to infants with documented lung surfactant immaturity, the decline in BPD among surfactant treated infants compared with controls was highly significant: 5/26 vs. 9/14 survivors for 28 days, $p < .0003$ (13).

In contrast clinical trials using calf lung surfactant extract have been less encouraging in terms of decreasing BPD. Enhorning et al. (14) reported 22/39 or 56% of infants treated at birth with this surfactant developed BPD, compared with 22/33 or 66% (not significant) of control infants. Shapiro et al. (15) reported an identical rate of BPD in surfactant treated and control groups (5/16; 31.3%), while Kwong and associates (16) reported that 6/14 cow surfactant treated infants vs. 9/13 control infants reported BPD. Studies using artificial phospholipids as surfactant also have not spared infants the complication of BPD.

Because of the possibility of an adverse response to heterologous surfactant preparations it remains essential to follow these infants for assessment of pulmonary function, for possible later onset "allergic" reactions or reactive airways, and for other possible undesirable effects of exposure to heterologous antigens such as immune complex mediated glomerulonephritis associated with complement activation.

Data from infants treated with human surfactant have not demonstrated any adverse response in terms of complement activation, deleterious immune complex formation, allergic disorders, or systematic abnormalities of pulmonary function throughout the first year. Nonetheless long-term follow-up studies are critical to determining the safety of intratracheally administered surfactant analogues. Although other heterologous surfactants; Surfactant TA, a Japanese surfactant derived of minced cow lung with added lipids; or Curosurf, a Swed-

Table 20.1. Effect of Surfactant on Complications of RDS and Prematurity

	Study (ref)									
	Hallman et al. (12)	Enhorning et al. (14)	Kwong et al. (16)	Shapiro et al. (15)	Merritt et al. (13)	Gitlin et al. (18)	Raju et al. (19)	SUM	% Total Infants	p-value
No. of Infants										
S	22	39	14	16	31	18	17	157		
C	23	33	13	16	29	23	13	150		
Pneumothorax										
S	1*	6	4	NA	2*	3	2	18	11.5	p < .02
C	7*	11	2	NA	7	13	6	46	30.7	
Pulmonary Interstitial Emphysema										
S	0*	3*	2	NA	1*	4	2	12	7.6	p < .01
C	5	13	5	NA	14	11	7	55	36.7	
Patent Dutus Arterious										
S	18	18	7	4	23	11	12	93	59.2	NS
C	19	19	4	2	24	15	3	86	57.3	
Total intraventricular Hemorrhage (IVH)										
S	10	11*	5	4	19	15	7	71	45.2	NS
C	15	20	4	2	20	17	8	86	57.3	
Grade III & IV IVH										
S	7	4	2	NA	8	6	5	32	20.4	NS
C	7	3	2	NA	9	6	5	32	21.3	
Severe Retinopathy of Prematurity										
S	0	2	1	NA	0	3	5	12	7.6	NS
C	2	0	1	NA	0	4	2	9	6.0	
Necrotizing Enterocolitis										
S	1	2	1	NA	2	2	1	9	5.7	NS
C	3	0	1	NA	4	1	0	9	6.0	
Bronchopulmonary Dysplasia										
S	2*	22	6	5	5*	4	9	53	33.7	NS
C	8	22	9	5	9	7	4	64	40.7	
Deaths										
S	3	2	1	3	5*	3	2	19	12.1	p < .02
C	6	7	2	5	15	6	6	41	31.3	

S = surfactant. C = control. NA = not available. NS = not significant. *p < .05 between surfactant and control.

ish porcine surfactant) are under clinical investigation, little or no data are available regarding their immunogenicity, although reports of clinical efficacy are encouraging (20).

Perhaps our goal is more complex. Clinicians want to provide temporary alleviation of surfactant insufficiency for a few days until the infant can make his own. By improving gas exchange exogenous surfactant allows us to decrease the intensity of our noxious therapies and cause less damage to the lung. It may also decrease protein leak into the air spaces (thereby preventing inactivation of endogenous surfactant), change the pressures in the interstitium (decreasing the gradient for efflux of fluid from the capillaries into the air sacculus), enhance reabsorption of fetal pulmonary fluid, and change the pattern of airway opening by maintaining terminal airway expansion and thus preventing the bronchiolar ballooning observed by Taghizadeh and Reynolds (21). All these physiologic changes may impinge on the pathogenesis of BPD, which we hope to prevent as an ultimate goal. What we can observe is decreased need for forced inspiratory oxygen pressure. To date treatment with human surfactant has been associated with significant reduction in BPD. As with any new therapeutic modality, extensive testing using other proposed surface active agents is a prerequisite before advocating their widespread use. It remains critical, however, for future clinical trials to include the occurrence of BPD as a critical outcome measure, if such new therapies are to have a real beneficial impact on infants.

References

1. Robillard E, Alarie U, Dagenais-Perusse D, Barie E, Guilbeault A. Microaerosol administration of synthetic beta-gamma-dipalmitoyl-L-alpha lecithin in the respiratory distress syndrome. Can Med Assoc J 1964;50:55–59.
2. Chu J, Clements JA, Cotton EK, Klaus MH, Sweet AY, Tooley WH. Neonatal pulmonary ischemia. Pediatrics 1967;40(suppl):709.
3. Enhorning G, Robertson B. Lung expansion in the premature rabbit fetus after tracheal disposition of surfactant. Pediatrics 1972;50:588–595.
4. Adams F, Towers B, Osher AB, Ikegami M, Fujiwara T, Nozaki M. Effects of tracheal instillation of natural surfactant in premature lambs. I. Clinical and autopsy findings. Pediatr Res 1978;12:841–848.
5. Cutz E, Enhorning G, Robertson B, Sherwood W, Hill D. Hyaline membrane disease: effect of surfactant prophylaxis on lung morphology in premature primates. Am J Pathol 1978;78:581–588.
6. Jobe A, Ikegami M, Glatz T, Yoshida Y, Diakomanolis E, Padbury J: Duration and characteristics of treatment of premature lambs with natural surfactant. J Clin Invest 1981;67:370–376.
7. Egan E, Dillon W, Zorn S. Fetal lung liquid absorption and alveolar epithelial solute permeability in surfactant deficient, breathing fetal lambs. Pediatr Res 1984;18:566–569.
8. Jobe A, Ikegami M, Jacobs H, Jones S, Conaway D. Permeability of premature lamb lungs to protein and the effect of surfactant on that permeability. J Appl Physiol: Respirat Environ Exercise Physiol 1983;55:169–176.
9. Nilsson R, Grossman G, Robertson B. Pathogenesis of neonatal lung lesions induced by artificial ventilation; evidence against the role of barotrauma. Respiration 1980;40:218–222.
10. Enhorning G. Attempts at prevention of hyaline membrane disease in the delivery room. In: Nelson GH, ed. Pulmonary development. New York: Marcel Dekker, 1985, pp 285–310.
11. Wilkinson A, Jenkins P, Jeffrey J. Two controlled trials of dry artificial surfactant: early effects and later outcome in babies with surfactant deficiency. Lancet August 10, 1985, pp 287–291.
12. Hallman M, Merritt TA, Jarvenpaa AL, et al., Exogenous human surfactant for treatment of

severe respiratory distress syndrome: a randomized prospective clinical trial. J Pediatr 1985;106:963–969.
13. Merritt TA, Hallman M, Bloom B, *et al*. Prophylactic human surfactant treatment: a randomized bicenter study demonstrating a reduction in mortality and bronchopulmonary dysplasia from respiratory distress syndrome in very preterm infants. N Engl J Med 1986;315:785–790.
14. Enhorning G, Shennan A, Possmayer F, Dunn M, Chen C, Milligan J. Prevention of neonatal respiratory distress syndrome by tracheal instillation of surfactant: a randomized clinical trial. Pediatrics 1985;76:145–153.
15. Shapiro D, Notter R, Morin F, *et al*. Double-blind, randomized trial of a calf lung surfactant extract administered at birth to very premature infants for prevention of respiratory distress syndrome. Pediatrics 1985;76:593–599.
16. Kwong M, Egan E, Notter R, Shapiro D. Double-blind clinical trial of calf lung surfactant extract for the prevention of hyaline membrane disease in extremely premature infants. Pediatrics 1985;76:585–592.
17. Konishi M, Fujiwara T, Shimada S, *et al*. Method of surfactant replacement therapy in RDS—multicenter randomized study for determination of the replacement dose. Shonika Rinsho. 1986;39:161–174.
18. Gitlin JD, Soll RF, Parad RB, *et al*. Randomized controlled trial of exogenous surfactant for the treatment of hyaline membrane disease. Pediatrics 1987;79:31–37.
19. Raju TNK, Vidyasgar D, Bhat R, *et al*. Double-blind controlled trial of single-dose treatment with bovine surfactant in severe hyaline membrane disease. Lancet 1987;*i*:651–656.
20. Robertson B, van Golde LMH, Batenburg JJ, eds. Pulmonary surfactant. Amsterdam, The Netherlands: Elsevier, 1984.
21. Taghizadeh A, Reynolds EOR. Pathogenesis of bronchopulmonary dysplasia following hyaline membrane disease. Am J Path 1976;82:241–253.

21

High-Frequency Ventilation

BRUCE R. BOYNTON AND IVAN D. FRANTZ III

Introduction

The use of intermittent positive pressure ventilation has dramatically reduced the neonatal mortality rate. However, it is now apparent that current methods of positive pressure ventilation are damaging to the immature lung and that their use is accompanied by frequent pulmonary injury. Bronchopulmonary dysplasia (BPD), one of the most serious of these sequelae, develops in about 20% of infants who are mechanically ventilated for respiratory distress syndrome (RDS) (1, 2). The pathogenesis of BPD is incompletely understood, but barotrauma from positive pressure ventilation is definitely instrumental. Several innovative therapies have been proposed to reduce the incidence and severity of BPD. Recently there has been widespread interest in several methods of ventilation that use rates much greater than those observed during normal breathing. These techniques, known collectively as high-frequency ventilation, can maintain adequate gas exchange in newborn infants with a variety of diseases, including RDS, pulmonary interstitial emphysema, and pneumonia (3). The inspiratory pressures required to maintain carbon dioxide elimination are reported to be lower during high-frequency ventilation than during conventional mechanical ventilation. Since the use of high inspiratory pressures is associated with barotrauma and BPD, these findings have raised hopes that high-frequency ventilation will be less damaging to the immature lung (4). This hypothesis has not been tested in neonates. Thus far studies of neonatal high-frequency ventilation have been limited either to short-term observation or to the rescue of critically ill infants. Therefore the question of whether treatment with high-frequency ventilation will prevent BPD cannot be answered at this time. In this chapter we discuss the different techniques that have been used for high-frequency ventilation, their clinical application in neonates, and the differences between classical and high-frequency pulmonary physiology relevant to ventilator induced lung injury.

Techniques for High-Frequency Ventilation

Four types of high-frequency ventilation have been studied in neonates: 1) high-frequency positive pressure ventilation (HFPPV); 2) high-frequency jet ventilation (HFJV); 3) high-frequency oscillatory ventilation (HFOV); and 4) high-frequency flow interruption (HFFI). Although all four techniques use rapid rates, they differ in circuit design, clinical use, potential complications, and mechanism of gas transport (Table 21.1).

High-Frequency Positive Pressure Ventilation

High-frequency positive pressure ventilation, the oldest method of high-frequency ventilation, was developed by Sjöstrand and his colleagues in the early 1970s while searching

Table 21.1. Tidal Volume, Rate, and Mode of Expiration for Four Methods of High-Frequency Ventilation

Technique	Tidal Volume	Rate (per min)	Expiration
High-frequency positive pressure ventilation	$>V_D$	60–150	Passive
High-frequency jet ventilation	$>V_D$	100–600	Passive
High-frequency oscillatory ventilation	$<V_D$	300–3,000	Active
High-frequency flow interruption	$<V_D$	300–1,800	Passive

V_D = anatomic dead space

for a ventilatory technique to eliminate respiratory synchronous changes in blood pressure (5). They later hypothesized that HFPPV might have other advantages over conventional ventilation, particularly its ability to maintain gas exchange at reduced peak-inspiratory pressures. HFPPV operates at frequencies between 60 and 150 per minute. Tidal volume probably is greater than anatomic dead space, although this has not been studied carefully. Expiration is entirely passive, as in conventional ventilation. The use of ventilatory rates of 60 to 150 per minute has become commonplace in the treatment of critically ill infants who are hypoxemic or hypercapneic despite appropriate conventional ventilation. These rates can be delivered by most neonatal ventilators or by manual ventilation with an anesthesia bag. Bland et al. used standard neonatal ventilators at rates of 60 to 110 per minute to treat 24 preterm infants with RDS (6). Twenty-two infants survived, four of whom developed BPD. Unfortunately there was no control group in this study, so it is impossible to determine whether HFPPV is superior to conventional ventilation. Heicher et al. compared HFPPV with conventional ventilation in a controlled trial of 102 neonates with RDS or pneumonia (7). The HFPPV group was ventilated at a rate of 60 per minute with a 0.5 second inspiratory time; the control group, at 20 to 40 per minute with a 1.0 second inspiratory time. There was no difference between the two groups in mean airway pressure, end-expiratory pressure, use of paralyzing drugs, arterial PO_2 or PCO_2, number of deaths, or cases of chronic lung disease. However, the HFPPV group was exposed to lower peak airway pressures and had fewer pneumothoraces than the controls (14% vs. 35%).

High-Frequency Jet Ventilation

High-frequency jet ventilation is the high-frequency ventilation technique used most frequently in adults. Pulses of gas are injected at high pressure through a small-diameter catheter placed in the upper airway (Fig. 21.1). Most jet ventilators operate at rates of 100 to 600 pulses per minute, the actual pulse lasting only 100 to 200 milliseconds (8). The jet pulse may entrain ambient air, which contributes to the final tidal volume. Other factors affecting tidal volume include size and position of the jet catheter, pulse duration, and driving pressure (9, 10). Tidal volume

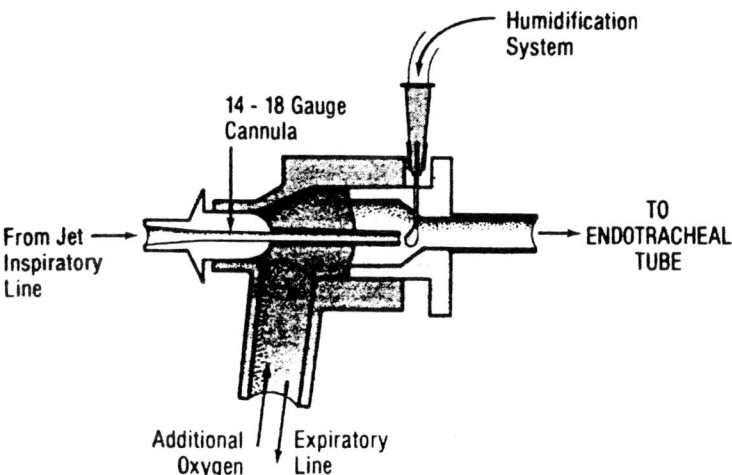

Figure 21.1. Diagram of a high-frequency jet ventilator. Pulses of gas enter the endotracheal tube through the jet cannula. Fresh gas may be entrained and expired gas is expelled through a second opening. (Reprinted, with permission, from Turnbull AD, Carlon G, Howland WS, Beattie EJ Jr. Ann Thorac Surg 1981;32:468–474.)

usually exceeds dead space during HFJV. Expiration is entirely passive, and air trapping and increases in functional residual capacity have been demonstrated.

Lung volume depends both on the amount of distending pressure applied and on the relationship between expiratory time and the expiratory time constant. Frantz and Close studied the effect of increasing inspiratory time on lung volume in rabbits ventilated with HFJV at 2 Hz (11). As the percentage of inspiratory time increased from 10% to 30% to 50%, lung volume increased from the relaxation volume to near total lung capacity. These changes in lung volume clearly increase the risk of pneumothorax and undesirable cardiovascular effects.

Pokora et al. used HFJV (260/min) to treat 10 neonates with intractable respiratory failure from RDS or pneumonia (12). Nine infants had bronchopleural fistulas or interstitial emphysema. Initiation of HFJV permitted a reduction in peak-inspiratory pressure, and air leaks improved in seven infants. However, only five infants survived. Three of the six patients treated for 20 hours or longer developed tracheal necrosis and airway obstruction from mucus plugs. The mechanism of airway injury is controversial but probably involves a combination of inadequately humidified gas and tissue trauma from the jet stream (13, 14). Subsequent improvement in equipment design may decrease these problems.

Carlo et al. compared HFJV (250/min) with conventional ventilation in 12 neonates with RDS (15). During HFJV the infants were able to maintain normal gas exchange even though peak-inspiratory pressure, mean pressure, and pressure amplitude were lower than during conventional ventilation. None of these studies has addressed the risk of developing BPD.

High-Frequency Oscillatory Ventilation

High-frequency oscillatory ventilation originated with the work of Lunkenheimer and his colleagues (16). While studying the effects of tissue oscillation on cardiac performance, these investigators noticed that transtracheal vibrations induced apnea but maintained normal gas exchange.

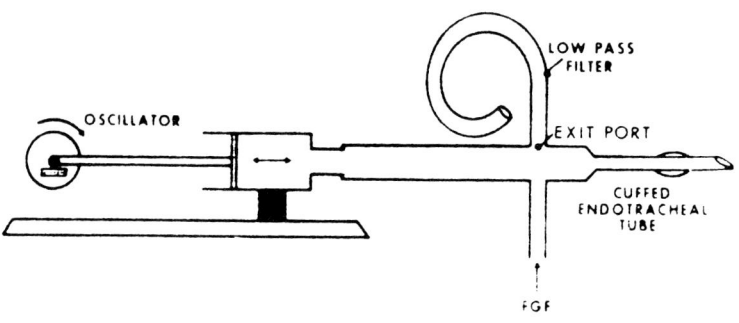

Figure 21.2. Diagram of a piston pump high-frequency oscillator. An electric motor and eccentric cam drive a piston and generate gas oscillations. Fresh gas enters the system through a high impedance side port (FGF). Expired gas exits through the low pass filter. (Reprinted, with permission, from Butler W, Bohn M, Bryan A, *et al.* Anesthesia and Analgesia 1980;59: 577–584.)

High-frequency oscillations can be produced by many techniques. Most systems in clinical use employ a piston pump driven by a rotary or linear motor (Fig. 21.2). Oscillators produce negative as well as positive pressure swings and thus actively assist in expiration. Because no gas flows through the oscillator itself, a bias flow is needed to add fresh gas to the circuit and remove expired gas. A low pass filter allows expired gas to leave the circuit while preventing attenuation of the high-frequency oscillations. High-frequency oscillators can operate at rates as high as 64 Hz, but frequencies of 12 to 20 Hz have been used most often in clinical work (17, 18). Tidal volumes are almost always less than dead space. Several investigators have reported increases in lung volume during HFOV (19, 20).

The mechanism of gas transport during HFOV is incompletely understood. Although bulk flow occurs during HFOV, convective processes alone cannot explain gas exchange when the tidal volume is less than dead space. Four basic processes may be involved in gas transport, but the relative importance of each is unknown. These processes are bulk flow by convection, convective streaming, convective mixing between lung units, and augmented diffusion.

Direct ventilation of some alveoli may take place even when the tidal volume is less than dead space (21). The length of pathways from the airway opening to the alveolus is not uniform throughout the lung. Alveoli with shorter path lengths may receive fresh gas by bulk flow with each ventilator cycle while more distal alveoli are hypoventilated. This mechanism must account for some fraction of gas transport during high-frequency ventilation, especially when the tidal volume is near dead space volume.

Convective streaming is another mechanism that may help to explain gas transport during high-frequency ventilation (21, 22). During streaming the flowing gas occupies only a fraction of the cross-sectional area of the airway. Therefore the gas penetrates more deeply than if the velocity profile was uniform across the airway.

There may be extensive inter-regional flow between distal lung units during high-frequency ventilation. Lehr and coworkers demonstrated asynchronous expansion of the pleura in an excised dog lung oscillated at frequencies of 15 and 30 Hz (23, 24). The magnitude of this asynchrony is sufficient for individual lung units to exchange gas with one another three times for each time the entire lung is cleared (25). Inter-regional gas

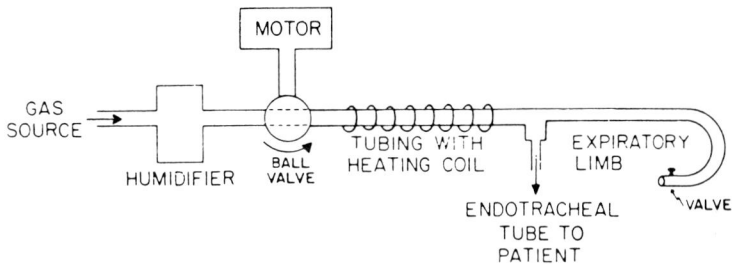

Figure 21.3. Diagram of the Emerson flow interrupter. Gas flow is repetitively interrupted by a motor driven ball valve. Mean airway pressure can be changed by adjusting the valve on the circuit's expiratory limb. (Reprinted, with permission, from Frantz ID III, Werthammer J, Stark AR. Pediatrics 1983; 71:483–488.)

mixing would promote homogenization of alveolar gas concentration and contribute to CO_2 elimination.

The transport mechanisms described thus far have been purely convective (*i.e.*, no radial mixing). However, convective transport may be coupled to diffusion. This process, known as augmented diffusion, was described first by Taylor (26) during unidirectional flow in long straight tubes and subsequently by Chatwin (27) during oscillatory flow. Fredberg has suggested that augmented diffusion contributes to gas transport during high-frequency ventilation (28). Simple molecular diffusion occurs during conventional ventilation and spontaneous respirations and is responsible for gas transport from the peripheral airways to the alveolus. During HFOV the to-and-fro movement of gas in the airways allows diffusion to take place over a much larger area thereby increasing the net dispersion of gas. Augmented diffusion is theoretically sufficient to explain gas transport during high-frequency ventilation.

It is most probable that gas transport during high-frequency ventilation involves all of these mechanisms, with the relative importance being dependent upon the species of animal, the relationship between tidal volume and dead space volume, and the particular experimental circumstances.

There are few clinical studies of HFOV in neonates. Marchak *et al.* demonstrated that HFOV could maintain gas exchange in infants with severe RDS (17). When the infants were switched from conventional ventilation to HFOV, the mean PCO_2 decreased from 52 to 44 torr and oxygenation improved, permitting a reduction in FiO_2. Boynton *et al.* combined HFOV with conventional ventilation to treat 12 neonates with respiratory failure who had inadequate gas exchange on conventional ventilation alone (18). Combined therapy improved ventilation in all infants and oxygenation in half. Eight infants survived, although all were thought to be dying before HFOV was started. BPD developed in five of the surviving infants. However, all of these infants had severe lung damage before starting HFOV, so it is difficult to determine whether high-frequency ventilation contributed to the pathogenesis.

High-Frequency Flow Interruption

High-frequency flow interrupters have similarities to both oscillators and jet ventilators (Fig. 21.3). Flow interrupters operate at frequencies similar to those used in HFOV, but there is no negative pressure phase, and exhalation is passive. Gas flow is interrupted by a solenoid valve or other device that partitions the flow into short bursts similar to those produced by jet ventilators. However, a jet catheter is not used, there is no gas entrainment, and the gas pulse enters the circuit proximal to the endotracheal tube. Tidal volumes are less than dead space. Frantz *et al.* used HFFI to ventilate 10 infants with RDS at rates of 12 Hz (29). Although mean pressure was approximately the same as during conventional ventilation, peak pressures were lower. Frantz *et al.* ventilated five additional infants with interstitial emphysema. Gas exchange improved in four of these infants, and tracheal pressure swings were less than those observed during conventional ventilation. Mean airway pressure and FiO_2 were unchanged. Resolution of interstitial emphysema occurred within 24 hours in two infants.

The Clinical Trial of High-Frequency Ventilation in Premature Infants

Thus far there are no published studies showing that high-frequency ventilation by any technique decreases the incidence of BPD. A 10-center collaborative study of the safety and efficacy of HFOV is now under way (30). Infants with birth weights between 750 and 2000 grams in respiratory failure will be randomly assigned to either HFOV or conventional ventilation during the first 24 hours of life and before 12 hours of conventional ventilation. The infant will remain on the ventilator to which he was randomized as long as mechanical ventilation is required unless gas exchange is inadequate. If this happens, the infant will be switched to the other type of ventilator. Infants with respiratory failure from RDS, pneumonia, or pulmonary hypertension are eligible for the study, but those with meconium aspiration, major congenital anomalies, and cyanotic congenital heart disease are specifically excluded. The outcome variable of most interest will be the relative frequency of chronic lung disease in the HFOV and conventionally ventilated groups. Chronic lung disease will be operationally defined as the need for supplemental oxygen on the 28th postnatal day together with abnormal chest radiographic findings persisting until the 28th day. Because only a fraction of ventilated infants develop BPD, a large sample size will be needed to detect a decrease in BPD incidence.

Airway Pressure During High-Frequency Ventilation

The distribution and magnitude of airway pressure during high-frequency ventilation is of great interest given the close association between barotrauma and BPD. During spontaneous respirations and mechanical ventilation at conventional frequencies, pressure is uniform throughout the lung. During high-frequency ventilation the situation is much more complex. To understand this topic it is necessary to differentiate between mean pressure and the amplitude of pressure excursions. In excised lungs mean pressure in the alveolus is approximately equal to that at the airway opening regardless of frequency (31). Mean pressure in the central airways is slightly lower. However, the amplitude of pressure excursions in the alveoli (P_{alv}) may exceed that in the trachea (P_{tr}) at frequencies near the resonant frequency of the lungs (Fig. 21.4) (32). At frequencies used in conventional ventilation, the ratio of P_{alv} to P_{tr} is approximately 1, while at frequencies much greater than the resonant frequency it is much less than 1. This amplification of P_{alv} increases with distending pressure but di-

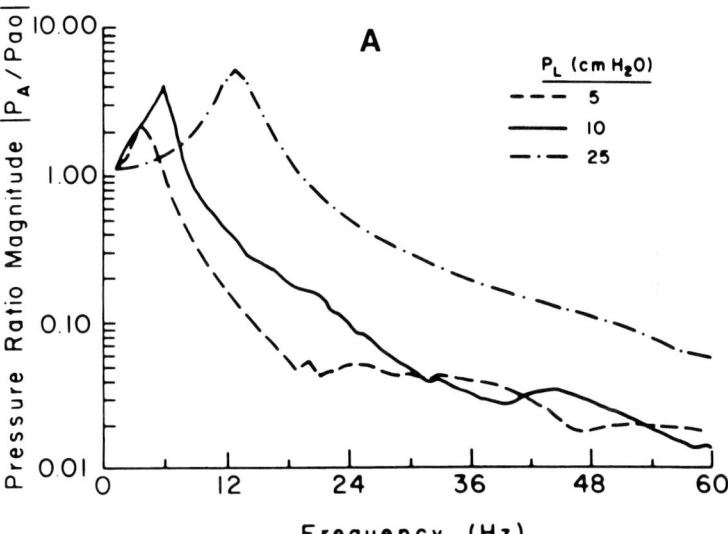

Figure 21.4. Ratio of pressure swings in alveoli (P_A) to those at the airway opening (Pao) in an excised dog lung at three transpulmonary pressures (P_L). (Reprinted, with permission, from Fredberg JJ, Keefe DH, Glass GM, Castile RG, Frantz ID III. J Appl Physiol 1984;57:788–800.)

minishes with increases in airway resistance and tidal volume. This pattern has been observed in dogs and rabbits, indicating that it does not depend on lung size (32, 33).

Alveolar pressure amplification has not been observed in studies of healthy, living rabbits oscillated using a complex waveform, although it has been predicted by a computer model of the canine respiratory system that included chest wall simulation (34, 35). In comparing these studies it is important to consider the location to which a reported pressure is referenced. In studies of excised lungs P_{alv} is referenced to the lung surface while studies in animals with closed chests reference P_{alv} to body surface. Fredberg has predicted that resonant amplification will be observed in animals with closed chests if both P_{alv} and P_{tr} are measured relative to pleural pressure (P_{pl}). If this proves true, the absence of resonant amplification of P_{alv} referenced to body surface is irrelevant because the pressure drop across the lung tissue ($P_{alv} - P_{pl}$) is the pertinent stress that deforms lung parenchyma and causes pneumothoraces and interstitial emphysema.

Very little is known about the magnitude and homogeneity of P_{alv} in diseased lungs. Fredberg and coworkers studied an open chest dog model after histamine aerosol challenge (36). Although the mean ratio of P_{alv} to P_{tr} at resonance was markedly reduced, those airways unresponsive to histamine exhibited enhanced resonant amplification. This suggests that in a lung with nonuniform distribution of resistance and compliance among parallel pathways, the least affected pathways may be subjected to the greatest pressure fluctuations. These pressures may exceed those reported in healthy and more homogeneous lungs. Because there is substantial ventilatory inhomogeneity in the surfactant deficient lung, similar processes may occur in infants with RDS during HFOV.

The optimum frequency for high-frequency ventilation is unknown and probably differs from system to system. At resonance, pressure excursions are at a minimum in the

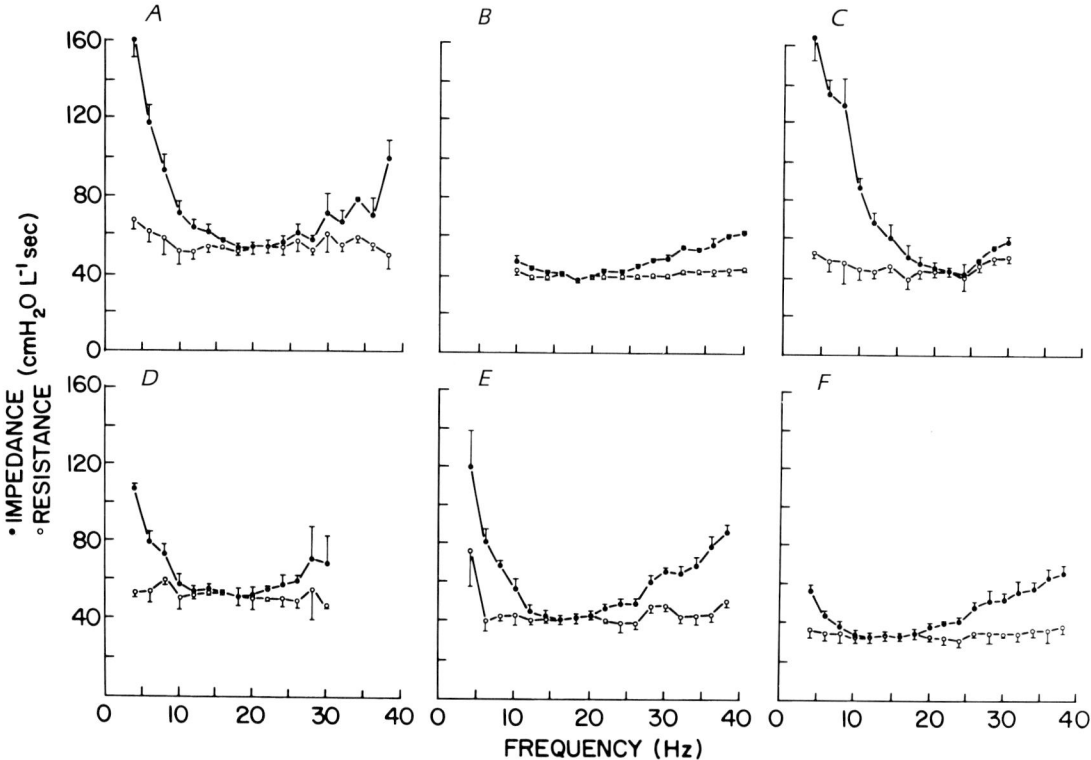

Figure 21.5. Oscillatory impedance (●) and resistance (○) as a function of frequency for 6 intubated neonates with respiratory disease. (Reprinted, with permission, from Dorkin HL, Stark AR, Werthammer JW, Strieder DHJ, Fredberg JJ, Frantz ID III. J Clin Invest 1983;72:903–910.

trachea and at a maximum in the alveoli. As frequency increases P_{tr} rises while P_{alv} falls. Thus the selection of an optimum frequency involves a trade-off between pressure exposure in the central and terminal airways. Fredberg has suggested that infants be ventilated at frequencies at least as high as their resonant frequency (32). At this frequency pressure cost per unit of oscillatory flow is at a minimum, and several investigators have shown that CO_2 elimination is proportional to oscillatory flow (37, 38).

Knowledge of the oscillatory mechanics of the neonatal respiratory system is limited. Dorkin and coworkers used forced oscillations to measure impedance and resonant frequency of six intubated infants with RDS (Fig. 21.5) (39). The resonant frequency of the respiratory system alone was calculated by subtracting endotracheal tube impedance from the impedance of the intubated infants. While the resonant frequency of the respiratory system alone was estimated to be greater than 40 Hz (the highest frequency studied), the intubated infants had resonant frequencies between 13 and 23 Hz. These frequencies are in the same range as those used in clinical trials (18, 29). However, the frequency spectrum of clinical importance may be quite different, because Dorkin's measurements were made at functional residual capacity. Since the infants were ill enough to require positive pressure ventilation with an end-expiratory pressure of 5 to 6 cm H_2O, it is reasonable to assume that they might have developed atelectasis when continuous distending pressure was withdrawn. Atelectasis would decrease tissue compliance and raise the resonant frequency of the lungs. On the other hand, in healthy excised lungs, resonant frequency increases with distending pressure (11). Thus the resonant frequencies reported by Dorkin and coworkers may be either higher or lower than those occurring during treatment with positive end-expiratory pressure, depending on the dominant process. Further research is needed to understand the effects of disease and distending pressure on resonant frequency.

Fredberg and coworkers have provided evidence that alveolar pressure may differ from tracheal pressure during HFOV (32). These pressure differences are the result of high flow rates through the relatively small cross-sectional area of the trachea. Allen and coworkers found inter-regional differences in mean alveolar pressure and alveolar pressure excursions (31, 40). In excised dog lungs P_{alv} in apical lobes exceeds P_{alv} in diaphragmatic lobes at low frequencies (2 to 8 Hz) regardless of tidal volume. At higher frequencies pressure swings in apical alveoli exceed those at the base at low tidal volumes whereas those at the base are greater when tidal volume exceeds dead space volume. Allen and coworkers hypothesized that these changes in the regional distribution of inspired gas are determined by the balance between unsteady inertia and convective momentum at central airway bifurcations. These findings suggest that manipulation of frequency and tidal volume might be used to control, to some degree, regional lung filling.

Accurate measurement of airway pressure during high-frequency ventilation is technically difficult. Measurements made at the airway opening or in the ventilator circuit may not be adequate estimates of pressure exposure in the central airways or alveoli. There are several possible sources of error. First, the pressure-measuring system may not have an adequate frequency response (41, 42). The transducers used to measure blood pressure may not be fast enough to record accurately the high-frequency phenomena. Furthermore the addition of catheters, connectors, and adaptors between the airway and transducer will degrade the frequency response even when the transducer itself is adequate.

Given an adequate pressure-measuring system, the location where measurements are made is also important (Fig. 21.6). Alveolar pressure is perhaps the most useful but cannot be measured directly in a clinical setting. However, mean alveolar pressure can be estimated by occluding the airway after disconnecting the ventilator and measuring relaxation pressure. At low rates tracheal pressure swings are a reasonable estimate of P_{alv} during HFJV. However, pressures measured near the jet cannula may be erroneous. During HFOV P_{tr} may underestimate P_{alv} at frequencies near resonance (32). Special endotracheal tubes are available that allow measurement of tracheal pressure through an intramural lumen that opens near the tube's tracheal tip and exits in a pigtail that can be connected to a pressure transducer (42). Some of these tubes have an adequate frequency response while others do not. Pressure swings measured at the airway opening

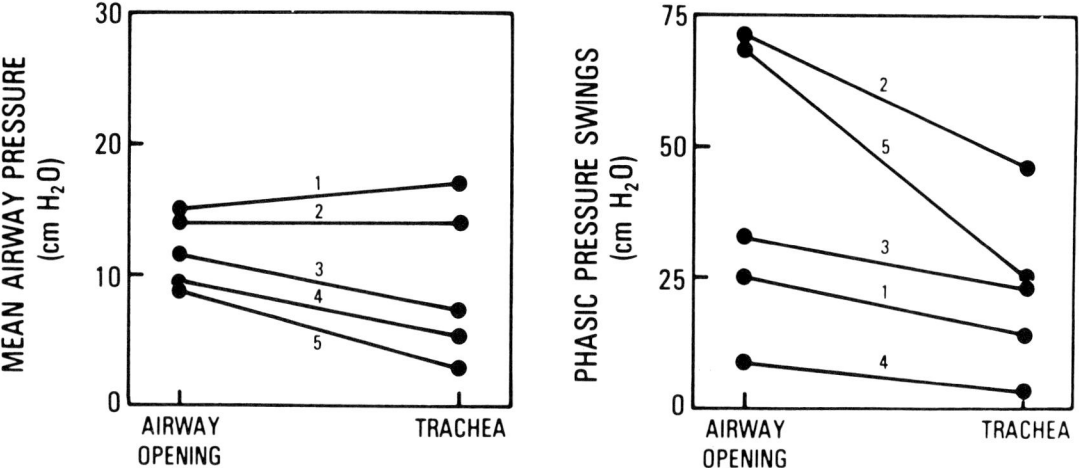

Figure 21.6. Mean airway pressure (*left*) and amplitude of pressure swings (*right*) are measured simultaneously at the airway opening and in the trachea of five neonates during high-frequency oscillation at 25 Hz. (Reprinted, with permission, from Boynton BR, Mannino FL, Meathe EA, Kopotic RJ, Friedrichsen G. Crit Care Med 1984;12:39–43.)

do not closely approximate those in the trachea or alveoli and should not be used as the sole estimate of pressure exposure.

Barotrauma and Effects on Surfactant

Pulmonary barotrauma may be defined as damage to the structural integrity of the lung tissue caused by a pressure differential (43). As we have discussed high-frequency ventilation may produce larger or smaller pressure fluctuations than conventional mechanical ventilation, depending upon frequency, distending pressure, and site of measurement. What is the evidence that high-frequency ventilation reduces the risk of barotrauma?

Hamilton and coworkers compared HFOV and conventional ventilation in rabbits made surfactant deficient by repeated saline lavage of the lungs (44). After lavage the rabbits were randomly assigned to either HFOV (15 Hz) or conventional ventilation matched for mean distending pressure. A 20 hour period of ventilation was planned, but all five rabbits assigned to conventional ventilation died before completion of the study. In contrast only one of the five animals assigned to HFOV died in less than 20 hours. At necropsy the lungs of all animals showed pneumonitis and changes in bronchial epithelium caused by pulmonary lavage. However, animals who received conventional ventilation developed diffuse hyaline membranes whereas those receiving HFOV did not. Hyaline membranes are believed to be a nonspecific response of the lung to injury and have been found in multiple pulmonary diseases. Militzer and coworkers performed a similar study using HFJV (240/min) (45). Adult rabbits were lavaged with saline until their PO_2 fell below 100 torr while breathing 100% oxygen. The rabbits were assigned to one of three groups: 1) conventional ventilation; 2) HFJV; or 3) conventional ventilation for 1 hour followed by HFJV. Four of five rabbits in group 1 died, and five of six in group 3 died. In contrast all four rabbits in the HFJV group survived. Hyaline membranes were found in 10 of the 11 animals in groups 1 and 3, but in only one of the four animals in group 2. The findings of these two studies suggest that HFOV and HFJV reduce the development of hyaline membranes, a nonspecific indication of barotrauma, in surfactant deficient lungs. Furthermore conventional ventilation in these studies produced extensive pulmonary damage after only a brief period of use.

High-frequency ventilation has been reported to be useful in treating several forms of air leak resulting from barotrauma, including pneumothorax, interstitial emphysema (29), bronchopleural fistula (46), and major airway disruption (47). These air leak syndromes occur in as many as one-third of all infants receiving mechanical ventilation for RDS, but their incidence during high-frequency ventilation is unknown. High-frequency ventilation does not completely prevent air leaks; they have been reported during all forms of high-frequency ventilation in clinical use. The increases in lung volume and high flow rates associated with HFJV may place patients at especially high risk for air leak (11).

Findings by Ackerman and coworkers suggest that combining conventional ventilator breaths or sighs with HFOV may cause interstitial emphysema (48). Using premature, surfactant deficient baboons, these investigators carried out brief crossover experiments comparing HFOV, HFFI, and conventional ventilation. Compared with conventional ventilation the high-frequency techniques improved oxygenation at lower airway-opening pressures. However, when high-frequency ventilation was prolonged beyond 6 hours, the animals developed diffuse atelectasis, hypoxemia, and hypercapnia. The use of intermittent mechanical breaths or periods of hand ventilation prevented atelectasis but caused extensive interstitial emphysema.

High-frequency ventilation does not appear to interfere with surfactant function or metabolism. Frantz and coworkers compared the quantity and function of surfactant recovered from pulmonary lavage of adult cats after a 4 hour period of HFFI, conventional ventilation, or spontaneous breathing (49). There was no difference among the three groups in assays of phosphatidylcholine or disaturated phosphatidylcholine. Surfactant function, as determined by surface balance measurements and pressure-volume curves, was similar in all groups. Truog and coworkers studied the effect of HFOV on pulmonary phospholipid concentration and function in immature primates with RDS (50). Disaturated phosphatidylcholine content of lung homogenates and alveolar lavage fluid was similar in animals treated with HFOV and those treated with conventional ventilation. Postmortem pressure-volume curves were also identical in the two groups.

Summary

High-frequency ventilation by any technique has not been proven superior to conventional ventilation for treating neonates with lung disease. Most clinical studies have been anecdotal, short-term, or restricted to critically ill infants. Studies of oscillatory mechanics suggest that alveolar pressure swings may be higher or lower with high-frequency ventilation than with conventional ventilation, depending upon the proximity of ventilatory frequency to the resonant frequency of the respiratory system. Studies of barotrauma in experimental animals suggest that high-frequency techniques are less damaging and may result in less BPD. A national collaborative study of HFOV is under way to test this hypothesis. The study of high-frequency ventilation has increased our understanding of mechanical ventilation and pulmonary physiology. The role for these techniques in clinical medicine is not yet clear.

References

1. Wung J-T, Koons AH, Driscoll JM, James LS. Changing incidence of bronchopulmonary dysplasia. J Pediatr 1979;845–847.
2. Lindroth M, Svenningsen NW, Ahlström H, Jonson B. Evaluation of mechanical ventilation in newborn infants. II. Pulmonary and neurodevelopmental sequelae in relation to original diagnosis. Acta Pædiatr Scand 1980;69:151–158.
3. Ackerman NB Jr, deLemos RA. High-frequency ventilation. In: Oski F, ed. Advances in pediatrics 1984. Chicago: Year Book Medical Publishers, 1984, pp 259–293.
4. Special conference report—high frequency ventilation for immature infants. Pediatrics 1983;71:280–287.
5. Sjöstrand U. Review of the physiological rationale for and development of high frequency positive-pressure ventilation (HFPPV). Acta Anaesthesiol Scand 1977;64(suppl):7–27.
6. Bland RD, Kim MH, Light MJ, Woodson JL. High-frequency mechanical ventilation in severe hyaline membrane disease—an alternative treatment? Crit Care Med 1980;8:275–280.
7. Heicher D, Kasting D, Harrod J. Prospective clinical comparison of two methods of mechanical ventilation of neonates: rapid rate and short inspiratory time vs slow rate and long inspiratory time. J Pediatr 1981;98:957–961.
8. Miodownik S. Technical implications of high frequency jet ventilation. In: Carlon GC, Lowland WS, eds. International symposium on high frequency ventilation. New York: Memorial Sloan-Kettering Cancer Center, 1983, pp 13–16.
9. Carlon G, Ray C, Peirri M, et al. High frequency jet ventilation. Chest 1982;81:350–354.
10. Keszler H, Klain M. Importance of position of jet orifice in high frequency jet ventilation (abstr). Crit Care Med 1982;10:234.
11. Frantz ID III, Close RH. Elevated lung volume and alveolar pressure during jet ventilation of rabbits. Am Rev Respir Dis 1985;131:134–138.
12. Pokora T, Bing D, Mammel M, Boros S. Neonatal high-frequency jet ventilation. Pediatrics 1983;72:27–32.
13. Ophoven JP, Mammel MC, Gordon MJ, Boros SJ. Tracheobronchial histopathology associated with high frequency jet ventilation. In: Carlon GC, Howland WS, eds. International symposium on high frequency ventilation. New York: Memorial Sloan-Kettering Cancer Center, 1983, pp 93–94.
14. Mammel MC, Ophoven JP, Lewallen PK, Gordon MJ, Sutton MC, Boros SJ. High-frequency ventilation and tracheal injuries. Pediatrics 1986;77:608–613.
15. Carlo WA, Chatburn RL, Martin RJ, et al. Decrease in airway pressure during high-frequency jet ventilation in infants with respiratory distress syndrome. J Pediatr 1984;104:101–107.
16. Lunkenheimer P, Rafflenbeul W, Keller H, et al. Application of transtracheal pressure oscillations as a modification of "diffusion respiration" (letter). Br J Anaesth 1972;44:627.
17. Marchak BE, Thompson WK, Duffty P, et al. Treatment of RDS by high frequency oscillatory ventilation: a preliminary report. J Pediatr 1981;99:287–290.
18. Boynton BR, Mannino FL, Davis RF, et al. Combined high-frequency oscillatory ventilation and intermittent mandatory ventilation in critically ill neonates. J Pediatr 1984;105:297–302.
19. Saari AF, Rossing TH, Solway J, Drazen JM. Lung inflation during high-frequency ventilation. Am Rev Respir Dis 1984;129:333–336.
20. Brusasco V, Beck KC, Crawford M, Rehder K. Resonant amplification of delivered volume

during high-frequency ventilation. J Appl Physiol 1986;60:885–892.
21. Drazen JM, Kamm RD, Slutsky AS. High-frequency ventilation. Physiol Rev 1984;64:505–543.
22. Haselton FR, Scherer PW. Bronchial bifurcations and respiratory mass transport. Science 1980;208:69–71.
23. Lehr J. Circulating currents during high frequency ventilation (abstr). Fed Proc 1980;39:576.
24. Lehr J, Butler JP, Westerman PA, et al. Photographic measurement of pleural surface motion during lung oscillation. J Appl Physiol 1985;59:623–633.
25. Allen JL, Fredberg JJ, Keefe DH, Frantz ID III. Alveolar pressure magnitude and asynchrony during high-frequency oscillations of excised rabbit lungs. Am Rev Respir Dis 1985;132:343–349.
26. Taylor GI. Dispersion of soluble matter in solvent flowing slowly through a tube. Proc Roy Soc Lond (Biol) 1953;219:186.
27. Chatwin PC. On the longitudinal dispersion of passive contaminant in oscillatory flows in tubes. J Fluid Mech 1975;71:513–527.
28. Fredberg JJ. Augmented diffusion in the airways can support pulmonary gas exchange. J Appl Physiol 1980;49:232–238.
29. Frantz ID III, Werthammer J, Stark AR. High-frequency ventilation in premature infants with lung disease: adequate gas exchange at low tracheal pressure. Pediatrics 1983;71:483–488.
30. Research Triangle Institute. High Frequency Intervention Trial (HIFI)—research protocol. Research Triangle Park: 1985.
31. Allen J, Frantz I, Fredberg J. Mean alveolar pressures during high frequency oscillations (abstr). Physiologist 1984;27:212.
32. Fredberg JJ, Keefe DH, Glass GM, Castile RG, Frantz ID III. Alveolar pressure nonhomogeneity during small-amplitude high-frequency oscillation. J Appl Physiol 1984;57:788–800.
33. Allen JL, Fredberg JJ, Keefe DH, Frantz ID III. Alveolar pressure magnitude and asynchrony during high-frequency oscillations of excised rabbit lungs. Am Rev Respir Dis 1985;132:343–349.
34. Frantz ID III, Close RH. Alveolar pressure swings during high frequency ventilation in rabbits. Pediatr Res 1985;19:162–166.
35. Jackson AC, Tabrizi M, Kotlikoff MI, Voss JR. Airway pressures in an asymmetrically branched airway model of the dog respiratory system. J Appl Physiol 1984;57:1222–1230.
36. Fredberg JJ, Ingram RH Jr, Castile RG, Glass GM, Drazen JM. Nonhomogeneity of lung response to inhaled histamine assessed with alveolar capsules. J Appl Physiol 1985;58:1914–1922.
37. Slutsky AS, Kamm RD, Rossing TH, et al. Effects of frequency, tidal volume, and lung volume on CO_2 elimination in dogs by high frequency (2–30 Hz), low tidal volume ventilation. J Clin Invest 1981;68:1475–1484.
38. Rossing TH, Slutsky AS, Lehr JL, Drinker PA, Kamm R, Drazen JM. Tidal volume and frequency dependence of carbon dioxide elimination by high-frequency ventilation N Engl J Med 1981;305:1375–1379.
39. Dorkin HL, Stark AR, Werthammer JW, Strieder DHJ, Fredberg JJ, Frantz ID III. Respiratory system impedance from 4 to 40 Hz in paralyzed intubated infants with respiratory disease. J Clin Invest 1983;72:903–910.
40. Allen JL, Frantz ID III, Fredberg JJ. Regional alveolar pressure during periodic flow—dual manifestations of gas inertia. J Clin Invest 1985;76:620–629.
41. Jackson AC, Vinegar A. A technique for measuring frequency response of pressure, volume, and flow transducers. J Appl Physiol 1979;47:462–467.
42. Boynton BR, Mannino FL, Meathe EA, Kopotic RJ, Friederichsen G. Airway pressure measurement during high frequency oscillatory ventilation. Crit Care Med 1984;12:39–43.
43. Kotas RV. Barotrauma to the developing lung. In: Bronchopulmonary dysplasia. Report of the 90th Ross Conference on Pediatric Research. Columbus, Ohio: Ross Laboratories, 1986.
44. Hamilton PP, Onayemi A, Smyth JA, et al. Comparison of conventional and high-frequency ventilation: oxygenation and lung pathology. J Appl Physiol 1983;55:131–138.
45. Militzer HW, Quan SF, Calkins JM, et al.

Effects of high frequency jet ventilation in a rabbit model of infant respiratory distress syndrome (IRDS) (abstr). Crit Care Med 1983;11:222.
46. Carlon GC, Ray C Jr, Klain M, McCormack PM. High-frequency positive-pressure ventilation in management of a patient with bronchopleural fistula. Anesthesiology 1980;52:160–162.
47. Turnbull AD, Carlon G, Howland WS, Beattie EJ Jr. High-frequency jet ventilation in major airway or pulmonary disruption. Ann Thoracic Surg 1981;32:468–474.
48. Ackerman NB, Kuehl TJ, Coalson JJ, *et al.* Distal airway rupture during high frequency ventilation (HFV) in the premature baboon with hyaline membrane disease (HMD) (abstr). Crit Care Med 1983;11:223.
49. Frantz ID III, Stark AR, Davis JM, *et al.* High-frequency ventilation does not affect pulmonary surfactant, liquid, or morphological features in normal cats. Am Rev Respir Dis 1982;126:909–913.
50. Truog WE, Standaert TA, Murphy J, *et al.* Effects of high-frequency oscillation on gas exchange and pulmonary phospholipids in experimental hyaline membrane disease. Am Rev Respir Dis 1983;127:585–589.

22

Pharmacologic Intervention: Use of the Antioxidant Superoxide Dismutase

WARREN ROSENFELD AND LUZMINDA CONCEPCION

Introduction

Definitive pharmacologic intervention for the prevention of bronchopulmonary dysplasia (BPD) may involve one or more of three basic strategies: 1) prevention of toxic challenges to the developing lung—*i.e.*, prevention of the formation of toxic oxygen radicals; 2) increased capacity to quench toxic radicals once they have been generated; or 3) prevention or diminution of toxic effects of elastases released by free radical injury.

Prevention of Free Radical Generation

Reduction of the duration of exposure to intermittent positive pressure breathing (IPPB), oxygen, and barotrauma may help to reduce the incidence of BPD. Instillation of surfactant (1), high-frequency ventilation (2), and support during severe ventilatory failure by extracorporeal membrane oxygenation (ECMO) (3) are three treatment modalities presently being investigated. Their efficacy and feasibility will soon be determined, and their effects on lowering the incidence of BPD can be evaluated.

These therapies may soon be a reality, and some believe that they will greatly reduce the incidence of BPD. In a recent report by Avery *et al.* (4) which surveyed eight major neonatal intensive care units throughout the country, the incidence of BPD was greater than 30% for patients of less than 1500 g with one exception, Columbia Babies Hospital. Use of nasal continuous positive airway pressure (CPAP) rather than intubation as initial treatment for even the smallest patients, avoidance of paralyzing agents, and the acceptance of PCO_2 greater than 50 mmHg (with pH > 7.20) apparently decrease the incidence of BPD. If BPD is an iatrogenic disease, lessening the challenges of IPPB and hyperoxia may have a major effect on its incidence. However, this disease may not be totally eliminated, especially in the very low birth weight (VLBW) group. While the effects of barotrauma and high oxygen concentrations on the lung can be limited, the exposure of the lung to low oxygen concentrations (*i.e.*, room air) may be toxic if free radical defenses are inadequate.

Free radical generation also occurs during conditions other than hyperoxia, thereby limiting the effectiveness of decreasing oxygen exposure to prevent BPD. Other mechanisms of free radical generation may continue to result in chronic lung changes in patients who require minimal ventilatory or oxygen therapy. This may be especially important in very premature and compromised neonates. Generation of superoxide radicals during reperfusion via the xanthine oxidase pathway may be an important source of superoxide radicals (5). This type of injury will undoubtedly continue and may even increase when the previously mentioned technologies are utilized to reestablish perfusion in compromised neonates. In addition the respiratory bursts of oxygen by macrophages and polymorphonuclear cells involved in host defenses against infection (6) may be another important source of free radical generation in neonates.

Increased Quenching of Free Radicals

The second strategy of defense, increased quenching of free oxygen radicals, has been studied both in animals and in premature humans. Numerous antioxidants are available:

A. Low molecular weight free radical scavengers
   1. Lipid soluble
      a. Vitamin E
      b. Ascorbic acid
      c. Beta-carotene
   2. Cytoplasmic: glutathione
B. Enzymatic free radical scavengers
   1. Superoxide dismutase (SOD)
      a. Cu-Zn SOD
      b. Manganese SOD
   2. Catalase
   3. Peroxidase
   4. Ceruloplasmin

Among known antioxidants, superoxide dismutase appears to be the most active (7) and is found in every cell that requires oxygen. Catalase removes H_2O_2, which is not a free radical but an oxidizing agent produced as a byproduct of O_2 metabolism. Other free radicals such as the hydroxyl radical (OH·) and singlet oxygen ($^1O_2$) will not be formed without generation of superoxide anion (O^-_2). Another antioxidant, vitamin E, has received wide attention in the neonatal literature as a potential treatment for BPD and retinopathy of prematurity (ROP) (8, 9, 10, 11), but clinical trials have failed to demonstrate its efficacy.

Superoxide dismutase (SOD) is found in all aerobic cells within both the cytosol and mitochondria. It has also been found in much lower concentrations in extracellular fluids (12). Human SOD has several different structures. Cu-Zn SOD, consisting of two identical amino acid chains liganded by two Cu^{++} and two Zn^{++} molecules, weighs 33,000 daltons and is found in the cytosol and free in the serum. Manganese SOD, which is made of four identical amino acid chains bound to four Mn^{++} molecules and weighing 82,000 daltons, is found within the mitochondria. Marklund (13) has also described a larger molecule of SOD bound to four Cu molecules and weighing 120,000 daltons which is found free in serum. However, this form of SOD has not been confirmed by other investigators. The evolution of two functionally similar enzymes with markedly different molecular and amino acid structures remains an unsolved question. However, each form of SOD is able to aid the transfer electrons within the mitochondria and cytosol, and on the cell membrane, preventing cell destruction due to free radical injury.

SOD's activity as an antioxidant has resulted in many investigations into its possible use in preventing free radical injury. Numerous investigators have demonstrated its protective effect. Intermittent exposure of rats to sublethal doses of oxygen (40%–85%) for 7 days increased their survival rate over that of nonexposed controls when both were exposed to 100% oxygen. This increased tolerance to 100% oxygen was accompanied by a 50% increase in lung SOD (14). This effect has been demonstrated in neonatal rats, mice, and rabbits, but similar experimental conditions did not induce either increased SOD or tolerance to 100% oxygen in hamsters or guinea pigs.

Pretreatment of rats with SOD prevented toxic changes in lung macrophages when exposed to hyperoxia (15) and prevented damage to lung cells as measured by pulmonary serotonin clearance (16). Intravenous injections of liposome entrapped catalase and SOD significantly increased survival time in rats from 70 to 119 hours and was associated with a decrease in pleural effusions (17). Changes in permeability of the pulmonary vasculature of dogs due to infusion of an inflammatory agent, α-naphthyl thiourea, was blocked by SOD infusion but not by catalase (18). A similar protective effect of SOD with heparin prevented increased lung permeability during air embolization in the sheep lung (19). Other routes of administration have also been attempted. Instillation of liposome-SOD and liposome-catalase into the trachea of rats resulted in increased tissue levels of the enzymes and increased survival from 11% to 93% and to 96%, respectively (20). A variety of animal models and routes of administration have been utilized to study SOD's antioxidant properties. While all have not been successful, a growing number of reports support SOD's potential role as a means to scavenge free radicals and prevent BPD.

Premature neonates may be particularly susceptible to the development of BPD secondary to free radical injury. They frequently require endotracheal intubation, IPPB, and high oxygen concentrations. In addition the premature may not have the antioxidant defenses to quench free oxygen radicals. Pulmonary antioxidant enzymes develop simultaneously with the development of the surfactant system, providing a total package to provide for extrauterine respiration and increased oxygen exposure (21, 22). Among these antioxidants SOD has been shown deficient in premature rabbits, rats, guinea pigs, and hamsters. Other studies have shown similar findings suggesting that human premature neonates are deficient for SOD (23, 24).

It has also been demonstrated that administration of dexamethasone stimulates the production of not only surfactant but also SOD. Frank and coworkers (25) have evaluated several possible mechanisms of surfactant and antioxidant stimulation and suggest both are stimulated by steroids but only surfactant production is blocked by β-adrenergic blockade (26). Further investigation will be required to evaluate the potential usefulness of steroid stimulation of SOD in preterm labor, the length of time needed to induce this antioxidant enzyme system, and the effectiveness of increased SOD levels in the prevention of BPD.

Pharmacology

SOD has been purified from a number of sources, most notably bovine liver (27). Its pharmacokinetics have been studied in a variety of species including mice, rabbits, dogs, monkeys, and humans. Absorption occurs from intravenous, intramuscular, subcutaneous, and intraperitoneal injections. Oral administration is ineffective. Intravenous injection results in first order kinetics, and half-life has been evaluated to be 6–8 minutes in the animal models studied. In rats subcutaneous, intramuscular, and intraperitoneal injections resulted in peak levels 1–2 hours following administration. SOD is excreted directly through the kidneys. More than two-thirds of radioactive SOD injected intravenously was recovered in the urine within 30 minutes, and nephrectomized rats had a serum half-life 10 times greater than normals. In adult humans intravenous injections resulted in a half-life of 25 minutes and 3–6 hours following intramuscular or subcutaneous injections. Doses of 0.36 mg/kg intramuscularly resulted in peak serum levels of 0.5 μg/mL at 2–5 hours postinjection.

The potential effectiveness of exogenously administered SOD has been questioned because of SOD's short half-life and its inability to enter cells. Some investigators have sought to overcome these problems by combining SOD with either liposomes or polyethylene glycols (PEG). Liposome encapsulation increased the half-life of intravenous SOD from 8 minutes to 42 hours (17). When combined with PEG, 36% of intravenous SOD remained in circulation 72 hours after injection (20).

In their studies of bovine SOD, Huber and Menander (27) suggested that exogenous SOD does not enter cells. This was also the conclusion of Shaffer, O'Neill, and Thibeault (29) during their evaluation of continuous subcutaneous infusion of SOD in rats. In their study serum levels rose by 26 times while intracellular levels rose only 6 times. The authors interpreted these results as SOD's failure to enter the cytosol. While this study does demonstrate tissue levels do not rise as rapidly as serum levels, they were 20% of serum concentrations. This increase may have therapeutic implications, although the authors did not find any beneficial effect under the conditions of this experiment.

Investigators have demonstrated that both liposome-SOD (30) and PEG-SOD enter cells. However, both liposomes and PEG have been associated with toxicity. Liposomes, alone or in combination with SOD, may increase susceptibility to infection. In *vitro,* decreased killing of *Staphylococcus aureus* by neutrophils incubated with liposomes has been demonstrated (31). *In vivo* inhibition of the clearance of *S. aureus* was demonstrated in rabbits who were treated with liposomes. PEG does not affect neutrophil function, but antigenicity to PEG with the development of antibodies and loss of activity of the enzyme to which it was conjugated has been demonstrated (32).

While numerous animal experiments have resulted in some variation in the effectiveness and pharmacokinetics of SOD, there has been human experience with SOD for treatment of diseases other than BPD. The bovine preparation of SOD (Ontoseen, Diagnostic Data, Inc., Mountainview, Calif.) has been studied in adults as an anti-inflammatory agent in rheumatoid arthritis, osteoarthritis, and radiation cystitis (27). These double-blind, controlled investigations have demonstrated that SOD does have anti-inflammatory properties which result in clinical improvement. This preparation has been approved for use in Europe and Japan and the incidence of allergic reactions has been infrequent.

Clinical Trials Utilizing SOD

Previous studies and observations showing the beneficial effect of SOD in protecting animals exposed to hyperoxia from developing BPD stimulated us to study the use of this enzyme in human premature infants. With FDA approval an initial study was undertaken to establish the safety and pharmacokinetics of systematic administration of bovine SOD to premature infants.

Nineteen premature infants with a mean birth weight of 1200 g and a mean gestational age of 29 weeks, with severe respiratory distress syndrome requiring FiO₂ greater than 0.7 at 24 hours of age, were included (33). Patients with other causes of respiratory distress including aspiration, sepsis, pneumonia, drug withdrawal, and major congenital anomalies were excluded. Each patient received an initial test dose of 0.1 mg/kg intradermally and was observed over a period of 1 hour for cutaneous or systemic reactions. If none occurred, a dose of 0.25 mg/kg was given subcutaneously every 12 hours. Baseline chest x-ray, complete blood count with platelet and reticulocyte count, sodium, potassium, glucose, creatinine, and urinalysis were obtained. These determinations were serially evaluated during, and for 2 to 3 days following, SOD administration. Coagulation profile, SGPT, and SGOT were obtained before, during, and after SOD administration. There were no significant changes in any of these laboratory evaluations during or after SOD therapy.

No abnormal reactions to the test dose were observed. Plasma levels of SOD were measured by thin-layer agarose gel electrophoresis with nitroblue tetrazolium (NBT) staining as described by Beauchamp and Fridovich (34). This method can differentiate between the endogenous human SOD and the exogenously administered bovine SOD. Exogenous SOD reached detectable levels in all patients at 1½ hours after dose 1 (mean 0.22 µg/mL), gradually rose to a peak at 4–8 hours (mean 0.37 µg/ml), and then reached a plateau over the remainder of the 12 hour interval. Mean levels remained between 0.2 and 0.36 µg/mL during the 12 hour interval between doses. Similar responses resulted following doses 2–5, with mean levels between 0.36 and 0.68 µg/mL. SOD is excreted via the kidneys, and the levels as expected

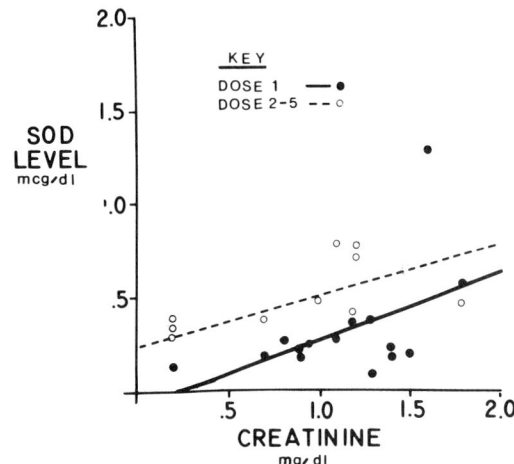

Figure 22.1. Relationship of serum creatinine and SOD levels 2 hours after dose 1 ($y = 0.37x - 0.07$, $r = 0.5043$, $p < .05$), and dose 2 ($y = 0.25x + 0.3$), $r = 0.6293$, $p < .05$).

correlated directly with serum creatinine levels (Fig. 22.1).

After demonstrating that bovine SOD could be administered safely and therapeutic levels could be achieved, a randomized double-blind trial of SOD for the prevention of BPD in premature infants with severe respiratory distress syndrome was conducted (35). Forty-five infants (mean birth weight 1154 g, mean gestational age 28.7 weeks) were enrolled; 21 received SOD, and 24 received placebo (saline solution). The treatment and placebo groups were comparable in birth weight, gestational age, sex ratio, Apgar scores, and other significant clinical characteristics. All infants were ventilator dependent with FiO₂ greater than 0.7 at 24 hours of age and were treated until they could be maintained in room air without ventilatory or CPAP support.

No plasma bovine SOD was detectable in any of the 21 patients prior to drug therapy. It was detectable in the plasma of all treated

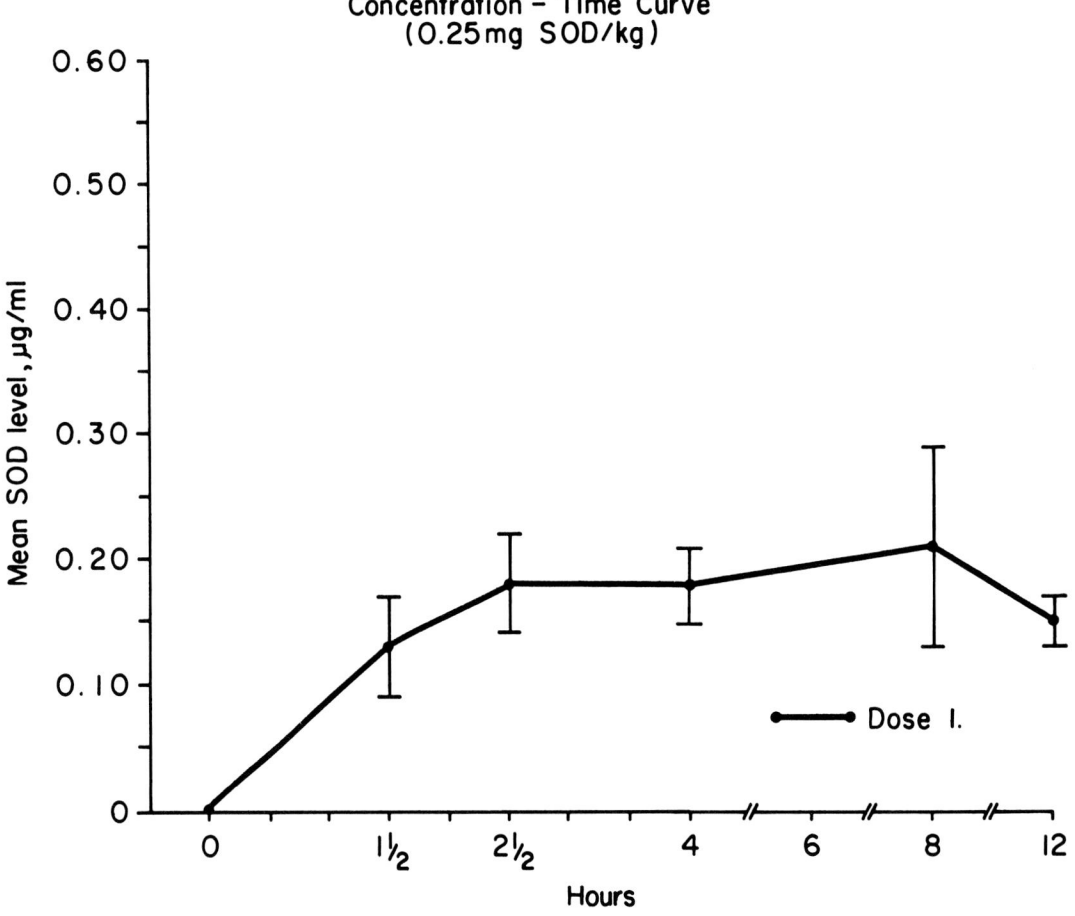

Figure 22.2. Concentration-time curve after dose 1 of superoxide dismutase (SOD) (0.25 mg/kg subcutaneous).

patients at 1½ hours after dose 1 (mean 0.15 µg/mL). Levels gradually rose, peaked at 8 hours (mean 0.21 µg/mL), and declined slowly at 12 hours (Fig. 22.2). The mean peak levels before dose 5 and dose 10 were 0.35 and 0.27 µg/mL, respectively. The levels rose slightly by 4 hours (0.40 and 0.43 µg/mL) and declined slowly over the next 8 hours (0.27 and 0.35 µg/mL) (Fig. 22.3). During this study there was no correlation of peak SOD plasma levels to serum creatinine concentration. However, in contrast to the previous study, serum creatinine levels did not rise to levels found in the initial group of patients. The drug was well tolerated, and there were no cutaneous or systemic reactions in the treatment group.

Of the original 45 patients, 31 survived and were discharged from the NICU. Seven patients in each treatment group died. Three of seven SOD and two of seven placebo nonsurvivors weighed less than 750 g at birth, and five

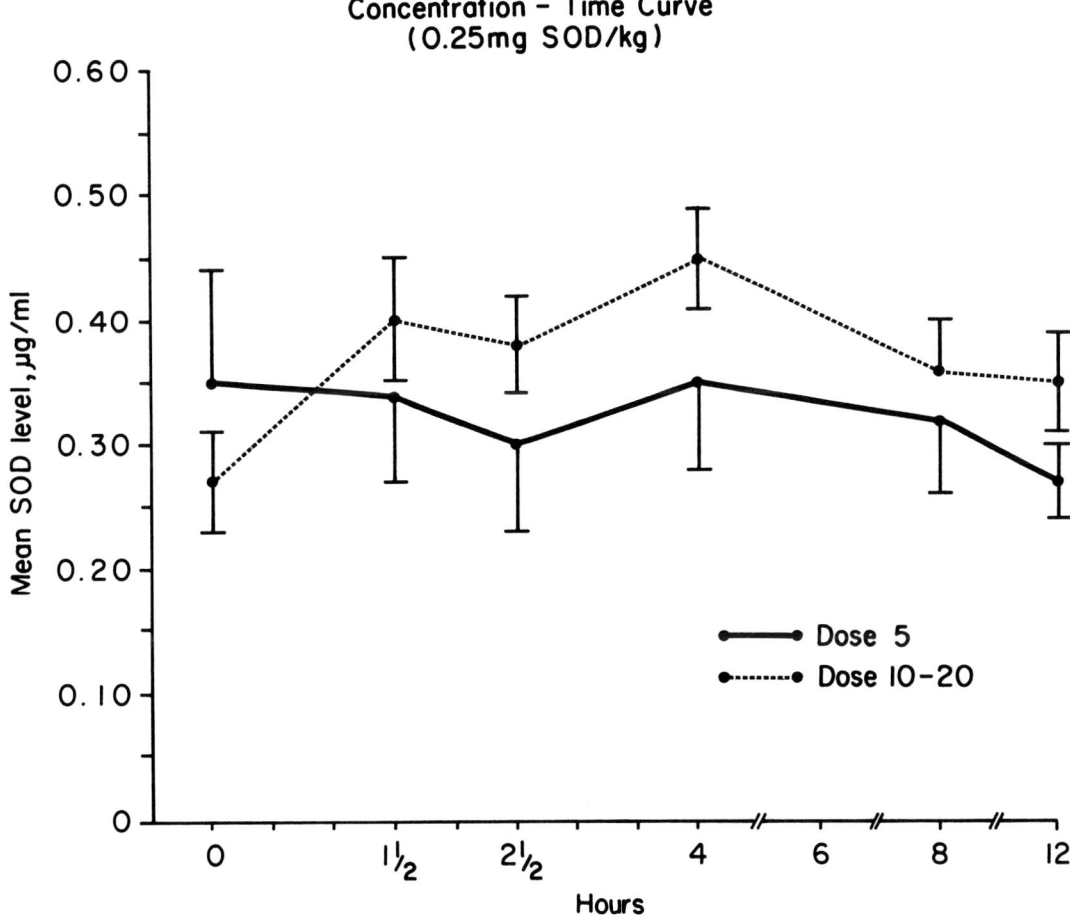

Figure 22.3. Concentration-time curve derived from samples taken after dose 5 and from one sample taken between doses 11 and 20.

in each group weighed less than 1000 g. The two patient groups had similar total number of days on intermittent mandatory ventilation and supplemental oxygen. The mean peak-inspiratory pressures during the first week, incidence and severity of patent ductus arteriosus or intraventricular hemorrhage were comparable in both groups. However, patients treated with SOD required fewer days of CPAP (4.9 vs. 9.7 days, $p < .03$). Radiologic evidence of BPD as determined by a pediatric radiologist blind to the therapy received, developed in 3 of 14 (21%) SOD patients compared with 12 of 17 (71%) control patients. This result is statistically significant ($p = .008$). Clinical signs of BPD (wheezing, pneumonia, theophylline use, and hospitalization for respiratory distress) were also significantly less, 3 of 14 (21%) SOD treated survivors compared with 11 of 17 (65%) control infants ($p = .019$).

The results of this preliminary therapeutic trial are encouraging. Concerns about the use of bovine protein are now moot with the production of pure human SOD by recombinant DNA techniques. This preparation is now available, and pending FDA approval, our group will soon be investigating its effectiveness. Questions of SOD's site of action (extracellular vs. intracellular) continue to be raised, and the ability of SOD to enter sites and its site of action (membranes vs. cytosol) require further study.

Although toxicity due to SOD has not been documented, the effect of antioxidant therapy on bactericidal activity of polymorphonuclear cells is of concern. In a prospective study of prevention of ROP with vitamin E (36), the treated group had a significantly higher incidence of sepsis and necrotizing enterocolitis. In addition this association was greatest in the most premature patients. Sherman et al. (37) reported the effects of the antioxidants catalase, deferoxamine, dimethyl thiourea, and quinacrine of chemiluminescence on microcidal activity against *Candida albicans*. While the latter two agents did decrease activity, catalase and deferoxamine did not. Tosi et al. (38) have specifically studied the effects of varying concentrations of human SOD on the respiratory burst of both neonatal and adult polymorphonuclear cells and their ability to kill three common neonatal pathogens (*E. coli*, *S. aureus*, group B *Streptococcus*). Ferricytochrome C reduction of both adult and neonatal cells was not affected in concentrations up to 1.0 μg/mL. However, at concentrations of 10 μg/mL activity was only 50% of control values, and at 100 μg/mL activity was only 12%–17% of controls. There were no significant differences between adult and newborn cells. Both adult and neonatal polymorphonuclear cells retained 99% of their killing activity against all three organisms despite incubation in serum with an SOD concentration of 100 μg/mL. SOD does not appear to diminish the cidal capacity of polymorphonuclear cells and on a theoretical basis can be used safely in neonates.

Dimunition of Toxic Effects of Elastases

This third strategy for prevention of BPD may also be possible. α_1-Protease inhibitor (α_1PI) will soon be employed in clinical trials in adult patients with deficiencies of this enzyme. If successful, it might be applied in neonates to neutralize elastases released during oxidant injury. However, this lack of defense does not appear to be a deficiency of α_1PI but rather a deficiency of activity of α_1PI (39, 40). One mechanism of inactivation of α_1PI is oxidation of the active methionine site. Therefore prevention of generation of free radicals with antioxidants (*i.e.*, SOD) may also be of benefit in host defenses. Theron and Anderson (41) demonstrated *in vitro* that the antioxidants (ascorbates, cysteine, and dapsone) preserved the elastase inhibitory capacity of α_1PI. Evaluation of α_1PI activity in lung tissue and lung effluent, but probably not in serum, during SOD administration will help to determine if antioxidant therapy is effective in reducing α_1PI inactivation.

References

1. Merritt TA, Hallman M, Holcomb K, et al. Human surfactant treatment of severe respiratory distress syndrome: pulmonary effluent indicators of lung inflammation. J Pediatr 1986;108:741–748.
2. Frantz I, Werthammer J, Stark A. High-frequency ventilation in premature infants with

lung disease: adequate gas exchange at low tracheal pressure. Pediatrics 1983;71:483–488.
3. Kirkpatrick B, Krummel T, Mueller D, Ormazald M, Greenfield L, Salzberg A. Use of extracorporeal membrane oxygenation for respiratory failure in term infants. Pediatrics 1983;72:872–876.
4. Avery M, Hurd S, Tooley W. Is chronic lung disease in prematurely-born infants preventable? Pediatr Res 1986;20:341A.
5. McCord JM. Oxygen-derived free radicals in postischemic tissue injury. N Engl J Med 1985;312:159–163.
6. Weiss SJ, LoBuglio A. Phagocyte-generated oxygen metabolites and cellular injury. Lab Invest 1982;47:5–18.
7. Halliwell B. Mechanisms accounting for the toxic actions of oxygen on living organisms: the key role of superoxide dismutase. Cell Biol Invest 1978;2:113–128.
8. Ehrenkranz R, Bonta B, Ablow R, Warshaw J. Amelioration of bronchopulmonary dysplasia after vitamin E administration. N Engl J Med 1978;299:564–569.
9. Ehrenkranz R, Ablow R, Warshaw J. Prevention of bronchopulmonary dysplasia with vitamin E administration during the acute stages of respiratory distress syndrome. J Pediatr 1979;95:873–878.
10. Saldanha R, Cepeda E, Poland R. The effect of vitamin E prophylaxis on the incidence and severity of bronchopulmonary dysplasia. J Pediatr 1982;101:89–93.
11. Knight M, Roberts RJ. Disposition of intravenously administered doses of vitamin E in newborn rabbits. J Pediatr 1986;108:145–150.
12. Freeman B, Crapo J. Free radicals and tissue injury. Lab Invest 1982;47:412–426.
13. Marklund SL. Clinical aspects of superoxide dismutase. Med Biol 1984;62:130–134.
14. Crapo J, Tierney D. Superoxide dismutase and pulmonary oxygen toxicity. Am J Physiol 1974;226(6):1401–1407.
15. Simon L. Protection against toxic effect of sustained hyperoxia on lung macrophages by superoxide dismutase. Clin Res 1980;28:432A.
16. Block ER, Fisher AB. Protection of hyperoxic-induced depression of pulmonary serotonin clearance by pretreatment with superoxide dismutase. Am Rev Respir Dis 1977;116:441.
17. Turrens J, Crapo J, Freeman B. Protection against oxygen toxicity by intravenous injection of liposome-entrapped catalase and superoxide dismutase. J Clin Invest 1984;73:87–95.
18. Parker JC, Martin MD, Rutili G, McCord J, Taylor AE. Prevention of free radical mediated vascular permeability increases in lung using superoxide dismutase. Chest 1983;5(suppl):52S–53S.
19. Flick M, Hoeffel J, Staul N. Superoxide dismutase with heparin prevents increased lung vascular permeability during air emboli in sheep. J Appl Physiol: Respirat Environ Exercise Physiol 1983;55(4):1284–1291.
20. Padmanabhan R, Gudapaty R, Liener IE, Schwartz B, Hoidal J. Protection against pulmonary oxygen toxicity in rats by the intratracheal administration of liposome-encapsulated superoxide dismutase or catalase. Am Rev Respir Dis 1985;132:164–167.
21. Frank L, Groseclose E. Preparation for birth into an O_2-rich environment: the antioxidant enzymes in the developing rabbit lung. Pediatr Res 1984;18(3):240–244.
22. Tanswell AK, Freeman B. Pulmonary antioxidant enzyme maturation in the fetal and neonatal rat. I. Developmental profiles. Pediatr Res 1984;18(7):584–587.
23. Yoshioka T, Sugive A, Shimaola T, et al. Superoxide dismutase activity in the maternal and cord blood. Biol Neonate 1979;36:173–180.
24. Rosenfeld W, Sahdev S, Zabaleta I, Jhaveri R. Measurement of human superoxide dismutase in neonates utilizing polyclonal antibodies. Pediatr Res 1986;20:209A.
25. Frank L, Lewis P, Sosenko I. Dexamethasone stimulation of fetal rat lung antioxidant enzyme activity in parallel with surfactant stimulation. Pediatrics 1985;75(3):569–574.
26. Sosenko I, Martinez M, Sio R, Frank L. Prenatal propranolol increases fetal rat lung disaturated phosphatidy L choline (DPSC) content but does not affect antioxidant enzyme development. Pediatr Res 1986;20:209A.
27. Huber W, Menander Huber K. Orgotein. Clin Rheum Dis 1980;6:465–498.

28. Pyatak P, Abuchowski A, Davis F. Preparation of a polyethylene glycol: superoxide dismutase adduct, and on examination of its blood circulating life and antiinflammatory activity. Res Commun Chem Pathol Pharmacol 1980; 29:113–127.
29. Shaffer S, O'Neil D, Thibeault D. High plasma concentration of superoxide dismutase (SOD) in hyperoxic neonatal rats fails to prevent chronic vascular pulmonary dysplasia. Pediatr Res 1986;20:440A.
30. Poste G, Bucana C, Raz A, et al. Analysis of the fate of systemically administered liposomes and implications for their use in drug delivery. Cancer Res 1982;42:1412–1422.
31. McDonald R, Berger E, White C, White J, Freeman B, Repine J. Effect of superoxide dismutase encapsulated in liposomes or conjugated with polyethylene glycol ion neutrophil bactericidal activity in vitro and bacterial clearance in vivo. Am Rev Respir Dis 1985;131: 633–637.
32. Tsuji J, Hirose K, Kasahara E, Naitoh M, Yamanoto T. Studies on antigenicity of the polyethylene glycol (PEG) modified uricase. Int J Immunopharmacol 1985;7:725–730.
33. Rosenfeld W, Evans H, Jhaveri R, et al. Safety and plasma concentrations of bovine superoxide dismutase administered to human premature infants. Dev Pharmacol Ther 1982;5:151–161.
34. Beauchamp C, Fridovich I. Superoxide dismutase: improved assay and an assay applicable to acrylamide gel. Anal Biochem 1971;44:276.
35. Rosenfeld W, Evans H, Concepcion L, Jhaveri R, Schaeffer H, Friedman A. Prevention of bronchopulmonary dysplasia by administration of bovine superoxide dismutase in preterm infants with respiratory distress syndrome. J Pediatr 1984;105:781–785.
36. Johnson L, Bowen F, Abbasi S, et al. Relationship of prolonged pharmacologic serum levels of vitamin E to incidence of sepsis and necrotizing enterocolitis in infants with birth weight 1,500 grams or less. Pediatrics 1985;75:619–638.
37. Sherman M, Roberts RL, Danielpour M, Stiehm E. Oxygen scavengers depress phagocytic defenses of neonatal lung. Pediatr Res 1986;20:440A.
38. Tosi M, Bruckner L, Rosenfeld W. Superoxide generation and killing of three important bacterial pathogens by neonatal neutophils: effects of exogenous superoxide dismutase. Pediatr Res 1986;20:393A.
39. Merritt TA, Cochrane C, Holcomb KE, et al. Elastase and α_1-proteinase inhibitor activity in tracheal aspirates during respiratory distress syndrome. J Clin Invest 1983;72:656–666.
40. Rosenfeld W, Concepcion L, Evans H, et al. Serial trypsin inhibitory capacity and ceruloplasmin levels in prematures at risk for bronchopulmonary dysplasia. Am Rev Respir Dis 1986;134:1229–1232.
41. Theron A, Anderson R. Investigation of the protective effects of antioxidants ascorbate, cysteine, and dapsone on the phagocyte-mediated inhibitor in vitro. Am Rev Respir Dis 1985;132:1049–1054.

Comments

William H. Northway, Jr.

The initial experimental clinical results using SOD are encouraging, but the antioxidant protection system is multifactorial and interactive, and more than one exogenous antioxidant may well be required for maximal protection. These could include not only SOD but also catalase, glutathione (mono or diethyl ester), vitamin E, and vitamin C. Infants fed parenterally may also require the sulfur-containing amino acids cysteine and methionine as well as the trace metals copper, zinc, manganese (components of SOD), and selenium.

23

Use of Steroids

RONALD L. ARIAGNO

Introduction

Bronchopulmonary dysplasia (BPD) is a complication primarily seen in infants weighing less than 1500 g at birth with severe respiratory distress who require mechanical ventilatory support and oxygen supplementation (1). The incidence of BPD is approximately 20% in the Stanford Intensive Care Nursery. The highest incidence (almost 50%) occurs in infants weighing less than 1000 g at birth, and in those infants who receive more than 2 weeks of mechanical ventilatory support (70%). Based on 45,000 cases of respiratory distress syndrome (RDS) per year with an 80% survival, we estimate that there may be 5000 to 7000 new cases of BPD (15% to 20% incidence) each year nationally. There is a 20% to 40% mortality in BPD patients in the first year. Approximately 67% of these die in the hospital prior to discharge, and 33% die after discharge home. Of the discharged infants who survive, 50% require rehospitalization (2–8).

This chapter will provide a brief review of the clinical diagnosis of BPD, the lung pathology in BPD, the pathogenesis of the factors involved and the potential therapies as a preparation for the discussion of human studies which suggest that steroid therapy may be effective in the management of BPD. Additionally, there will be a review of the potential toxicity of glucocorticoid therapy (animal and human data), animal studies of pulmonary oxygen toxicity and steroid effects. Finally, the pharmacology of steroids and management of pituitary-adrenal suppression will be discussed.

The Clinical Diagnosis of BPD

There are varying criteria used for the diagnosis of BPD (9–11). Originally the diagnosis was based primarily on roentgenographic findings (9). However, more recently, Toce *et al.* have suggested a clinical and roentgenographic scoring system for assessing BPD (see Tables 23.1 and 23.2) (10). The National Institutes of Health Clinical Centers, for a collaborative clinical trial in high-frequency ventilation on preterm infants to prevent BPD, defined BPD as a need for supplemental oxygen and evidence of abnormal chest radiographs for more than 28 days after birth. Several factors are important in the pathogenesis of BPD: prematurity (lung immaturity), mechanical ventilation with positive airway pressure and lung trauma, oxygen toxicity, the duration of assisted ventilation and oxygen therapy, hyaline membrane disease or RDS, persistent fetal circulation, patent ductus arteriosus, pulmonary air leak, interstitial emphysema, and pulmonary infection (3–6, 8, 12).

Lung Pathology in BPD

A brief review of the lung pathology will be helpful in understanding the potential role of glucocorticoid therapy in the management of BPD. The entire pulmonary system: airways

Table 23.1. Clinical Scoring System for Bronchopulmonary Dysplasia

Variable	Normal	Mild (1)	Moderate (2)	Severe (3)
Respiratory rate (no./min)	40	40–60	61–80	>80
Dyspnea (retractions)	0	Mild	Moderate	Severe
FiO_2 requirements to keep PaO_2 50–70 torr	.21	.21–.30	.31–.50	>.50
$PaCO_2$ (torr)	45	46–55	56–70	>70
Growth rate (g/d)	25	15–24	5–14	<5

(Reprinted, with permission, from Toce SS, Farrell PM, Leavitt RA, et al. Clinical and roentgenographic scoring systems for assessing bronchopulmonary dysplasia. Am J Dis Child 1984;138:581–585. Copyright 1984, American Medical Association.)

parenchyma, and pulmonary vasculature are extensively involved in advanced BPD (see Table 23.3). The airway pathology is characterized by a necrotizing bronchiolitis, squamous metaplasia, increase in smooth muscle, bronchiolar fibrosis, and increase in mucous and macrophages. Parenchymal changes include poor alveolar development, interstitial fibrosis and edema, atelectasis, increase in inflammatory cells, and necrosis of alveolar cells. The vessel abnormalities are arteriolar thrombosis, increase in muscle of arterioles, medial hypertrophy, degenerative changes of the intima, and adventitial fibrosis. Furthermore the lungs have increased infiltration of neutrophils, increased elastase, decreased antiproteases, as well as increased mediator-containing cells (5a, 13). Bronchial alveolar lavage fluid studies from BPD patients show cellular abnormalities which re-

Table 23.2. Radiographic Severity of Bronchopulmonary Dysplasia

Variable	Score		
	0	1	2
Cardiovascular abnormalities	None	Cardiomegaly	Gross cardiomegaly, RVH or enlarged pulmonary artery
Hypertension	+	++	+++
Emphysema	None	Scattered small abnormal lucencies	One or more large blebs or bullae
Fibrosis/interstitial abnormalities	None	Few streaks; interstitial prominence	Many dense strands
Subjective	Mild disease	Moderate disease	Severe disease

(Reprinted, with permission, from Toce SS, Farrell PM, Leavitt RA, et al. Clinical and roentgenographic scoring systems for assessing bronchopulmonary dysplasia. Am J Dis Child 1984;138:581–585.)

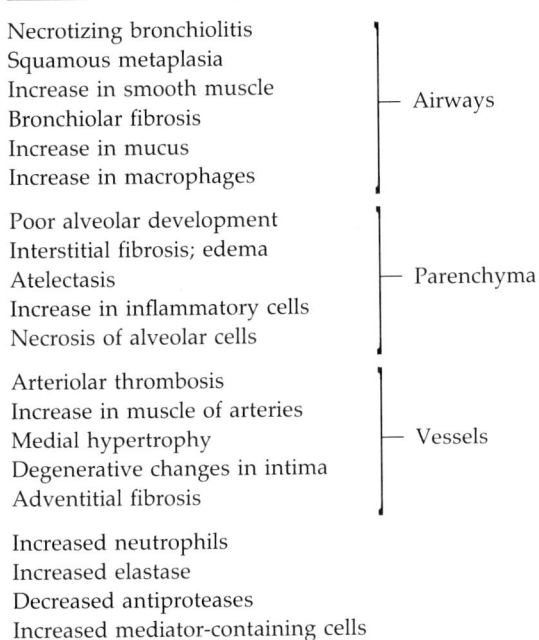

Table 23.3. Pathology of the Lung in Bronchopulmonory Dysplasia

(Reprinted with permission of Ross Laboratories, Columbus, OH 43216, From Ninetieth Ross Conference on Pediatric Research, p127, © 1986 Ross Laboratories.)

flect the microscopic findings of BPD patients who have died. Sobonya et al. (14) have reported the long-term effects on lung development in a 34 month old child who died from BPD and had markedly abnormal lung morphology and enlargement of air spaces. Alveolar growth was severely impaired, and this infant had fewer alveoli (19×10^6) than a term infant (24×10^6) and age matched controls ($123-214 \times 10^6$). The small airways were relatively well preserved in both size and number. The architecture of the lung fissuration was quite abnormal, probably as a result of postnatal asynchronized growth. There was marked medial thickening of the muscular pulmonary arteries, with muscular arteries extending out to the ascinar level. There was also cardiac enlargement of both the right and left ventricles and pulmonary vascular changes of hypertension.

Pathogenesis, Factors Involved and Potential Therapies

Recently Goetzman (12) published an excellent overview of the current understanding of BPD (see Table 23.4). Although the pathogenesis of BPD is complex and our understanding is incomplete, the four elements presented in Goetzman's pathogenic scheme are clear: susceptible host, acute lung injury, secondary lung injury, and abnormal healing.

Various pharmacologic approaches have been considered in the prevention and/or management of BPD (5, 6). Merritt et al. (11) have reported respiratory cytopathology from tracheobronchial aspirates of preterm infants who had a diagnosis of RDS after 10 days of supplemental oxygen and mechanical ventilation. These infants had cytopathology consistent with abnormal healing and the development of BPD. Corticosteroid therapy may be most useful during this stage of the pathogenesis of BPD (11, 12). Although available data from two human controlled trials would suggest that steroid treatment may improve lung function and permit "weaning" from mechanical ventilation, there are many unknowns about the clinical use of this treatment (15, 16). The benefits of the therapy may be offset by multiple potential adverse effects such as sepsis and hypertension. In some cases there may also be a prolonged dependence on steroids to sustain the improvement in lung function. The risk-benefit analysis of this treatment is still under study.

Table 23.4. Proposed Pathogenesis of, Factors Involved in, and Therapies for Bronchopulmonary Dysplasia

Proposed Pathogenesis	Factors Involved	Potential Therapies
Susceptible host	Premature birth Genetic predisposition Fetal asphyxia Fetal infection	Prenatal care Antenatal care Intrapartum care
+ Acute lung injury	Surfactant deficiency Barotrauma Infection	Surfactant replacement Decr. inflation pressure Decr. bacterial damage
+ Secondary lung injury	Oxidants Proteolytic enzymes	Antioxidants Antiproteases
+ Abnormal healing	Hyperoxia/hypoxia Vitamin A deficiency Interstitial fibrosis	Monitoring oxygenation Vitamin A Anti-inflammatory and antifibrotic agents
BPD		Supportive Care

Decr. = decrease
(Reprinted with permission, from Goetzman BW. Understanding bronchopulmonary dysplasia. Am J Dis Child 1986;140:332–334. Copyright 1986, American Medical Association.)

Furthermore the optimal timing of treatment, dose, duration, and the indication for use of steroids in premature infants with chronic lung disease is unclear.

Human Studies Suggesting Effectiveness of Steroid Therapy in the Management of Bronchopulmonary Dysplasia

Since 1983 multiple studies have looked at the effect of steroids on the ventilator dependent infant with BPD (15–24). Many of these studies were retrospective and uncontrolled (see Table 23.5). There have been two randomized prospective studies published on a small number of patients (15, 16). Mammel et al. (16) reported a double-blind, crossover randomized study in which the data were analyzed sequentially. The six infants in this study had a mean gestational age of 29 weeks and mean birth weights of 1049 g. The infants were 30–36 days postnatal age, and all the patients were ventilator dependent at the start of the study.

During the first part of the study, the infants received 0.5 mg/kg per day of dexamethasone intravenously for 3 days, and during the second 3 days, intravenous normal saline. All six infants were weaned from mechanical ventilation at a mean time of 7.4 ± 3.6 days (range 3–12 days) following the

USE OF STEROIDS

Table 23.5. Use of Steroids in Bronchopulmonary Dysplasia

Study (ref)	Design	No. Patients	Results	Comments
Pomerance & Puri (17)	Retrospective, uncontrolled	10	2/10 – Weaned 8/10 – ↓ PIP	Multiple complications, sepis, NEC, ↑ BP, osteo, pneumothorax
Grylack et al. (18)	Retrospective, uncontrolled	13	8/13 – ↓ A-aO$_2$ 9/13 – ↓ Vent Tx	↑ BP, glucosuria
Kramer & Hultzan (19)	Uncontrolled	11	11/11 – ↑ C$_L$ ↓ A-aO$_2$ ↓ Vent Tx	Multiple complications
Shick et al. (20)	Retrospective, uncontrolled	23	13/23 – ↓ A-aO$_2$ ↓ PCO$_2$	Prednisone, no mention of complications
Mammel et al. (16)	Double-blind, crossover, randomized	6	6/6 – ↓ A-aO$_2$ ↓ PIP ↓ Vent Tx	Sequential analysis—study terminated after only 6 patients; 5/6 had sepsis
Avery et al. (15)	Prospective controlled	14	7/7 – ↑ C$_L$ 7/7 – Weaned	Sequential data analysis; dynamic compliance improved; minimal complications
Mammel et al. (22)	Uncontrolled, prospective	8	8/8 – Weaned 8/8 – ↓ FiO$_2$	"Control" group had less significant lung disease
Ariagno et al. (23)	Controlled, double-blind, prospective	21	6/10 – Weaned (dex.) 1/11 – Weaned (control)	Respiratory system compliance improved in dex. group. There appears to be a greater risk of sepsis (2/10) and ↑ BP (3/10) in the dex. group.

↓ = decrease; ↑ = increase; A-aO$_2$ = alveolar-arterial oxygen gradient; BP = blood pressure; C$_L$ = pulmonary compliance; Dex. = dexamethasone; FiO$_2$ = fraction of inspired oxygen; NEC = necrotizing enterocolitis; Osteo = osteomyelitis; PCO$_2$ = arterial carbon dioxide tension; PIP = peak inspiratory pressure; Vent Tx = ventilatory therapy.

start of dexamethasone treatment. After the initial 3 days of dexamethasone, it was tapered over the next 1–5 months. Infection was a significant complication. Five infants had infections while receiving steroids. In all infants the responsible organisms were coagulase negative staphylococci. One infant developed subacute bacterial endocarditis. All of the infants had a central venous catheter when the infection was diagnosed. Three of the six infants survived. Although pulmonary function was not measured in this study, dexamethasone induced clinical improvement and successful weaning from mechanical ventilation occurred. They concluded that dexamethasone decreased the need for mechanical ventilation and oxygen therapy. However, they felt that steroid treatment could not be recommended without further study of patient selection, dosage schedule, short- and long-term side effects, and the mechanism of its action.

The second prospective controlled trial of dexamethasone therapy in BPD was by Avery et al. (15). The purpose of their study was to test if dexamethasone caused improvement in lung function and permitted weaning of respirator dependent babies within 72 hours of steroid treatment. Seven matched consecutive pairs of infants with BPD who were ventilator dependent and not responding to conventional therapy were admitted to this study. All of the infants who entered this study had a diagnosis of RDS, were refractory from weaning from the respirator after 2 weeks, and had chest radiograph findings of Stages II and III BPD. None of the infants had a symptomatic patent ductus arteriosus, congenital heart disease, sepsis, or pneumonia, and they had not received intravenous lipids for at least 24 hours. None of the infants could be successfully weaned from the ventilator during the preceding 5 days despite fluid restriction and diuretics. Infants who were older than 6 weeks of age were excluded from the study. The mean gestational ages of the control and experimental groups were 27.6 and 28.5 days, respectively, with mean birth weights of 942 ± 227 g and 961 ± 138 g, respectively. The postnatal age at entry into the study was 27 ± 13 days and 24 ± 7 days, respectively. In order to control for the effect of birth weight, the infants were stratified by weight into three categories: <1000 g, 1000–1250 g, and 1251–1500 g. The experimental group was given dexamethasone sodium phosphate 0.5 mg/kg per day intravenously in two divided doses. This dosage was continued for 72 hours, then reduced to 0.3 mg/kg per day for 72 hours and thereafter decreased by 10% of the current dose every 3 days until a dose of 0.1 mg/kg was reached.

Thereafter the drug was given for an additional week and then discontinued.

The primary outcome in this study was weaning from the respirator within 72 hours. Success in weaning from the ventilator in one of the pair (matched dexamethasone and control infant) and failure by the other was considered evidence of benefit for the successful regimen. The data were analyzed sequentially. Pulmonary compliance was recorded before therapy and after 48–72 hours. The dynamic pulmonary compliance was determined using an esophageal balloon to measure transpulmonary pressure and a Fleisch pneumotachograph to measure air flow. All compliance studies were performed while the baby was intubated. For those babies who could be weaned, the final compliance study was done prior to extubation. The study was considered completed when there were seven matched consecutive pairs that favored the dexamethasone and weaning from the respirator. The mean compliance in the control and study infants before the study was similar 0.53 ml/cm H_2O/kg ± 0.12 SD and 0.54 ± 0.1 SD, respectively. After treatment control infants were 0.58 ml/cm H_2O/kg ± 0.24, compared with the study infants of 0.86 ml/cm H_2O/kg ± 0.21. The outcome and morbidity data are shown in Table 23.6.

Three infants in the treatment group died of pulmonary related deaths. One control infant died of sepsis and one of respiratory failure. Interestingly the median hospital stay in days was greater in the study infants (86 vs. 62). There were no significant differences in mortality or long-term outcome. However, the authors point out that since the clinical team was free to use dexamethasone after the acute trial, it was not possible to evaluate the long-term outcome, since dexamethasone

Table 23.6. Outcome and Morbidity of Infants in a Controlled Trial of Steroid Treatment for Bronchopulmonary Dysplasia

Outcome	Study Infants		Control Infants	
Survival	5/8	63%	6/8	75%
Sepsis	3/8	38%	2/8	25%
Hypertension	1/8	13%	0/8	0%
Hyperglycemia	1/8	13%	1/8	13%
Median stay				
No. of days	86		62	
Range	31–161		17–157	

(Reproduced by permission of Pediatrics, from Avery GB, Fletcher AB, Kaplan M, Brudno S. Controlled trial of dexamethasone in respirator-dependent infants with bronchopulmonary dysplasia. Pediatrics 1985;75:106–111. Copyright 1985.)

could be used liberally in both groups of infants after the acute trial. They concluded that the study provides evidence for acute improvement of lung function with dexamethasone when it is used in the early stages of BPD and that the increase in lung compliance was achieved within 48–72 hours. They hypothesized that this was due to a reduction in lung water and increased synthesis and depolyment of surfactant and improvement in airways resistance. The authors also concluded that further controlled studies of a different design were required to delineate complications of this therapy and to determine the optimal time, dosage, and indications for using steroids in preterm infants with chronic lung disease. They cautioned that the risks and benefits must be studied carefully to ensure that the cure was not worse than the disease.

At Stanford we have been conducting a double-blind trial to study infants less than 1500 g at birth who were ventilator dependent and not weaned from mechanical ventilation at 3 weeks of age (23, 24). The mean gestational age and birth weight were 27 ± 2 weeks and 956 ± 159 g in the dexamethasone and 27 ± 2 weeks and 875 ± 228 g in the placebo group. This study is still in progress and is designed to look at the acute clinical effects as well as the subacute and long-term complications of dexamethasone use. Twenty-one infants were randomized into parenteral dexamethasone or placebo groups. Infants in the dexamethasone group received 1 mg/kg the first day, and 0.5 mg/kg per day for 6 days. All the infants were intubated during these studies. The total respiratory system compliance was measured prior to, and at the end of, the 1 week treatment period. Compliance was calculated from pneumotachograph and airway pressure measurements during mechanical inflation. The total respiratory system compliance measured was similar at pretreatment, 0.52 ± 0.12 ml/cm H_2O/kg in the dexamethasone group, and 0.51 ± 0.21 in the placebo group. The post-treatment mean compliance was improved ($p < .05$) 0.64 ± 0.13/ml/cm H_2O/kg in the dexamethasone treated vs. 0.47 ± 0.19 ml/cm H_2O/kg in the placebo group. Sixty percent of the dexamethasone treated infants and 9% of the placebo group were extubated within 8 days following the start of treatment. There were five deaths—three in the dexamethasone group and two in the placebo group—and all were associated with BPD and intractable respiratory failure with the exception of one control infant who had a sudden death due to a pulmonary embolism of unknown etiology. Although the birth weights were similar in the two groups, the proportional weight gain (weight on day 7/weight on day 0) during the treatment was greater in the placebo infants

Table 23.7. Possible Toxic Effects of Glucocorticoid Therapy during Pregnancy

First Author	Species	Steroid	Duration (days)	Estimated Dose (mg/kg/d)	Effect
Wellman	Rabbit	Cortisone	2–7	4	↓ Placental mitosis; ↑ senescence of placenta
Wong	Mouse	Dexamethasone	1	1–4	↓ Maternal-fetal glucose transfer
Fainstat	Mouse, rabbit	Cortisone	4–5	60	↑ Cleft palate, fetus
Glaubach	Mouse	Cortisone	6–20	10	↑ Fetal death; ↓ birth weight; ↑ neonatal death
Lee	Rabbit	Cortisone	7	4	↑ Pancreatic islet maturation and degeneration, fetus
Carson	Rabbit	Cortisol	1	—	↓ Lung growth, fetus

(Reprinted, with permission, from Taeusch HW. Glucocorticoid phophylaxis for respiratory distress syndrome: a review of potential toxicity. J Pediatr 1975;87:617–623.)

($p < .003$). The proportional weight gain during the week after treatment was similar in both groups. Two infants in the dexamethasone group had gram negative infections (one had necrotizing enterocolitis). Four in each group had hyperglycemia defined as a glucose level greater than 150 mg% in two successive determinations. Three in the dexamethasone group had systemic hypertension defined as a blood pressure greater than 80/45 mm of mercury. One placebo group infant had a gastrointestinal hemorrhage. We concur with the previous studies at this time that dexamethasone therapy appears to improve compliance and facilitates weaning from mechanical ventilation. However, there may be a greater risk of sepsis and hypertension and decreased growth during the dexamethasone exposure. Before steroid therapy can be recommended, more data are needed to evaluate the risk-benefit balance and long-term effects of this therapeutic modality.

Potential Toxicity of Glucocorticoid Therapy

Animal Data

Taeusch has written a review of the potential toxicity of glucocorticoid prophylaxis in which both animal and human data are cited (25) (Tables 23.7 and 23.8). During pregnancy steroid exposure has been shown to cause decreased lung growth and birth weight in the rabbit (26) as well as increased neonatal deaths in the mouse (27). The possible toxic effects in the newborn animal include decreased antibody responses, decreased brain and body weight, decreased locomotor activity, decreased dendritic branching and central nervous system cholesterol (Table 23.8). Taeusch concluded from this review that although the effects of long-term high-dose steroid therapy have been well studied in adults, the long-term effects of pharmaco-

Table 23.8. Possible Toxic Effects of Glucocorticoid Therapy on the Newborn

First Author	Species	Steroid	Estimated Dose (mg/kg/day)	Duration (days)	Effect
Schapiro	Rat	Cortisol	100	1	↓ Antibody responses; ↓ brain and body weight; ↓ locomotor activity; ↓ dendritic branching; ↓ CNS cholesterol
Winick	Rat	Cortisone	100	1	↑ Running: ↓ organ DNA
Howard	Mouse	Corticosterone	–	5	↓ CNS DNA; ↑ CNS malfunction
Taylor	Rat	Corticosterone	250m	5	↓ Abnormal glucose metabolism
Branceni	Rat	Prednisolone	1500	1, 2	↓ Immune response; ↑ thymic involution. Blocks circadian rhythm of corticoid secretion
Krieger	Rat	Dexamethasone	0.1		↑ Pulmonary susceptibility to O_2 toxicity
Bean	Rat	Endogenous glucocorticoids	–		
Gallagher	Rat	Cortisone	–	1	↓ Pinocytosis

(Reprinted, with permission, from Taeusch HW. Glucocorticoid prophylaxis for respiratory distress syndrome: a review of potential toxicity. J Pediatr 1975;87:617–623.)

logic doses of glucocorticoids in the human fetus during the third trimester are not well documented. No examples of fetal or maternal risks have been documented to date in humans that would obviate the potential benefit of this form of therapy.

In one study increased pulmonary susceptibility to oxygen toxicity was seen in the newborn rat (28). Weichsel (29) has reported potential neurologic hazards in animals when glucocorticoids are used during the perinatal period. Shapiro (30) has noted that the administration of 1 mg of cortisol acetate in the newborn rat affected its somatic growth as well as brain weight, brain chemistry, behavior, and the ontogeny of cerebral cortical dendritic spines. Cotterrell et al. (31) injected doses of 0.2 mg cortisol acetate in rats in the first 4 days of life and found less incorporation of radioactive thymidine into cerebral and cerebellar DNA at 5 days of age. The rat's cerebellum, which increases its DNA (cell number) 8–10 fold in the first 21 days of life, was shown by Weichsel (29) to undergo 46% depression of DNA content by 12 days of age following a 0.6 mg dose of hydrocortisone acetate given on the day of birth. The activity of thymidine kinase, an enzyme considered essential for incorporation of thymidine into DNA and regulation of DNA synthesis during development, was depressed from day 3 to day 6 of life, prior to the time of decline in the steroid induced growth suppression. These data suggest that glucocorticoids in pharmacologic doses may have an inhibitory effect on the biochemistry of brain and somatic growth during early development. Salas and Schapiro (32) showed retardation in the appearance and organization of evoked responses in rat sensory cortex and in animals treated with cortisol on the first day of life. Howard and Benjamins (33) found that when corticosteroid pellets (1.1 to 1.6 mg corticosteroid per gram of body weight) were implanted at 2–3 days postnatal life in the rat, there was a severe deficit of cerebral DNA by 15 days of age, which persisted for 6 months. Since postnatal cerebral DNA synthesis in the rat is represented predominantly by glial formation, they concluded that corticosteroids may interfere with multiplication of glia or disrupt the neural interaction of glia and their potential dendritic or axonal surface relationships. They also found an 11% reduction in sulfatide, a relatively specific marker for myelin, which was consistent with the reduction of oligodendrocytes associated with the DNA deficit.

Ulrich *et al.* (34) noted increased norepinephrine and serotonin in the medial hypothalamus at age 30 days in rats given 1 mg of hydrocortisone at birth. The changes in biogenic amine levels may relate to alterations in endocrine function and control of circadian periodicity. Krieger (28) was able to suppress the circadian periodicity of plasma corticosterone (the naturally occurring cortisone in the rat at 30 days of age) by injecting dexamethasone 2–4 days after birth. A similar dose administered 2 weeks after birth had no effect. The interaction of steroid hormones with target cells in brain tissue appeared to influence neuroendocrine physiology and behavior. Howard and her colleagues have demonstrated remarkable behavioral changes in mice beyond the period of steroid administration (35–37). The mice had less ability to stand on a slowly rotating bar and difficulty crossing a space between a cord and a narrow surface. These results suggested lasting impairment in fine motor control compatible with interference with cerebral function secondary to a 25% reduction in cerebellar DNA. Furthermore these mice showed poor initial adjustment to a maze, less activity in an open field, and other behaviors suggestive of abnormalities in emotional reactivity. Weichsel (30) concluded from his review that perinatal hormone therapy during critical periods of brain development was capable of exerting irreversible immediate effects on brain cell division and differentiation, which could result in late or long-term physiologic behavioral effects.

Human Data

Despite a variety of serious sequelae noted in fetal or newborn animals treated with glucocorticoids, there are few data regarding adverse effects during human development. Silverman *et al.* (38) were the first to describe adverse effects in infants who received ACTH therapy in an attempt to prevent retrolental fibroplasia (RLF). In this study premature infants were treated for 9–27 days at 2 weeks to 3 months of postnatal age. Somatic growth essentially stopped during the treatment period, but catch-up growth occurred in all infants after the steroid was stopped. Infection did not appear to be increased.

A series of papers has been published from McGill University on preterm infants exposed to postnatal steroids (39–42). The initial paper was published by Baden *et al.* (39) regarding a controlled trial of hydrocortisone therapy or placebo in infants with RDS. The mean gestational age and birth weight were 32 weeks in both and 1730 ± 134 g and 1767 ± 121 g, respectively, in the hydrocortisone and placebo groups. The infants received 15 mg/kg of hydrocortisone parenterally on admission to the study, and 12 hours later. The plasma cortisol levels before treatment were 27.2 ± 2.5 µg/100 mL and 29.9 ± 3.8 µg/100 mL in the hydrocortisone and placebo groups, respectively. At 1 hour the level of cortisol was 700 µg% in the treated group compared with 25 µg% in the placebo. The authors found no beneficial effects of steroid treatment on the clinical management of RDS when it was started within the first 24 hours of life and continued for 72 hours.

In 1973 Taeusch et al. (40) published pathologic data on 16 babies, from the Baden et al. study group, who died within 2 months of birth. Eight had been treated with steroids and eight with placebo. A moderate to severe degree of intraventricular hemorrhage was recorded in six of seven infants in the steroid group. One infant in the placebo group showed a moderate degree of intracerebral and intraventricular hemorrhage. The authors hypothesized that the bleeding in most cases may have started from the terminal veins, since all cases in the steroid group had associated hemorrhage in the periventricular areas of the lateral ventricles. With one exception all thymus weights in the steroid group were below the normal mean, and the adrenals in the steroid group were all within -1 SD mean of normal weights (all except one fell below the mean). There were no statistical differences in lung, liver, adrenal, thymus, heart, or spleen pathology attributed to steroid treatment.

Fitzhardinge et al. (41) reported follow-up studies on 13 infants from the original Baden et al. study who received hydrocortisone intravenously in the first 24 hours of life as therapy for RDS compared with 13 placebo infants. No difference was found in the rate of growth, head size, or body length at 1 year of age. Steroid therapy was not associated with an increased rate of infection. The mean developmental quotient (Griffiths Developmental Scale) was 95.4 in the steroid group and 97.9 in the placebo group. The difference was not significant. There were differences in the subtests for gross motor development (with a mean score for the steroid group being 93 compared with 104 for the control; $P < .05$). It is known that cerebral and cerebellar replication in the rat continues for 3 weeks postnatally, whereas most neuronal division in humans ends by birth. In the premature infant brain, however, especially prior to 36 weeks' gestation, the situation may be similar to the rat at term as far as the rate of DNA synthesis and the susceptibility of mytotic interference by steroids.

Many of the patients in the steroid and the placebo groups reported by Fitzhardinge et al. had physiologic hypogammaglobinemia. All the patients had an absolute number of lymphocytes exceeding 1000 per cubic millimeter. In response to phytohemagglutinin (PHA) test, a 50% blastogenesis and at least a threefold increase in thimidine incorporation was seen. Complement levels (C_3 and C_4) were decreased to 90–150 mg% and 20–40 mg%, respectively. Fifteen percent of neutrophils from both groups took up nitroblue tetrazolium, and there was an increase of 2–3 fold after stimulation. The authors concluded that the immune competence in the steroid group appeared to be within normal limits.

A more recent paper from the original study of Baden et al. was published by Gunn et al., in 1981 (42). They reported follow-up at 4 years of age in 12 children from the steroid group and 10 from the placebo group. The immune competence was reassessed at 5 years of age. The mean weight, height, and head circumference were similar in the two groups at 4 years of age, and the psychometric results were not significantly different, the mean IQ was 100.7 ± 10.8 in the steroid group and 108 ± 11.3 in the control group. Preschool and primary scale of intelligence by Gestalt (scored according to Koppitz) or the Rutger's scale showed no significant differences between the two groups at 4 years of age. Electroencephalogram (EEG) abnormalities were seen in both groups.

The immunologic data were interesting, however, in that patients who received steroids had a significantly lower percentage of T lymphocytes 63% vs. 69%. The number of infections between 1 and 5 years of age was greater in the steroid group, with eight of 11 patients having otitis or x-ray proven pneumonia, compared with only two of seven patients in the control group having otitis. The authors concluded that even brief therapy with corticosteroids in infants may result in lasting immunologic impairment.

Mammel *et al.*, in a follow-up uncontrolled study of eight infants treated with dexamethasone for RDS, reported that at 1 year adjusted age, all dexamethasone treated infants (n = 8) compared with a selected group of nontreated infants had similar 1 year Bayley scores (22). The treated infants received dexamethasone at 3 weeks of age for 1 week with a dose of 0.5 mg/kg per day intravenously. Bone age determined by wrist radiographs was 11.6 months (adjusted age) in dexamethasone treated infants compared with 12.6 months in controls. All the dexamethasone treated infants were alive, well, and living at home. None required oxygen supplement or diuretic therapy.

The long-term effects of antenatal dexamethasone administration (maternal dose 5 mg intramuscularly every 12 hours up to 20 mg) from the Collaborative Group on Antenatal Steroid Therapy were published in 1984 (43). There were no statistical differences between the placebo and steroid groups with regard to head circumference or neurologic abnormalities at 9, 18, and 36 months. The mental developmental and psychomotor developmental indices of the Bayley scores at 9 and 18 months and the general cognitive index or any subscales of the McCarthy scale of children at 36 months also indicated comparable development within the two groups. The treatment effect on developmental outcomes was considered for sex, race, and socioeconomic group. The results of the developmental test were significantly influenced by socioeconomic levels, which were controlled in the analysis. The study concluded that no detectable growth, physical, motor, or developmental deficiencies were seen within the first 3 years of life that could be attributed to dexamethasone therapy in mothers just prior to delivery.

In summary, there appear to be short-term benefits of dexamethasone therapy in the management of BPD for infants who are ventilator dependent. Further data are required to analyze the potential risks for the acute benefits (Tables 23.9 and 23.10). Although there are some data reviewed above on the long-term effects, further delineation is needed. No risks have been documented in human beings that would obviate further evaluation of this form of therapy.

Animal Studies of Pulmonary Oxygen Toxicity and Steroid Effects

Many investigators have used animal models to investigate pulmonary oxygen toxicity (44–54) as well as steroid effects (48–50, 55)

Table 23.9. Later Effects of Perinatally Administered Steroids on Animals and Man

First Author	Animal	Steroid	Route	Dose and Duration	Age*	Adverse Effects
Motoyama	Rabbit	Cortisol	IM mother	30 mg/kg/d × 3d	3 d a.p.	↑Fetal death, ↓body & lung weight
Motoyama	Rabbit	Cortisol	Fetus & sac	1 mg	3 d a.p.	↓Length and weight
Carson	Rabbit	Hydrocortisone	IM fetus	2 mg	2 d a.p.	↓Lung weight, 12% reduction in cell number
Cotterrell	Rat	Cortisol	Intraperit.	0.2 mg q.d. × 3 d	1–4 d p.p.	↓Body weight 50%, ↓brain weight 30% Inhibition of cell division Reduced brain cell number: cerebrum–20% cerebellum–30%
Shapiro	Rat	Cortisol	IM	0.50 mg	1 d p.p.	Delayed CNS maturation
Howard	Mice	Corticosterone	Subcut.	40% in cholesterol pellets—removed at 14 days	2 d p.p.	Impaired gross motor coordination
Silverman	Human	ACTH	IM	1.7–20 mg/kg/d for 9–27 d	Premature infants	Impaired growth in weight and length during administration
De Lemos	Human	Methylprednisolone	IV	40 mg q.i.d. × 3 d	1 mo & older (meningitis)	Increased incidence of residual CNS damage
Altman	Human	Cortisone	IM	25–50 mg q.6.hr	Premature with RDS	Nil
Ewerbeck	Human	Prednisolone	IV	20–40 mg/kg/d	Premature with RDS	Increased incidence of CNS damage
Taeusch	Human	Hydrocortisone	IV	12.5 mg/kg q.12.hr × 2	12 hr p.p.	Increased incidence of intraventricular hemorrhage

*a.p., antepartum; p.p., postpartum.
(Reproduced by permission of Pediatrics, from Fitzhardinge PM, Eisen A, Lejtenyi C, Metrakos K, Ramsay M. Sequelae of early steroid administration to the newborn infant. Pediatrics 1974;53:877–883. Copyright 1974.)

Table 23.10. Potential Late Adverse Effects of Steroids

Central nervous system
  Impaired development
Growth
  Decreased growth potential
Immunologic
  Thymolymphatic cellular depletion
  Prolonged impairment of immunologic responsiveness
  Increased infections and decreased life span

For specific problems see Gunn T, Reece ER, Metrakos K, Cole E. Depressed T cells following neonatal steroid treatment. Pediatrics 1981;67:61–67.

(Table 23.11). It is generally known that oxygen at high concentrations is toxic and that prolonged exposure of animals to hyperoxia alters the mechanical properties of the lung. These studies have been stimulated by the recommendation that corticosteroids should be used in the treatment of adult respiratory distress syndrome as well as in chronically ventilator dependent infants with BPD. It is important to recognize in these studies that the experiments may involve adult or newborn animals and that the concentrations of oxygen and the durations of exposure vary. The methodologies used in evaluating lung mechanics are also variable and it is important to take this into consideration when various studies are compared. In some studies the lungs are evaluated with pressure volume maneuvers on inflation, others during deflation. Since inspiratory and expiratory compliance may differ, the method of evaluation should be noted. The pressure-volume changes during an expiratory compliance show the elastic recoil of the respiratory system. Measurements of elastic recoil and inspiratory compliance usually demonstrate an inverse relationship, so that a subject with interstitial restrictive lung disease may have increases in recoil (expiratory compliance) and decreases in compliance (inspiratory) (56, 57). This phenomenon is called hysteresis which is the failure of a system to follow identical paths of response upon application and withdrawal of a forcing agent.

Hysteresis normally occurs in the respiratory system, and in the normal lung it is mainly due to surface properties and alveolar recruitment (58, 59). In the review of animal studies that follows, the compliance measurements may have been done with air or saline. Those studies that used the saline method would have the least hysteresis and reflect tissue effects primarily (58, 59). In the preparation of the lungs for study, some investigators degassed the lungs, either by using 100% oxygen before the animal was sacrificed or by using a vacuum technique. Some investigators have pointed out that degassing injured lungs artifactually augments the decrease in compliance because it is difficult to reinflate the lungs once they are totally collapsed (48). In summary, the details of the methodology are important for understanding the significance of these studies and for interpreting and comparing their data.

Newborn Studies

In the newborn rat, lung saccule septation usually occurs between 4 and 14 postnatal days (55). Bucher and Roberts (51) have shown that hyperoxia from 6 to 12 days markedly impairs alveolar development and decreases secondary septal development by 88%. In this study the compliance (air) on deflation was decreased (lung recoil decreased), or the lungs were less "stiff."

Massaro et al. (55) treated neonatal rats from days 4 to 13 with 1 μg per day of dexamethasone and found that saccule septation and the alveolar surface area were markedly decreased. In these studies the lungs were degassed, and no difference in compliance was noted using a saline inflation technique. An air inflation study was not done; therefore it was not possible to determine whether there was a surfactant deficiency (with a surfactant deficiency the compliance may be decreased during air inflation, but unchanged during saline inflation).

We have recently studied the effect of dexamethasone treatment after 2 weeks of pulmonary oxygen toxicity in newborn mice (48). The mice were continuously exposed to hyperoxia (80% oxygen) or humidified air from birth. The mice received dexamethasone treatment (0.1, 1, or 5 mg/kg/day, subcutaneously) from day 14 through day 18. Lung compliance was measured on day 18 after sacrifice with pentobarbital. The lungs were not degassed, and air pressure–volume measurements were made. Increased compliance (air) on deflation (lung recoil increased) was seen following hyperoxia and there was no improvement with dexamethasone treatment. The lung water was decreased in hyperoxic animals receiving dexamethasone, 1 or 5 mg/kg per day. The volume density of the cellular component of the interstitial tissue in both the air and oxygen exposed animals was decreased by dexamethasone treatment. The decrease in lung wet weight and lung water in the dexamethasone treated and oxygen exposed mice was not accompanied by a significant decrease in the thickness of the blood-air barrier or change in the barrier's three components: the epithelial cells, the endothelial cells, and the basal lamina tissue between them. We hypothesized that this change was due to a loss of fluid from the interstitium, which was not reflected in the other components of the blood-air barrier. Our data agree with those of Sahebjami and coworkers (50), who have also demonstrated a decrease in lung edema and pleural effusion in the adult rats who received a single dose of 9-alpha-fluoromethylprednisolone after 48 hours of more than 95% oxygen.

The average alveolar size was increased in our oxygen exposed mice, which has also been demonstrated in adult male rats (52). However, we did not demonstrate any significant differences in lung volume at 18 cm of water pressure and the lung volume measured by the fluid displacement method. Therefore we did not conclude that there was evidence of air trapping. The enlargement of the alveoli seen in our neonatal hyperoxic exposed mice may be due to a reduction in alveolar septation. The alveolar enlargement seen in the hyperoxic exposed mice was unaffected by dexamethasone treatment.

As was seen in the study by Riley et al. (52), the increase in lung collagen with oxygen exposure may in part explain the increased compliance on deflation (i.e., increased lung recoil). Since saline pressure-volume measurements or measurements of pulmonary system surfactant were not done, we could not differentiate tissue from surface active factors. There is some evidence that a change in compliance following hyperoxia exposure may be attributable to a derangement of the surfactant system (53, 54). The decrease in lung water and improvement in the blood-air exchange surface area induced by dexamethasone may be beneficial in chronic pulmonary oxygen toxicity. The potential improvement for lung mechanics is less clear from the animal studies. These

Table 23.11. Animal data on Pulmonary Oxygen Toxicity and Steroid Effects

Animal	Study (ref)	O$_2$ Percent (duration)	Steroid (dose, t, duration)	Lungs Degassed	Compliance Change	Air Method Infl.	Air Method Defl.	Saline Method Infl.	Saline Method Defl.	Comments
I. Neonatal rat	1. Massaro et al. (55)	—	1 μg/d (d 4–13) Dex.	+	0			x		1. Saccule septation (usu. occurs 4–14th postnatal day) impaired; alveolar surface area decreased.
	2. Bucher & Roberts (51)	40->90% (6–12 d)	—	+	↓		x			2. Alveolar development impaired (secondary septal development decreased by 88%).
Rabbit	3. Ward & Roberts (53)	95% (birth–48 hr)	—		↓ (0)*	x	(x)			3. Airway surfactant decreased in hyperoxia exposed female rabbits; compliance on inflation decreased in male & female.
	4. Ward & Roberts (54)	>95% (birth–48 hr)	—		↑ (↓)*	(x)	x			4. Airway sufactant decreased. Compliance on inflation decreased and on deflation increased (viz., lung recoil increased).
Mice	5. Ariagno, et al. (48)	80% (birth–14 d)	1 or 5 mg/kg/d (d 14–18) Dex.		↑		x			5. Compliance on deflation increased in hyperoxia. Dex. had no effect on the compliance. Lung water decreased and lessening of decrease in blood-air exchange surface area in hyperoxia dex. treated group.

Animal	Study (ref)	O_2 Percent (duration)	Steroid (dose, t, duration)	Lungs Degassed	Compliance Change	Air Method Infl.	Air Method Defl.	Saline Method Infl.	Saline Method Defl.	Comments
II. Adult mice	6. Gross (47)	>98% (2–3 d)		+	↓		x			6. Decreased compliance on deflation with hyperoxia. *Degassing artifactually augmented the decrease in compliance.*
	7. Gross & Smith (49)	>98% (60–72 hr)	10 mg/kg/d Methylpred. (7 d prior to O_2)		↓ (0)*		x		(x)	7. Decreased compliance on deflation (less lung recoil) in hyperoxia (greater decrease in steroid treated). Saline compliance on deflation was the same in the steroid and saline pretreated hyperoxia group.
Male rats	8. Riley et al. (52)	90–95% (60 hr)	—		↑			x		8. Lung volume and collagen content increased with hyperoxia; saline compliance on inflation was increased in hyperoxia.
Rats	9. Sahabjami et al. (50)	98% (96 hr)	0.5 mg 9 α-Fluoromethylpred. (after O_2)		↓ (0)*		x		(x)	9. Compliance on deflation decreased at low pres. and incr. at pres. > 20 cm H_2O in hyperoxia. Lung volume improved with steroids. Compliance on deflation with saline or air unimproved with steroids.

* See Method of measurement in "( )"
Defl. = deflation; Dex. = dexamethasone; Infl. = inflation; -pred. = prednisone; t = time; 0 = no change; ↑ = increase; ↓ = decrease; + = yes.

studies are in contrast to the clinical studies, in which compliance appears to increase following steroid treatment. In a clinical setting compliance is measured with an air inflation method. We found no improvement in compliance on inflation in mice. Most of the animal reports summarized above (47–51, 53–55) have measured compliance on deflation, so an increase would indicate increased lung recoil. If compliance on inflation were analyzed, a decrease in compliance may have been seen.

The studies of Ward and Roberts (53, 54) in the newborn rabbit would best represent what appears to occur clinically. Newborn rabbits exposed to more than 95% oxygen for 48 hours had decreased compliance noted on inflation. In our studies of infant mice, although dexamethasone did have significant side effects such as decreasing body weight, thymus weight, and brain weight, at a daily dose of 1 mg/kg or more, there also were beneficial effects such as the reduction of lung water (48). If the latter occurred in human infants with BPD, it would improve pulmonary function and could be beneficial in the clinical management of infants who are ventilator dependent.

Adult Studies

In the adult male rat lung volume and collagen content have been shown to be increased after hyperoxia. Hyperoxia exposure also has an effect on decreasing the surfactant in the airway (52). When methylprednisolone at a daily dose of 10 mg/kg was given for 7 days prior to hyperoxia, and then every 3 days after the oxygen was started in adult mice, Gross and Smith (49) found a decrease in compliance on deflation (less lung recoil) in the steroid treated lungs compared with the controls and no change in the saline deflation curve. Although the authors suggested that the methylprednisolone may have an unfavorable effect on the surfactant system in oxygen toxicity by accentuating the inhibition of the phospholipid synthesis, a decreased lung recoil is not consistent with this hypothesis. There were more deaths in their hyperoxic exposed steroid treated mice. After 10 days of oxygen exposure, there was a 40% mortality in the steroid group, compared with 12% in the control group.

Sahebjami et al. (50) exposed adult rats for 96 hours to 98% oxygen and gave the rats 0.5 mg of 9-alpha-fluoromethylprednisolone intramuscularly. The lungs of the steroid injected rats accepted more air than those from rats given a placebo, whether expressed as absolute volume or as milliliter per gram of lung wet weight. The lungs from rats in all groups exposed to hyperoxia had a greater residual volume than lungs from rats exposed to air. The compliance on deflation measured after degassing the lungs was decreased below a distending pressure of 20 and increased above 20 cm H_2O. The lungs from steroid injected rats in hyperoxia accepted more air than the placebo group. The authors concluded that steroids increase the absolute volume of air accepted by the lung during recovery from hyperoxia, but the compliance on deflation with air or saline was not improved. They hypothesized that the 9-α-fluoromethylprednisolone accelerated the recovery from hyperoxia, and improved alveolar volume by either increasing the rate of resolution of the alveolar fluid exudate or decreasing the formation of alveolar fluid. The pressure-volume curves with volume expressed as percentage of maximum lung volume indicated that there was decreased compliance in deflation (less lung recoil) and retention of air at distending pressures less than 20 cm H$_2$O. This increased retention of air may be due to narrowing of the bronchioles secondary to secretions or edema. Interestingly, in related studies in this paper, rats treated with diuretics had less residual air present.

Pharmacology of Steroids

The adrenal cortex synthesizes a number of classes of steroids, the glucocorticoids, mineral corticoids, and progestogens with 21 carbon atoms, androgens with 19 carbon atoms, and estrogens with 18 (60). Cortisol (hydrocortisone), a typical glucocorticoid, is produced by the adrenal cortex in amounts of approximately 12.5 mg/m^2 per day (range 6.3–16.5 mg/m^2/d) under normal conditions, and 90% or more is reversibly bound to corticosteroid-binding globulin and albumin in the circulation (61–63). Only the unbound plasma cortisol is considered physiologically active (64). Cortisol is metabolized mostly by the liver, and the metabolites are excreted by the kidney and the liver. Approximately one-third of these can be measured as urinary 17-hydroxy-corticosteroids (17-OHCH) (64, 65). The secretion of cortisol is under the direct control of adrenal corticotrophic hormone (ACTH) in the pituitary, which is under feedback control by plasma cortisol concentrations in both normal and pathologic states. A hypothalamic factor, corticotrophin releasing factor, stimulates ACTH and is affected both by negative feedback from plasma cortisol concentration and by neural stimuli from elsewhere in the central nervous system. These neural stimuli are the origin of the adrenal stress response (61).

The pharmacologic effects of the glucocorticoids are numerous and widespread (66) (Table 23.12). They influence carbohydrate, protein, and lipid metabolism, electrolyte balance, and the functions of the cardiovascular system, the kidney, skeletal muscle, nervous system, and other organs and tissues. The pharmacologic effects include decreased uptake and utilization of glucose, with a tendency for hyperglycemia and glucosuria as well as increased glucogeonesis and glycogen deposition in the liver. They also influence insulin responses. There are multiple effects on protein metabolism, including a negative nitrogen balance with tissue protein depletion and an effect on the mobilization and uptake of amino acids for peripheral tissue. Fatty acid synthesis is inhibited in the adipose tissue as is the mobilization of fatty acids. Furthermore the glucocorticoids provide the capacity to resist many types of noxious stimuli in the environment.

Other important effects include resistance to stress, ability to excrete water loads, suppression of the hypothalamic pituitary adrenal axis, suppression of growth in children, and involution of the thymus and lymphoid tissue, and anti-inflammatory effect and inhibition of granuloma formation. Glucocorticoids have a striking effect on the distribution of various pools of leukocytes in the body. Neutrophils that are normally marginated on the capillary in various tissues can re-enter the circulation. There is impairment of the chemotaxis activity which has been seen *in vitro* for neutrophils and monocytes following exposure to corticosteroids, perhaps as a result of the stabilization of lysosymes.

Some of the biologic actions of the corticosteroid potency can be quantified. Table 23.13 gives the relative potency of natural and synthetic corticosteroids. The plasma half-life and biologic half-life are also given. The biologic half-life is measured by suppres-

Table 23.12. Pharmacologic Effects of Glucocorticoids

In Vitro or Animal Studies	Changes in Humans
Metabolic effects	
Carbohydrate effects	
Decreased uptake and utilization of glucose	Hyperglycemia
Increased gluconeogenesis	Glucosuria
Liver glycogen deposition	
Anti-insulin effect	Anti-insulin effect
Protein effects	
Negative nitrogen balance	Negative nitrogen balance
Tissue protein depletion	Antianabolic effect
Decreased uptake and mobilization of amino acids from peripheral tissue	Increase in plasma amino acids
Increased uptake of amino acid	
Synthesis of protein by the liver	
Fat metabolism	
Inhibition of fatty acid synthesis by adipose tissue	
Mobilization of fatty acids from adipose tissue	Fatty acid mobilization
Other effects	
Increased resistance to stress	Increased resistance to stress
Restoration of ability to excrete a water load	Restoration of ability to excrete a water load
Suppression of HPA axis	Suppression of HPA axis
Suppression of growth	Suppression of growth
Lymphoid tissue and thymus involution	Neutrophilic granulocytosis
	Eosinopenia, lymphocytopenia, and monocytopenia
Inhibition of granuloma formation	Anti-inflammatory effect

(Reprinted, with permission, from Morris HG. Pharmacology of Corticosteroids in asthma. In: Middleton E Jr, Reed CE, Ellis EF, eds. Allergy: principles and practice. 2nd ed. St. Louis: The C. V. Mosby Co., 1983.)
HPA = hypothalamic pituitary axis.

sion of the hypopituitary adrenal function (67).

A dose of glucocorticoids may be physiologic or pharmacologic. Steroids may be given as replacement therapy or may be used therapeutically in nonendocrine diseases. Among the very few suggested indications for other than replacement use of glucocorticoids in the infant are hemangiomatosis and BPD (67). Some authors who recently reviewed the use of steroids in BPD (3, 4) caution that further study of the efficacy and risks is needed before this treatment can be recommended. Several mechanisms have been suggested for the improvement in lung function (5b, 15, 16, 62, 66, 68–86) in BPD ventilator dependent infants (Table 23.14). No data from human infant studies to date have documented any of these modes of action; however, increased surfactant synthesis, a reduction in pulmonary edema, and a decrease in polymorphonuclear recruitment

Table 23.13. Pharmacology of the Corticosteroids

Corticosteroids	Glucocorticoid Equivalent Dose (mg/m^2/d)	Relative Activity or Potency			$T_{1/2}$(hr)	
		Gluco-corticoid	Mineralo-corticoid	Anti-inflammatory	Plasma	Biologic
Short-acting						
Cortisol(hydrocortisone)	20	1	1	1	1.5	8–12
Cortisone	25	0.8	0.8	0.8	0.5	8–12
Prednisone	5	4	<1	4	3	12–36
Prednisolone	5	4	<1	4	2	12–36
Intermediate-acting						
triamcinolone	4	5	0	5	5	
Long-acting						
Betamethasone	0.6	25	0	25		
Dexamethasone	0.75	30	0	25	3–4	36–54
9-Alpha-fluorocortisol	0	0	20	10		
Deoxycorticosterone acetate(DOCA)	0	0	20	0		

(Reprinted, with permission, from Roberts RJ, ed. Drug therapy in infants. Philadelphia: WB Saunders, 1984, p 297.)

to the lung could explain the acute reduction in the lung stiffness and improvement in compliance that has been seen in the clinical studies to date. The possible complications of steroid therapy, which have been reviewed by Rimza (87) (see Table 23.15) are extensive and involve the eye, central nervous system, gastrointestinal, renal, muscular, endocrine, and metabolic systems. As has been reviewed earlier in this chapter, there is also concern about late effects of corticosteroid therapy (see Tables 18.9 and 18.10). At this time the optimal steroid dose and timing of therapy for BPD are unknown. The published controlled studies have used long-acting glucocorticoids—namely, dexamethasone given parenterally at a daily dose of 0.5 mg/kg for several days to 1 week, and in some cases the dose was tapered slowly over a period of several weeks. Responses to therapy have been seen within 72 hours; however, the necessity for longer duration of therapy and the incidence of recurrence of symptoms when the effects have decreased is unknown.

Management of Pituitary-Adrenal Suppression Secondary to Corticosteroid Therapy

Pituitary-adrenal suppression secondary to brief high-dose long-acting steroid therapy may be minimal; however, this important question also needs study (61). Byyny (88) has written that the adrenal cortex lags behind the recovery of the pituitary after withdrawal of corticosteroids. The basal ACTH levels increase before the adrenal cortex is capable of responding. On this basis it can usually be assumed that complete recovery has occurred when the adrenal gland is capa-

Table 23.14. Potential Beneficial Effects of Steroids on Lung Function

Gross
  Reduction in pulmonary edema (71, 48, 50)
  Reduction of bronchial edema and bronchospasm (15, 66)
  Decrease in collagen deposition in tissues (72, 73)
Cellular
  Polymorphonuclear effects
    Decrease in polymorphonuclear recruitment to lung (74, 75)
    Decreased breakdown of granulocyte aggregation with improvement in pulmonary microcirculation (76, 77)
  Stabilization of cell and lysosomal membranes (78)
Biochemical
  Increased surfactant synthesis (79, 80)
  Increase in lung antioxidant activity (80)
  Enhancement of β-adrenergic activity (81)
  Prostaglandin effects (82)
    Inhibition of prostaglandin and leukotriene synthesis (83, 84, 85, 88)
    Enhancement of prostaglandin E_2 degradation (5b, 86)
    Increased prostaglandin I_2 levels (5b, 86)

Table 23.15. Complications of Steroid Therapy

Ophthalmologic
  Posterior subcapsular cataracts
  Glaucoma
  Reactivation of herpes keratitis
Central Nervous System
  Pseudotumor cerebri
  Psychiatric disturbances and dependency
Hematopoietic system
  Leukocytosis, neutrophilia, monocytopenia, lymphopenia, eosinopenia
  Purpura
Gastrointestinal system
  Pancreatis
  Peptic ulcer (?)
  Fatty infiltration of the liver
Renal system
  Nephrocalcinosis
  Nephrolithiasis
  Uricosuria
Musculoskeletal system
  Myopathy
  Osteoporosis and fractures
  Aseptic necrosis of bone
Endocrine and metabolic
  Diabetes
  Adrenal insufficiency
  Growth failure
  Hyperlipidemia
  Lipomatosis
  Hypocalcemia
  Hypokalemic alkalosis
  Sodium retention and hypertension

(Reprinted, with permission, from Rimza RE. Complications of corticosteroid therapy. Am J Dis Child 1978;132:806.)

ble of cortisol secretory response after a brief pulse of exogenous ACTH. Chamberlain and Meyer wrote that the tendency to cause suppression correlates with the potency of the glucocorticoid activity (61). The duration of ACTH suppression produced by corticosteroids is determined by the circulating half-life and other factors such as tissue half-life. Although the circulating half-life of dexamethasone is only approximately 200 minutes, this long-acting glucocorticoid suppresses secretion of ACTH for over 48 hours. Other factors in addition to circulating half-life determine the duration of ACTH-suppressing effects, and the half-life of steroid in the tissue is probably more important. A classic study by Graber et al. in 1965 (89) showed the pattern of recovery in adults who received high-dose steroid therapy for 1 year. First there was recovery of ACTH secretion, and then some time later, after the adrenal has been stimulated sufficiently, there was a return of adequate corticosteroid production. The time separating adrenal recovery and pituitary recovery has not been clearly defined, but these authors and others suggest that it ranges from several days to several months in adults but may differ in infants or children. There is general agreement that pituitary recovery is the most limiting factor.

Chamberlain and Meyer (61) suggest that the determination of whether suppression is present can be evaluated in the following manner: the cortisol concentration can be used in screening as an indicator of pituitary-adrenal integrity. If there is a low value (<10 $\mu g/100$ ml), it can be concluded that adrenal function is suppressed. Cortisol can be measured at baseline and following ACTH. A baseline in plasma cortisol of at least 10 $\mu g/100$ mL and a cortisol greater than 30 $\mu g/100$ mL 2 hours after ACTH is considered a normal result. The response to ACTH generally indicates the patient's ability to respond to physiologic stress. A study comparing ACTH test results with cortisol levels during and after major surgery showed that the correlation between the two is excellent. Cortisol concentration less than 10 $\mu g/100$ mL is evidence of hypothalamic pituitary adrenal suppression. If the baseline cortisol concentration is normal, the steroid may be stopped, and in 2 weeks ACTH testing can be done to document normal adrenal function. Until a normal response to ACTH stimulation is obtained, supplemental steroid should be given at the time of stress. Oral short-acting steroid should be used during withdrawal in order for endogenous corticosteroid production to be stimulated during the recovery period.

Mammel et al. (22) have published the results of cosyntrophin (synthetic ACTH) testing in ventilator dependent infants who received intravenous dexamethasone, 0.5 mg/kg daily for 7 days (mean age 22 ± 7 days at start) with tapering of the dose over 2 weeks. At a mean age of 2.8 months, the mean 1 hour cortisol increase after ACTH stimulation was 25 $\mu g/dL$. We have also evaluated adrenal responsiveness in ventilator dependent preterm infants with BPD (90). In our study parenteral dexamethasone or placebo were used in a double-blind trial at 3 weeks of age. The infants were randomized into 7 day parenteral dexamethasone or placebo treatment trial groups. Infants in the dexamethasone group received 1 mg/kg on day 1 and 0.5 mg/kg daily for the remaining 6 days. The baseline cortisol was measured prior to starting the treatment trial (day 0), at the end of the trial (day 7), and 10 days after the trial (day 17). On day 0 there were similar cortisol levels of 11.8 $\mu g/dL$ ± 8 and 11.6 ± 4 in the placebo and dexamethasone groups, respectively. On day 7 the placebo group had 7.6 ± 5 $\mu g/dL$ and the dexamethasone group 2.6 ± 1.3 $\mu g/dL$; and on day 17, 11.2 ± 10.8 $\mu g/dL$ and 10.8 ± 8.9 $\mu g/dL$, respectively. The cortisol response was measured 30 minutes following an ACTH (α-1-24 corticotrophin) stimulation test using 36 $\mu g/kg$ infused intravenously over 2 minutes (91–94). The cortisol measurements were made by radioimmunoassay. There was no significant difference in response to the ACTH stimulation test on days 0, 7, and 17 within or between the dexamethasone and placebo groups. These preliminary data suggest that the adrenal responsiveness to ACTH stimulation is unaffected by 7 days of parenteral dexamethasone therapy. The significantly decreased baseline cortisol level at day 7 may represent short-term suppression of the hypothalamic pituitary control of cortisol secretion. We concluded that there was no long-term adverse effect on the control of cortisol after 1 week of high-dose dexamethasone.

Summary

Clinically, steroids have been randomly used in the management of BPD during acute, subacute, and chronic phases. Currently there are prospective data to indicate that long-acting corticosteroids, namely dexamethasone, may be helpful in the management of the ventilator dependent BPD patient at approximately 3 weeks of age. The mechanism of improvement in these patients is unknown; however, the acute increase in lung compliance would favor decrease in lung edema and neutrophil infiltration, and an increase in surfactant. The most serious of the short-term side effects are increased risk of infection and hypertension. The long-term outcome of these infants to date seems to be unaffected by the glucocorticoid exposure; however, further data are needed. At this time the use of steroids in the treatment of BPD should still be considered experimental, and further data are required regarding indications, dose, duration of treatment, and risk-benefit balance before it can be recommended as a clinical routine.

References

1. Smith DW, Stevenson DK, Sunshine P, Northway W, Ariagno RL. Predominance of bronchopulmonary dysplasia in infants less than 1500 gm at birth. Am Rev Respir Dis 1983;127: 212A.
2. US Department of Health and Human Services, Public Health Service, National Institutes of Health. Chapter 7, Chronic obstructive respiratory disorders. NIH Publication No. 86-2107, August 1986, pp 50–55.
3. Bancalari S, Gerhardt T. Bronchopulmonary dysplasia. Pediatr Clin N Am 1986;33:1–23.
4. Shannon DC, Epstein M. Bronchopulmonary dysplasia. In: Thibeault DW, Gregory GA, eds. Neonatal pulmonary care. 2nd ed. Norwalk, Conn: Appleton-Century-Crofts, 1986, pp 697–707.
5. Farrell PM, Taussig LM, eds. Bronchopulmonary dysplasia and related chronic respiratory disorders. Report of the 90th Ross Conference on Pediatric Research. Columbia, Ohio: Ross Laboratories, 1986 pp 1–150.
5a. Taussig LM. Long-term management and pulmonary progress in bronchopulmonary dysplasia. In: Farrell PM, Taussig LM, eds. Bronchopulmonary dysplasia and related chronic respiratory disorders. Report of the 90th Ross Conference on Pediatric Research. Columbus, Ohio: Ross Laboratories, 1986, p 127.
5b. Thompson TR. Bronchopulmonary dysplasia: treatment with dexamethasone. In: Farrell PM, Taussig LM, eds. Bronchopulmonary dysplasia and related chronic respiratory disorders. Columbus, Ohio: Ross Laboratories, pp 121–126.
6. National Heart, Lung, and Blood Institute. Workshop on Bronchopulmonary Dysplasia. J Pediatr 1979;85:815–919.
7. Koops BL, Abman SH, Accurso FJ. Outpatient management and follow-up of bronchopulmonary dysplasia. Clin Perinatol 1984;11:101–122.
8. O'Brodovich HM, Mellins RB. Bronchopulmonary dysplasia. Am Rev Respir Dis 1985;132: 694–709.
9. Northway WH Jr, Rosan RC, Porter DY. Pulmonary disease following respirator therapy of hyaline membrane disease: bronchopulmonary dysplasia. N Engl J Med 1967;276: 357–368.
10. Toce SS, Ferrell PM, Leavitt RA, *et al.* Clinical and roentgenographic scoring systems for assessing bronchopulmonary dysplasia. Am J Dis Child 1984;138:581–585.
11. Merritt TA, Stuard IS, Pusia J, *et al.* Newborn tracheal aspirate cytology: classification during respiratory distress syndrome and bronchopulmonary dysplasia. J Pediatr 1981;98: 949–956.
12. Goetzman BW. Understanding bronchopulmonary dysplasia. Am J Dis Child 1986;140: 332–334.
13. Bonikos DI, Bensch KG, Northway WH Jr, Edwards DK. Bronchopulmonary dysplasia: the pulmonary pathologic sequel of necrotizing bronchiolitis and pulmonary fibrosis. Hum Pathol 1976;7:643–666.
14. Sobonya RE, Logwinoff MM, Taussig LM, Theriault A. Morphometric analysis of the

15. Avery GB, Fletcher AB, Kaplan M, Brudno DS. Controlled trial of dexamethasone in respirator-dependent infants with bronchopulmonary dysplasia. Pediatrics 1985;75:106–111.
16. Mammel MC, Green TP, Johnson DE, Thompson TR. Controlled trial of dexamethasone therapy in infants with bronchopulmonary dysplasia. Lancet 1983;1:1356–1358.
17. Pomerance JJ, Puri A. Treatment of severe neonatal bronchopulmonary dysplasia with dexamethasone. Pediatr Res 1982;16:359A
18. Grylack LL, Scanlon KB, Scanlon JW. Corticosteroid treatment of fourteen newborns with bronchopulmonary dysplasia. Clin Res 1979;27:819A.
19. Kramer LI, Hultzan C. The role of steroids in early bronchopulmonary dysplasia (BPD). Pediatr Res 1978;12:546A.
20. Shick CB, Goetzman BW, Smith LE, Wennberg RP. Corticosteroid responsiveness in chronic lung disease of prematurity. Pediatr Res 1981;15:680.
21. Stokes DM, Izner W. Effect of corticosteroids on postnatal lung function. Pediatr Res 1982;16:363A.
22. Mammel MC, Fiterman C, Coleman JM, Boros SJ. Dexamethasone in bronchopulmonary dysplasia: acute effects and long-term outcome. Clin Res 1985;33:114A.
23. Ariagno RL, Sweeney TJ, Baldwin RB, Inguillo R, Martin D. Dexamethasone effects on lung function and risks in three week old ventilator dependent preterm infants. Am Rev Resp Dis 1987;135:A125.
24. Ariagno RL, Baldwin RB, Inguillo D, Martin D. Lung function post dexamethasone in ventilator dependent preterm infants < 1500 gm birth weight. Am Rev Respir Dis 1986;133:A207.
25. Taeusch HW. Glucocorticoid prophylaxis for respiratory distress syndrome: a review of potential toxicity. J Pediatr 1975;87:617–623.
26. Carson S, Taeusch HW Jr, Avery M. Inhibition of lung cell division after hydrocortisone injection into fetal rabbits. J Appl Physiol 1973;34:660–663.
27. Glaubach S, Antopol W, Graff S. Excessive doses of cortisone in pregnant mice: effect on development and survival of the fetus and newborn, and on maternal breast tissue. Bull NY Acad Med 1951;27(6):398.
28. Krieger D. Circadian corticosteroid periodicity: critical period for abolition by neonatal injection of corticosteroid. Science 1972;178:1205–1207.
29. Weichsel ME. The therapeutic use of glucocorticoid hormones in the perinatal period: potential neurologic hazards. Ann Neurol 1977;2:364–366.
30. Shapiro S. Some physiological, biochemical and behavioral consequences of neonatal hormone administration: cortisol and thyroxin. Gen Comp Endocrinol 1968;10:214–228.
31. Cotterrell M, Balaga R, Johnson AL. Effects of corticosteroids on the biochemical maturation of rat brain: postnatal cell formation. J Neurochem 1972;19:2151–2167.
32. Salas M, Schapiro S. Hormonal influences upon the maturation of the rat brain's responsiveness to sensory stimuli. Physiol Beh 1970;5:7–11.
33. Howard E, Benjamins JA. DNA, ganglioside and sulfatide in brains of rats given corticosterone in infancy, with an estimate of cell loss during development. Brain Res 1975;92:73–87.
34. Ulrich R, Yuwike A, Geller E. Effects of hydrocortisone on biogenic amine levels in the hypothalamus. Neuroendocrinology 1975;19:259–268.
35. Howard E. Increased reactivity and impaired adaptability in operant behavior of adult mice given corticosterone in infancy. J Comp Physiol Psychol 1973;85:211–220.
36. Howard E. Absence of effects of corticosterone given at 22 days. Dev Psychobiol 1976;9:25–29.
37. Howard E, Granoff DM. Increased voluntary running and decreased motor coordination in mice after neonatal corticosterone implantation. Exp Neurol 1968;22:661–673.
38. Silverman W, Day R, Blod F. Inhibition of growth and other effects of ACTH in premature infants. Pediatrics 1951;8:177–191.
39. Baden M, Bauer CR, Colle E, Klein G, Taeusch HW, Stern L. A controlled trial of hydrocortisone therapy in infants with respiratory distress syndrome. Pediatrics 1972;50:526–534.

40. Taeusch HW, Wang NS, Baden M, Bauer M, Stern L. A controlled trial of hydrocortisone therapy in infants with respiratory distress syndrome. II. Pathology. Pediatrics 1973;52: 850–854.
41. Fitzhardinge PM, Eisen A, Lejtenyi C, Metrakos K, Ramsay M. Sequelae of early steroid administration to the newborn infant. Pediatrics 1974;53:877–883.
42. Gunn T, Reece ER, Metrakos K, Cole E. Depressed T cells following neonatal steroid treatment. Pediatrics 1981;67:61–67.
43. Collaborative Group on Antenatal Steroid Therapy. Effects of antenatal dexamethasone administration in the infant: long-term follow-up. J Pediatr 1984;104:259–267.
44. Pappas CTE, Obara H, Bensch KG, Northway WM Jr. Effect of prolonged exposure to 80% O_2 on the lung of the newborn mouse. Lab Invest 1983;48:735–748.
45. Bonikos DI, Bensch KG, Northway WM Jr. Oxygen toxicity in the newborn. The effect of chronic continuous 100% exposure on the lungs of newborn mice. Am J Pathol 1976;85: 623–650.
46. Beckman DL, Weiss HS. Hyperoxia compared to surfactant washout on pulmonary compliance in rats. J Appl Physiol 1969;26:700–709.
47. Gross NJ. Mechanical properties of mouse lungs: effects of vacuum degassing on normal hyperoxic and irradiated lungs. J Appl Physiol 1981;51:391–398.
48. Ariagno RL, Sweeney TE, Northway WH, et al. Dexamethasone decreases lung water without affecting lung compliance in infant mice raised in 80% oxygen environment. Am Rev Respir Dis 1986;133:A108.
49. Gross NJ, Smith DM. Methylprednisolone increases the toxicity of oxygen in adult mice. Am Rev Respir Dis 1984;129:805–810.
50. Sahebjami H, Jacob G, Massaro D. Influence of corticosteroid on recovery from oxygen toxicity. Am Rev Respir Dis 1974;110:566–571.
51. Bucher JR, Roberts RJ. The development of the newborn rat lung in hyperoxia: a dose-response study on lung growth, maturation, and changes in antioxidant enzyme activities. Pediatr Res 1981;15:999–1008.
52. Riley DJ, Berg RA, Edelman NH. Prevention of collagen deposition following pulmonary oxygen toxicity in the rat by cis-4-hydroxy-L-proline. J Clin Invest 1980;65:643–651.
53. Ward J, Roberts RJ. Hyperoxia effects on pulmonary pressure: volume characteristics and lavage surfactant phospholipid in the newborn rabbit. Biol Neonate 1984;46:139–148.
54. Ward JA, Roberts RJ. Vitamin E inhibition of the effects of hyperoxia on the pulmonary surfactant system of the newborn rabbit. Pediatr Res 1984;18:329–334.
55. Massaro D, Teich N, Moxwell S, Massaro GD, Whitney P. Postnatal development of alveoli-regulation and evidence for a critical period in rats. J Clin Invest 1985;76:1297–1305.
56. Dawson A. Elastic recoil and compliance. In: Clausen JL, ed. Pulmonary function testing guidelines and controversies, chapter 18. New York: Academic Press, 1982, pp 193–204.
57. Collier CR. Elastic recoil and compliance. In: Wilson AF, ed. Pulmonary function testing indications and interpretations, chapter 9. San Francisco: Grune and Stratton, 1985.
58. Hoppin FG Jr, Stishert JC, Greaves JA, Lai Y-L, Hildebrandt J. Lung recoil: elastic and rheological properties. In: Fishman AP, Macklem PT, Mead J, Geiger SR, eds. Handbook of physiology, section 3. The respiratory system, vol. 3. Mechanics of breathing, part 1. Bethesda, Md: American Physiological Society, 1986, pp 195–215.
59. Agostoni E, Hyatt RE. Chapter 9, Static behavior of the respiratory system. In: Fishman et al., eds. Handbook of physiology, section 3. The respiratory system, vol. 3. Mechanics of breathing, part 1, pp 113–130.
60. Haynes RC Jr, Murad F. Adrenocorticotropic hormone: adrenocortical steroids and their synthetic analogs; inhibitors of adrenocortical steroid biosynthesis. In: Gilman AG, Goodman LB, Rall RW, Murad F, eds. The pharmacological basis of therapeutics. 7th ed. New York: Macmillan, 1985, pp 1459–1489.
61. Chamberlin P, Meyer WJ. Management of pituitary-adrenal suppression secondary to corticosteroid therapy. Pediatrics 1981;67: 245–251.

62. Kenny FM, Preeyasombat C, Migson CJ. Cortisol production rate. II. Normal infants, children and adults. Pediatrics 1966;37:34–42.
63. Slaunwhite WR Jr, Sandberg AA. Transcortin: a corticosteroid-binding protein of plasma. J Clin Invest 1959;38:384–391.
64. Hellman L, Bradlow HL, Adesman J, et al. The fate of hydrocortisone-4-C^{14} in man. J Clin Invest 1954;33:1106–1115.
65. Migeon CJ, Sandberg AA, Decker HA, et al. Metabolism of 4-C^{14} cortisol in man: body distribution and rates of conjugation. J Clin Endocrinol Metab 1956;16:1137–1150.
66. Morris HG. Pharmacology of corticosteroids in asthma. In: Middleton E, Reed CE, Ellis EF, eds. Allergy: principles and practice. St. Louis: CV Mosby, 1983, pp 593–611.
67. Roberts JJ. Drug therapy in infants. Philadelphia: WB Saunders, 1984, pp 297–299.
68. Chang SW, King TE. Corticosteroids. In: Chesniach RM, ed. Drugs for the respiratory system. Orlando, Fla: Grune and Stratton, 1986, pp 77–138.
69. Thompson EB, Lippman ME. Progress in endocrinology and metabolism: mechanism of action of glucocorticoids. Metabolism 1974;23:159–202.
70. Axelrod L. Glucocorticoid therapy. Medicine 1976;55:39–65.
71. Shasby DM, Fox RB, Harods RN, Repine JE. Reduction of edema of acute hyperoxic lung injury by granulocyte depletion. J Appl Physiol: Respirat Environ Exercise Physiol 1982;52:1237–1244.
72. Aronon L. Effects of glucocorticoids on fibroblasts. In: Baxter JD, Rousseau GG, eds. Monograph on endocrinology. New York: Springer-Verlag, 1979, pp 327–340.
73. McNelis B, Cutroneo K. A selective decrease of collagen peptide synthesis by dermal polysome isolated from glucocorticoid-treated newborn rats. Molec Pharmacol 1978;14:1167–1175.
74. Fox RB, Hoidal JK, Brown DM, Repine JE. Pulmonary inflammation due to oxygen toxicity: involvement of chemotactic factors and polymorphonuclear leukocytes. Am Respir Dis 1981;123:521–523.
75. Hammerschmidt DE, White JG, Craddock PR, Jacob HS. Corticosteroids inhibit complement-mediated granulocyte aggregation. A possible mechanism for their efficacy in shock states. J Clin Invest 1979;63:798–803.
76. Skubitz KM, Craddock PR, Hammerschmidt DE, August JT. Corticosteroids block binding of chemotactic peptide to its receptor on granulocytes can cause disaggregation of granulocyte aggregates in vitro. J Clin Invest 1981;68:13–20.
77. Kusajima K, Wax SD, Webb WR. Effects of methyl-prednisolone on pulmonary microcirculation. Surg Gynecol Obstet 1974;139:1–5.
78. Wilson JH. Treatment or prevention of pulmonary cellular damage with pharmacologic doses of corticosteroid. Surg Gynecol Obstet 1972;134:675–681.
79. de Lemos RA, Shermeta DW, Knelson JH, Kotas R, Avery ME. Acceleration of appearance of surfactant in the fetal lamb by administration of corticosteroids. Am Rev Respir Dis 1970;102:459–461.
80. Frank L, Lewis P, Sosenko I. Dexamethasone stimulates fetal rat antioxidant enzyme activity in parallel with surfactant stimulation. Pediatr Res 1984;18:391A.
81. Barnes P, Jacobs M, Roberts J. Glucocorticoids preferentially increase fetal alveolar-adrenoreceptors: audioradiographic evidence. Pediatr Res 1985;18:1191–1194.
82. Mathe AA, Hedqvist P, Stranberg K, Leslie CA. Aspects of prostaglandin function in the lungs. N Engl J Med 1977;296:850–855 (part 1);910–914 (part 2).
83. Gryglewski RJ, Panczenko B, Kosbut R, Grodzinaka L, Ocepkiewicz A. Corticosteroids inhibit prostaglandin release from profused lungs of sensitized guinea pigs. Prostaglandins 1975;10:343–355.
84. Hong SCL, Levine L. Inhibition of arachadonic acid release from cells as the biochemical action of anti-inflammatory corticosteroids. Proc Nat Acad USA 1976;73:1730–1734.
85. Russo-Marie F, Duval D. Dexamethasone-induced inhibition of prostaglandin production does not result from a direct action on phospholipase activities but is mediated through a steroid-inducible factor. Biochim Biophys Acta 1972;712:177–185.
86. Moore PK, Hoult JRS. Anti-inflammatory ste-

roids reduce tissue PG synthetase activity and enhance PG breakdown. Nature 1980;288: 269–270.
87. Rimza ME. Complications of corticosteroid therapy. Am J Dis Child 1978;132:806–810.
88. Byyny RL. Withdrawal from glucocorticoid therapy. N Engl J Med 1976;295:30–32.
89. Graber AL, Ney RL, Nicholson WE, Island DP, Liddle GW. Natural history of pituitary-adrenal recovery following long-term suppression with corticosteroids. J Clin Endocrinol Metab 1965;25:11–27.
90. Ariagno RL, Wilson DM, Inguillo D, Martin D. The effect of dexamethasone on adrenal responsiveness in ventilator dependent preterm infants with bronchopulmonary dysplasia. Am Rev Respir Dis 1987;135: in press.
91. Arad I, Landau H. Adrenocortical reserve of neonates born of long term, steroid treated mothers. Eur J Pediatr 1984;142:279–280.
92. Thomas J, Murphy JF, Dyas J, Ryall M, Hughes IA. Response to ACTH in the newborn. Arch Dis Child 1986;61:57–60.
93. Ohrlander S, Gennser G, Nilsson KO, Eneroth P. ACTH test to neonates after administration of corticosteroids during gestation. Obstet Gynecol 1977;49:691–694.
94. Okuno A, Nishimura Y, Kawarazaki T. Changes in plasma 11-hydroxy-corticosteroids after ACTH, insulin and dexamethasone in neonatal infants. J Clin Endocrinol 1972;34: 516–520.

ACKNOWLEDGMENTS

This work was supported in part by grant RR-81 from the General Clinical Research Centers Program of the Division of Research Resources, National Institutes of Health, by grant HL-34118, and by grant HL 30394 from the National Institutes of Health. My gratitude to Mrs. Mary Clausen for her patience and expertise in word programming and typing.

Comments

William H. Northway, Jr.

Steroid drugs appear to be increasingly used in the Intensive Care Nursery when infants are being weaned from prolonged artificial ventilation. Their clinical benefit is not yet convincingly supported by the results of controlled clinical trials and animal studies. Anecdotal accounts of the effectiveness of steroids should not be sufficient to establish their use as accepted treatment particularly when they may produce significant deleterious side effects. If steroids are used during weaning or at various stages of chronic lung dysfunction, they should be used with great caution and in such a way that the short and long term results and risks of treatment are clear.

V

Outcome of Bronchopulmonary Dysplasia

24

Growth and Neurodevelopmental Outcome of Infants Who Had Bronchopulmonary Dysplasia

ELSA J. SELL AND YVONNE E. VAUCHER

Introduction

In this chapter we review both published and unpublished data from two neonatal intensive care units in Tucson, Arizona, pertaining to growth and development in infancy and early childhood of children who had bronchopulmonary dysplasia (BPD).

Growth

Growth is adversely affected in infants who have BPD, and the degree of growth delay is related directly to the severity and duration of disease. Acceleration of length, accompanied by a smaller increase in rate of weight gain, is usually seen within a few months of improvement in pulmonary function (1). Decreased work of breathing, adequate oxygenation, and/or reduction in oxygen consumption have been postulated as mechanisms responsible for the improvement in growth (1, 2).

Although growth rates increase with age, infants with BPD remain relatively small. In infants at 2 years of age adjusted for prematurity both Markestad and Yu reported mean weight, length, and head circumference in the third to 10th, 10th to 25th, and 50th percentiles, respectively. As in other premature infants head growth was least affected, but for weight alone 67% of these infants were in less than the 10th percentile (1), and for both length and weight 25% were in less than the third percentile (3). Northway noted that 29% of BPD survivors had length and/or weight below the third percentile at 3 years of age (4).

Several studies have compared growth in infants who had BPD with controls matched for birth weight and gestational age. Vohr *et al.* found no difference between BPD and control infants by 2 years of age (5). However, Meisels *et al.* reported persistent delay in growth of BPD infants, with weight, length, and head circumference of less than the 10th percentile in 67%, 53%, and 29%, respectively, compared with 35%, 25%, and 17% of control infants at 2 years of age (6). Sauve and Singhal reported that more children with BPD had weight, length, head circumference, and arm muscle mass at or below the fifth percentile than did age matched controls (7). Differences in growth outcome may relate to the severity and chronicity of BPD in each study.

Our unpublished data also demonstrate persistent growth delay throughout early childhood. We reviewed data from over 1300 premature children born at less than 37 weeks' gestation by exam between 1976 and 1981 (the population is described in the section on follow-up). Mean growth percentiles for our RDS group corresponded closely to

Table 24.1. Mean Growth Percentile in Subjects Who Are Average for Gestational Age

No. of Subjects (RDS/BPD)	Chronologic Age							
	4 mo	8 mo	12 mo	18 mo	24 mo	36 mo	48 mo	60 mo
	192/69	137/60	163/66	111/41	117/45	111/37	87/22	65/17
Head Circumference								
RDS	25	31	38	43	44	43	48	42
BPD	9	15	19	28	21	26	25	29
p value	<.0001	<.0001	<.0001	<.001	<.0001	<.001	<.001	NS
Length								
RDS	16	29	35	33	34	40	38	37
BPD	4	10	13	22	24	26	31	26
p value	<.0001	<.0001	<.0001	<.02	<.02	<.02	NS	NS
Weight								
RDS	14	18	23	25	32	34	31	34
BPD	3	5	6	12	17	19	20	20
p value	<.0001	<.0001	<.0001	<.01	<.0001	<.001	NS	NS

NS = not significant

those reported by Ross *et al.* for very low birth weight (VLBW) infants 3–4 years of age—31%, 39%, and 30%, for length, weight, and head circumference (8). Mean growth percentiles for BPD subjects who were average for gestational age (AGA) were significantly below those of AGA infants who had only respiratory distress syndrome (RDS) through 36 months (Table 24.1). The head circumference remained significantly smaller at 48 months. As expected head growth was the best preserved, and weight was the least well preserved. The age at which growth percentiles stabilized (*i.e.*, catch-up growth completed) in both groups was between 18 and 36 months.

We found that the variables most predictive of growth were earlier growth parameters (Table 24.2). Thus prior weight explained 70%–85% of the variance in subsequent weight after 8 months, and prior length and/or weight explained 51%–69% of the variance in length between 8 and 48 months. The explained variance in head circumference by prior head measurement ranged from 62% to 81% between 8 and 24 months; thereafter the explained variance ranged from 33% to 50%, and other variables contributing included birth weight and length. BPD contributed to the explanation of the variance for only one measurement (*i.e.*, 24 month head circumference), indicating that the presence or absence of BPD was not an important factor contributing to later growth in this population of premature infants. Thus our data on infants with BPD that was not extremely severe indicate

Table 24.2. Multiple Regression Analysis of Factors Influencing Growth

Dependent Variable	R^2	Independent Variable	Beta
Weight			
4 mo	.35	Birth length	.59
8 mo	.46	4 mo weight	.68
12 mo	.70	8 mo weight	.84
18 mo	.69	12 mo weight	.83
24 mo	.73	18 mo weight	.85
36 mo	.76	24 mo weight	.87
48 mo	.71	36 mo weight	.65
60 mo	.85	48 mo weight	.92
Length			
4 mo	.32	Birth weight	.56
8 mo	.51	Birth length	.47
		4 mo head circumf.	.34
12 mo	.64	8 mo length	.80
18 mo	.57	12 mo length	.76
24 mo	.59	18 mo length	.77
36 mo	.51	24 mo length	.50
		24 mo weight	.28
48 mo	.69	36 mo length	.59
		36 mo weight	.32
60 mo	.97	48 mo length	.95
		APIB reflex cluster	.36
		48 mo neurologic	.23
Head circumference			
4 mo	.35	Birth head circumf.	.59
8 mo	.62	4 mo head circumf.	.58
		Birth length	.30
12 mo	.70	8 mo head circumf.	.84
18 mo	.81	18 mo head circumf.	.90
24 mo	.75	18 mo head circumf.	.79
		BPD	−.21
36 mo	.30	24 mo head circumf.	.54
48 mo	.55	36 mo head circumf.	.35
		Birth length	.88
		APIB hypertonic reflexes	−.33
		Birth weight	−.61
60 mo	.37	Birth length	1.0
		Duration of labor	−.29
		Birth weight	−.67

Because all data points were not available for each age, pairwise deletion of missing data was performed along with the regression analysis. Perinatal variables included birth weight, gestation, Apgar scores, intrauterine growth, length of ventilation support. APIB variables included clusters as defined by Lester (habituation, orientation, motor, state range, regulation, autonomic, and reflex) along with hypertonicity score (reflexes = 3) and laterality score (the number of reflexes scored differently between right and left sides) (36). Maternal variables included maternal age and number of medical diseases.

An independent variable was retained only if, in addition to statistical significance, it contributed to an increase in the square of the multiple correlation coefficient (R^2) of at least 5%. The beta value is the standarized regression coefficient.

that they remain significantly smaller on a long-term basis primarily because of their size at birth.

The impact of suboptimal head growth upon developmental outcome may be the most significant aspect of growth retardation, since head circumference directly reflects brain mass (9). Although neuronal division is complete long before the third trimester, neuronal migration and organization, glial proliferation, and dendritic multiplication are active processes during the third trimester and early infancy. Interference with brain growth during this period may significantly influence long-term brain function. For instance chronic, severe malnutrition during infancy restricts ultimate brain growth, even after adequate nutrition has been restored, and is associated with developmental delay (10).

Deceleration or arrest of head growth has been reported when AGA very low birth weight infants received less than 85 kcal/kg daily (11). Poor growth was related to both duration of mechanical ventilation and parenteral nutrition. Most importantly a decline in long-term catch-up potential occurred with prolonged inadequate caloric intake. Motor, but not cognitive, development was significantly lower (more than 1 SD below the mean) at 1 year adjusted age on the Bayley Scales in infants with caloric deprivation of more than 4 weeks as neonates (11).

Gross and Eckerman also reported the adverse effect of poor postnatal head growth on long-term neurodevelopmental outcome at 2 years of age (12). Among VLBW infants who were normocephalic at birth, 32% of those with less good head growth during the nursery stay had either cognitive or motor development below 80 at 15 months of adjusted age; in contrast, very few (≤3%) with adequate postnatal head growth had similarly low developmental scores. They also compared long-term outcome by good versus poor head growth over the first 6 weeks of life (13). Normal early postnatal growth was associated with normal developmental outcome and was similar to that in socioeconomically matched term controls. VLBW infants with poor developmental outcome had a significantly lower rate of head growth during the first 6 weeks; these children had experienced delayed enteric feeds, took longer to regain birth weight, and had slower weight gain thereafter. The rate of early head growth was thus proposed as an important summary index of severity and duration of neonatal illness and poor nutrition (13). Marks *et al.* noted that the impact of neonatal illness is most profound upon the somatic growth of the smallest, least mature infants (*i.e.*, those at greatest risk for BPD and malnutrition), with short-term catch-up being less good in all growth parameters, even after resolution of acute illness (14).

Head circumference alone may be a strong predictor of developmental outcome in preterm infants. Hack and Breslau noted that head circumference at 8 months of adjusted age, regardless of subsequent catch-up in head growth, was the single best predictor of IQ at 3 years in VLBW infants after controlling for biologic, medical, and socioeconomic factors (15). In their study 5/30 infants with poor brain growth had BPD; four of the five remained less than 2 SD below the mean at 8 months of adjusted age. Developmental outcome was normal in two, mild to moderately abnormal in two, and severely abnormal in one of the five with BPD and poor brain growth; all were normal neurologically. Ross *et al.* also found that head circumference at 3 years, but not length or weight, was significantly associated with IQ at 3–4 years of age (8). Whereas the mean head circumference percentile was 44% for developmentally normal survivors, it was 23% for those with an abnormally low IQ. In contrast Eilers *et al.* found no relationship between early school performance and head circumference at discharge in infants weighing less than 1250 g at birth, although 52% of this group required special education in order to perform at grade level (16). This latter result is not unexpected in view of other findings of high prevalence of educational problems among premature infants (17–20).

Nutritional Factors Affecting Growth

While provision of optimal nutrition for the infant with BPD is an important goal, it is often extraordinarily difficult to achieve. Efforts to provide adequate caloric intake to sustain good somatic growth may be thwarted by the need to limit fluid intake. Caloric expenditure may be increased by the greater work of breathing or increased oxygen consumption (1, 2). Chronic mild hypoxemia may result in poor growth, even when caloric intake is thought to be adequate.

Common feeding problems include recurrent vomiting with or without gastroesphogeal reflux, poor suck, or inadequate physical stamina necessary to sustain regular nipple feeds (2, 3). Repeated insertion of a gavage tube is often poorly tolerated, especially by older infants, resulting in agitation, crying, and hypoxemia. Leaving a nasogastric tube in place occludes a portion of the nasal airway and increases resistance to air flow in an already compromised infant (21). While nasojejunal feedings may eliminate vomiting, diminished utilization of fat occurs because of the reduced delivery of lingual lipase (22). Occasionally measures such as central hyperalimentation or placement of a gastrostomy are necessary to achieve an anabolic state and to enhance growth.

Skeletal growth may be impaired by rickets that in the most severe form can cause pathologic fractures and chest wall deformity which may further impair pulmonary function (23). Profound and prolonged hypochloremia associated with failure to thrive and poor somatic growth has been reported in both healthy neonates and infants with BPD (24, 25). An unusual pattern of growth deceleration occurs in this condition, with head growth being affected more severely than weight. Both rickets and hypochloremia have been associated with chronic use of furosemide, presumably because the drug promotes calcuria and blocks chloride reabsorption in the renal tubule (24).

Environmental and Psychosocial Considerations

The considerable effort directed toward achieving sufficient caloric intake to allow lung and brain growth is to little avail if the needed energy is promptly expended through constant agitation, prolonged crying, or other excessive physical exertion. This degree of upset is accompanied by hypoxemia, which is in turn associated with poor physical growth (1). The effects of disturbed sleep-wake cycles, constant assault by bright lights and noise, and both emotional and environmental deprivation are largely unexplored in this group of patients but are likely to have an adverse effect upon both physical growth and mental health (1, 26, 27).

Infants with severe BPD are often temperamental, irritable, easily upset, and difficult to console. They are acutely sensitive to their caregiver's frustration or negative feelings. The soothing effect of a calm and loving nurse or parent upon such infants is dramatic. On the other hand havoc is often wrought between caregiver and infant when temperament and expectations are mismatched, leaving both physically and/or emotionally exhausted. Unfortunately nursing assignments often fail to take these important interpersonal considerations into account. Instead these infants may be assigned to staff who may be inexperienced, easily frustrated, or emotionally unable to cope with them, or who, despite the best of skills and intentions, are overburdened by the conflicting demands of their other patients. Every effort should be made to identify primary care nurses who will consistently invest themselves in an individual infant's 24-hour-a-day care. In that capacity the primary nurse educates less experienced staff who share the care and provides consistent input and contact with the family. An occupational or physical therapy assessment and/or behavioral assessment can be very helpful in pointing out ways to identify stress cues, set limits to handling, and encourage positive rather than negative social interaction.

While sedatives may be useful as adjunctive therapy, they should not be used on a regular basis as a substitute for complete nursing care. Chronic use of such drugs may result not only in dependence and signs of withdrawal, which increases agitation, but also in disrupted normal sleep rhythms and sucking patterns (28). It is preferable to first provide physical comfort (holding, rocking, bundling, sucking), prevent hypoxemia, reduce extraneous and multiple sensory inputs, avoid overstimulation, and identify the cause of agitation. Waterbeds (29, 30), sheep-skin mattress covering (31), and non-nutritive sucking during gavage feeding (32, 33) are some techniques that have been associated with enhanced growth in healthy preterm infants. Those modalities may be effective by calming and consoling the infant with BPD, thereby reducing unnecessary energy expenditure.

The process of gavage or nipple feeding, which may occur as often as eight times per day, is frequently an unpleasant experience for the infant. As noted above active resistance to passing a gavage tube, exhaustion from the effort of nippling, lack of adequate oxygen supplementation, fussiness limiting intake, and vomiting due to agitation or gastroesophageal reflux occur commonly. Each infant requires an individualized approach to feeding, designed to maximize caloric intake and minimize caloric loss; this approach should then be consistently used with each feeding by every caregiver, whether nurse or parent.

Careful attention must also be paid to the surrounding physical environment. Hospitalized infants need not be denied age appropriate sensory and fine motor experience, although poor exercise tolerance and muscle weakness may especially hinder gross motor development. The use of a large oxygen tent or nasal cannula allows greater mobility and flexibility in positioning, thus facilitating normal play with toys and reciprocal social interaction. These infants should also be encouraged to develop normal patterns of sleep and wakefulness, by reducing noncontingent ambient noise, avoiding unnecessary or frequent intrusions, dimming lights at night and intermittently during the day for "quiet time," and allowing the infant to sleep undisturbed for long periods, especially at night. We have seen infants with chronic agitation and sleeplessness ("ICU psychosis") whose behavior and medical status improved dramatically after appropriate adjustment of the surrounding physical environment.

Ideally the chronically ill infant with BPD should be cared for at home if adequate medical care can be provided by the family. If hospital care is necessary, however, efforts should be made to develop a special ward or room where as much attention can be devoted to these environmental and social needs as to the pulmonary needs. Unfortunately optimal care of these infants is necessarily labor intensive and costly and thus not likely to be enthusiastically supported by cost-conscious administrators. It is well to remember, however, that improvement in pulmonary function and ultimate hospital discharge are closely tied to physical growth, which is in turn inextricably linked to both nutrition and psychosocial health.

Early Outcome

Little has been written about neonatal development of infants with BPD and whether that correlates with later outcome. In an unpublished study we followed a group of infants with BPD (n = 131) and compared them with a group of premature infants with RDS only (n = 265) and with a group of premature infants without significant pulmonary disease (n = 51). Behavioral ability was measured with the preliminary form of the Assessment for Preterm Infant Behavior (APIB) as described by Sell et al. (34). Gestational age and growth parameters for these groups are given in Table 24.3. The controls and those having RDS were larger and more mature at birth than those with BPD. The group with BPD had poorer behavioral performance, even though they were older when tested.

The infants with BPD were less socially responsive to animate and inanimate stimuli, were not as cuddly, were more easily upset (e.g., peak of excitement, rapidity of buildup, irritability, state lability), had less skill in self-quieting as well as being less consolable, and had higher tone and lower hand-to-mouth ability. Overall those with BPD had poorer self-organization and were not as robust for the examination as the other two groups. Multiple regression analysis identified only one APIB variable (total reflex score) for which some of the variance (R^2 = .29) was explained by the selected perinatal variables. The lack of identifiable factors to explain behavioral characteristics and the less optimal performance in infants with BPD may be interpreted as meaning that the behavioral qualities observed were intrinsically, rather than extrinsically, determined.

We have evaluated neonatal behavior of another 69 premature infants born during 1984–1986 to validate the above observations on groups that were more similar in birth weight (control = 1204 g; RDS = 1084 g, BPD = 1054 g) and gestational age (control = 29.5 wk; RDS = 29.2 wk; BPD = 28.1 wk). A more recent and published version of the APIB (35) was used for this unpublished behavioral study. There were 13 control infants, of whom one required ventilation for apnea; 34 infants with RDS only (mean duration of ventilatory assistance 10.1 days; mean duration of oxygen 23.7 days); and 22 infants with BPD (mean duration of ventilatory assistance 41.7 days; mean duration of oxygen 90.6 days, with 12 being discharged home on oxygen). At the time of behavioral assessment, the group with BPD was significantly larger (control = 2170 g; RDS = 1904 g; BPD = 2518 g) and older (control = 7.7 wk; RDS = 8.3 wk; BPD = 11.7 wk). There was a trend

Table 24.3. Neonatal Behavior of Infants Less Than 37 Weeks' Gestational Age

Variable	Controls* (51 subjects)	RDS* (265 subjects)	BPD* (131 subjects)	Significance Level of Group Compared	Group†
Birth					
Gestational age (wk)	34.1	32.3	30.0	$p<.0001$	A,C
	1.7	2.4	2.7		
Weight (g)	1904	1656	1311	$p<.0001$	A,C
	574	563	513		
Length (cm)	43.5	42.0	38.5	$p<.0001$	A,C
	4.1	5.3	4.5		
Head circumf. (cm)	30.9	29.0	26.7	$p<.0001$	A,C
	2.5	3.2	3.2		
Behavior Test					
Age (d)	24.8	38.0	73.7	$p<.001$	A,C
	14	28	25		
Gestational age (wk)	37.6	37.7	40.5	$p<.0001$	A
	2.4	3.8	3.4		
Weight (g)	2128	2137	2440	$p<.001$	A
	345	390	583		
Length (cm)	45.6	45.1	46.9	$p<.003$	B
	.27	.30	.32		
Head circumf. (cm)	32.6	32.2	32.7	NS	
	.19	.22	.25		
Duration hospitalization					
ICU (d)	5.6	18.5	46.4	$p<.0001$	A,C
	7.0	16.4	26.4		
	(range 0–56d)	(range 0–101d)	(range 6–224d)		
Intermediate Care (d)	20.4	24.2	48.4	$p<.0001$	A
	13.2	15.1	31.5		
	(range 0–79d)	(range 0–113d)	(range 0–263d)		

* Values given are mean and standard deviation.
† A = BPD vs. other two groups; B = BPD vs. RDS; C = RDS vs. controls.
NS = not significant

for the BPD group to also be gestationally older at behavioral testing, but that was not significant.

A brief description of the APIB follows to help the reader unfamiliar with this tool. The APIB exam is administered very similarly to the Neonatal Behavioral Assessment Scale (NBAS) for term infants (36); the items are grouped into packages according to the amount of handling given the infant and the degree of difficulty. Package I consists of habituation items administered during sleep (flashlight shined over eyes, rattle and bell shaken 6 inches from the baby). Package II contains uncovering and turning over. Package III contains the reflexes tested with the baby in supine position (*e.g.*, grasps, passive movements of arms and legs). Package IV and V include the more aversive reflexes that require movement of the infant and more handling (*e.g.*, pull to sit, tonic neck reflex, and Moro reflex). Package VI contains six orientation items that are usually administered with the infant held in the examiner's lap. The unique feature of the APIB is that it measures the infant's level of organization, self-regulation, and use of examiner help. The level of organization before, during, and after each package is scored on four different subsystems (physiologic, motoric, state, and regulatory) and attention-interaction during orientation.

Preliminary analysis of the subsystems data showed a trend for the BPD group to complete the entire exam less frequently. They also had poorer motor organization after package I and during package IV, poorer physiologic control during both package IV and package V, and greater difficulty with regulation during package III and package IV than the RDS subjects. Although fewer differences were found on individual behavioral responses than in our first study, it was significantly more difficult to elicit animate auditory and inanimate visual responses from the infants with BPD, they made less effort to respond to inanimate visual items, and they smiled less often. This study suggests that infants with BPD have greater difficulty in organization and regulatory control.

Als *et al.* developed an individualized behavioral and environmental intervention for VLBW infants at risk of developing BPD (27). Their hypothesis was that the respiratory and functional ability of the VLBW infant with BPD could be improved by prevention of inappropriate sensory stimuli. They compared eight infants who received intervention with eight control infants; all were similar in birth weight (<1250 g), gestational age (<28 wk), severity of respiratory disease in the first 10 days, incidences of intraventricular hemorrhage and patent ductus arteriosus, and socioeconomic status. The infants were observed behaviorally at 10, 20, and 30 days after birth, and at 36 weeks and 40 weeks after conception. The infants who received caregiving intervention to reduce inappropriate sensory input had significantly shorter durations of ventilatory and oxygen supports and were able to take all feedings by nipple sooner. The following outcome measures were also significantly better in those who had received the intervention: 1) behavioral regulation 1 month postconception as measured with the APIB; 2) cognitive and motor development at 3, 6, and 9 months postconception as measured with the Bayley Scales; and 3) behavioral regulation at 9 months postconception. These findings suggest that behavioral status and environmental events are relevant issues in the NICU for infants at risk of developing BPD. It will be important to see if the findings of Als *et al.* can be replicated in their expanded study and in other NICUs. If that is possible, individualized behavioral and environmental intervention could be added to other regimens currently used in the care of infants with BPD. Behavioral intervention will not be easily achieved, because most NICUs are noisy, brightly lit, and have a continuously high activity level; nor will caregivers find it easy to plan handling maneuvers around the baby's readiness and recovery after procedures. However, it may well be worth the effort for adult caregivers to learn more sensitive methods of interacting contingently with infants in NICUs.

Later Neurodevelopmental Outcome

In the studies of later neurologic and developmental outcome of children who had BPD, the definition of BPD almost uniformly included 1) assisted ventilation during the first week of life, 2) supplemental oxygen for more than 28 days to maintain adequate oxygenation, and 3) radiographic evidence as defined by Northway's criteria (37). Early studies were primarily descriptive. Harrod found no infants with severe developmental handicap (38); it should be noted that these infants were born in a period when there were very few survivors with BPD. Northway *et al.* in 1979 documented severe developmental handicap in 34% of their population (4). More recent papers on outcome are summarized in Table 24.4. Markestad and Fitzhardinge followed 20 children who had RDS and BPD to at least 2 years of age (1). During the neonatal period pulmonary air leaks, patent ductus arteriosus, and apnea were frequent problems. Five patients (25%) had mean Bayley scores below 85; two of those remained severely retarded, and two others had accelerated development between 18 and 36 months. A similar improvement in development was not seen in the 15 children who initially scored within the normal range. The five children with low Bayley scores had prolonged need for oxygen supplementation and hospitalization, and recurrent apnea; their other perinatal variables and their socioeconomic status (SES) were similar to those of the children who had normal development. All had normal electroencephalograms, and none had seizures beyond the neonatal period.

Vohr *et al.* compared three groups of VLBW infants who were similar in mean birth weight, gestational age, and socioeconomic status (5). The groups were defined by the length of oxygen administration and chest radiographic changes. The 25 with mild pulmonary disease and less than 21 days of oxygen had no BPD. The two groups with severe disease received more than 21 days of oxygen; eight had no BPD, and 26 had BPD. Developmental ability was similar in all groups at 12 months, but cognitive skills were lower in those with BPD at 24 months. Neurologic disability was present in 8/21 (38%) of the BPD group, 1/6 (17%) of the RDS group, and 2/22 (9%) of those with short oxygen requirements. When the neurologic abnormality in the BPD group was related to severity of BPD, 8/13 (62%) with Stage III to IV BPD had neurologic deficits, in contrast to only 3/9 (33%) of those with Stage I to II. Eleven (52%) of the BPD group were abnormal neurologically and/or developmentally; it is not known if there was developmental improvement concomitant with resolution of pulmonary disease.

Mayes *et al.* followed 11 infants with BPD, four of whom had RDS, and seven of whom did not (39). Developmental scores were corrected for gestational age. Delay was defined as a developmental quotient or IQ less than 80 and was present in eight of 10 testable children; the 11th was thought by the primary physician to be delayed.

Yu et al.'s study of VLBW infants (3) documented completely normal outcome in only 9/16 (38%); prediction of the disabilities was not possible from the available perinatal data. Goldson also followed a small number of children with severe BPD (Northway Stage IV) and compared them to a group with milder BPD (Northway Stage III) or no BPD (40). Infants were excluded if they had clinical evidence of intracranial hemorrhage, seizures, neonatal neuropathology, cicatricial or vision-compromising retrolental fibroplasia, or sensorineural hearing deficits. The children were seen at 2 years chronologic age, and the scores were not adjusted for prematurity. Only 1/8 (13%) of those with no or mild BPD had a mental score below 84, whereas 8/9 (89%) of those with severe BPD had a mental score below 84. The differences in motor scores were not significant, although the severe BPD group had a higher incidence of pathologic findings on a neuromotor assessment.

Sauve and Singhal followed 141 infants with BPD and 66 controls who had received assisted ventilation during the first week of life and supplemental oxygen for fewer than 16 days; the controls had no radiographic evidence of BPD (7). The control and BPD groups were matched for year of birth and birth weight groups of large ranges (i.e., 500–1500 g, 1501–2500 g, and >2500 g). Follow-up was at 4, 8, and 12 months' adjusted age, and yearly thereafter until a maximum age of 8 years. The neurodevelopmental results were based on the most recent (oldest) follow-up assessment. There were no differences between groups on the mean Bayley Mental Development Index and the McCarthy General Cognitive Index or in the percentage with developmental scores in the abnormal range, or cerebral palsy. Five children who had BPD and one control child have profound neurosensory hearing loss and wear hearing aids. There was a higher frequency of retinopathy of prematurity diagnosed among the BPD group in the NICU (71.7% vs. 34.1% for controls) and at follow-up (40% vs. 20%) ($p < .001$). Although abnormal speech assessments were described in 31 (22%) of the children who had BPD, it was not specified if that represented language delay or abnormalities in articulation or voice quality.

Meisels et al. recently compared 20 infants with RDS and 17 with BPD, matched by sex, parity, family configuration, and socioeconomic status at 12–18 months after hospital discharge (6). The infants did not have other major perinatal problems. Follow-up was scheduled for age in months after hospital discharge, to control for the potential impact of differing lengths of time in the home environment. The developmental scores were also corrected for the degree of prematurity. The infants with BPD were not smaller or younger than those with RDS only. One infant with a neurologic problem had RDS and hypotonia. More of those who had BPD had Bayley scores below 85 on both the MDI (35% vs. 5% for RDS) and the PDI (47% vs. 10% for RDS). Regression analysis showed that the explained variance (R^2) in developmental measures was in the range of 13%–47%, and that BPD contributed more than birth weight or gestational age to the variance.

Berman et al. found that 5 of 10 infants

Table 24.4. Neurodevelopmental Outcome of Infants with Bronchopulmonary Dysplasia

Study (ref)	Year Birth	Birth Weight (g)*	Gestational Age (wk)*	No. Subjects	Years Followed	Developmental Outcome†	Neurologic Abnormality	Sensory Deficits
Markestad & Fitzhardinge (1)	1974–76	1661 (830–2600)	31.1 (25–36)	20	2 post-term	18 mo-mean MDI & PDI = 88.9 (50–101.5) 5/20 scores <85	1 with hydrocephalus	1-severe myopia (ROP), 2-strabismus only, 0-sensorineural hearing loss
Vohr et al. (5)	1975–77	1100 (610–1500)	29 (27–33)	21	2	12 mo-corrected MDI = 80 (SD 25) 24 mo-corrected MDI = 65 (SD 16, 3 (14%) with MDI <60	24 mo-8/21 (38%)	
Mayes et al. (39)	1974–78	RDS 1353 (1020–2000) Non-RDS 961 (709–1162)	30 (28–33) 28 (26–30)	11	2–5	8/10 (80%) had DQ or IQ < 80, 1 other delayed (not formally tested)		2-blind (ROP)
Yu et al. (3)	1977–80	<1500	—	16	2 post-term	9 (38%) normal neurodevelopmental outcome 7 (29%) developmental, neurologic, and/or sensory handicap)	3 (19%) with CP	2 sensorineural hearing loss (1 of those blind with ROP)
Goldson (40)	1976–79	868 (650–1100)	27 (26–31)	9	2	Not adjusted for prematurity, mean MDI = 75 (range 57–92), mean PDI = 70 (range 37–101)		None

Study	Years	Birth weight (g)	Gestational age (wk)	N	Age at follow-up	Developmental outcome	Neurologic outcome	Other
Sauve & Singhal (7)	1975–82	See text	69% < 29	141	Maximum of 8	Mean MDI = 88.6 (SD 23.6), mean McCarthy GCI = 98.2 (SD 18.5), abnormal development in 34%	15 (10.6%) with CP	119/166 (71.7%) with ROP in NICU 20/141 (14.2%) with ROP in follow-up
Meisels et al. (6)	1980–82	1291 (SD 5.9)	30.1 (SD 2.8)	17	12 and 18 mo post hospital discharge	Mean MDI = 86.1 (SD 13.7), mean PDI = 90.1 (SD 17.1), REEL language quotient = 90.6	None abnormal	

† MDI = Bayley Scales Mental Developmental Index; PDI = Bayley Scales Psychomotor Developmental Index.
* Numbers in parentheses are ranges.

Table 24.5. Early Developmental Outcome

Age Group and Index*	Controls†	RDS†	BPD†	Significance Level of Groups Compared	Groups‡
12 mo	(28)	(141)	(78)		
MDI	101	93	79	$p < .0001$	A
MDI-corrected	118	117	108	$p < .05$	A
PDI	88	82	66	$p < .0001$	A
PDI-corrected	103	101	90	$p < .001$	A
18 mo	(20)	(117)	(53)		
MDI	104	97	83	$p < .0001$	A
MDI-corrected	116	112	102	$p < .01$	A
PDI	101	90	78	$p < .0001$	A,C
PDI-corrected	110	102	93	$p < .01$	A
24 mo	(23)	(124)	(63)		
MDI	98	96	86	$p < .01$	A
MDI-corrected	102	106	96	$p < .05$	B
PDI	101	91	85	$p < .05$	A,C
PDI-corrected	106	100	94	NS	

    MDI = Bayley Scales Mental Developmental Index; PDI = Bayley Scales Psychomotor Developmental Index; corrected = corrected for gestational age at birth.
    † Numbers in parentheses are total number of subjects in the respective age groups.
    ‡ A = BPD vs. other two groups; B = BPD vs. RDS; C = RDS vs. controls.
    NS = Not significant

with BPD required therapy or special school assistance because of motor delay or moderate to severe developmental delay (41).

In our unpublished study of premature infants of less than 37 weeks, there were no differences in neurologic outcome among groups, with 68%–79% being normal. There were significant differences in development during the first 2 years of life (Table 24.5) but few thereafter. Explained variance of the developmental scores was in the range of 18%–40% at 12 months, 54%–64% at 18 months, 69%–72% at 24 months, and 28%–39% at 3 and 4 years. Variables included in the regression analysis were the APIB exam, prior developmental assessment, maternal education, and perinatal variables. RDS, BPD, and maternal education did not contribute to explanation of the variance; prior developmental ability was the strongest predictor. The frequency of normal neurologic and developmental exams as defined by uncorrected Bayley MDI and PDI scores of 84–116 were as follows: 1) 12 months, control 12/21 or 57%,

RDS 53/120 or 44%, BPD 9/65 or 13.9%; 2) 18 months, control 10/18 or 56%, RDS 50/85 or 59%, BPD 11/41 or 26.8%; 3) 24 months, control 11/13 or 85%, RDS 53/86 or 61.6%, BPD 14/41 or 34.2%; 4) 36 months, control 8/9 or 89%, RDS 58/75 or 77%, BPD 17/25 or 68%. Thus as the children with BPD became older, their developmental abilities were more similar to those who had either no pulmonary disease or only RDS. This could represent catch-up for the degree of prematurity but must be interpreted cautiously because it is possible that infants with suboptimal development dropped out of follow-up in later years. We unfortunately do not have those data available at present. It should also be noted that we followed very few infants who were hospitalized in the NICU beyond 6 months; those infants have the most severe BPD, and others have shown them to experience greater developmental delays and a higher frequency of neurologic problems.

Summary

Currently available data are inconsistent with respect to future growth and neurodevelopmental abilities of premature children who had all but the most severe degree of BPD. Some investigators, but not all, have found that early growth percentiles were lower in premature infants with BPD. Early catch-up in growth occurs between 24 and 36 months of age; whether there is additional catch-up growth after 5 or 6 years of age is not known. Adequacy of early head growth may be an important predictor of long-term developmental outcome, as is also shown in premature infants without BPD.

There is evidence that infants with BPD have less behavioral organization and regulatory skills in the neonatal period, possibly secondary to repeated noxious stimuli experienced in the NICU. Studies on premature infants in general have documented improvement in early growth with various intervention programs. One intervention study that began at 10 days of age in infants at risk for developing BPD showed that reduction of inappropriate sensory stimuli decreased the duration of both assisted ventilation and oxygen administration, decreased time on gavage feedings, and improved behavioral regulation and developmental outcome in the first year of life.

The frequency of abnormal neurologic exams ranged from 0% to 38%, and the prevalence of developmental problems varied from 14% to 80%, with most in the range of 30% to 60%. All but one study were on pre-school-age children, so we do not know what school-age outcome will be. Factors that were related to outcome status included having BPD, severity of the pulmonary disease, and prior developmental ability. More detailed statistical analyses of data have been limited by the small number of subjects in most studies. Whether the results from children with BPD born in the 1970s are applicable to those born in the later 1980s is doubtful; the latter are smaller and more immature, receive different ventilatory and nutritional support, and experience more complications that may influence future growth and development.

References

1. Markestad T, Fitzhardinge PM. Growth and development in children recovering from bronchopulmonary dysplasia. J Pediatr 1981; 98:597–602.
2. Koops BL, Abman SH, Accurso FJ. Outpatient management and follow-up of bronchopulmonary dysplasia. Clin Perinatol 1984;11:101–122.
3. Yu VYH, Orgill AA, Lim SB, Bajuk B, Astbury

J. Growth and development of very low birth-weight infants recovering from bronchopulmonary dysplasia. Arch Dis Child 1983;58: 791–794.
4. Northway WH. Observations on bronchopulmonary dysplasia. J Pediatr 1979;95:815–818.
5. Vohr BR, Bell EF, Oh W. Infants with bronchopulmonary dysplasia. Growth pattern and neurologic and developmental outcome. Am J Dis Child 1982;136:443–447.
6. Meisels SJ, Plunkett JW, Roloff DW, Pasick PL, Stiefel GS. Growth and development of preterm infants with respiratory distress syndrome and bronchopulmonary dysplasia. Pediatrics 1986;77:345–352.
7. Sauve RS, Singhal N. Long-term morbidity of infants with bronchopulmonary dysplasia. Pediatrics 1985;76:725–733.
8. Ross G, Lipper EG, Auld PAM. Physical growth and developmental outcome in very low birth weight premature infants at 3 years of age. J Pediatr 1985;107:284–286.
9. Winick M, Rosso P. Head circumference and cellular growth of the brain in normal and marasmic children. J Pediatr 1969;74:774–778.
10. Rosso P, Winick M. Relation of nutrition to physical and mental development. Pediatr Ann 1973;2:33–43.
11. Georgieff MK, Hoffman JS, Pereira GR, Bernbaum J, Hoffman-Williamson M. Effect of neonatal caloric deprivation on head growth and 1-year developmental status in preterm infants. J Pediatr 1985;107:581–587.
12. Gross ST, Eckerman CO. Normative early head growth in very-low-birth-weight infants. J Pediatr 1983;103:946–949.
13. Gross SJ, Oehler JM, Eckerman CO. Head growth and developmental outcome in very low-birth-weight infants. Pediatrics 1983;71: 70–75.
14. Marks KH, Maisels MJ, Moore E, Gifford K, Friedman Z. Head growth in sick premature infants—a longitudinal study. J Pediatr 1979; 94:282–285.
15. Hack M, Breslau N. Very low birth weight infants: effects of brain growth during infancy on intelligence quotient at 3 years of age. Pediatrics 1986;77:196–202.
16. Eilers BL, Desai NS, Wilson MA, Cunningham MD. Classroom performance and social factors of children with birth weights of 1,250 grams or less: follow-up at 5 to 8 years of age. Pediatrics 1986;77:203–208.
17. Drillien CM, Thompson AJM, Burgoyne K. Low-birthweight children at early school-age: a longitudinal study. Dev Med Child Neurol 1980;22:26–47.
18. Kitchen WH, Ryan MM, Rickards A, et al. A longitudinal study of very low-birthweight infants. IV. An overview of performance at 8 years of age. Dev Med Child Neurol 1980;22: 172–188.
19. Gunn TR, Lepore E, Outerbridge EW. Outcome at school-age after neonatal mechanical ventilation. Dev Med Child Neurol 1983;25: 305–314.
20. Sell EJ, Gaines JA, Gluckman C, Williams E. Early identification of learning problems in neonatal intensive care graduates. Am J Dis Child 1985;139:460–463.
21. Stocks J. Effect of nasogastric tubes on nasal resistance during infancy. Arch Dis Child 1980;55:17–21.
22. Roy RN, Pollnitz RP, Hamilton JR, et al. Impaired assimilation of nasojejunal feeds in healthy low-birth-weight newborn infants. J Pediatr 1977;90:431–434.
23. Glasgow JFT, Thomas PS. Rachitic respiratory distress in small preterm infants. Arch Dis Child 1977;52:268–273.
24. Perlman JM, Moore V, Siegel MJ, Dawson J. Is chloride depletion an important contributing cause of death in infants with bronchopulmonary dysplasia? Pediatrics 1986;77:212–216.
25. Roy S, Arant BS. Hypokalemic metabolic alkalosis in normotensive infants with elevated plasma renin activity and hyperaldosteronism: role of dietary chloride deficiency. Pediatrics 1981;67:423–429.
26. Powell GF, Brasel JA, Blizzard RM. Emotional deprivation and growth retardation simulating idiopathic hypopituitarism. I. Clinical evaluation of the syndrome. N Engl J Med 1967;276:1271–1278.
27. Als H, Lawhorn G, Brown E, et al. Individualized behavioral and environmental care of the VLBW preterm infant at high risk for bronchopulmonary dysplasia: NICU and de-

28. Kron RE, Litt M, Phoenix MD, Finnegan LP. Neonatal narcotic abstinence: effects of pharmacotherapeutic agents and maternal drug usage on nutritive sucking behavior. J Pediatr 1976;88:637–641.
29. Kramer LI, Pierpont ME. Rocking waterbeds and auditory stimuli to enhance growth of preterm infants: a preliminary report. J Pediatr 1976;88:297–299.
30. Korner AF. The use of waterbeds in the care of preterm infants. J Perinatol 1986;6:142–147.
31. Scott S, Cole T, Lucas P, Richards M. Weight gain and movement patterns of very low birthweight babies nursed on lambswool. Lancet 1983;2;1014–1016.
32. Bernbaum JC, Pereira GR, Watkins JB, Peckham GJ. Nonnutritive sucking during gavage feeding enhances growth and maturation in premature infants. Pediatrics 1983;71:41–45.
33. Field T, Ignatoff E, Stringer S, et al. Nonnutritive sucking during tube feedings: effects on preterm neonates in an intensive care unit. Pediatrics 1982;70:381–384.
34. Sell EJ, Luick A, Poisson SS, Hill S. Outcome of very low birth weight (VLBW) infants. Neonatal behavior of 188 infants. Dev Behav Pediatr 1980:1(2):78–85.
35. Als H, Lester BM, Tronick EZ, Brazelton TB. Towards a systematic assessment of preterm infants' behavior. Appendix: manual for the assessment of preterm infants behavior (APIB). In: Fitzgerald HE, Lester BM, eds. Theory and research in behavioral pediatrics, vol 1. New York: Plenum, 1982, pp 35–132.
36. Brazelton TB. Neonatal behavioral assessment scale. 2nd ed. Philadelphia: JB Lippincott, 1984.
37. Northway WH Jr, Rosan RC, Porter DY. Pulmonary disease following respirator therapy of hyaline membrane disease: bronchopulmonary dysplasia. N Engl J Med 1967;276:357–368.
38. Harrod JR, L'Heureux P, Wangensteen OD, Hunt CE. Long-term follow-up of severe respiratory distress syndrome treated with IPPB. J Pediatr 1974;84:277–286.
39. Mayes L, Perkett E, Stahlman MT. Severe bronchopulmonary dysplasia: a retrospective review. Acta Paediatr Scand 1983;72:225–229.
40. Goldson E. Severe bronchopulmonary dysplasia in the very low birth weight infant: its relationship to developmental outcome. Dev Behav Pediatr 1984;5(4):165–168.
41. Berman W, Katz R, Yabek SM, Dillon T, Fripp RR, Papile L. Long-term follow-up of bronchopulmonary dysplasia. J Pediatr 1986;109:45–50.

Comments

Bruce R. Boynton

There is now abundant evidence that infants with BPD are smaller than infants without BPD of the same chronological age. There are several possible explanations for this:

1. Infants with BPD may have lower birthweights than infants without BPD. The risk of BPD increases with decreasing birthweight so that infants with low birthweight may be overrepresented in groups of infants having BPD.
2. Infants with BPD may receive inadequate calories for normal growth. These infants expend a large number of calories in breathing because of their rapid respiratory rate and expiratory flow limitation. Thus, they have increased caloric needs. To make matters worse, their inability to tolerate large amounts of fluid limits the number of calories that can be supplied. Feeding problems may further reduce caloric intake.
3. The pathophysiology of BPD may limit growth velocity. Growth is impaired in many other chronic diseases of childhood, although the mechanism by which growth is affected is often incompletely understood. Infants with BPD frequently have a chronic intermittent hypoxemia. It

is possible that chronic tissue hypoxia might limit growth velocity. Unfortunately, there is as yet no practical method for assessing the long-term adequacy of tissue oxygenation. Growth velocity of infants with BPD usually increases as pulmonary function improves.

4. There may be other factors that interfere with the growth of infants with BPD. For example, the environment in which we care for critically ill infants may adversely affect growth. We know very little about the effects of noise, bright lights, changes in personnel, and painful stimuli to which infants with BPD are exposed. The psychosocial dwarfism reported among older children with abnormal home environments may have its counterpart in the intensive care nursery.

Unfortunately, we have little knowledge about the relative importance of these various factors. Even less is known about the influence of BPD on development. The results of published developmental studies are inconclusive partly because of inconsistency in eliminating the effects of confounding variables such as gestational age, interventricular hemorrhage, seizures, or differences in medical management. More research is needed on the effects of malnutrition, chronic hypoxemia, and environmental stress on the developing brain.

25

Pulmonary Status of Infants and Children with Bronchopulmonary Dysplasia

GREGORY P. HELDT

Introduction

Bronchopulmonary dysplasia (BPD) is a chronic condition that represents delayed resolution of acute neonatal lung injury. It is difficult to define and has changed in character during the last 20 years, primarily because the nature of the acute neonatal lung injury and its treatment have changed. Smaller babies are now surviving the most severe lung disease. It is expected that the resolution of the neonatal lung disease is quite different in the 600 gram baby who survives 3 months of mechanical ventilation, which is more typical of the smallest survivors in 1986, than in the larger infants who survived during the past two decades. In addition new forms of therapy such as surfactant replacement and high-frequency oscillatory and jet ventilation will probably improve survival of infants with the most severe lung disease, but the treatment itself may further complicate the acute lung disease and the course of its resolution.

Many methods of pulmonary function testing used in older subjects have been adapted for investigating the pulmonary status of premature infants. These investigations must account for the size of the lungs at the time of study. The classical measurements used to describe the status of the airway and lung parenchyma are now being expanded to include studies of the function of the respiratory muscles and the pulmonary circulation. Another factor that may drastically alter the course of the resolution of acute neonatal lung injury is viral pneumonitis. Recent developments for diagnosis of viral infections and assessing the biochemical mediators of lung injury and repair may become potent indirect tests of "pulmonary function" in the future.

This chapter describes the status of pulmonary function in infants and children with BPD. I will not detail the recent work regarding new forms of therapy, the pathogenesis of BPD, or other diagnostic tools such as biochemical analysis of amniotic fluid or airway secretions. Rather, I will review the physiologic investigations so as to provide a better understanding of the cardiopulmonary status of these infants and children.

Methods of Investigation

Many of the basic methods used to evaluate infants with BPD have been adapted from standard pulmonary function testing. These include assessment of overall gas exchange, pulmonary mechanics, distribution of ventilation, and tests of small and larger airway function. In addition to the classical methods, the study of mechanics of breathing must include that of respiratory muscle function, with special attention given to the function of the diaphragm and chest wall.

Overall Gas Exchange

Overall gas exchange has become easier to assess since the introduction of continuous skin surface oxygen (1) and carbon dioxide (2) electrodes. Although these methods are used routinely in the intensive care situation, they tend to underestimate the PaO_2 and overestimate the $PaCO_2$ in infants beyond 10 weeks of chronological age (3). Pulse oximetry, which has been improved recently, allows the noninvasive estimation of oxygen saturation (4). The interpretation of oxygen saturation data must account for all the variables that may change the shape or position of the deoxyhemoglobin dissociation curve (5). This method appears to be reliable and will probably supersede the use of skin surface PO_2 measurements, especially when used to adjust the rate of delivery of supplemental oxygen to infants on chronic oxygen therapy.

The Mechanical Properties of the Lungs

The classical concept for describing the mechanics of the lung is based on a model in which elements having compliance, resistance, and inertance are connected in series. The resistive term includes one term for the laminar and another for the turbulent pressure drop in the system due to gas flow in and out of the respiratory system. During breathing the pressure across the respiratory system due to these three elements can be described by the following classical equation of motion:

$$\Delta P_{tp} = \frac{1}{C} \times \Delta V_L + R1 \times \dot{V}_L + R2 \times \dot{V}_L^2 + I \times \ddot{V}_L$$

This equation can be used to describe the pressure drop (ΔP_{tp}) across any fluidic system which has the equivalence of capacitance (compliance) (C), resistance (laminar, R1, and turbulent, R2), and inertance (I), and where the volume (V_L) is known. Early studies of respiratory mechanics in adults showed that the inertance accounts for less than 5% of the change in transpulmonary pressure with breathing (6). Recent studies in mechanically ventilated animals (whose trachea and airways are similar in size to those of human newborns) indicate that most of the inertance of the system is in the gas in small-diameter endotracheal tubes, especially at rapid rates of ventilation (7). Thus the inertance is usually ignored in this type of analysis.

The measurement of mechanics depends upon the measurement of the transpulmonary pressure (ΔP_{tp}) and the flow of gas ($\dot{V}_L$) during breathing. Transpulmonary pressure can be estimated by measuring the difference between the airway pressure and the pressure in the mid-thoracic esophagus. The esophageal pressure is measured with a fluid filled feeding catheter (8) or a catheter whose tip is covered with a deflated, thin-walled latex balloon (9). Its position must be carefully checked before making the measurements (10). The flow of gas is measured with a pneumotachograph, which is attached to the infant's endotracheal tube or to a face mask (11). The flow is integrated or differentiated using analog or digital methods for performing these calculations (12).

The compliance to which most authors refer is the dynamic compliance. It is most easily calculated by dividing the tidal volume by the change in transpulmonary pressure at points of zero flow during the respiratory cycle. At these points, since there is no airway flow, the second and third term on the right side of the equation of motion are equal to zero. Furthermore, assuming that the contribution of inertance is negligible, the change in transpulmonary pressure under these circumstances represents that due to compliance.

Measurement of the total respiratory system compliance has been advocated as advantageous to that of dynamic compliance (13). This method uses airway occlusions to produce point of zero flow. During airway occlusion there is no resistive pressure drop across the airways, and the pressure measured in the airway is equal to the elastic recoil pressure of the lungs and chest wall. By measuring the amount of volume change prior to the airway occlusion and the elastic recoil (airway occlusion) pressure, it is possible to construct a quasistatic pressure-volume curve for the respiratory system (14). This measurement is performed in intubated, ventilated patients who are presumed to have completely relaxed respiratory muscles. It may also be performed in older infants who are not intubated, in whom the Hering-Breuer reflex inhibits respiratory muscle activity for a short time during airway occlusion (15). The compliance calculated by this method is different from the dynamic compliance, since it is a static measurement, and since it represents the stiffness of the entire respiratory system.

The second method of measuring the static compliance of the respiratory system is with a weighted spirometer (16). The infant breathes through a mask into and out of a miniature spirometer which has a recirculation system and CO_2 absorber. Additional oxygen is added to this closed system to replace that which the patient consumes, so that a stable baseline recording is obtained. A weight is then added to the bell of the spirometer to increase the airway pressure. The increase in airway pressure is measured, and the corresponding increase in the end-expiratory lung volume is measured from the spirometer tracing. The static compliance is then calculated by dividing the change in end-expiratory lung volume by the change in airway pressure. This compliance is yet another way to express the stiffness of the entire respiratory system, which may differ from the dynamic compliance of the lungs.

The most widely used parameter for pulmonary resistance is the mid-volume resistance, which is measured at points of equal lung volume in the middle of inspiration and expiration (17). The instantaneous flow is measured at these points with a pneumotachograph. The difference in transpulmonary pressure is measured between these points, which is assumed to be a purely resistive loss, since the lung volume is the same at these points. (This assumes that the first term on the right side of the equation of motion equals 0 and that the inertial loss also equals 0; terms 3 and 4 are combined.) The resistance is equal to the difference in transpulmonary pressure at those points, divided by the sum of the inspiratory and expiratory flows. This measurement of total pulmonary resistance is the sum of the resistance to breathing during inspiration and expiration. A statistical method has also been used (18), relating the pressure, flow, and integrated flow (volume) signals using a multiple linear regression to solve the equation of motion. This method can be used to calculate the resistance separately during inspiration and expiration.

A third method of measurement of pulmonary resistance is obtained indirectly by the measurement of the time constant of the emptying of the lung during a relaxed expiration. The flow-volume loop thus obtained is the basis for a number of methods of assessing pulmonary function. Normally the lungs and respiratory system empty in an exponential fashion since the lungs' elastic recoil pressure, which is the major driving force for expiration, is proportional to lung volume. The curve of the lung volume versus time is therefore an exponential curve. Advantage is taken of this concept in constructing curves relating the expiratory flow and the volume expired. Since passive expiration is an exponential curve, the plot of the derivative of the function (flow) versus the function (volume) is a straight line. Thus, in conjunction with the airway occlusion method, the flow of gas out of the lungs after release of the airway occlusion results from passive exhalation. The lung volume data thus measured as a function of time can be fit to an exponential curve using a computer program, or the slope of the expiratory flow-volume curve can be used to calculate the time constant graphically. The time constant, being the product of the resistance and compliance, can then be divided by compliance of the respiratory system, as measured during the airway occlusions (14), to compute the resistance. This method has been used in mechanically ventilated patients as well as in spontaneously breathing infants in whom expiration is inhibited by the Hering-Breuer reflex due to occlusion of the airway.

These methods measure the resistance of the entire respiratory system. One of the oldest methods, body plethysmography, measures the airways resistance (19). The subject (usually 6 years of age or older) is seated in a sealed box and breathes on a mouthpiece attached to a tube which passes through the box. The tube contains an airway occluder and pneumotachograph. During inspiration the subject's body expands, and the gas in the box is slightly compressed. The pressure in the box is calibrated against changes in the volume of the body, by adding known amounts of gas with a calibrating syringe. At the midpoint of a breath the airway is occluded, and airway pressure is recorded while the subject voluntarily makes small panting respiratory efforts. From the slope of the plot of the change in the mouth pressure versus box pressure, the thoracic gas volume (TGV), or the total volume of gas in the thorax which is subjected to the airway pressure change (by way of either open airways or surrounding lung parenchyma), can be determined. Plots of transairway pressure versus flow are then constructed, which allows for the computation of airway resistance. This method has been applied to children (20) but requires their cooperation for successful studies. Similar studies have been performed in newborns, but success depends on the skill of the operator (21, 22). Although the method provides nearly simultaneous measurements of airways resistance and lung volume in a most elegant fashion, it is not applicable to acutely ill infants or uncooperative young children.

The absolute volume of the lungs may also be measured by equilibrating it with an inert gas such as helium or neon during quiet breathing. This may be performed in infants by connecting a rebreathing bag to the airway at the end of expiration (23). The baby breathes into and out of the bag, and the gas in the lungs equilibrates with the bag's contents. The content of inert gas lost from the bag is computed by measurement of the concentration of the gas before and after equilibration. The functional residual capacity (FRC) is computed as the change in content of the inert gas before and after equilibration, divided by the gas concentration after equilibration. This method has been adapted to newborns and older patients during mechanical ventilation (24).

A number of methods have been devised to localize the source of airway obstruction, whether in the large central airways or in the smaller peripheral airways. The flow volume loop described above is a plot of expiratory airway flow as a function of expired lung volume. The flow rates during the first half of expiration are limited primarily by the effort of the subject and by the resistance of the large airways. The flow rates in the last half or third of expiration are thought to reflect more the contribution of the small airways. In diseased lungs the airways collapse at a higher lung volume than in normal lungs, and expiratory flow rates are reduced during mid or late expiration. This technique may be useful in differentiating damage to the trachea or large bronchi due to prolonged endotracheal intubation from obstruction in the lower airways. With patience the peak-expiratory flow rate may be measured during large spontaneous breathing efforts, and can be used to detect tracheal obstruction, such as stenosis (25). Since infants cannot voluntarily perform the maximal expiratory flow maneuver, a "squeeze" plethysmograph ("Hammersmith jacket") has been devised to assist expiration (26), especially at lung volumes near FRC. This inflatable, jacket-like device fits around the torso and is inflated to a pressure of 50–80 cm H_2O early in expiration, gently squeezing the infant and assisting expiration. The parameter calculated from this technique is the flow rate at the FRC of the breath immediately preceding the "squeeze", or V_{FRC}, as shown in Figure 25.1, thought to be a reproducible indicator of large airway flow limitation. The combined

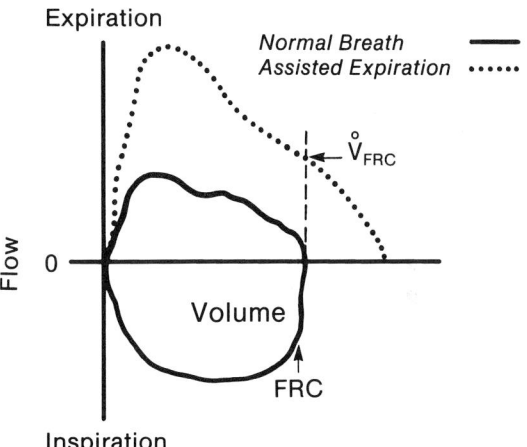

Figure 25.1. Flow-volume loops during normal quiet breathing (solid line) and during an assisted expiration (dotted line). The flow rate at FRC ($\dot{V}_{FRC}$) is a reproducible indicator of airways obstruction.

use of these measurements may be useful in separating damage to the trachea and large airways associated with treatment with high-frequency jet ventilation (27), from the more distal airway and lung parenchymal damage of BPD.

Another technique used to differentiate between obstruction of large and small airways makes use of having the subject breathe mixtures of helium and oxygen (HeO_2). Flow in large airways is more turbulent than that in small airways, which is nearly laminar. The fluidic pressure loss due to turbulent flow is more dependent upon the density of gas than that due to laminar flow, which is more dependent on viscosity. Turbulent flow resistance accounts for about 25% of the resistance of the airways. When patients breathe HeO_2 mixtures rather than nitrogen-oxygen mixtures, the airway resistance is decreased, since the turbulent flow resistance is decreased with the decreased respired gas density (28, 29). Thus by comparing flow rates

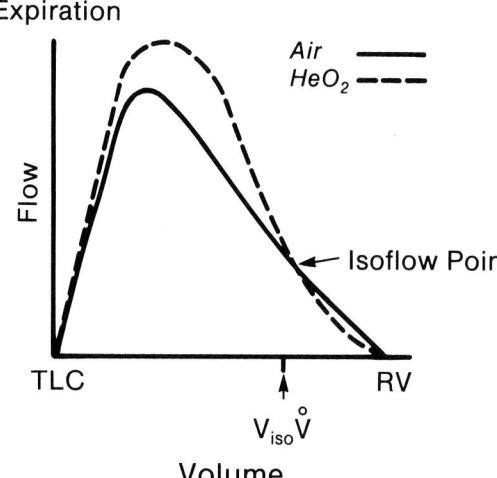

Figure 25.2. Flow-volume loops during air (solid line) and Heliox (dotted line) breathing. The volume of isoflow ($V_{iso}\dot{V}$) is an indicator of obstruction in small airways.

measured during HeO_2 breathing with those measured during air breathing, the resistance of the small airways can be assessed. A parameter useful in describing the difference between HeO_2 and air breathing is the volume of iso-flow, $V_{iso}\dot{V}$, which is the lung volume at which the expiratory flow is the same whether the subject is breathing air or a HeO_2 mixture (Fig. 25.2). The higher the $V_{iso}\dot{V}$, the greater the contribution of the small airways to the overall expiratory resistance.

Work of Breathing and Respiratory Muscle Function

Patients with airways obstruction and decreased compliance have an increase in the work of breathing. The work of breathing is classically calculated as the pressure-volume work performed on the lungs, or the area during inspiration under the pressure-volume curve. The diaphragm is the infant's primary respiratory muscle. The classical computation of the work of breathing underestimates the pressure-volume work actually performed by the diaphragm. Infants have a highly compliant chest wall (30), which presents a mechanical disadvantage to the diaphragm. In adults and older children the diaphragm contracts and applies traction on the rib cage, which provides an upward and expansive inspiratory force on the lower ribs. The abdominal contents thus act like a fulcrum for the diaphragm to apply a lever-like force on the lower ribs. If the chest wall is highly compliant, such as in the preterm infant, or if the diaphragm is flattened due to obstructive lung disease, the contraction of the diaphragm pulls the rib cage inward. Thus some of the volume displacement with contraction of the diaphragm is expended in collapsing the chest wall, rather than in inflating the lungs.

The volume displacement of the diaphragm in preterm infants has been quantitatively estimated by partitioning the pulmonary ventilation between that which is produced (or lost) by the chest wall and diaphragm, using an inductance plethysmograph. Two bands of the inductance plethysmograph estimate separately the volume changes of the chest wall and abdomen, and a weighted sum of the volume change of each is statistically fitted to the volume change of the lungs (Fig. 25.3). The diaphragm in many infants must make a tidal volume displacement greater than the volume change of the lungs, due to the volume lost by the collapse of the chest wall. This volume displacement can amount to up to 175% of the tidal volume change of the lungs (31). In addition the diaphragm must work against two pressures: the intra-

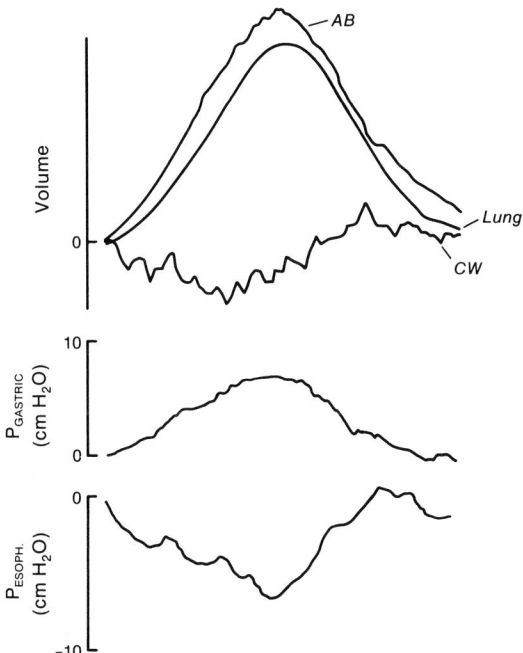

Figure 25.3. Tracing showing change in abdominal (diaphragmatic), chest wall, and lung volume, and gastric and esophageal pressures. Paradoxical chest wall movement during inspiration causes greater abdominal (diaphragmatic) volume displacement than that of the lungs.

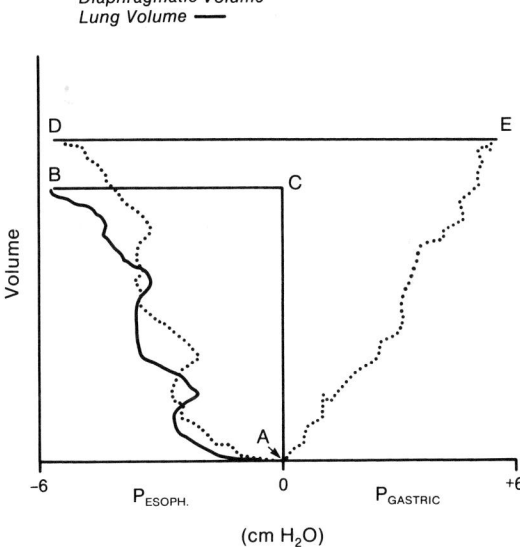

Figure 25.4. Pressure-volume relationship of the lungs (solid line) and diaphragm (dotted lines) during inspiration. Work performed on the lungs (area ABC) is less than that performed by the diaphragm (area ADE) because of chest wall distortion and the work performed on the abdomen.

pleural pressure, which becomes more negative on inspiration, and the intra-abdominal pressure, which becomes more positive on inspiration. Thus the pressure-volume work can be several times greater than that performed on the lungs (32), as shown in Figure 25.4.

Status of Infants During Early Recovery

Numerous investigations using these methods have been performed in preterm infants during early recovery from respiratory distress syndrome (RDS). The first month is a critical time wherein most infants either recover nearly normal cardiopulmonary function or develop signs of increased pathology.

Some of the earliest observations about the pathophysiology of BPD described abnormalities of blood gas tensions. Infants who develop BPD have been noted to have lower oxygen and higher carbon dioxide tensions in the arterial blood (33, 34). These abnormalities may persist throughout the first year of life. Early investigations point to a number of physiologic mechanisms for deficient overall gas exchange including atelectasis (35), intrapulmonary venous admixture (36), maldistribution of ventilation (37), and pulmonary hypoperfusion (38). In addition preterm infants appear to be less responsive to hypercarbia (39), which may explain, at least in part, their higher arterial PCO_2 values during early recovery. The improved oxygenation of most infants with BPD when they are given even minute amounts of enriched oxygen to breathe confirms that some fraction of the ventilation goes to areas with decreased ratios of ventilation to perfusion. The overall gas exchange status at 1 month of age, however, is not predictive of subsequent outcome (40). Furthermore a direct correlation between overall gas exchange during multiple points in the course of BPD and measures of pulmonary mechanics has not been made.

The derangements in the mechanics of breathing during RDS can be severe, but they resolve in infants who do not develop BPD. The preterm infant is born with lower dynamic and static lung compliances (41, 42), higher airway and total pulmonary resistances (43, 44), and a lower FRC (33) and thoracic gas volume (45) than full-term infants. These infants have prototypic restrictive lung disease. In babies with uncomplicated respiratory distress syndrome, the mechanics of breathing improve and become normal by the time they are ready for discharge. The FRC of most preterm infants increases linearly with length during early recovery (33). The specific compliance, or the dynamic compliance divided by the FRC, is unchanged with growth. Thus in infants with uncomplicated RDS, it appears that the lung parenchyma grows at a rate which is proportional to its volume and has a relatively normal mechanical status, in spite of the infant's prematurity.

Measurements of lung compliance in infants with BPD suggest several pathophysiologic mechanisms that complicate early recovery from RDS. The dynamic compliance of infants who develop BPD is markedly reduced early in the course of lung disease (44, 46). Infants with the lowest dynamic compliances during acute RDS are also those who are most prone to develop pulmonary air leaks, a complication associated with BPD (37). The static compliance of the lungs of infants with BPD, as measured using the weighted spirometry method, has been found to be reduced (16), although not to as great a degree as the dynamic compliance is. It has been proposed that the measurement of total respiratory system compliance (a parameter which is similar to the static compliance), performed in the first 8 hours of life, may be a predictor of outcome (47); however, it has also been shown that the static compliance increases in the first 5 postnatal days, even in term infants (48, 49), probably because of absorption of lung fluid (50, 51). Part of the reduction in the dynamic compliance during the first days of RDS is probably at least in part due to clearance of pulmonary edema. For example the dynamic compliance of infants improves with the resolution of pulmonary edema after the closure of the patent ductus arteriosus (52, 53). Another factor may be the mechanical heterogeneity of the lungs. The observation that lung compliance may be improved with bronchodilators (54, 55) and the observed frequency dependency of compliance suggest that gas is trapped behind airways with increased airway resistance because there is inadequate time for regional emptying of the lungs. The greater the regional heterogeneity of resistance and compliance of the lung units, the greater the dependency of the compliance on the respiratory frequency. The lung is also heterogeneous in terms of overall gas exchange, in that there is evidence for maldistribution of ventilation (see above, 37). Thus the observed frequency dependent inequality of ventilation, associated with overdistention of parts of the lungs, contributes to the reduced dynamic compliance. Finally, the fibrosis that develops during chronic resolution of RDS, as seen in histologic sections, may decrease both the dynamic and the static compliance (56).

The total pulmonary and airway resistances are increased demonstrably even before the diagnosis of BPD is established. It has been suggested that the total pulmonary resistance may be elevated even on the first day of life in infants who subsequently develop BPD (44). This has been corroborated by studies in very low birth weight infants (less than 750 g) at a mean age of 4.8 days (57). The early measurement of expiratory resistance may be of greater value in identifying infants at increased risk than that of total pulmonary resistance, because the large airways may be dilated by the positive airway pressure of the mechanical ventilator during inspiration. The inspiratory resistance is lower than the expiratory resistance, and is dependent upon the rate of mechanical ventilation (58). The value of this resistance measurement during acute RDS for predicting BPD, however, is confounded by factors such as lung fluid shifts, dynamic lung volume changes with therapy, leaks around the endotracheal tube (59), or acute airway inflammation.

In infants with established BPD the total pulmonary and airway resistances are significantly increased (43, 46) relative to those in premature infants during uncomplicated convalescence. The elevated resistance decreases with the resolution of early BPD in infancy (43, 46), and appears to be acutely decreased by inhaled bronchodilators, theophylline, furosemide, or a combination of acute therapies (54, 55, 60). The course of the decrease in resistance, however, should be studied in larger populations in which bronchodilator or diuretic therapies are strictly controlled.

Expiratory flow rates have been shown to be increased at 75%, 50%, and 25% of the expiratory volume of infants with BPD after the administration of bronchodilators (61) and with the administration of oxygen (62). The maximal observed flow rate at FRC or $\dot{V}_{max}FRC$, derived from the "squeeze" method, has been shown to be lower in infants with BPD than in controls, indicating large airways disease (61). These findings are similar to those in bronchiolitis, which has serious implications for the future pulmonary status of these infants (see below).

Investigations attempting to localize the source of the airways obstruction suggest that both large and small airways are obstructed. Infants, when given HeO_2 mixtures to breathe, have lower total pulmonary resistance and work of breathing (63). The decrease in resistance is not as great as that following the administration of bronchodilators or furosemide (54, 55, 60). The effect of bronchodilators in relaxation of the large airways has not been demonstrated in normal infants (64, 65). The histologic appearance of hypertrophied smooth muscle in the airways of infants with BPD, however, (56) is consistent with the observed effect of bronchodilators on airway resistance. The $V_{iso}\dot{V}$ is increased in children with BPD which implicates obstruction in small airways (57). Therefore there is physiologic evidence of obstruction of both large and small airways, which is consistent with the histologic appearance of hyperplasia of the smooth muscle of large airways and dysplasia of the epithelium of the small airways at the level of the respiratory bronchioles.

Infants appear to have pulmonary hyperinflation both on physical examination and on chest x-ray. Studies of lung volume, however, using both inert gas equilibration and body plethysmographic techniques, have shown a decrease in FRC during the first 8 months of life (33, 43, 55). Important questions have been raised as to the technical validity of the plethysmographic method of study used in infants with bronchiolitis, who also have manifestations of hyperinflation, but whose lung volumes measured by this method have also been found to be low or normal (66, 67). The underestimation of the lung volumes may be due to the great deal of maldistribution of ventilation and obstruction of distal airways, which prevents transmission of alveolar pressures to the mouth during airway occlusion. This physiologic "error" is consistent with the fibrous scarring of airways seen on histologic sections of the lungs of infants dying of bronchiolitis and, to some degree, BPD. The tissue content of the lungs of infants who have either bronchiolitis or BPD may be greater for a given amount of alveolar gas, which may make the lungs appear radiographically larger than their actual gas content. Moreover in longitudinal studies it was found that the FRC of infants approached normal by the time the infants were well into recovery at 7 to 22 months of age (43). Chronic airway obstruction may persist into early childhood and be more accurately reflected by increased values of functional residual capacity and residual volumes (see below).

The decreased compliance and increased resistance (whether in the large or small airways) causes the infant to increase his respiratory effort. Esophageal pressure swings (which estimate intrapleural changes) during quiet tidal breathing are commonly in excess of 20 cm of water. The oxygen consumption of BPD patients has been shown to be 25% greater than that of infants who were matched for age and weight (68). This increase in overall oxygen consumption, if attributed to the work of breathing, represents a three- or fourfold increase in the work of breathing over that of controls. It has been stated, however, that the computed work of breathing does not account for the increase in the oxygen consumption seen in these patients, or for the lack of growth commonly seen in these infants, even when they are given "adequate" calories for growth (63). Distortion of the chest wall is an important cause of the increased work of the diaphragm, even in preterm infants whose lung mechanics may be normal. Chest wall distortion may be especially pronounced in infants with BPD for a number of reasons. Many are malnourished, with wasting of their respiratory muscle mass. Those treated with chronic diuretics may have osteopenia, with structural rib cage weakness and even rib fractures (69). The distortion of the chest wall may also be associated with inspiratory inhibitory reflexes, which may further increase the respiratory rate and the work of breathing (70). The estimated work of the diaphragm in preterm infants (31, 32) is not dissimilar from that calculated for adults in respiratory failure when corrected for body weight (71).

The increased work of the diaphragm may lead to an additional problem for the infant with BPD. The diaphragm may be called upon to work so excessively that it fatigues. Muscular fatigue is associated with frequency spectral changes in the electromyogram of skeletal muscle (72, 73). Fatigue of the diaphragm has been demonstrated by this method in adults during loaded breathing (74), and it may occur during apneic episodes in preterm infants (75). The weakness and susceptibility of fatigue of the diaphragm may be enhanced by the depletion of potassium and chloride ions caused by diuretic therapy and its associated metabolic alkalosis (76). This may contribute to the prolonged need for intermittent mandatory ventilation for many patients with BPD during early recovery from RDS. It may also contribute to apnea in infants after discharge, which may be a vital factor in the increased incidence of sudden infant death syndrome in infants with BPD (77). It may also account for the acute CO_2 retention commonly seen in these infants during viral illnesses, which frequently complicates later recovery. Evidence suggests that the contractility of the diaphragm, like skeletal muscle, may be improved by theophylline therapy (78). This may in part explain the improved respiratory status of apneic infants treated with theophylline, since improved performance of the respiratory muscles may prevent the formation of atelectasis. Theophylline therapy, however, has not been shown to be helpful in improving the endurance of skeletal or respiratory muscle (79), and so the long-term effects and overall advantage of theophylline in infants with BPD from a respiratory muscle standpoint remain in question. Bronchodilation, however, is a major factor in the treatment of infants with BPD, not unlike patients with asthma, which may be the primary indication for the use of theophylline. "Endurance training" of the respiratory muscles during weaning from mechanical ventilation, either during acute RDS or later during respiratory illness, may be helpful in providing the endurance necessary for prolonged extubation (80). Studies of respiratory muscle function are being actively pursued to describe the basic physiology and its practical application for optimizing the care of these infants.

Status of Older Infants and Young Children

There is little information regarding the pulmonary status of children with BPD between 9 months and 4 to 5 years of age, since there are few methods to assess pulmonary function in this age group. Future studies of children at these ages will be especially interesting since the lungs increase in volume severalfold during this period of time. The marginal gas exchange and radiographic abnormalities in many infants resolve during this period, and virtually all infants attain a normal pattern of somatic growth (81). Spirometry has been performed in children 4 years of age after they have completed a program of training (82), and will undoubtedly be applied to infants with BPD. Knowledge about this transition period will undoubtedly improve as methods for studying the pulmonary function of young children improve.

Status of School-Age Children

A number of early investigations described the pulmonary status of school-age survivors of RDS who had been treated in the late 1960s and 1970s. Cross-sectional studies of spirometry using routine pulmonary function methods confirmed that the cardiopulmonary function of the average school-age survivor treated for RDS 15 to 20 years ago was normal (83). Later studies suggested not only that spirometry was normal (84), but that the distribution of ventilation, as assessed by inert gas washout, becomes normal by school age (37). A cross-sectional study assessed the exercise performance of premature infants at school age, and no group abnormalities were detected, even in infants who had been mechanically ventilated (85). Of the children in this study, however, three had CO_2 retention on exercise and maldistribution of ventilation; all three of these children had air leaks during their early course of RDS. These studies are supported by a recent report of a cross-sectional study with excellent follow-up (86) which showed that finding lung disease in school-age survivors is difficult, especially when the presence of asthma is considered. Moreover the children with abnormal spirometric studies were also those who had more frequent episodes of wheezing and chronic respiratory symptoms during the first years of life.

More recently investigations have centered on smaller numbers of survivors and controls matched for age and gestational age, with and without RDS. Oxygenation is impaired in some children with BPD even at school age (87). Other studies have reported residual abnormalities consistent with airway obstruction: elevated residual volumes, functional residual and total lung capacities (37, 87, 88). The observed obstruction is at least partially reversible by inhaled bronchodilators. Reactive airways disease is a feature of older survivors, as evidenced by increased sensitivity to the nonspecific bronchial challenge with aerosols of methacholine (87). Moreover infants who develop BPD have more frequent family histories of asthma than premature infants who survive and do not develop BPD (89). Preliminary data on a large group of infants, representing a cross-section of survivors 5 to 10 years of age and controls, have demonstrated significant airway reactivity to exercise challenge, independent of a family history of asthma (90). Other authors have detected evidence of abnormalities of the small airways using sensitive testing, as reflected in the $V_{iso}\dot{V}$ (87). Further study will be necessary in the coming decade to assess the present therapy using these specific indicators of small airways disease to examine adequately the survivors of prematurity, especially in comparing those treated with mechanical ventilation and matched controls with less severe disease.

Factors That Complicate the Assessment of Children with Bronchopulmonary Dysplasia

A complication of severe BPD in infants is pulmonary vascular disease and cor pulmonale. This complication, which is difficult to assess, may have profound implications for the morbidity and mortality of infants with BPD. Studies of infants with severe BPD using cardiac catheterization have documented high mean pulmonary arterial pressures, even when left ventricular end-diastolic pressures are normal (91, 92). This is consistent with the autopsy findings of pulmonary arterial muscular hypertrophy (56, 93, 94) and organizing mural thrombi (94). The finding that right ventricular hypertrophy persisted in the most severely affected school-age survivors suggests that fixed medial hypertrophy is present (34). Modern echocardiographic assessment is helpful. The ratio of the pre-ejection period to the right ventricular ejection time (95) has correlated well with values obtained from cardiac catheterization data and the more subjective clinical assessment, but is not well correlated with measured pulmonary arterial pressures (91). However, it is useful in identifying infants with moderate or severe elevation of pulmonary arterial pressures. In addition it has been suggested that there may be areas of irregular necrosis and hypertrophy of the myocardium (94) consistent with the echodense regions seen in the ventricular walls on the echocardiograms of some patients (96). However, hemodynamic measurements made in a small number of children suggest that the right ventricular end-diastolic pressure and right ventricular contractility may be normal, even in patients with high mean pulmonary arterial pressures (91). Furthermore it is encouraging that the pulmonary vessels may be dilated by proper administration of supplemental oxygen, with a significant lowering of mean pulmonary arterial pressure (92), even in cases of severe pulmonary hypertension. The evaluation of infants with pulmonary hypertension and cor pulmonale thus remains empirical. Further studies will be necessary to define the effect of the pulmonary vascular disease on the overall cardiopulmonary status of these children. The message is clear, however, that adequate treatment with supplemental oxygen may be preventative or at least may partially alleviate the increased pulmonary vascular resistance seen in the most severely affected patients.

A second factor complicating the evaluation of infants with BPD is their tendency to contract viral infections of the lower respiratory tract during the first year of life. Viral infections have a profound effect on lung function (97). The small infant who is intubated and ventilated is extremely susceptible to pulmonary infections, even with the best newborn intensive care. Many infants develop an early interstitial pattern on their chest x-rays with hyperinflation while they are being mechanically ventilated, which rapidly progresses to chronic lung disease with hyperinflation and intermittent atelectasis, without laboratory confirmation by the clinician of the diagnosis of viral pneumonitis. In older infants even a single bout of bronchiolitis may have profound implications for the development of small airways disease (98). The combination of small airways damage due to the viral infection and the trauma induced by mechanical ventilation and high inspired oxygen tensions may in fact produce the most severe pathology in infants with the most intractable course of pulmonary disability. Rapid diagnostic techniques for viral pneumonitis (99), as well as early incorporation of tests for small airways obstruction and subsequent follow-up in the pre-school-age survivors of prematurity, will be necessary before making conclusions about the long-term pulmonary status of the survivors of prematurity. Only controlled, prospective studies will allow the separation of the effects of BPD from those of viral illnesses on the pulmonary status of older infants and young adults, because of the proven inadequacies of even well-performed retrospective studies (100, 101).

Summary

The further development and application of specific tests for evaluation of the young infant and older survivors of RDS may allow us to identify features of the treatment for RDS that prolong recovery, thus producing BPD. Therapeutic modalities such as exogenous surfactant replacement and high-frequency oscillatory and jet ventilation will require the close assessment of the function of the lungs of these infants to define and possibly prevent untoward complications. The past three decades have more or less defined the survivability of the prematurely born infant; during the next decades we may define their ultimate outcome.

References

1. Huch R, Huch A, Albani M, et al. Transcutaneous PO_2 monitoring in routine management of infants and children with cardiorespiratory problems. Pediatrics 1976;57:681.
2. Hansen TN, Tooley WH. Skin surface carbon dioxide tensions in sick infants. Pediatrics 1979;64:942.
3. Rome ES, Stork EK, Carlo WA, Martin RJ. Limitations of transcutaneous PO_2 and PCO_2 monitoring in infants with bronchopulmonary dysplasia. Pediatrics 1984;74:217.
4. Fanconi S, Doherty P, Edmonds JF, Barker GA, Bohn DJ. Pulse oximetry in pediatric intensive care: comparison with measured saturations and transcutaneous oxygen tension. J Pediatr 1985;107:362.
5. Wilkinson AR, Phibbs RH, Heilbron DC, Gregory GA, Versmold HT. In vivo oxygen dissociation curves in transfused and untransfused newborns with cardiopulmonary disease. Am Rev Respir Dis 1980;122:629.
6. Mead J. Measurement of inertia of the lungs at increased ambient pressure. J Appl Physiol 1956;9:208.
7. Perez-Fontan JJ, Heldt GP, Gregory GA. Resistance and inertia of endotracheal tubes used in infants during periodic flow. Crit Care Med 1985;13:1052.
8. LeSouef PN, Lopes JM, Muller N, Bryan AC. Influence of chest wall distortion on esophageal pressure. J Appl Physiol 1983;55:353.
9. Beardsmore CS, Helms P, Stocks J, et al. Improved esophageal balloon technique for use in infants. J Appl Physiol 1980;49:735.
10. Baydur A, Behrakis PK, Zin WA, Jaeger M, Milic-Emili J. A simple method for assessing the validity of the esophageal balloon technique. Am Rev Respir Dis 1982;126:788.
11. Muller NL, Zamel N. Pneumotachograph calibration for inspiratory and expiratory flows during HeO_2 breathing. J Appl Physiol 1981;51:1038.
12. Heldt GP, Targett RC, McIlroy MB. A microcomputer-based data acquisition system for physiological studies of the newborn. In: Harris JR, Bahr JP, eds. The use of computers in perinatal medicine. New York: Praeger, 1982
13. Thomson A, Elliott J, Silverman M. Pulmonary compliance in sick low birthweight infants. Arch Dis Child 1983;58:891.
14. Olinsky A, Bryan AC, Bryan MH. A simple method of measuring total respiratory system compliance in newborn infants. S Afr Med J 1976;50:128.
15. Kirkpatrick SML, Olinsky A, Bryan MH, Bryan AC. Effect of premature delivery on the maturation of the Hering-Breuer inspiratory inhibitory reflex in human infants. J Pediatr 1976;89:1010.
16. Tepper RS, Pagtakhan RD, Taussig LM. Noninvasive determination of total respiratory system compliance in infants by the weighted-spirometer method. Am Rev Respir Dis 1984;130:461.
17. Geubelle F, Senterre J. Methods of investigation of the mechanics of breathing in artificially ventilated newborn. Biol Neonate 1970;16:35.
18. Roy R, Powers SR, Kimball WR. Estimation of respiratory parameters by the method of covariance ratios. Comput Biomed Res 1974;7:21.
19. Dubois AR, Botelho SY, Bedell GN, Marshall R, Comroe JH Jr. A rapid plethysmographic method for measuring thoracic gas volume: a comparison with the nitrogen washout method for measuring functional residual capacity in normal subjects. J Clin Invest 1956;35:322.
20. Polgar G, Promadhat V. Pulmonary function testing in children. Techniques and standards. Philadelphia, Pa: Saunders, 1971
21. Auld PAM, Nelson NM, Cherry RB, et al. Measurement of thoracic gas volume in the newborn infant. J Clin Invest 1963;42:476.
22. Stocks J, Godfrey S. Specific airway conductance in relation to postconceptional age in infancy. J Appl Physiol 1977;43:144.
23. Krauss AN, Auld PAM. Measurement of functional residual capacity in distressed neonates by helium rebreathing. J Pediatr 1970;77:228.
24. Heldt GP, Peters RM. A simplified method to determine functional residual capacity dur-

25. Harrison M, Heldt GP, Gregory GA, DeLorimer A. Resection of a distal tracheal stenosis in a baby with agenesis of the lung. J Pediatr Surg 1980;15:938.
26. Taussig LM. Maximal expiratory flows at functional residual capacity: a test of lung function for young children. Am Rev Respir Dis 1977;116:1031.
27. Boros SJ, Mammel M, Coleman JM, et al. Neonatal high-frequency jet ventilation: four years' experience. Pediatrics 1985;75:657.
28. Despas PJ, Leroux M, Macklem PJ. Site of airway obstruction in asthma as determined by measuring maximal expiratory flow breathing air and a helium-oxygen mixture. J Clin invest 1972;51:3235.
29. Gelb AF, Maloney PA, Klein E, Aronstam PS. Sensitivity of volume of isoflow in the detection of mild airway obstruction. Am Rev Resp Dis 1975;112:401.
30. Gerhardt T, Bancalari E. Chest wall compliance in full-term and premature infants. Acta Paediatr Scand 1980;69:359.
31. Heldt GP, McIlroy MB. The dynamics of the chest wall in preterm infants. J Appl Physiol 1987;62:170.
32. Heldt GP, McIlroy MB. Distortion of the chest wall and the work of the diaphragm in preterm infants. J Appl Physiol 1987;62:164.
33. Bryan MH, Hardie MJ, Reilly BJ, Swyer PR. Pulmonary function studies during the first year of life in infants recovering from the respiratory distress syndrome. Pediatrics 1973;52:167.
34. Harrod JR, L'Heureux P, Wangenstein OD, Hunt CE. Long-term follow-up of severe respiratory distress syndrome treated with IPPB. J Pediatr 1974;83:277.
35. Strang LB, McLeish MH. Ventilatory failure and right-to-left shunt in newborn infants with respiratory distress. Pediatrics 1961;28:17.
36. Corbet AJS, Ross JA, Beaudry PH, Stern L. Ventilation-perfusion relationships as assessed by aAD_{N_2} in hyaline membrane disease. J Appl Physiol 1974;36:74.
37. Watts JL, Ariagno RL, Brady JP. Chronic pulmonary disease in neonates after artificial ventilation: distribution of ventilation and pulmonary interstitial emphysema. Pediatr 1977;60:273.
38. Chu L, Clements JA, Cotton EK, Klaus MH, Sweet AY, Tooley WH. Neonatal pulmonary ischemia. I. Clinical and physiological studies. Pediatrics 1967;40(2):709.
39. Rigatto H, Brady JP. Periodic breathing and apnea in preterm infants. I. Evidence for hypoventilation possibly due to central respiratory depression. Pediatrics 1972;50:202.
40. Truog WE, Jackson JC, Badura RJ, Sorensen GK, Murphy JH, Woodrum DE. Bronchopulmonary dysplasia and pulmonary insufficiency of prematurity. Am J Dis Child 1985;139:351.
41. Cook CD, Sutherland JM, Segal S, et al. Studies of respiratory physiology in the newborn infant. III. Measurement of mechanics of respiration. J Clin Invest 1957;36:440.
42. Cook CF, Cherry RB, O'Brien D, Karlberg P, Smith CA. Studies of respiratory physiology in the newborn infant. I. Observations on normal premature and full-term infants. J Clin Invest 1955;34:175.
43. Ahlstrom H. Pulmonary mechanics in infants surviving severe neonatal respiratory insufficiency. Acta Paediatr Scand 1975;69:69.
44. Desai NS, Cunningham MD, Boyer DJ, et al. Predisposing pulmonary dynamics from birth for infants with bronchopulmonary dysplasia. Clin Res 1983;31:908A.
45. Auld PAM, Nelson NM, Cherry RB, Rudolph AJ, Smith CA. Measurement of thoracic gas volume in the newborn infant. J Clin Invest 1963;42:476.
46. Morray JP, Fox WW, Kettrick RG, Downes JJ. Improvement in lung mechanics as a function of age in the infant with severe bronchopulmonary dysplasia. Pediatr Res 1982;16:290.
47. Simbruner G, Coradello H, Lubec G, Pollak A, Salzer H. Respiratory compliance of newborns after birth and its prognostic value for the course and outcome of respiratory disease. Respiration 1982;43:414.
48. Nelson NM. Neonatal pulmonary function. Pediatr Clin N Am 1966;13:769.

49. Mortola JP, Fisher JT, Smith B, Fox G, Weeks S. Dynamics of breathing in infants. J Appl Physiol 1982;52:1209.
50. Milner AD, Saunders RA, Hopkins IE. Effects of delivery by caesarean section on lung mechanics and lung volume in the human neonate. Arch Dis Child 1978;53:545.
51. Milner AD, Yvas H. Lung expansion at birth. J Pediatr 1982;101:879.
52. Naulty CM, Horn S, Conroy J, Avery GB. Improved lung compliance after ligation of patent ductus arteriosus in hyaline membrane disease. J Pediatr 1978;93:682.
53. Yeh TF, Thalji A, Luken L, Lilien L, Carr I, Pildes RS. Improved lung compliance following indomethicin therapy in premature infants with persistent ductus arteriosus. Chest 1981;80:698.
54. Rooklin AR, Moomjian AS, Shutack JG, Schwartz JG, Fox WW. Theophylline therapy in bronchopulmonary dysplasia. J Pediatr 1979;95:882.
55. Kao LC, Warburton D, Platzker ACG, Keens TA. Effect of isoproterenol inhalation on airway resistance in chronic bronchopulmonary dysplasia. Pediatrics 1984;73:509.
56. Rosan RC. Hyaline membrane disease and a related spectrum of neonatal pneumopathies. Perspect Pediatr Pathol 1975;2:15–60.
57. Goldman SL, Gerhardt T, Sonni R, *et al*. Early prediction of chronic lung disease by pulmonary function testing. J Pediatr 1983;102:613.
58. Perez-Fontan JJ, Heldt GP, Targett RL, Willis MM, Gregory GA. Dynamics of expiration and gas trapping in rabbits during mechanical ventilation at rapid rates. Crit Care Med 1986;14:39.
59. Perez-Fontan JJ, Heldt GP, Gregory GA. The effect of a leak around the endotracheal tube on the mean tracheal pressure during mechanical ventilation. Am Rev Respir Dis 1985;132:339.
60. Kao LC, Warburton D, Sargent LW, Platzker ACG, Keens TG. Furosemide acutely decreases airways resistance in chronic bronchopulmonary dysplasia. J Pediatr 1983;103:624.
61. Motoyama EK, Fort MD. Evidence of bronchial reactivity in premature infants with bronchopulmonary dysplasia. In: Bronchopulmonary dysplasia and related chronic respiratory disorders. Report of the 90th Ross Conference on Pediatric Research. Columbus, Ohio: Ross Laboratories, 1986, pp 53–59.
62. Teague WA, Heldt GP, Tooley WH. Hypoxia causes bronchoconstriction of infants with chronic lung disease. Pediatric Res 1986;20:443A.
63. Wolfson MR, Bhutani VK, Shaffer TH, Bowen FW. Mechanics and energetics of breathing helium in infants with bronchopulmonary dysplasia. J Pediatr 1984;104:752.
64. Phelan PD, Williams HE. Studies of respiratory function in infants with recurrent asthmatic bronchitis. Aust J Paedtr 1969;5:187.
65. Rutter N, Milner AD, Hiller EJ. Effect of bronchodilators on respiratory resistance in infants and young children with bronchiolitis and wheezy bronchitis. Arch Dis Child 1975;50:719.
66. Godfrey S, Beardsmore CS, Maayan C, Bar-Yishay E. Can thoracic gas volume be measured by infants with airways obstruction? Am Rev Respir Dis 1986;133:245.
67. Castile RG. More problems with Boyle's law—or "Vtg or not Vtg, that is the question." Am Rev Respir Dis 1986;133:184.
68. Weinstein MR, Oh W. Oxygen consumption in infants with bronchopulmonary dysplasia. J Pediatr 1981;99:958.
69. Venkataraman PS, Han BK, Tsang RC, Daugherty CC. Secondary hyperparathyroidism and bone disease in infants receiving long-term furosemide therapy. Am J Dis Child 1983;137:1158.
70. Hagan R, Bryan AC, Bryan MH, Gulston G. Neonatal chest wall afferents and regulation of respiration. J Appl Physiol 1977;42:362.
71. Field S, Kelly SM, Macklem PT. The oxygen cost of breathing in patients with cardiorespiratory disease. Am Rev Respir Dis 1982;126:9.
72. Schweitzer TW, Fitzgerald JW, Bowden JS, Lynne-Davies P. Spectral analysis of human inspiratory diaphragmatic electromyograms. J Appl Physiol 1979;46:152.
73. Lynne-Davies P. Diaphragmatic electromyographic studies. The application of frequency

74. Gross D, Grassino A, Ross WRD, Macklem PT. Electromyographic pattern of diaphragmatic fatigue. J Appl Physiol 1979;46:1.
75. Muller N, Gulston G, Cade D. Diaphragmatic muscle fatigue in the newborn. J Appl Physiol 1979;46:688.
76. Patel H, Yeh T-F, Jain R, Pildes R. Pulmonary and renal responses to furosemide in infants with Stage III-IV bronchopulmonary dysplasia. Am J Dis Child 1985;139:917.
77. Werthammer J, Brown ER, Neff RK, Taeusch W. Sudden infant death syndrome in infants with bronchopulmonary dysplasia. Pediatrics 1982;69:301.
78. Aubier M, DeTroyer A, Sampson M, Macklem PT, Roussos C. Aminophylline improves diaphragmatic contractility. N Engl J Med 1981;305:249.
79. Belman MJ, Sieck GC, Mazur A. Aminophylline and its influence on ventilatory endurance in humans. Am Rev Respir Dis 1985;131:226.
80. Nickerson BG. Bronchopulmonary dysplasia. Chronic pulmonary disease following neonatal respiratory failure. Chest 1985;87:529.
81. Vohr BR, Bell EF, Oh W. Infants with bronchopulmonary dysplasia. Growth pattern and neurologic and developmental outcome. Am J Dis Child 1982;136:443.
82. Strope GL, Helms RW. A longitudinal study of spirometry in young black and young white children. Am Rev Respir Dis 1984;130:1100.
83. Lamarre A, Linsao L, Reilly BJ, Swyer PR, Levison H. Residual pulmonary abnormalities in survivors of idiopathic respiratory distress syndrome. Am Rev Respir Dis 1973;108:56.
84. Mansell AL, Driscoll JM, James LS. Pulmonary follow-up of moderately low birth weight infants with and without respiratory distress syndrome. Am Rev Respir Dis 1985;131:A249.
85. Heldt GP, McIlroy MB, Hansen TN, Tooley WH. Exercise performance of the survivors of hyaline membrane disease. J Pediatr 1980;96:995.
86. Stahlman M, Hedvall G, Lindstrom D, Snell J. Role of hyaline membrane disease in production of later childhood lung abnormalities. Pediatrics 1982;69:572.
87. Smyth JA, Tabachnik E, Duncan WJ, Reilly BJ, Levison H. Pulmonary function and bronchial hyperactivity in long-term survivors of bronchopulmonary dysplasia. Pediatrics 1981;68:336.
88. Wheeler WB, Castile RA, Brown ER, Wohl MEB. Pulmonary function in survivors of prematurity. Am Rev Respir Dis 1984;129:A218.
89. Nickerson BF, Taussig LM. Family history of asthma with bronchopulmonary dysplasia. Pediatrics 1980;65:1140.
90. Zaglul HF, Heldt GP, Tooley WH. Lung function in long-term survivors of HMD. Presented at Congresso Argentino de Pediatria, Cordoba, Argentina, September 1986.
91. Berman W Jr, Yabek SM, Dillon T, Burstein R, Corlew S. Evaluation of infants with bronchopulmonary dysplasia using cardiac catheterization. Pediatrics 1982;70:708.
92. Abman SH, Wolfe RR, Acurso FJ, Koops BL, Bowman CM, Wiggins JW Jr. Pulmonary vascular response to oxygen in infants with severe bronchopulmonary dysplasia. Pediatrics 1985;75:80.
93. Taghizadeh A, Reynolds EOR. Pathogenesis of bronchopulmonary dysplasia following hyaline membrane disease. Am J Pathol 1976;82:241.
94. DeSa DJ. Myocardial changes in inmature infants requiring prolonged ventilation. Arch Dis Child 1977;52:138.
95. Hirschfeld SS, Meyer RA, Schwartz DC, et al. The echocardiographic assessment of pulmonary artery pressure and pulmonary vascular resistance. Circulation 1975;52:642.
96. Way RC, DeSa D, Watts J, Manning C. Echocardiographic recognition of myocardial scars in premature infants. Clin Invest Med 1983;6(suppl 1):41.
97. Samet JM, Tager IB, Speizer FE. The relationship between respiratory illness in childhood and chronic airflow obstruction in adulthood. Am Rev Respir Dis 1983;127:508.
98. Kattan M, Keens TG, Lapierre J-G, Levison

H, Bryan AC, Reilly BJ. Pulmonary function abnormalities in symptom-free children after bronchiolitis. Pediatrics 1977;59:683.
99. Jalowalski A, England BL, Temm CJ, *et al.* Rapid detection of respiratory syncytial virus in nasal epithelial specimens from infants and children by peroxidase-antiperoxidase assay. J Clin Microbiol, 25:722–725, 1987.
100. Goddard KE, Broder G, Wenar C. Reliability of pediatric histories. A preliminary study. Pediatrics 1961;28:1011.
101. Watkins CJ, Burton P, Leeder S, Sittampalam Y, Weaver AMJ, Wiggins R. Doctor diagnosis and maternal recall of lower respiratory illness. Int J Epidemiol 1982;11:62.

Comments

Bruce R. Boynton

Most testing of pulmonary function in infants with BPD has been restricted to tests of pulmonary mechanics. There are several reasons for this. Infants with BPD have important disturbances of mechanical function that correlate with the severity of their clinical illness. Mechanical tests are inexpensive, noninvasive, and relatively simple to carry out. Furthermore there is a vast experience with the interpretation of such tests in adults with obstructive pulmonary disease. However, alterations in pulmonary mechanics are not the only disturbances of clinical significance in BPD and may not even be the most important ones. Our knowledge of pulmonary gas exchange in BPD is limited to cursory assessments of overall PO_2, PCO_2, and oxygen saturation. Yet there is evidence that infants with BPD have complex disturbances in pulmonary gas exchange. The dramatic increase in arterial PO_2 with minute increases in F_iO_2 suggests the presence of a large population of respiratory units with low ratios of ventilation to perfusion. The regional distribution of ventilation and perfusion also may be dramatically affected by changes in F_iO_2, even in children who have become asymptomatic. These and other disturbances in gas exchange are poorly understood. Future understanding depends on the development of new study techniques or the modification of existing techniques for use in infants.

26

Prevention of Bronchopulmonary Dysplasia: The Challenge

WILLIAM H. NORTHWAY, JR.

In any review of the possibilities for prevention of bronchopulmonary dysplasia (BPD) in the immature infant, it is important to emphasize that BPD is a disease process that does not occur naturally in this infant population. BPD begins in a setting of premature birth and significant respiratory difficulty. The injury and repair seen in BPD are associated with the use of efficient artificial ventilation and supplemental oxygen therapy to treat the initial underlying respiratory distress. Any complication of prematurity, such as persistent patent ductus with congestive heart failure, or of therapy, such as pulmonary interstitial emphysema, which increases the degree of respiratory distress, will prolong artificial ventilation and oxygen therapy and contribute to the development and severity of BPD.

A reduction or elimination of premature births would be the single most important intervention for reducing the incidence of BPD or eliminating the disease. Without the respiratory disorders associated with premature birth, primarily respiratory distress syndrome (RDS), which initiate the requirement for artificial ventilation and supplemental oxygen therapy, the incidence of BPD would be significantly reduced. The challenge to reducing premature birth is partly a scientific and partly a socioeconomic problem. Just as obstetricians played a major role in the development of improved care for the newborn infant, so too the discipline of obstetrics (perinatology) can play an important role in the prevention of BPD.

The etiology of premature birth is complex. In his model for studying the pathogenesis of low birth weight infants, Miller identified four major categories of significant extrinsic associated conditions: 1) environmental factors, such as high altitude and exposure to toxins; 2) fetal factors including multiple births, congenital malformations, intrauterine infections, and inborn errors of metabolism; 3) medical complications of pregnancy, such as toxemia of pregnancy and severe chronic maternal disease; and 4) adverse maternal practices including cigarette smoking, lack of prenatal care, and delivery before 16 years of age (1). When he analyzed a group of 972 infants, Miller found that the incidence of low birth weight babies was 37.9% in the fetal category, 18.5% in the medical complication category, and 9.6% in the adverse maternal practices category. All three incidences were significantly higher than the 1.8% incidence of low birth weight infants in pregnancies without these factors.

Medical complications of pregnancy and fetal factors leading to premature delivery can be reduced by advances in medical science. Reduction of adverse maternal practices requires educational and sociopolitical action. Premature births are less common in countries where careful attention is paid to prenatal care of the mother and infant (2). The provision of good prenatal care for all pregnant women offers not only the opportunity to detect maternal medical problems but also the possibility of early diagnosis of fetal dysmaturity and malformations by the use of ultrasound and diagnostic amniocentesis. Earlier accurate diagnosis of fetal problems can lead to therapeutic intervention with agents to increase lung maturation such as glucocorticoids, or in some instances to termination of pregnancy. The increasing trend toward identification of mothers at risk for complications of pregnancy (including identifying those likely to deliver prematurely and considering their transportation to major medical centers specializing in perinatal care) is an important step in improving the chances of survival for the prematurely born infant and decreasing the incidence of BPD.

Once an infant is born prematurely, prevention of BPD rests initially upon preventing the development of primary respiratory distress. While prevention of RDS is of major importance, careful attention to clearing the tracheobronchial tree of aspirated meconium and other material immediately following delivery can significantly decrease the severity of meconium aspiration pneumonia. The use of artificial human surfactant (see Chapter 20, by Merritt and Hallman) has the potential for reducing the severity of RDS, if not eliminating it as a significant respiratory problem for the premature infant. Initial clinical trials using surfactant derived from human amniotic fluid appear to have demonstrated a reduction in BPD (3, 4). These results are encouraging considering that only three doses of the human surfactant were used in the treatment regimen. As Merritt points out a surface active human nonantigenic surfactant ought to function best when administered as early in the course of the development of RDS as possible and should be delivered so as to provide as uniform a deposition as possible for as long as is necessary. The goal of this therapy from the point of view of prevention of BPD would be to reduce the airway pressure and duration of artificial ventilation and the duration and concentration of the supplemental oxygen required to treat the RDS.

Efforts made to prevent or reduce the incidence of BPD have in fact been successful, as demonstrated in Table 26.1. The incidence of BPD in infants weighing more than 1500 grams at birth has fallen from 27% in 1962–1965 to 9% in 1984 and 1985 ($.05 > p < .10$). Such a decrease in incidence of BPD would be considered a major success were it not for the significant increase in the number of premature infants weighing less than 1000 g treated with artificial ventilation and supplemental oxygen for longer than 24 hours and their associated high incidence (50%–55%) of BPD. The major factors in the reduction of the incidence of BPD in the premature infant weighing more than 1500 g included lowering of the acceptable standard for peripheral oxygenation in premature infants, the development of continuous positive airway pressure and positive end-expiratory pressure artificial ventilation techniques, closure of the symptomatic patent ductus arteriosus, and reduction of the level of the supplemental oxygen concentration and peak airway pressure during artificial ventilation. Although these technical improvements in therapy have also resulted in improved survival of premature infants weighing less than 1000 g at birth, their incidence of BPD has been very high.

Prevention of BPD in these very low birth weight infants may require not only early supplementation with exogenous human surfactant to correct a deficiency related to

Table 26.1. Stage IV Bronchopulmonary Dysplasia in Infants Treated for RDS

Year Treated and Weight Group	BPD/RDS (%)		
	Survivors	Nonsurvivors	Total
1962–65			
≤1000 g	0/0 (0)	0/3 (0)	0/3 (0)
1001–1500 g	1/2 (50)	2/5 (40)	3/7 (43)
>1500 g	3/11 (27)	3/11 (27)	6/22 (27)
Overall	4/13 (31)	5/19 (26)	9/32 (28)
1984			
≤1000 g	8/14 (57)	2/6 (33)	10/20 (50)
1001–1500 g	6*/24* (25)	3/7 (43)	9/31 (29)
>1500 g	4/51* (8)	1/3 (33)	5/54 (9)
Overall	18/89 (20)	6/16 (38)	24/105 (23)
1985			
≤1000 g	9/16 (56)	2/4 (50)	11/20 (55)
1001–1500 g	6/26 (23)	2/4 (50)	8/30 (26)
>1500 g	4*/42* (10)	0/4 (0)	4/46 (9)
Overall	19/84 (23)	4/12 (33)	23/96 (24)

All infants born at Stanford University Medical Center or transferred to it who were treated with intermittent positive pressure ventilation and O_2 for longer than 24 hours are included. From 1979 all infants treated with IPPV also received continuous positive airway pressure. By chi-square calculations the decreases in incidence of BPD in infants weighing more than 1500 g at birth in 1984–85, compared with 1962–65, have a p value between .05 and .10. The overall incidence of BPD in severe RDS is not significantly different.

*One death after initial discharge.

prematurity, RDS, but also early supplementation with multiple antioxidants. The natural increase in antioxidant protection is developmentally regulated, and maturation of this protection appears to parallel the maturation of the surfactant system (see Chapter 6, by Wispe and Roberts). While superoxide dismutase and other antioxidant protective activity increases with oxygen exposure in most newborn animals, it should be noted that the animals exposed were not prematurely born (5–9). The response of the premature infant weighing less than 1500 g to oxygen stress of a continuing nature is unclear and may well be inadequate (see Chapter 22, by Rosenfeld and Concepcion). At the least it would seem reasonable to attempt to maintain "normal" levels of activity of antioxidant protection in the face of continuing supplemental oxygen challenge. In this regard nutritional factors such as vitamin E, vitamin C, and β-carotene need to be provided as part of the management of the premature infant prone to develop BPD. Because natural antioxidant protection is multifactorial, it is unlikely that a single totally protective exogenous antioxidant will be developed or that nutritional factors alone will be sufficiently protective.

Prevention of BPD may continue to depend on further development of artificial ventilation techniques such as high-frequency positive pressure ventilation, high-frequency jet ventilation, and high-frequency oscillation, but these newer ventilation techniques have not yet been proven to be superior to artificial ventilation techniques currently being used to treat very low birth weight premature infants (see Chapter 21, by Boynton and Frantz). Prevention of pulmonary interstitial emphysema is highly desirable, since as a complication it increases the need for augmented artificial ventilation pressures and increased concentrations of supplemental oxygen. It is unclear, however, that these newer methods of artificial ventilation can in fact reduce the incidence of pulmonary interstitial emphysema and, at the same time, continue to ventilate successfully the very low birth weight premature infant.

While closure of the symptomatic patent ductus arteriosus probably contributed to decreasing the incidence of BPD (see Chapter 13, by Cotton), it is unclear that prophylactic medical or surgical closure of the patent ductus arteriosus in very low birth weight infants will further decrease the incidence of BPD. The desire to prevent the development of symptomatic patent ductus arteriosus by either medical or surgical means to reduce the incidence of BPD points out the current difficulty in identifying the early stages of development of BPD and predicting the eventual outcome of very low birth weight infants.

Since none of the current or proposed therapeutic interventions to prevent BPD is without risk, better means of identifying the earliest stages of developing BPD are needed. Closer monitoring of early pulmonary function, automated recording of duration and concentration of supplemental oxygen in the early stages of therapy, and a more widespread use of tracheal aspirate cytology, and biochemical analysis early in the course of treatment of premature infants predisposed to develop BPD (see Chapter 4, by Neave, and Chapter 22, by Rosenfeld and Concepcion), correlated with the eventual clinical outcome, might result in more precise criteria for earlier diagnosis. The possibility of using biochemical markers to identify early pulmonary fibrosis in BPD has been raised with the description of increased serum galactosylhydroxylysyl glucosyltransferase activity and serum procollagen type III amino-terminal propeptide concentration measured in adult patients with acute interstitial lung fibrosis (10). It may be that serum biochemical markers of lung inflammation will be developed which will also contribute to the multifactorial prediction of the development of BPD.

With reduction in peak airway pressures and supplemental oxygen concentrations since 1967, there has been a modification of the clinical and radiographic progression of the disease (see Chapter 12, by Edwards), but the underlying pathology of BPD has not changed (see Chapter 3, by Bonikos and Bensch). The chest radiograph remains a hallmark of the later stages of the disease, but it was not originally, and is not now, a sensitive indicator for the early development of the disease. Earlier identification of BPD will depend on pulmonary physiologic, biochemical, and ventilatory parameters and their correlation with development of the chronic phases of the disease, in which diagnostic radiology will play a significant role.

BPD in premature infants is potentially preventable. If it is recognized as a costly alternative to providing improved prenatal care to reduce premature delivery and its associated respiratory difficulties, it may be possible to effect sociopolitical change that would make available prenatal care to all pregnant women in the United States who do not now receive it. For those infants who are born prematurely in spite of such care, early replacement therapy of surfactant deficiency may alleviate the major cause of respiratory difficulty, which initiates the artificial ventilation and supplemental oxygen therapy leading to the development of BPD. Early identification of the development of BPD prior to diagnostic radiographic changes of the late stages is essential if interventional therapies such as administration of exogenous antioxidants to prevent oxygen toxicity are to be used selectively to prevent the development of BPD. Continuing efforts to decrease peak airway pressures during artificial ventilation or to eliminate artificial ventilation by the use of extracorporeal membrane oxygenation would seem to have less promise than correction of fundamental deficiencies in the immature infant that predispose to the development of BPD.

References

1. Miller HC. A model for studying the pathogenesis and incidence of low-birth-weight infants. Am J Dis Child 1983;137(4):323–327.
2. Avery ME. Can RDS be eradicated in respiratory distress syndrome. In: Raivo KO, Hallman N, Kouvalainen K, Valimaki I, eds. New York: Academic Press, 1984.
3. Hallman M, Merritt TA, Jarvenpaa AL, et al. Exogenous human surfactant for treatment of severe respiratory distress syndrome: a randomized prospective clinical trial. J Pediatr 1985;106:963–969.
4. Merritt TA, Hallman M, Bloom B, et al. Prophylactic treatment of very premature infants with human surfactant. N Engl J Med 1986;315:785–790.
5. Bucher JR, Roberts RJ. The development of the newborn rat lung in hyperoxia: a dose-response study of lung growth, maturation, and changes in antioxidant enzyme activities. Pediatr Res 1981;15:999–1008.
6. Frank L, Bucher JR, Roberts RJ. Oxygen toxicity in neonatal and adult animals of various species. J Appl Physiol: Respirat Environ Exercise Physiol 1978;45:699–704.
7. Warshaw JB, Wilson CW III, Saito Kotara, Prough RA. The responses of glutathione and antioxidant enzymes of hyperoxia in developing lung. Pediatr Res 1985;19:819–823.
8. Yam J, Roberts RJ. Oxygen-induced lung injury in the newborn piglet. Early Hum Dev 1980;4:411–424.
9. Frank L, Auto AP, Roberts RJ. Oxygen therapy and hyaline membrane disease: the effects of hyperoxia on pulmonary superoxide dismutase activity and the mediating role of plasma or serum. J Pediatr 1977;90:105–110.
10. Anttinen H, Terho EO, Myllyla R, Savolainen E. Two serum markers of collagen biosynthesis as possible indicators of irreversible pulmonary impairment in farmer's lung. Am Rev Respir Dis 1986;133:88–93.

Index

ACTH. *See* adrenal corticotrophic hormone
ARDS. *See* adult respiratory distress syndrome
APIB. *See* Assessment for Preterm Infant Behavior
acidosis, 237, 314–15, 317, 333
adrenal corticotrophic hormone (ACTH), 393, 395–97
adrenergic agonist aerosols, beta 2, 296–98
adrenoceptor, beta, 298
adult respiratory distress syndrome (ARDS), 12, 121, 122, 147, 148, 150, 165, 168, 169, 171, 191, 388
aerosolized dipalmitoyl phosphatidycholine, 343
agonists, beta 2, 296–98, 307, 312,
"air leak," pulmonary, 27, 90, 192, 193, 194, 237, 315, 333, 412. *See also* pulmonary air leak syndrome
airways and alveoli, 44–45
albuterol, 297, 298, 312
aldasterone, 287–88
"alveolar wash mechanism," 138
"alveolitis," 169
American Academy of Pediatrics Committee on Environmental Hazards, 320
amniocentesis, 440
amrinone, 260
anaphylaxis, 304
anascara, 195
antibiotics, 336
anticholinergic agents, 308, 312
antigens, 301, 302, 304, 345, 347
antigen, HLH-A, 179
anti-inflammatory agents, 293–312
antioxidant systems, 103–14, 169, 238, 275, 365–74, 441, 443
    enzymatic, 103–10, 179
    nonenzymatic, 110–14
    See also oxygen
antiprostanoids, 149
antiproteases. *See* protease-antiprotease mechanism
Apgar score, 209, 211
apnea, 193, 312, 319, 321, 324, 347, 431
ascorbic acid, 366. *See also* vitamin C
asphyxia, 333
Assessment for Preterm Infant Behavior (APIB), 409, 411, 416
asthma, 201, 212, 270, 293, 296, 300, 302, 305, 307, 308, 431, 432

Assessment of Preterm Infant Behavior (APIB), 320
asymmetric bronchopulmonary dysplasia, 205
atelactasis, 34, 36, 37, 81, 118, 120, 161, 163, 164, 167, 188, 190, 199, 200, 212, 213–14, 216, 235, 359, 361, 376, 427, 431, 433
atropine, 306–8
    and PBD, 308
    clinical trials with, 307–8
    mechanism of action of, 306–7
    pharmacology of, 307
azotemia, 317, 326

BPD. *See* bronchopulmonary dysplasia
Bagellardus a flumine, P., 6
"barker syndrome," 162
barotrauma, 27–29, 39, 44, 45, 79–101, 162, 168, 179, 235, 236, 237, 238, 244, 314, 344, 356, 360–61, 365
    animal models of, 89–90
    and chronic lung disease, 96
    effects of on large airways, 87–89
    effects of on small airway of immature lung, 81–83
    and HMV, 95–96
    and muscle relaxants, 93–94
    and small airway perturbation in immature animal lung, 83–85
    and surfactant deficiency, 85–87, 94–95
    and types of mechanical ventilation, 90–93
Bayley Mental Development Index (MDI), 413, 416
Bayley Scales of Infant Development, 26, 319, 321, 411, 412
Bayley Scales Psychomotor Developmental Index (PDI), 413, 416
beclomethasone, 307
Bell, Alexander Graham, 7
Berlin Charite Hospital, 5
Berlin Exposition, 5
Bernoulli equation, 206, 256
Bert, Paul: *La Pression Barometrique*, 8
Bird Mark VII respirator, 11, 12
blood vessels, 43–44
bombesin, 43
Bonnaire, A., 8
Boston Children's Hospital, 9
bradycardia, 316, 321, 324

Braun, Egon, 7
breath sounds, 181
bronchiolitis, 24, 36, 45, 171, 212, 236, 376, 429, 430, 433
bronchitis, 212
bronchodilators, 293–312, 428, 429
bronchopulmonary dysplasia (BPD)
    and antioxidant systems, 103–16, 365–74
    and barotrauma, 79–101, 360–61
    and bronchodilators, 293–312
    clinical presentation of, 179–84
    complications and associations of, 211–26
    connective tissue in, 122–23
    and cor pulmonale, 251–60
    diagnostic criteria of, 19–21
    and diuretic therapy, 277–88
    epidemiology of, 19–30
    four stages of, 19, 33–39, 161
    and high-frequency ventilation, 351–64
    growth and neurodevelopment after, 403–20, 431–33
    historical perspectives in, 3–13
    and home respiratory care, 331–37
    and laboratory study, 161–76
    and lung damage, 117–27, 154–55
    natural history of, 24–26
    and nursing care, 313–28
    and patent ductus arteriosus, 235–49, 317
    pathogenesis of, 26–29, 33–52
    prevalence and incidence of, 21–24
    prevention of, 29, 439–43
    and pulmonary edema, 143–59
    and pulmonary function, 263–75, 421–38
    and RDS, 19–20, 33, 59–78, 117–27, 143–59, 161–71, 187–93, 270–75, 343–48
    and radiology, 185–234
    and steroids, 375–402
    and surfactant, 131–41, 343–48, 360–61
    tracheal aspirate cytology in, 59–78
bronchodysplasia alba, 206–8
Budin, Pierre Constant, 4
bronchospasm, 293, 298, 301

"C" fibers, 303
CMV. See cytomegalovirus
CPAP. See continuous positive airway pressure
Candida, 212, 372
cardiomegaly, 199–200, 204, 206, 211, 236

carotene, beta-, 113–14, 366, 442
catalase, 40, 107–9, 126, 366–67, 372, 374
catheterization, cardiac, 257–59
Center for Premature Infants at Hopital des Infants Baudeloque, 3
ceruloplasmin, 366
Champneys, F. H., 6–7
chest physiotherapy (PT), 317
chest shape deformity, 221–23, 430
child abuse, 221
chlorothiazide, 283–84, 287
cholelithiasis, 185, 223–24, 283, 286
collagen, 49–50, 120, 122, 125, 161, 236
colloid osmotic pressure, 147
Columbia Babies Hospital, 365
compliance, lung, 88, 112, 118, 120, 193, 206, 236, 244, 265–66, 270, 277, 279, 293, 300, 308, 315, 316, 343, 380, 381, 388, 388–92, 395, 422–31
    weighted spirometer measurement of, 266
    See also surfactant
congenital heart disease, 186
congestive heart failure, 66, 214–15, 277, 281, 291, 317, 439
continuous positive airway pressure (CPAP), 79, 88, 91, 190, 334, 365, 440
Coolidge, W. D., 9–10
Cooney, Martin, 5
cor pulmonale, 218, 251–61, 281, 296, 332, 432, 433
    evaluation of, 253–59
    pathophysiology of, 251–53
    treatment of, 259–60
corticosteroid therapy, 139, 377, 393–97
cortisol, 393, 397
cosintrophin (synthetic ACTH), 397
cromoglycate, 307
cromolyn sodium, 300–6, 312
    in BPD, 306
    adverse reactions and toxicity of, 303–4
    clinical effectiveness of, 304–5
    mechanisms of action of, 301–3
    nebulizer solution of, 305–6
    pharmacokinetics of, 303
Curosurf, 347
Curschman's spirals, 67–68, 76
cyanosis, 331
cysteine, 374
cystic fibrosis, 171, 201, 209, 210, 211
cytomegalovirus (CMV), 202–3, 204

DAD. *See* diffuse alveolar damage
DTPA. *See* diethylenetriaminepentacetate
deferoxamine, 372
demineralization, 218, 221
Denucé, P. Berceau, 4
Denver Developmental Screening Test, 26
De Paul, J. A. H., 6
developmental quotient, the, 25
dexamethasone, 127, 299, 300, 367, 375–82, 384, 386, 389, 395
diethylenetriaminepentacetate (DTPA), 125
diffuse alveolar damage (DAD), 164–69
digitalis, 260
digoxin, 260
dimethyl thiouria, 372
displacement of bilirubin from albumin binding sites, 283, 286–287
diuretic therapy, 277–91, 293, 299–300, 323, 325, 326, 430
    chlorathiazides, 287
    furosemide, 277–87
    spironolactone, 287–88
dopamine, 317
Doppler echocardiagraphy, 249, 256
dypsnea, 183

ECF-A. *See* eosinophil chemotactic factor
ECG. *See* electrocardiogram
E. coli, 169
echocardiography, 254–59, 317
    Doppler, 249, 256
    motion-mode (M-mode), 256
    and right-sided pre-ejection period (RPEP), 255
    and right ventricular ejection time (RVET), 255
elastase. *See* neutrophil elastase
elastin degradation products (demosines), 125
elastin, 49–50, 121, 122, 125
electrocardiogram (ECG), 253
electrodes, carbon dioxide, 422
electrolytes and fluid imbalance, 283, 285
emphysema, 36, 45, 49–50. *See also* focal emphysema; pulmonary interstitial emphysema
enterocolitis, 235, 236, 372
environment, influence on growth, 407–9. *See also* stress reduction
eosinophil, 301
eosinophil chemotactic factor (ECF-A), 301
epidemiology, 19

epinephrine, 303
erythromycin, 296
extracorporeal membrane oxygenation (ECMO), 89–90, 96, 365
extracorporeal shock wave therapy (ESWL), 285
extravascular pressures, 147–48

FRC. *See* functional residual capacity
FVC. *See* forced vital capacity
Fell-O'Dwyer ventilating apparatus, 6–7
fibroblasts, 36, 122–23
fibronectin, 122–23, 125
fibrosis, 36, 44, 45, 47, 120, 156, 165, 166, 169, 190, 200, 293, 376, 429, 442
focal emphysema, 205–6, 216; *See also* emphysema; pulmonary interstitial emphysema
forced vital capacity (FVC), 296
fractures, 220–21
functional residual capacity (FRC), of lung, 92, 93, 94, 263–64, 269, 293, 353, 359, 424–25, 428
furosemide, 218, 223, 224, 277–87, 323, 407, 429
    effects on BPD, 278–79
    indication and recommended dosage of, 280–82
    mechanism of action of, 278–79
    pharmacology of, 277–78
    side effects of, 282–87
gastroesophageal reflux, 201, 212–13, 319, 322, 323, 324
globulins, alpha 1, 121
glucocorticoid therapy, 375–97, 440
glutathione, 108, 366, 374
glutathione disulfide, 108
glutathione peroxidase, 40, 108–9
glutathione reductase, 108–9
glutathione S-transferases, 109–10
Gueniot, M., 4
glycolipid accumulation, 118, 120

HFFI. *See* high-frequency flow interruption
HFJV. *See* high-frequency jet ventilation
HFOV. *See* high-frequency oscillation ventilation
HFPPV. *See* high-frequency positive pressure ventilation
HFV. *See* high-frequency ventilation
HLA-A2 phenotype, 68

HMD. *See* hyaline membrane disease
"hazy lung," 206
Hering-Breuer reflex, 423, 424
hernia, inguinal, 225
Hess, Julius H., 6
Heubner, Otto, 5
high-frequency flow interruption (HFFI), 355–56, 360
high-frequency jet ventilation (HFJV), 352–53, 359, 360, 421, 425, 442
high-frequency oscillation ventilation (HFOV), 168, 183, 353–55, 359, 360–61, 441, 442
high-frequency positive pressure ventilation (HFPPV), 351–52, 442
high frequency ventilation (HFV), 29, 84, 95–96, 237, 275, 351–62, 365, 375, 377
    airway pressure during, 356–60
    and alveolar pressure, 356–59
    and amplitude of pressure, 356
    and barotrauma, 360–61
    and clinical trial in premature infants, 356
    and resonant frequency, 356–59
    and tracheal pressure, 356–59
    See also high-frequency flow interruption; high-frequency jet ventilation; high-frequency oscillation ventilation; high-frequency positive pressure ventilation; ventilation, artificial
Hippocrates, 6
histiocytes, 65–66
home respiratory care, 331–39
    and outpatient follow-up, 335
    and oxygen therapy, 332–35
Hook, Robert, 6
Hopital des Infants Malades, 3, 4
hyaline membrane disease (HMD), 3–4, 9, 10–11, 68, 70, 71, 145, 148, 150–151, 152, 154, 161, 163, 235, 236, 244, 360, 375, 432
hydrochlorothiazide, 287
hydrocortisone therapy, 384–86
hypercalciuria, 282, 283–85, 287
hypercapnia, 361
hypercarbia, 182, 183, 185, 331, 427–28
hyperinflation, 36, 164, 199, 200, 204, 344, 430, 433
hyperoxia, 365, 367, 368, 386–93. *See also* oxygen
hyperparathyroidism, secondary, 283, 285–86
hyperplasia, endothelial, 36, 45
hypertension, pulmonary, 22, 26, 41, 215, 251, 253, 254–57, 277, 281, 300, 315, 332, 377, 433
hypertrophy
    left ventricular, 215–16
    medial, 36, 41, 376, 432
    right ventricular, 215, 251
    pulmonary arterial muscular, 432
    smooth muscle, 212, 236, 270, 277, 293, 376, 429
hypochloremia, 285
hypokalemia, 285, 287
hyponatremia, 285
hypoperfusion, pulmonary, 427
hypotension, 316
hypoventilation, 283, 285
hypoxia, 25, 41, 44, 49, 89–90, 96, 103, 106–7, 108, 109. 112, 114, 118, 120, 147, 171, 182, 185, 251, 252, 261, 264, 313, 319, 331, 352, 361. *See also* oxygen
hysteresis, 388

IPPV. *See* intermittent positive pressure
idiopathic pulmonary fibrosis (Hamman-Rich syndrome), 201
"immature lung syndrome," 193
incubators, 4–6
indomethacin, 237, 238–46, 317
infants
    future development of those with BPD, 403–20, 427–33
    premature, care of, 4–6
    pulmonary status of BPD, 421–38
    very low birthweight (VLBW), 22–24, 242, 365, 404, 406, 411, 412, 413, 440–41, 442
    See also PALM babies; premature birth
inflammation, cell. *See* lung
inspiratory to expiratory time ratio (I:E), 92
intermittent positive pressure (IPPV), 3–4, 6–7, 11, 20–21, 27, 29–30, 88, 161, 163, 336, 343, 351, 365
intravascular hydrostatic pressure, 145–47, 148–49, 155, 165
intrapulmonary venous admixture, 427
intravascular protein osmotic pressure, 145–47
ipratropium bromide, 307
isoetharine, 297
isoproterenol, 297, 303

INDEX

Klebsiella, 169
Kaiserin-Auguste-Victoria-Haus, 6

Lavoisier, A. L., 8
lecithin, 134, 136
Lefebvre, Professor Jacques, 3
lesions, central airway, 216–18
leukocytes, 154–55, 302, 306. *See also* polymorphonuclear leucocytes (PMNs)
ligation, PDA, 237, 239, 242
lipid peroxidation, 179
lung, the
    immature, 81–85
    inflammation and injury of, 45–49, 117–127, 154–55
    and fluid, 143–59
    growth and maturation, 40–43
    pathology in BPD, 375–78
    structure and mechanics of, 79–81, 422–27
    volume, 263–64, 422–27
lymphangectasia, 201

MDI. *See* Bayley's Mental Development Index
McCarthy General Cognitive Index, 413
macrophages, 34, 49, 121, 122, 125, 154, 168, 306, 366, 367, 376
maldistribution of ventilation, 427
manometry, esophageal, 266
Marchant, M. Soins, 5
Maternité and the Clinique Tarnier, 4–5, 6
maximal expiratory flows, lung, 272
meconium aspiration syndrome, 186
Medical Center Hospital in San Antonio, 169
Menkes' kinky-hair syndrome, 221
Merritt's classification of cells, 60–68
metabolic alkalosis, 283, 285
metaphasia, 164, 236, 376
metaplasia, 34, 36, 60–62, 161, 163–64
metaproproterenol, 297, 298, 307
methionine, 374
methylprednisolone, 392
Milne-Edwards, H., 4
milrinone, 260
mixing index (MI), of intrapulmonary gas, 264
monocytes, 121, 125
motion, equation of, 422
mucus secretion, 67–68, 118, 376

muscle relaxants, 93–94
myelination, 318

NBAS. *See* Neonatal Behavioral Assessment Scale
NICU. *See* neonatal intensive care units
National Heart, Lung, and Blood Institute: *Pediatric Respiratory Disorders*, 183
National Institutes of Health, 11, 162, 185
National Institutes of Health Clinical Centers, 375
Neonatal Behavioral Assessment Scale (NBAS), 318, 320, 411
Neonatal Intensive Care Unit at Vanderbilt University Hospital, 235, 242, 243, 244
neonatal intensive care units (NICUs), 314–28, 411–12, 413, 417
nephrolithiasis, 282, 283, 284, 287, 291
neutrophil chemotactic activity, 301
neutrophil elastase, 49–50, 124–25, 154, 306. *See also* protease-antiprotease system; protease inhibitor
neutrophils, 48, 60, 66–67, 121, 123–24, 126, 131, 154, 306, 368, 376, 393
New England Journal of Medicine, 12
9-alphafluoromethylprednisolone, 389, 392
nursing care, 313–27
    and the acutely ill ventilated child, 314–15
    and BPD, 313–14
    and detection of ventilation complications, 316
    and developmental issues in BPD, 318–22
    and discharge planning, 326–27
    and nutrition in BPD, 323–25
    and PDA, 317
    and stimulus reduction, 322–23
    and suctioning in BPD, 317–18
    and weaning from ventilation, 315–16
nutritional deficiencies, 236, 313, 323–25, 406, 407, 430, 441–442

O'Dwyer, J., 7
oliguria, 317
osteogenesis imperfecta, 221
osteopenia, 218–20, 283, 430
osteoporosis, 219, 224
ototoxity, 283, 286, 291
oximetry, pulse, 422

oxygen
  continuous skin surface, 422
  free radicals, 103–14, 162, 236, 237, 238, 244, 365–67
  supplemental, 3–4, 7–9, 10–12, 20–21, 29, 37, 60, 62, 65, 94, 182, 183, 237, 244, 259–60, 299, 326, 332–34, 343, 439, 440–41
  toxicity of, 8, 26–29, 29–30, 37, 39–43, 70, 139, 154, 162, 182, 192–93, 235, 314, 375, 386–93, 443

PDA. *See* patent ductus arteriosus
PMN. *See* polymorphonuclear neutrophilic leucocytes
PALM babies (premature infants with accelerated lung maturity), 193–94, 203
palmitic acid, 131
pancuronium, 315, 316
pancuronium bromide paralysis, 195
partial expiratory flow-volume, 267–70
patent ductus arteriosus (PDA), 19, 37, 66, 152, 235–49, 287, 291, 317, 371, 375, 380, 411, 412, 439, 440
  and BPD, 236–39
  closure of, 239–45, 428, 442
  left to right shunt through, 19, 44, 159, 179, 181, 183, 186, 188, 189, 190, 194, 197, 204, 206, 236, 248, 249, 317, 344
  management of the symptomatic, 245–46
Patterson, Carl V. S., 10
peptide, arial naturetic, 291
perfused microvascular surface area, 151–54
periostitis, "physiologic," 221
permeability, high alveolar-capillary, 118, 144–56, 165
persistent interstitial pulmonary emphysema (PIPE), 96
phenobarbital, 296
phenytoin, 296
Philip's equation, 29
phosphatidyglycerol, 131, 134, 135, 181, 193
phosphatidylinositol, 131, 134, 135
phosphatisylcholine, 131, 137
phospholipids, 131, 132–39, 194
pituitary-adrenal suppression, 375, 395–97
plasma protein osmotic pressure, 118
plasminogen activator, 125
plethysmography, 266, 424, 425, 426, 429, 430
  "squeeze method," 425, 429

pneumotachography, 422, 423
pneumonia, 20, 24, 186, 190, 194–96, 200, 201, 208–9, 211–13, 347
pneumomediastinum, 37, 85, 91, 202
pneumonitis, 186, 188, 189, 360, 421
pneumothorax, 37, 85, 91, 93–94, 194, 202, 205, 315, 316, 360
polymorphonuclear neutrophilic leukocytes (PMNs), 49, 123, 124, 168, 169, 366, 372, 394–95. *See also* leucocytes
Porter, David, 3
premature birth, 4–6, 29, 185, 193–96, 218, 271, 367, 413–17, 439–40. *See also* infants; PALM babies
prevalence and incidence, measures of disease frequency, 21–24
Priestly, Joseph, 7
prostanoids, 261
protease, alpha$_1$, inhibitor, 49, 121–22, 126, 372. *See also* neutrophil elastase; protease-antiprotease mechanism
protease-antiprotease mechanism, 117–26, 169
  changes in after lung injury, 120–22, 154
  and connective tissue in BPD, 122–23
  and lung inflammation, 123–27
  and lung injury in ARDS, 120
  and lung injury in the newborn, 117–20
protein fluid, 143–45, 148–49, 150, 156, 159, 344
proteolysis, autolytic, 120
Pseudomonas aeruginosa, 169, 212
pulmonary air leak syndrome, 27. *See also* "air leaks"
pulmonary edema, 33, 44, 138, 143–59, 204, 206, 236, 237, 249, 277, 281, 290, 291, 294, 317, 323, 326, 376, 389, 428
  evidence of in RDS and BPD, 143–45
  and mechanisms of formation in HMD and BPD, 145–55
  significance of in RDS and BPD, 155–56
pulmonary function, neonatal, 263–75
  and airway function, 266–70
  and compliance, 265–66
  and distribution of ventilation, 264–65
  and early prediction of BPD, 270–72
  and lung volume, 263–64
pulmonary hypoplasia, 194–96
pulmonary infection, 37, 162, 169, 182, 183, 202–3, 375, 433
pulmonary interstitial emphysema (PIE), 19, 37, 49–50, 79, 85–87, 89, 90, 94, 95, 96, 118,

INDEX

120, 168, 179, 188–89, 190, 192–93, 200, 315, 316, 361, 375, 439, 442. *See also* emphysema; focal emphysema
pulmonary permeability to water and solutes, 149–51

RDS. *See* respiratory distress syndrome
radiology, diagnostic, 9–10, 19, 20, 70–71, 185–226
    and complications and associations of BPD, 211–225
    and radiographic progression of BPD, 186–97
    and stage IV BPD, 187–211
rales, 236
reactive airway disease, 24, 25, 36–37, 41–43, 117, 179, 264, 266, 293, 306, 311–12, 432
recombinant DNA, 372
renal calcifications, 224–25, 282, 283
resistance, pulmonary. *See* compliance; lung; surfactant
respiratory distress syndrome (RDS), 19, 28, 29, 37, 40, 59–76, 117, 120, 132–39, 143–59, 161, 162–63, 186–92, 252, 263, 270, 300, 413–17, 427, 428
respiratory frequency, 181
retinol, 126
retinopathy of prematurity, 366, 413
retractions, 182, 236, 268, 326, 331, 335
retrolental fibroplasia (RLF), 8, 384
rickets, 218–20, 283, 286
Roentgen, Conrad, 9
Rosan, Dr. Robert, 3
Rotch, Thomas: *The Diagnosis of Disease in Early Life by the Roentgen Method*, 9
Royal Humane Society, 6
Rubner, Max, 5

salbutamol, 303, 308
Serratia, 169
serum biochemical markers, 442
Smith, J. Lorrain, 8
sphingomyelin, 134, 136
spirometry, 266, 423, 431
spironolactone, 287–88
stage IV, BPD, 197–201
Standard Nomenclature of Disease, 9
Stanford Intensive Care Nursery, 375
Stanford University Medical Center, 11, 12

Staphylococcus epidermidis, 238
Starling's equation, 145
stenosis, subglottal, 216–17, 334, 425
steroids, 196, 298–300, 367, 375–402
    and animal studies of oxygen toxicity, 386–93
    and BPD, 374–86
    pharmacology of, 393–96
stress reduction, 321–22
    auditory, 322
    environmental, 322
    olfactory, 323
    tactile, 322–23
    visual, 322
suction, 317–18
sudden infant death syndrome, 138–139, 209, 215, 293, 431
"suicidal binding," 109, 113–14
Sunshine, Dr. Philip, 3
superoxide dismutase (SOD), 40, 105–7, 126, 127, 238, 365–74, 441
    clinical trials with, 368–72
    Cu-Zn, 366, 374
    and diminution of elastase toxicity, 372
    liposome, 366
    manganese, 366, 374
    pharmacology of, 367–68
    polyethylene glycol (PEG), 368
    and prevention of free radical generation, 365–67
surfactant, 81, 131–41, 148, 151, 193, 360–61, 367, 381, 394
    deficiency in, 10, 28, 29, 44–45, 46, 83–87, 90, 118, 120, 131–39, 154, 159, 162, 167, 179, 186, 189, 249, 317, 360–361, 389, 392, 443
    materials and methods in analysis of, 132–33
    and patients on ventilators, 132–39
    therapy, 29, 74, 94–95, 183, 204–5, 343–48, 421, 440
    See also compliance
Surfactant TA, 347
syntactic development, theory of, 320
syphilis, congenital, 221

Tc-DTPA. *See* technetium diethylenetriaminepentacetate
tachycardia, 321, 331

tachypnea, 143, 179, 182, 183, 236, 265, 268, 331, 336
Tarnier, Stephane, 4–5
technetium diethylenetriaminepentacetate (Tc-DTPA), 149–51
terbutaline, 297
theophylline, 288, 293–96, 305, 312, 325, 429, 431
    pharmokinetics of, 294–96
    toxicity of, 296
thiazides, 287
thoracic gas volume (TGV), 424, 428
thrombocytopenia, 317
thrombosis, arteriolar, 376
thymidine kinase, 383
tocopherol
    alpha-, 110–13, 126
    gamma-, 110
tracheal aspirate cytology, 59–78, 197
    and Curschmann's spirals, 67–68
    and histocytes, 65–66
    and hyaline membrane debris, 68
    and mucus, 67–68
    and neutrophils, 66–67
    and other techniques, 68–76
    progressive changes in, 60–65
    and surfactant composition, 131–38
    technical considerations of, 59–60
tracheitis, 334
tracheoesophageal fistula, H-type, 201
tracheomalacia, 334
tracheostomy, 333, 334, 337
transpulmonary pressure, 422

ultrasound, 440
University of California at San Diego Medical Center, 193, 208
uric acid, 114
urolithiasis, 282, 283

VLBW. *See* infants: very low birthweight
ventilation, artificial, 10–12, 37, 71, 90–94, 132–39, 155, 159, 162, 179–84, 191–92, 202, 203–4, 236–38, 244, 298–300, 314–18, 331–39, 344, 347, 375, 425, 439, 440
    continuous positive airway pressure (CPAP), 79, 88, 91, 190, 334, 365, 440
    intermittent positive pressure (IPPV), 3–4, 6–7, 11, 20–21, 27, 29–30, 88, 161, 163, 336, 343, 351, 365
    and mean airway pressure, 91–92, 180, 356
    negative pressure, 181
    and peak inspiratory pressure (PIP), 28, 91, 93, 299, 440, 442
    positive end-expiratory pressure (PEEP), 79, 84, 91, 93, 94, 96, 168, 440
    and pressure waveforms, 92–93
    and tidal volumes, 92–93, 94
    and ventilation rates, 92–93
    See also high-frequency ventilation
Vesalius, Andreas, 6
Villermé, M. M., 4
vitamin A, 239
vitamin C, 113, 374, 441. *See also* ascorbic acid
vitamin E, 110–12, 238, 366, 374, 441

"weaning effect," 189
wheezing, 269–70, 294, 306, 331, 336, 432
"whiteout," radiographic, 189–90
Wilson-Mikity syndrome, 20, 186, 201, 202
Workshop on Bronchopulmonary Dysplasia, 162, 182, 185

x-rays, 9–10, 70

Yllpo, Arvo H., 6